Orthopaedic Management
in Childhood

Orthopaedic Management in Childhood

BY THE STAFF OF THE DEPARTMENT OF
ORTHOPAEDIC SURGERY AT THE
ROYAL CHILDREN'S HOSPITAL, MELBOURNE
COMPILED AND EDITED BY

PETER F. WILLIAMS FRCS FRACS

Senior Orthopaedic Surgeon
Royal Children's Hospital, Melbourne and
Senior Associate, Department of Paediatrics
University of Melbourne

Blackwell Scientific Publications
OXFORD LONDON
EDINBURGH BOSTON MELBOURNE

© 1982 by
Blackwell Scientific Publications
Editorial offices:
Osney Mead, Oxford OX2 0EL
8 John Street, London WC1N 2ES
9 Forrest Road, Edinburgh EH1 2QH
52 Beacon Street, Boston,
  Massachusetts 02108, USA
99 Barry Street, Carlton
  Victoria 3053, Australia

All rights reserved. No part of this
publication may be reproduced, stored
in a retrieval system, or transmitted,
in any form or by any means,
electronic, mechanical, photocopying,
recording or otherwise
without the prior permission of
the copyright owner

First published 1982

Printed in Great Britain at the
Alden Press, Oxford
and bound at
The University Press, Cambridge

DISTRIBUTORS

USA
  Blackwell Mosby Book Distributors
  11830 Westline Industrial Drive
  St Louis, Missouri 63141

Canada
  Blackwell Mosby Book Distributors
  120 Melford Drive, Scarborough
  Ontario M1B 2X4

Australia
  Blackwell Scientific Book Distributors
  214 Berkeley Street, Carlton
  Victoria 3053

British Library Cataloguing in Publication Data

Orthopaedic management in childhood.
  1. Pediatric orthopedic
  I. Williams, Peter F.
  617'.3'008805   RD732.3.C48

ISBN 0-632-00879-2

Contents

Contributors, vi
Preface, vii
Acknowledgements, viii
Further Reading, ix

1 Orthopaedic Management in Childhood, 1
2 The Infant, 9
3 The Toddler, 88
4 The Child, 117
5 The Adolescent, 248
6 Fractures and Dislocations, 280
7 Bone Tumours, 353
8 Some Generalised Disorders with Orthopaedic Implications, 399
9 Reflections on the Practice of Surgery, 459

Index, 474

Contributors

PETER F. WILLIAMS FRCS FRACS
Senior Orthopaedic Surgeon

MALCOLM B. MENELAUS FRCS FRACS
Chief Orthopaedic Surgeon

D.R.V. DICKENS MBBS FRACS
Associate Orthopaedic Surgeon

W.G. COLE MSC FRACS
Associate Orthopaedic Surgeon

STAFF OF OTHER DEPARTMENTS

W.H.J. COLE MSC DA FFARACS
Senior Anaesthetist

DAVID J. HILL MRACP
Rheumatologist

Contributors are members of the staff at the Royal Children's Hospital, Melbourne, Victoria 3052, Australia.

Preface

The practice of orthopaedic surgery can be learnt in a variety of ways but there is no substitute for personal experience. Even though it is said that experience is not a transferrable commodity, it is nevertheless possible for those who have it to make it available to those who have not. If this practice were a science it would only be necessary to consult a manual to find out how to fix any given problem. Unfortunately for the student, orthopaedic practice conforms more to an art than a science and logical decisions are only possible if the facts are considered in the light of the patient with his infinite variety of hopes, fears and expectations.

There are several encyclopaedic text books available from which all the facts about orthopaedic disorders can be obtained. The volume of these facts and the wide variety of available methods of treatment make it difficult to select the correct management for a given patient. This small book does not set out to compete in any way with the more comprehensive texts. Our aim has been to provide the reader with one form of management which is of proven value rather than to catalogue all the available methods of treatment. Moreover we have tried in so far as it is possible to describe the management of the patient rather than the treatment of the disease. This advice represents the practice of orthopaedics at the Royal Children's Hospital in Melbourne and is based on the experience gained from the care of a huge number of children with orthopaedic disorders.

Acknowledgement is also given to many teachers in other countries who have added their store of experience to ours over many years.

The resulting mixture is suitable for orthopaedic residents and it is suggested that, if taken regularly, it should produce an orthopaedic consultant who will be able to combine science with sensitivity and efficiency with compassion.

Acknowledgements

Although this book has been written by members of the Staff of the Royal Children's Hospital, this effort has only been possible because of the invaluable assistance provided by members of other departments within the Hospital.

We are particularly indebted to Mrs Carol Rochester who typed the manuscript many times, the medical artist, Mrs Vivienne James and the staff of the department of Visual Aids. Dr Valerie Mayne, Director of Radiology and Dr Fred Jensen, her Deputy, provided most of the radiographs from their files. Many others helped in minor ways and to all of those people we acknowledge our gratitude.

Further Reading

APLEY A. G. (1968) *A System of Orthopaedics and Fractures*, 3rd edn. Butterworths, London.
BLOUNT W. P. (1955) *Fractures in Children*. Williams & Wilkins, Baltimore.
ILLINGWORTH R. S. (1979) *The Normal Child: Some Problems of the Early Years and their Treatment*, 7th edn. Churchill Livingstone, Edinburgh.
ILLINGWORTH R. S. (1980) *The Development of the Infant and young Child, Normal and Abnormal*, 7th edn. Churchill Livingstone, Edinburgh.
LOVELL W. W. & WINTER R. B. (1978) *Pediatric Orthopaedics*, 2 vol. Lippincott, Philadelphia.
MENELAUS M. B. (1980) *The Orthopaedic Management of Spina Bifida Cystica*, 2nd edn. Churchill Livingstone, Edinburgh.
MOE J. H. et al (1978) *Scoliosis and Other Spinal Deformities*. W.B. Saunders, Philadelphia.
RANG MERCER (1966) *Anthology of Orthopaedics*. Churchill Livingstone, Edinburgh.
RANG MERCER (1974) *Children's Fractures*. Lippincott, Philadelphia.
SAMILSON R. L. (1975) *Orthopaedic Aspects of Cerebral Palsy*. Lippincott, Philadelphia.
SHARRARD W. J. W. (1971) *Paediatric Orthopaedics and Fractures*. Blackwell Scientific Publications, Oxford.
TACHDJIAN M. O. (1972) *Pediatric Orthopedics*. W. B. Saunders, Philadelphia.

CHAPTER 1

Orthopaedic Management in Childhood

Child psychology, 2

Handicaps, 2
Effect on the child

The consultation, 4
Examination and diagnosis
Communication

Definition of terms, 8

The 20th Century has seen tremendous advances in therapeutics—our ability to cure diseases has become so great that medicine over the period has tended to become mechanistic. The doctors have rather lost sight of the patient in their enthusiasm to investigate, diagnose and cure. Nearly a hundred years ago, Hugh Owen Thomas the founder of British Orthopaedic Surgery made the following observation: 'The crying evil of our art in these times, is the fact that much of our surgery is too mechanical, our medical practice too chemical and there is a harkening to interfere, which thwarts the inherent tendency to recovery possessed by all persons not actually dying.'

Over that same period medical education has stressed the scientific approach and little attempt has been made to explore the art of medicine. The modern text book of orthopaedic surgery takes little account of the patient in planning management or designing surgical operations. Teachers in general have tended to avoid discussing such things either because they considered the subject as irrelevant or perhaps for fear of being considered unmanly. In more recent times, it has become apparent that many disorders cannot be understood unless the emotional, intellectual and sociological aspects of the patient are considered. Although the behavioural sciences have studied the psychological mechanisms involved, a detailed knowledge of this is not necessary to the practising physician or surgeon. Rather, he should have an awareness of the problem so that he will want to seek out this additional information and interpret and use it with sensitivity. With children this approach is even more necessary, for the child is often unable or unwilling to discuss his emotional conflicts which may have a direct bearing on his response to treatment.

In summary therefore, the practice of orthopaedics in childhood depends upon two factors. Firstly, an accurate knowledge of the facts of orthopaedics, especially the natural history of disease and the reaction of the body to injury and disease. Secondly, an understanding of the needs of children, namely the child–parent–society interaction; this will determine how all the patients are to be handled, what treatment is best undertaken, and whether the treatment is likely to be effective.

CHILD PSYCHOLOGY

Children are very susceptible to the influence of emotional conflicts and because they find difficulty in discussing these things with adults, they are more likely to express their worries and fears in the form of some psychosomatic disorder. Asthma, enuresis, abdominal pains and headaches are some of the more common manifestations but disorders of gait, backache and various aches and pains are also often encountered in orthopaedic practice. In adolescence, true hysterical manifestations are far from rare.

Early last century, a distinguished physician wrote, 'It is more important to know what sort of patient has the disease than what sort of disease the patient has.' This is especially true in paediatric practice where the surgeon must train himself to consider the pathology of the whole person.

In attempting to find a solution to any given problem it is paramount firstly to determine what exactly is bothering either the child or his parents, and what they expect to achieve from treatment. In many consultations the surgeon will have great difficulty in finding the answer to these questions and, on these occasions, it may seem that the parents are deliberately avoiding saying what it is that really worries them. Often the basis of their concern is some stray remark made by a neighbour which has sown the seed of doubt. The experienced surgeon can often guess what turmoil is going on in the child or his parents and, by discussing this point early on in the consultation, can defuse the whole issue so that the consultation can proceed in a more relaxed atmosphere.

HANDICAPS

'The moment in which they learn their child is handicapped, whether at birth or by later illness or accident, must be for many parents one of the watersheds of life'. Recently, one mother expressed this belief when she said, '. . .the worst day was the day of A's birth—my whole life was changed by that day. From the day of her birth, all our life is finished.' The feelings of parents are a mixture of inadequacy at their failure to reproduce normally, and guilt arising from a suspicion that the handicap is a punishment for some sin committed. It is aggravated by their lack of knowledge of the extent of the handicap and their inability to help.

It follows that a line of communication must be established very soon after birth and that the mother receives accurate and truthful information regarding the abnormality and its likely outcome, and what can be expected from treatment. As maternity hospital staff and general practitioners often do not have sufficient knowledge to do this, both parents should have access to a specialist as soon as possible. The information given must be sympathetic, simple, accurate and, if possible, biased to the optimistic. It may have to be repeated almost word for word a few days later as parents absorb very little of the first interview. Later, it is often helpful to bring the parents into contact with another family with a similar problem or to introduce them to lay literature on the subject. Fortunately, doctors have spent more time and effort in educating the public through the mass media; this has had the effect also of changing community attitudes so that parents of handicapped children no longer have the same feeling of shame at the reaction of others or the dread of being pitied. The surgeon who establishes a good initial rapport with child and parent, will be amply rewarded by their continuing loyalty and the end result for all concerned is likely to be better because of it.

EFFECT ON THE CHILD

The effect of the handicap on the parents is very much related to the effect on the child. As early as 1928, Allan and Pearson stated that '... the child seems to adopt the same attitude to his disability that his parents do. If they worry about it, so does he, if they are ashamed of it he will be sensitive too, if they regard it in an objective manner he will accept it as a fact and not let it interfere with his adjustment.' Most parents need counselling to make them aware of how important their attitudes and feelings are in influencing the child's development and behaviour. This process may be aided by arranging meetings with other parents with similar problems, either singly or in groups. At the same time, the parents need help to understand the 'child's eye view' of their handicap and their environment.

When a child has an accident

After the initial shock has worn off, the child should be encouraged to talk about how it happened since the more open the discussion the less likely he will develop hidden fears and nightmares. He may even learn from it and add this to his store of experience. If the young child is admitted to hospital his mother should be with him for as much time as possible in the first few days. The mother herself will require support especially in the case of head injury, and it is essential that the surgeon explain that full recovery is the rule rather than the exception. Neither child nor parent are particularly interested in the details or duration of treatment—only the end result.

The child in hospital

Hospitalisation involves removal of the child from the home and family and is a traumatic event at any age. If a child is admitted to hospital without adequate thought and preparation, serious and permanent emotional disturbance may result.

Separation of a mother from her newborn baby for any reason interferes with bonding—a process of maternal–infant interaction which normally occurs in the neonatal period. Bonding is now regarded as of great importance for normal mother–child relationships and subsequent satisfactory emotional development in the child. Thus, should the newborn require hospitalisation, the mother should spend as much time as possible with her baby and preferably 'live-in'. It is well established that rejection by the mother of her newborn infant may follow separation even for quite short periods of time. This is particularly relevant to infants with congenital malformations who may require multiple admissions.

Hospitalisation in the toddler period is particularly traumatic as no amount of explanation will relieve the anxiety of separation at this age. Toddlers never really settle down in hospital, they cry incessantly until in despair they finally withdraw, lying silently, quietly sobbing and gazing at the ceiling. When such a toddler is discharged from hospital the parents will almost invariably note behavioural problems which may last for many weeks. These usually involve disturbances of sleep pattern, feeding problems and temper tantrums. It is clear that such infants, if they must be admitted to hospital, should have a parent with them—optimally for the whole period of hospitalisation.

In the older age child, proper preparation for planned hospitalisation is necessary. Most children after the age of about 5 years will accept a reasonable explanation for their hospitalisation. The explanation must be given in simple terms, the child reassured that visiting will be regular, and that he will soon be home again. Failure to adequately prepare young children for hospital even in this age group is again followed by behavioural problems on discharge.

Long term hospitalisation or repeated admissions to hospital can similarly result in emotional disturbance unless adequate preparation has been undertaken. In addition to the provision of emotional support, these children require adequate play facilities and, as they become older, facilities for education. It will thus be clear that occupational therapists, medical social workers, and school teachers will play a very important part in the orthopaedic team if the children are going to mature fully.

THE CONSULTATION

To the parent, and to a lesser extent the child, the first consultation is often a very unnerving experience. They are worried and fear the worst. It follows that the surgeon must do his best to put them at ease and this may require a minute or two talking about something quite irrelevant. Country people particularly like to have the fact recognised that they have come a long way for the visit. Children are put at ease by being talked with (not at), using their christian name and given a smile. Older children, especially those approaching adolescence, are very sensitive about their appearance and do not like being accused of being too fat, too thin, or too short in stature. History taking in this context is not very different to any other consultation, but it is important to separate the observations of the parents from what they have been told so that one can clearly define the problem. It should be possible in most cases to reduce the problem to a single word, be it pain, instability, stiffness, appearance, or fear. Each of these will probably require a different solution.

EXAMINATION AND DIAGNOSIS

Examination of the child follows the same general principles as those used in the adult, but there are two fundamental differences. Firstly, whereas the adult almost always co-operates fully to help the examiner, this *co-operation* must be sought for in the child. This is especially so in the infant where special ruses are often required. Often co-operation can best be obtained in the infant if examined on the mother's lap or nursed in her arms, while a feeding bottle will often convert a struggling babe to one that is readily examined. This is especially important in the neonatal examination of hip dislocation which may easily be missed in the struggling infant. Cold hands and rough handling must be avoided at all times. In examining the toddler and young child, co-operation is equally important and careful handling of the situation in the early stages is essential lest the opportunity be lost. A constant stream of irrelevant conversation aids the process of undressing and it is always wise to leave the underpants on in the first instance. Many young children are initially surprisingly modest and will refuse to walk naked until some degree of rapport has been established. The second major difference is that young children, even when fully co-operating, are unable to describe their disability or even localise it with any accuracy. It is for this reason that *observation* to detect wasting or swelling, and to determine the type of limp and its source must be much keener when examining the child. Remember that observations made by the parents are usually accurate and helpful. In the diagnosis of limp, the skills of the examiner will be put to their most severe test and this subject will be discussed in greater detail in Chapter 4.

In all problems concerning the lower limbs and especially the feet, examination of the footwear is essential and is likely to give much valuable information that may not be gained in any other way. If a shoe wears normally, the foot is almost certainly plantigrade whereas even a minimal amount of hindfoot varus will often produce catastrophic shoe wear and distortion of the upper.

COMMUNICATION

Use of simple terms

The problems of paediatric examination and diagnosis may seem difficult but those of communication of ones findings and opinions to the parents are, at times, impossible. The patient or parent frequently misunderstands medical vocabulary or, worse still, places the wrong interpretation upon it so that the message received may be quite different to what the doctor intended. The use of simple terms is thus mandatory although, at the initial consultation, one should especially avoid the use of terms such as arthritis, tumour, spastic, cripple and so on as these will almost certainly be interpreted as meaning something much worse than intended.

Defining the natural history of the condition

Many children brought in for an orthopaedic consultation have variations of posture (e.g. knock knees) which make them appear different from their parents but which are within the range of normality for their age. It is of little use telling the parents that their child is normal without backing this up with a short discussion on the natural history of leg development in the child. It will then be possible for them to reconcile how their child can be normal yet appear abnormal and understand why treatment is unnecessary.

Treatment versus no treatment

In many situations treatment is not indicated because the natural history of the condition indicates that it will grow towards normality, e.g. bowlegs in the toddler. Sometimes the natural tendency seems to need a little help to achieve success and some simple method of splinting such as a Denis Browne night splint is indicated. Surprisingly enough it is much more difficult to convince parents that treatment is unnecessary than it is to prescribe a complicated, costly, and lengthy regime of active treatment. Even after a lengthy explanation that treatment is not needed, some parents will sum up the situation by saying 'So there is nothing you can do for our child.' This leaves the doctor no alternative but to go over the whole ground again—to repeat that there are dozens of things he can do for the child but that, in view of the good prognosis, there is nothing that he should do. Some surgeons take the view that most parents want treatment for their child so they oblige by prescribing some innocuous device such as a Thomas heel to keep them happy. This can be criticised on many counts but mainly because the initial premise is incorrect. Most parents are more interested in being convinced that treatment is unnecessary than in carrying out useless treatment.

The whole question of reassurance is a difficult one but, because it is so often required, the technique should be studied by all those engaged in paediatric practice. From what has already been said it will be obvious that the phrase 'There is nothing wrong' does not reassure. Even when a mother's anxiety about her child arises from not knowing the range of normal variation, there is something wrong if it is only her worrying. Similarly, the advice 'Don't worry' will fall on barren ground unless supported by an adequate explanation of the facts. Finally, it is well to remember that 'Words are not so effective as the way they are said.'

If treatment is indicated because it is known that time and growth cannot correct the fault, it is necessary to discuss the various possibilities and your reason for selecting any particular method. The parents may have a preference for some particular method and this may be allowed but they should always be given advice by the expert as to his preferred choice. It is unfair to suggest a number of different alternatives and expect the parents to make the choice. The prognosis, both with and without treatment, should be defined as accurately as possible and an attempt made to allay any unjustified fears.

Maternal treatment

It is commonly suggested that mothers should be instructed how to carry out stretching and moulding at home to overcome minor deformity, such as talipes calcaneus and infantile wry neck. I believe the practice should be discouraged because the treatment is unlikely to be effective unless performed at least to the point of discomfort and no mother is likely to do this; because the babe does not want to feel that every time her mother appears she is likely to have her neck wrung or her foot twisted; and because the majority of the conditions selected for this form of treatment will recover spontaneously anyway.

Genetic counselling

Whilst the practising orthopaedic surgeon cannot be expected to have a detailed knowledge of genetics, nevertheless he should be aware of the existence of heritable possibilities in any disorder that he diagnoses and alert the parents accordingly. Often the parents will be the first to raise the possibility especially those who have some disorder themselves or who have just produced a child with a disorder. They will want to know the chances that a future child of theirs will be affected and whether the child will pass the disorder on to his own children. In these circumstances, they should be referred to a medical geneticist who can usually give an accurate assessment of the situation. The need for accurate genetic counselling has become even more important now that prenatal diagnosis is possible with many important conditions (e.g. spina bifida) and selective abortion may be indicated.

DEFINITION OF TERMS

In developmental paediatrics and the orthopaedic surgery associated with this, many of the terms are used loosely and interchangeably. In order to promote better understanding and communication, it is important that these terms be defined and used precisely.

Defect—an abnormality of structure from any cause. The adjectival form *defective* is commonly used to describe loss of function when no actual structural defect is present. In these circumstances it is preferable to describe the loss of function as an impairment rather than a defect.

Malformation—an abnormal development or formation of part of the body. This implies that the defect is of congenital origin.

Deformity—any deviation from the normal shape and form. It is often used as a synonym for malformation but, strictly speaking, the term should be restricted to describe a change which has occurred to a part *after* birth. A deformity may be postural and fully corrigible (e.g. a drop foot) or it may be fixed and rigid. This rigidity may be due to contracture of soft tissue, to deformity of bone, or to a combination of both.

Disability—any abnormality which interferes with function.

Handicap—a disability which is sufficiently severe to impede development, activities, expectations and employment. It is important to realise that the presence of a malformation, defect, or deformity does not necessarily imply an impairment of function. Similarly, a disabled child may be taught or may learn to bypass his disability so that in practical terms he is no longer handicapped.

Handicapped, disadvantaged, deprived—Sheridan has made a clear distinction between these terms which often have a legal significance. In contrast to a handicapped child, a disadvantaged child is one who is subjected to a continuing inadequacy of materials, educational and emotional assistance which will result in his failing to achieve his inherent potential. A deprived child is one who is deprived of a normal home life and may on this account require custodial care.

CHAPTER 2

The Infant

Terminology

Acquired conditions seen in the neonate, 11
Diagnosis in the neonatal period; Birth fractures; Obstetrical paralysis; Neonatal sciatic paralysis; Acute septic arthritis of infancy

BIRTH DEFECTS AND THEIR CLASSIFICATION, 15

Packaging defects, 16

Malformations (manufacturing defects) presenting at birth, 19
Congenital talipes equinovarus (congenital club foot); Congenital dysplasia and dislocation of the hip

Spina bifida, 40
Definitions; Multiple system involvement; The causes of deformity; Problems resulting from skin anaesthesia and bone fragility; Management; The foot; The knee; The hip; Spinal surgery in spina bifida

Congenital vertical talus, 59

Proximal femoral focal deficiency, 65
Classification; Management

Congenital absence of the fibula, 72
Classification; Management

Angular deformities of the tibia, 76

Pseudarthrosis of the tibia, 79

Congenital absence of the radius (radial club hand), 80

Congenital pseudarthrosis of the clavicle, 83
Management

Supernumerary toes (polydactyly), 84

Syndactyly, 85

Congenital hemiatrophy and hemihypertrophy, 85
Hypertrophy

Chapter 2

The majority of newborn infants are born normally and are normal at birth. However, up to 40 births in every 1000 have a malformation—many of these are insignificant but approximately ten will be important and require active treatment. In recent times so much publicity has been given to the effect of drugs, smoking, insecticides, and many other noxious influences, on the developing fetus that expectant mothers are only too aware of the possibilities of having a malformed child. Each newly born babe must be carefully examined to exclude not only obvious anomalies of the musculoskeletal system but also anomalies appearing in other systems, particularly the heart. If a malformation is identified the parents should be told about it, an accurate prognosis and an outline of the necessary treatment given. As has been mentioned already, this can usually be given only by a specialist who should be brought into the picture as soon as possible, if possible on the first day of the child's life. The initial advice should always err on the side of optimism and if there are any particularly unpleasant features, these are best left out of the first consultation. The mother who has just given birth to a child with a club foot is only interested in the answer to three questions: Will he walk? Will he have to wear a boot? Will he be able to play sport? The surgeon may tend to discuss the length and complexity of treatment but the mother has little interest in this—she is only concerned with the outcome of treatment. The experienced surgeon will recognise this fact and provide answers to the relevant questions before the mother asks them.

TERMINOLOGY

Some confusion exists as to the use of descriptive terms. In order to clarify this for the reader the following notes may be useful.

Foot—the various joints in the foot and ankle have their own movements and their corresponding deformities. Table 2.1 sets out the correct usage of the terms.

In addition there are two terms used to describe the arch in the midfoot: *planus*

Table 2.1 Terminology of foot and ankle movement.

Joint	Movement	Deformity
Ankle	Dorsiflexion	Calcaneus
	Plantar flexion	Equinus
Subtalar	Inversion	Varus
	Eversion	Valgus
Midtarsal	Abduction	Abductus
	Adduction	Adductus
	Pronation	–
	Supination	–

if it is too low and *cavus* if it is too high. The big toe is said to lie in *valgus* if it points away from the midline and *varus* if towards it.

Knee—the knee is said to be in valgus when knock kneed and in varus when bandy. If hyperextended, the knee is in recurvatum (back knee).

Hip—the following terms are commonly used:
Coxa vara—decreased neck shaft angle.
Coxa valga—increased neck shaft angle.
Coxa magna—enlargement of the head.

Elbow—valgus and varus are used in a similar fashion to the knee.

ACQUIRED CONDITIONS SEEN IN THE NEONATE

Apart from congenital malformations, there are three conditions which may involve the orthopaedic surgeon in the neonatal period: birth fracture, obstetrical paralysis, osteomyelitis and septic arthritis. The important features of these will be considered before proceeding to a detailed description of birth defects.

DIAGNOSIS IN THE NEONATAL PERIOD

Every newborn baby is examined systematically in order to discover any congenital defect; however, as these are frequently multiple, the full picture may not emerge for some time. It is therefore necessary to carry out repeated examinations as opportunities present. During the stay in hospital a baby is one of many in a nursery and important symptoms and signs may be ignored.

HISTORY

The history may be somewhat vague during this period but the following areas should be explored.

Family history. A family history of congenital bone fragility or other transmissible diseases is sought.

Obstetrical history. Abnormal delivery may be associated with bone or nerve damage.

Injections. If the babe has had any injections, local signs could be due to either sepsis, haematoma, or nerve damage resulting from that injection.

Nursery infection. Any recent infections in the nursery should be noted and the particular organisms identified. The importance of this is that it may be possible to commence therapy before a bacteriological control is obtained.

EXAMINATION

The baby as a whole. This is particularly important and the overall condition may indicate that the baby is or is not ill. The presence of fever is important but it must be remembered that, even in the presence of bone sepsis, neonates rarely, if ever, have a raised temperature. A general examination is carried out for evidence of trauma or of sepsis particularly in the skin, umbilicus, nail areas, and other bones.

Local examination. The following observations are particularly important and many are likely to be noticed by the mother or an observant nurse: the baby may not move one or other limb or may cry when one particular limb is handled; a deformity may be present; or there may be tenderness, swelling or alteration in the colour of the limb.

BIRTH FRACTURES

In general, two groups can be recognised: the baby may be otherwise normal but difficult manipulations during delivery may have resulted in a fracture (especially in the femur, humerus, clavicle and skull); on the other hand, there may be a congenital bone fragility (osteogenesis imperfecta) and in this case one or more fractures may be present in association with a completely normal delivery. In the neonatal period fractures may occur if the baby is dropped or is subjected to physical maltreatment. Only the simplest possible treatment is required and considerable deformity can be accepted in the knowledge that it will rapidly correct. A collar and cuff is used for humeral fractures and simple wooden splints, well padded, are used for the femur, forearm and tibia.

OBSTETRICAL PARALYSIS

Traction on the brachial plexus during delivery may result in varying degrees of paralysis in the upper limb. This is most likely to occur when one shoulder becomes trapped behind the symphysis pubis and attempts are made to free this by traction on the head. There may be associated injuries such as fracture of the clavicle and separation of the upper humeral epiphysis. The diagnosis is usually fairly obvious at birth due to the abnormal posture of the limb and by the absence of movement. Three main types are seen.

UPPER ARM TYPE (ERB-DUCHENNE)

This results from injury to the upper trunk at Erb's point, i.e. the junction of the fifth and sixth cervical roots. The arm takes up the typical porter's tip posture by the side of the body. The elbow is a little flexed and the forearm pronated.

Examination will reveal paralysis of the deltoid, elbow flexors, and brachioradialis. Since the adductors and medial rotators of the shoulder remain innervated there is a tendency to develop an internal rotation deformity of the shoulder. The prognosis is good, although there may occasionally be some residual disability.

WHOLE ARM TYPE

All the cords of the plexus may be involved to give complete paralysis of the limb. The arm is also anaesthetic except for the medial side of the upper arm which is supplied by the intercosto brachial nerve. This type is much less common but has a much worse prognosis.

LOWER ARM TYPE

Here the predominant injury is to the last two roots of the plexus so that there is paralysis of the intrinsic muscles of the hand and a Horner's syndrome is also present. The prognosis is poor.

Treatment

Bracing in abduction—the so-called 'Statue of Liberty' position—was popular for many years but, unless used with great care this position may give rise to dislocation of the shoulder or late dislocation of the radial head. The necessary bracing is also difficult to fit and maintain and there is little evidence that the position contributes much to recovery.

For the first few days the limbs should be rested in a small collar and cuff sling to allow the local reaction around the nerves to settle down and any shoulder injury to become stable. Passive movements can then be instituted and several times a day the shoulder, elbow and wrist are put through a full range of passive movement. The mother can be taught how to do this and continue the regime when she returns home. No further recovery can be anticipated after the end of the first year. In older children, if the degree of fixed medial rotation is an embarrassment either to function or appearance, surgical correction may be indicated. This can be achieved either by tendon transplantation to restore lateral rotation as described by L'Episcopo or, in older children, lateral rotation osteotomy of the humerus.

Late posterior dislocation of the radial head may occur and is difficult to prevent. A somewhat increased range of rotation in the forearm may be obtained in those near maturity by resection of the radial head.

NEONATAL SCIATIC PARALYSIS

Sciatic paralysis occurring immediately after birth has now become a rarity since the discovery that it was caused by the injection of drugs into the umbilical cord to combat birth asphyxia. The paralysis may be complete or partial, but the lateral popliteal portion is the most commonly involved. Recovery is unusual but restoration of muscle balance below the knee may be possible by transfer of the tibialis posterior forwards to the dorsum of the foot. Shortening of the limb commonly occurs and may require correction by epiphysiodesis.

ACUTE SEPTIC ARTHRITIS OF INFANCY

Although now very uncommon, this condition still exists and, because it may be life threatening and is extremely destructive locally, it is important that the diagnosis be established quickly and proper treatment instituted. The hip and knee joints are those most commonly infected, although the shoulder and ankle may also be involved. The condition usually starts with sepsis around the umbilicus or in the skin and a metaphyseal osteomyelitis focus is established. If an abscess forms it may rupture into a joint and, in the case of the hip, this may lead to not only destruction of the epiphysis but also dislocation of the joint. The problem presents in some instances as an acute septicaemia and the involvement of the joint may not be suspected until quite late in the pathological process when an abscess forms and presents subcutaneously. In others, the general symptoms may be quite minor, consisting merely of malaise, slight fever and failure to gain weight or possibly loss of weight. Such infants may have no pyrexia, a normal white cell count, and a normal erythrocyte sedimentation rate. The patient commonly does not move the affected limb although restriction of movement at the affected joint is slight; this surprising mobility of a joint full of pus is most frequently seen at the knee.

RADIOLOGICAL APPEARANCES

In the early stages, radiographs may show soft tissue distension and, in the case of the hip, some degree of displacement. Subsequently, evidence of osteomyelitis in the femoral neck or above the acetabulum will become evident.

Early treatment

General treatment of the baby. A few infants show such disturbance and are so severely ill that the initial treatment is directed towards maintaining life by fluid balance and a high blood level of antibiotics. In addition, attention is directed firstly to the feeding—a secondary dyspepsia may be present and necessitate the use of a different milk mixture or of intravenous feeding. The haematological status is reviewed with particular reference to the haemoglobin level. It is unlikely that transfusion would be required but the administration of iron may be indicated. The second point that should be considered is that of vitamin intake.

Treatment of the infection with relevant antibiotics. Bacteriological control may be obtained by culture of a cutaneous focus or from the site of sepsis by joint aspiration or incision. Note that blood culture is only positive in a relatively small percentage of cases compared to infections occurring in the older child. Details of antibiotic therapy are considered on page 139.

Local treatment. Once the diagnosis is established, arthrotomy should be undertaken, the joint washed out, the skin only closed and the limb immobilised in some form of plaster. In the case of the hip, this will require a double hip spica with the hip in abduction, flexion and internal rotation. Drainage tubes with or without suction are not necessary.

COURSE OF THE DISEASE

In the case of the hip, a number of different changes may occur: 1 complete recovery with only some residual coxa magna; 2 dislocation with survival of the head; 3 destruction of the capital epiphysis with the femoral neck more or less in the acetabulum; 4 destruction of the epiphyseal plate with fibrous union occurring between the neck and head. In the case of the knee and ankle, dislocation does not occur but there may be destruction of all or part of the epiphysis on one side of the joint.

If dislocation occurs at the hip, is discovered early, and the joint infection adequately treated, it should be possible to replace the femoral head in the acetabulum by gentle manipulation and a good result may be obtained after a period of immobilisation. If dislocation is not discovered until late in the course of the disease or after the child has recovered from the infection, then the chances of successful reduction and retention are very poor. Even if the hip can be adequately reduced by some means, subsequent growth is often unsatisfactory and late subluxation and dysplasia are the rule. If the capital epiphysis has been destroyed, a severe leg length discrepancy will ensue. The pseudarthrosis of the hip will often retain good function and be painless for many years—often until the third or fourth decade—before pain necessitates intervention.

BIRTH DEFECTS AND THEIR CLASSIFICATION

Broadly speaking, defects can be divided into two major groups:

Packaging defects—those caused by faulty intra-uterine posture. By definition, these deformities are fully corrigible and tend to resolve spontaneously after removal from the package. The effect of growth is always towards restoring normality so that active treatment is usually not indicated. Occasionally this is not so: secondary contractures occur and a little help may be needed at birth and for a few weeks afterwards to ensure complete correction (e.g. genu recurvatum).

Manufacturing defects—those caused by maldevelopment of the fetus. These are permanent unless modified by treatment and, even when corrected by treatment, many have a tendency to grow back to the abnormal.

PACKAGING DEFECTS

Normal posture at birth

At birth, the normal babe lies on its side with arms and legs flexed. If placed on his back he rolls over to one side and if prone, the head turns to the side to allow unrestricted breathing. The normal infant exhibits a number of variations from, say, a normal 2-year-old, variations which have been brought about by the way in which the babe has been folded up and by the curvature of the uterine wall. The spine shows a C-shaped kyphosis rather like a banana, but this curve is fully mobile and, when stimulated, the babe will readily throw the spine into full extension. Other features include: 1 the hips cannot be fully extended but should abduct fully in the flexed position; 2 the knees often lack 20° of extension whereas the ankles usually allow excessive motion especially into dorsiflexion; 3 the tibia has a distinct outward curve (varus) and also a little inward twist (internal tibial torsion); 4 the feet tend to be held in equinovarus so that the soles of the feet face one another; 5 the upper limbs do not show any remarkable features at birth although the hands may be held clenched for the first month or so.

An attempt should always be made to estimate *muscle tone* based on posture—this is determined by the distribution of muscle tone and observation will usually suggest whether flexor or extensor tones predominates. Range of motion—this is excessive in hypotonia and restricted in hypertonia. Muscle consistency—gentle squeezing between finger and thumb will give quite an accurate estimate of muscle tone.

Variations of normal posture at birth

METATARSUS ADDUCTUS

This term is used to describe the foot in which there is a pure adduction of the forefoot on the hindfoot. The most striking feature is the big toe which swings out into varus leaving a wide gap between it and the second toe. The abductor hallucis constantly overacts to produce a prehensile big toe so that the foot almost resembles a hand. These feet are fully mobile and tend to grow towards normality although this correction may not be complete for several years. The posture is perpetuated by prone sleeping and resolution is aided by preventing this and, at a later date, by wearing shoes.

Occasionally, these feet develop some fixed deformity and correction by serial plaster casting will be indicated. Rarely a foot which commences life as a true

The Infant 17

metatarsus adductus seems to merge into a rigid metatarsus varus (page 167), with supination of the forefoot and cavus of the midfoot. In these, plantar release is required.

POSTURAL TALIPES EQUINOVARUS

At birth, one or both feet may resemble a moderately severe club foot. However, this condition will easily correct and overcorrect. If overcorrection is possible, treatment is unnecessary but, if the foot will only correct to the plantigrade position, it is usually wise to treat it like a club foot for a brief period using either strapping or plaster casts. Once overcorrected, there is little tendency to relapse so that prolonged splintage is unnecessary.

POSTURAL TALIPES CALCANEOVALGUS

When the foot has been packaged folded up against the leg, it appears at birth lying in calcaneus and valgus (Fig. 2.1). Again, spontaneous recovery is the rule, although in extreme cases with some fixed deformity, serial splinting for a few weeks will allay the anxiety of the parents and hasten correction. When these children begin walking, the affected foot may assume a more valgus posture but this will always resolve with simple measures such as the provision of suitable boots.

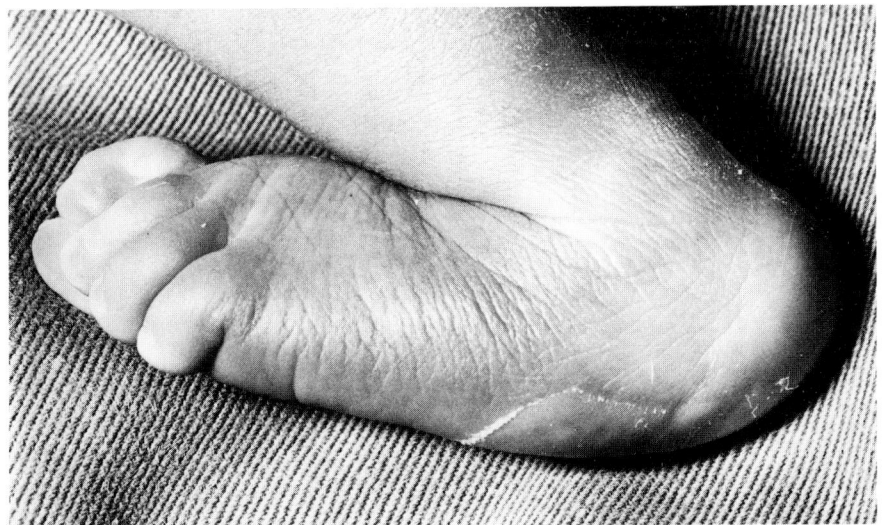

Fig. 2.1 Talipes calcaneus in the newborn. The foot is folded up against the front of the tibia. Most of these will resolve without treatment; in a few, recovery can be assisted by a short period of splinting.

18   Chapter 2

GENU RECURVATUM

This condition is very uncommon but nearly always follows a breech presentation. It appears that, in utero, the leg or legs have been folded up against the front of the body with the feet resting on the shoulders. The appearance at birth is rather alarming as the anterior surface of the knee is represented by a deep hollow and the femoral condyles are very prominent behind. There is an increased range of extension, and flexion is always limited by contracture of the quadriceps of varying degree. Although this deformity may correct spontaneously, it is best treated by serial splinting from birth. A well padded aluminium strip is bound to the anterior aspect of the leg with adhesive tape and this can be bent in situ every day until knee flexion of 90° has been obtained. This position is held for a month after which full correction will develop naturally.

EXTERNAL ROTATION OF THE HIP

When the babe lies supine, one leg may lie in external rotation and this is obviously occurring at the hip joint (Fig. 2.2). Examination will show that the

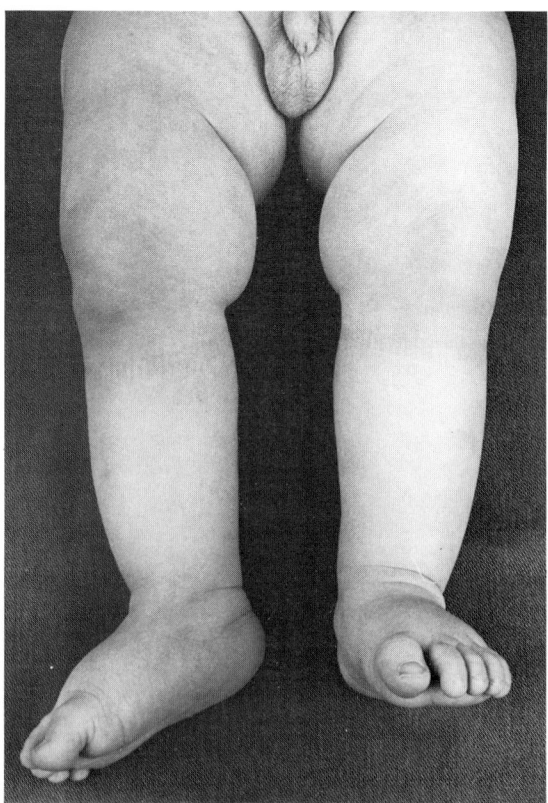

Fig. 2.2   A baby with external rotation at the right hip due to faulty intra-uterine packaging.

affected hip has an excessive range of external rotation and a limited range of internal rotation compared to the other side. The hip is otherwise normal both clinically and radiologically. This posture may persist for a year or more so that the toddler will walk with one foot turned out. Complete resolution without treatment is the rule but a protracted explanation to the parents may be anticipated.

INFANTILE POSTURAL SCOLIOSIS

Scoliosis is not usually recognised at birth unless attention is drawn to it by the presence of plagiocephaly or asymmetry of the rib cage anteriorly. The curve is long and C-shaped and fully corrigible. Neurological features are absent as are any radiological changes. Resolution is usually complete without treatment within the first year.

PLAGIOCEPHALY

Asymmetry of the vault of the skull is fairly common—the anterior portion of one side and the posterior portion of the opposite side are developed more than their counterparts so that the long axis of the skull is not in the sagittal plane but deflected to one side. There is no impairment of cerebral function and the condition can be regarded as a minor cosmetic disability most of which will resolve in the first two years. In some, the asymmetry persists in minor degrees but the hair obscures it almost entirely. Whilst most are due to intra-uterine moulding, some are acquired after birth in association with sternomastoid torticollis.

MALFORMATIONS (MANUFACTURING DEFECTS) PRESENTING AT BIRTH

CONGENITAL TALIPES EQUINOVARUS (CONGENITAL CLUB FOOT)

INCIDENCE

Congenital talipes equinovarus is the commonest congenital abnormality of the foot, occurring in about 1 per 1000 live births. It is twice as common in boys and may be uni- or bilateral.

ANATOMICAL FEATURES

The deformity in club foot is a combination of equinus, varus, adductus and cavus. The degree of each deformity is variable but all are rigid and incapable of being corrected manually. The reason for this lack of corrigibility is due to changes in the bones, skin, ligaments and tendons.

BONE AND JOINT CHANGES

The primary deformity is a dislocation of the talonavicular joint so that the forefoot is mounted on the hindfoot at almost a right-angle. Despite the fact that there is greatly increased medial deviation of the neck of the talus, the head of this bone is palpable on the outer side of the foot. It is fundamental to the understanding of club foot to appreciate how this occurs. The talus is locked in the ankle mortice and cannot rotate—the rest of the foot rotates around it. The navicular moves around to lie on the medial side of the neck of the talus and, in this position, it is in contact with the medial malleolus (Fig. 2.3). At the same time, the os calcis rotates medially and inverts so that, when seen from above, its long axis will now be the same as that of the talus. This latter feature is easily shown radiologically.

Because the foot is directed medially at right-angles to the plane of the knee, it might appear that tibial intorsion is present. This is usually not so and this fault

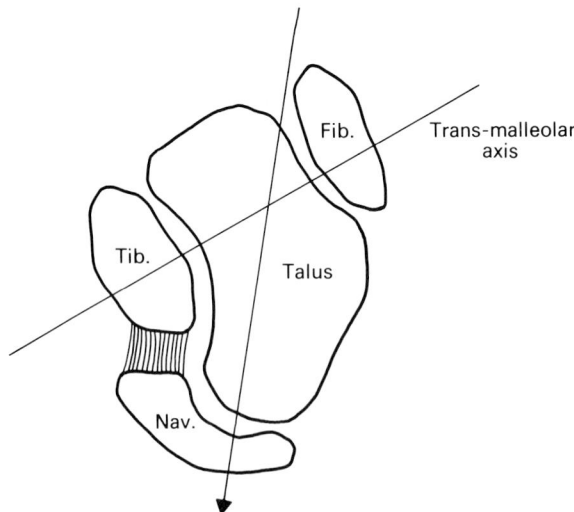

Fig. 2.3 Some of the features of the pathology of congenital talipes equinovarus. The vertical arrow indicates the direction in which the foot points. Note that the body of the talus, lying between the tibial and fibular malleoli, is directed much more laterally than this arrow. There is medial angulation on the neck of the talus so that the articular surface of the head of the talus is directed medially and lies just anterior to the medial malleolus. The navicular is subluxated medially relative to its normal relationship to the head of the talus and is bound to the medial malleolus by a 'knot'.

must be recognised as any de-rotation performed above the ankle will not correct the basic dislocation in the foot.

SOFT TISSUE CHANGES

Although all tissues at the back and medial side are contracted, it should be appreciated, if release surgery is contemplated, that some are more important than others.

Posterior contractures—the triceps surae muscle is the most important contracture and the posterior capsule of the ankle the least important barrier to correction. The posterior fibres of the deltoid ligament and the posterior talofibular ligament often prevent full correction.

Medial contractures—the talonavicular subluxation is firmly fixed by contractures involving the tibialis posterior tendon, the anterior fibres of the deltoid ligament, the bifurcate, and the spring ligament. All these structures demand release during surgical correction. The subtalar joint is held in varus by the contracted deltoid ligament, the subtalar capsule and the interosseus ligament.

Plantar contractures—the abductor hallucis is the main contracture but the plantar fascia and ligaments may be affected.

CLINICAL FEATURES

The classical appearance of a club foot is easy to recognise at birth but the examiner must first determine that the deformity is rigid. If slight pressure produces a plantigrade or valgus foot, the diagnosis is postural talipes and no further treatment is necessary. If the foot will not correct it is useful to record the degree of rigidity as this will often determine the plan of treatment. The more rigid the foot, the more likely it is that surgical release will be required.

RADIOLOGICAL FEATURES

The diagnosis of congenital talipes equinovarus is a clinical one and for the most part x-rays merely confirm the obvious. However, x-ray examination can record the degree of deformity or correction and also reveal the presence of degenerative changes which may influence the choice of treatment. This is particularly so in the older child.

In the neonate and small child where there may be difficulty in appreciating talonavicular displacement, x-rays cannot help as the navicular bone is unossified at this age; again we must rely on clinical evaluation. As a general rule, examination of the footwear will provide a more accurate parameter of correction or lack of it than will the x-ray examination. In regard to the radiology of club foot it is necessary to take at least two standard views and prerequisites to success are a willing subject and a skilled radiographer.

Antero-posterior. The foot is plantarflexed 30° at the ankle and the tube angled 30° to the perpendicular. Lines are drawn through the centre of the long axis of the talus (parallel to the medial border) and through the long axis of the calcaneus (parallel to the lateral border). The angle so formed is called the talocalcaneal angle and the normal variation is 20–40° (see Fig. 2.4).

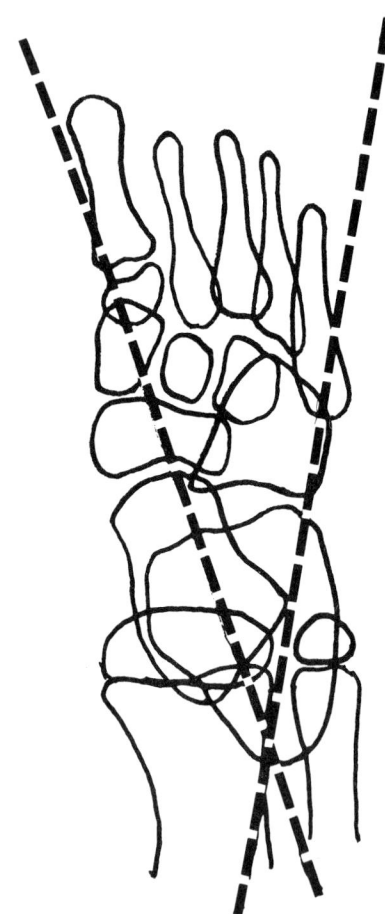

Fig. 2.4 The talocalcaneal angle is measured in an antero-posterior x-ray.

Lateral. The child is positioned lying on the affected side with knee flexed and the lateral malleolus and 5th metatarsal in contact with the cassette. The foot is forced into dorsiflexion either manually or with a translucent splint. Lines are drawn through the midpoint of the head and body of the talus and along the bottom of the calcaneus. The talocalcaneal angle so formed has a normal range of 35–50° (Figs. 2.5 & 2.6). The club foot range is between 35° and −10°.

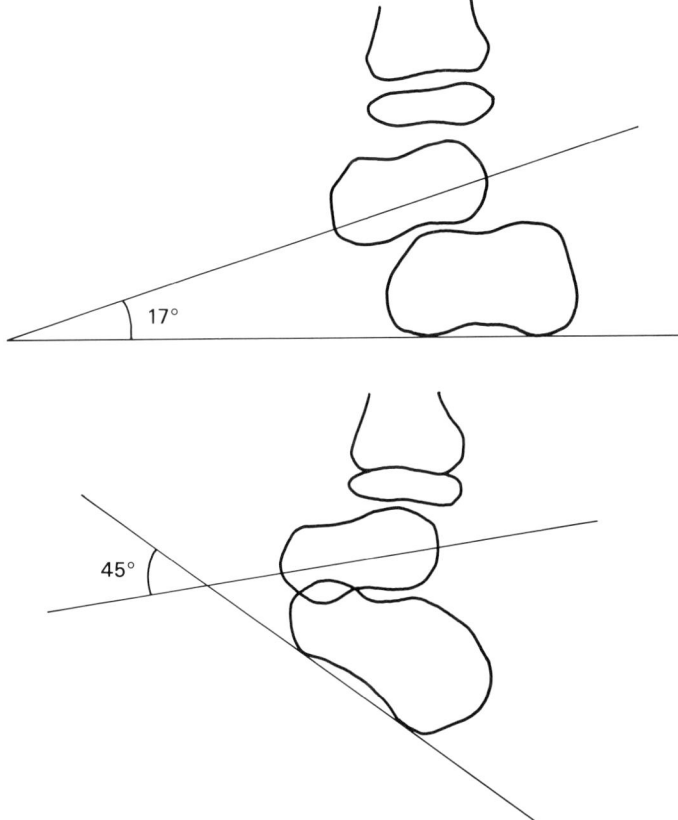

Figs. 2.5 & 2.6 (*Top*) The talocalcaneal angle in the lateral view in a normal foot. (*Bottom*) The talocalcaneal angle in a club foot.

TREATMENT

The aim of treatment is to produce, by the simplest means, a plantigrade, painless mobile foot which will not relapse during growth. Hippocrates summed up the position neatly although his advice was largely disregarded until very recent times. He said, 'in a word, as wax is moulded, the parts must be brought to their natural position . . . adjusting them with the hands and bandaging them in the same position, but putting them in position with delicacy and not violently.'

Many methods of treatment are available but the guiding principle should be to select a method which will not damage articular cartilage. In the young foot, the cartilage is the most delicate tissue and the ligaments the strongest, so that any application of force is more likely to damage cartilage and crush bone than to stretch any soft tissue. Once damaged in this way, stiffness is inevitable and stiff feet always relapse.

The actual method selected will also be influenced by the age of the child, previous treatment, and by economic and geographic considerations. The skill of the surgeon is also very relevant for unskilled treatment may produce a foot which is in fact worse than one entirely untreated. Regardless of the method used, the corrected position must be maintained for a long period in plaster to allow the bones to grow to a normal shape and to allow fibrous tissue to mature.

Correction of club feet has traditionally been conservative using various splints or serial casts and there is no doubt that good results can be obtained in this way. However, the method is time consuming, tends to produce incomplete or vicarious correction, and is associated with a high relapse rate. Surgical correction if carried out meticulously and followed by adequate after-care will give better results but should only be attempted by those surgeons constantly involved in this type of work. The trend has been to early surgery but there is general agreement that, in the newborn, a trial of conservative treatment is always indicated.

Primary treatment of the newborn foot

A wide variety of methods is available but the two most commonly used are Denis Browne splintage and serial casting.

DENIS BROWNE SPLINTAGE

This method is convenient and effective but requires considerable skill and experience. Because the splints are commonly used incorrectly the technique as advocated by Denis Browne is described here in some detail. The materials required and method of application are as follows.

1 A pair of splints made out of aluminium sufficiently soft that the metal can be bent with the fingers.
2 An aluminium bar and wing nuts (Fig. 2.7)
3 A reel of white zinc oxide adhesive plaster 1 inch wide.
(Elasticised strapping should not be used.)
4 A supply of tincture Benzoin Co.
5 White adhesive felt $\frac{3}{16}$th inch (5 mm) thick.

Stage I. The shin is first painted with tincture of Benzoin which increases the adhesion of the strapping and protects the skin. Two pieces of adhesive felt are cut: one is about $\frac{3}{4}$ inch (2 cm) square and is placed under the base of the fifth metatarsal; the other is a strip $\frac{3}{4}$ inch wide and 3 inches (8 cm) long—this is applied to the outer half of the heel and then up the outer side of the leg.

Stage II. An assistant (or the mother) holds the splint by the protruding bolt between the index and forefingers and applies the sole plate to the sole of the foot

The Infant

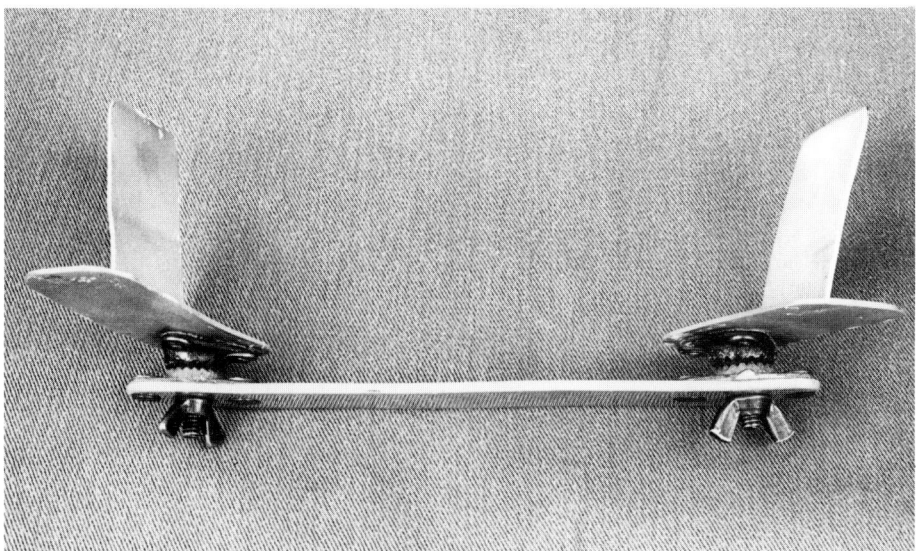

Fig. 2.7 The Denis Browne splint used for the correction of talipes in the infant. The foot pieces are made of soft aluminium so that they can be bent to increase the degree of correction.

and the felt pads. This will only be possible if the vertical part of the splint is allowed to stand well out from the leg.

Stage III. Non-stretch adhesive strapping 1 inch (2.5 cm) wide is started by attaching it to the sole plate just under the little toe and it is then passed twice around the forefoot. Note that the strapping must pull off the reel freely otherwise there is a tendency to apply it too tightly.

Stage IV. The third turn (3) passes across the front of the ankle from lateral to medial side, then round the heel but *not* round the corner of the splint.

Stage V. The fourth turn (4) follows a similar course to the third across the ankle but then crosses the corner of the splint. Now the foot is secured to the foot plate and the vertical part of the splint becomes a lever by which the foot can be inverted or everted and, to a certain extent, dorsiflexed.

Stage VI. The vertical part of the splint is now approximated to the side of the leg against the felt strip. If this is obviously exerting too much pressure, the angle between the foot plate and the vertical plate can be decreased by bending the metal.

Chapter 2

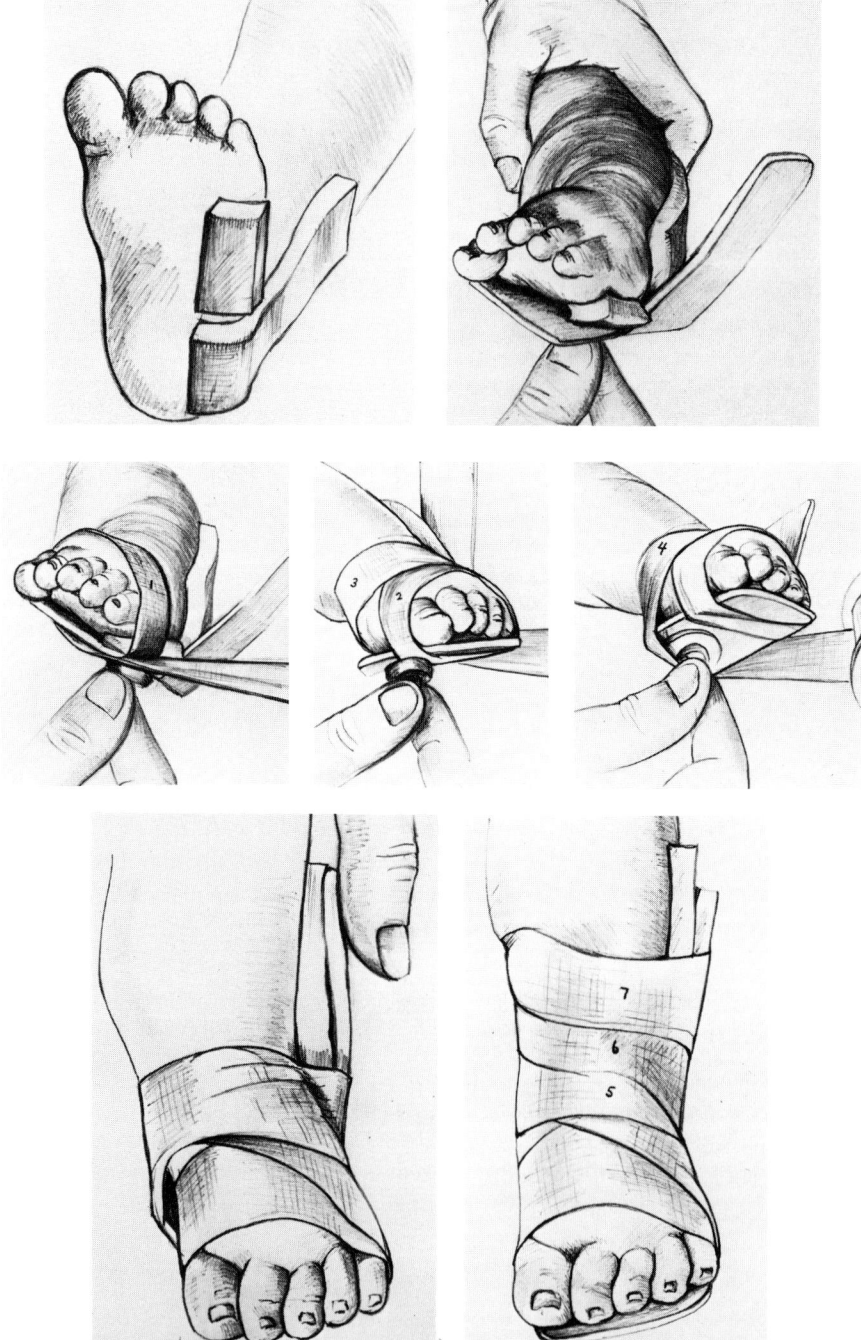

Figs. 2.8–2.14 Stages I–VII in the application of a Denis Browne splint.

Stage VII. The last three turns (5, 6, 7) are now applied. If the circulation is arrested by this manoeuvre they are removed and the plate allowed to swing out from the leg. After a few minutes it is returned to the leg and the strapping re-applied more loosely.

Finally the bar is attached to the two splints with wing nuts. For the first two applications it may be necessary to have the felt turned inwards towards each other for the first 24 hours. The mother can then be instructed to turn them out about 20° without fear of obstructing the circulation.

It is our usual practice to apply the splint as soon as the feet are first seen, to repeat this after 5–7 days and then every 10–14 days. Once full overcorrection is obtained, the splints need renewal every 14–21 days until the child is approximately 4 months of age. By the time the foot is large enough to accept a removable sleeping splint which consists of two small boots attached to a bar. This should be retained until the child begins to walk, when further splintage should be unnecessary.

The circulation of the toes is now checked. Some degree of blueness is acceptable but if the toes are white the last three turns are removed and the side piece allowed to swing out. Circulation will return at once and after an interval the position of the side piece can be restored without prejudice to the circulation.

At the first application it may not be possible to fit the bar immediately and it can therefore be left off for 24 hours. When it is finally placed into position the feet are allowed to take up whatever position appears to produce least discomfort, and this will usually be with both feet internally rotated. The mother is then instructed to undo the wing nut and turn the foot into external rotation a few degrees each day. The splints are re-applied firstly at weekly intervals and then, when correction has been obtained, at fortnightly intervals. At about the age of 4 months, the foot will be big enough to accept a small pair of bootees attached to a bar and this is worn as a night splint until the child commences walking.

SERIAL CASTING

This is perhaps the most commonly used method but again skill is required to make a cast which is not too tight that it will produce pressure sores yet not so loose that it falls off. The leg is covered in stockinette (Fig. 2.15) and the mother or a nurse holds the foot in a position of maximum correction while the cast is applied (Fig. 2.16). There should be no prior manipulation and the whole exercise should be painless. The cast is changed at weekly intervals until overcorrection is obtained and this position is then retained for several months. A removable night splint can then be used, at least until the child begins to walk.

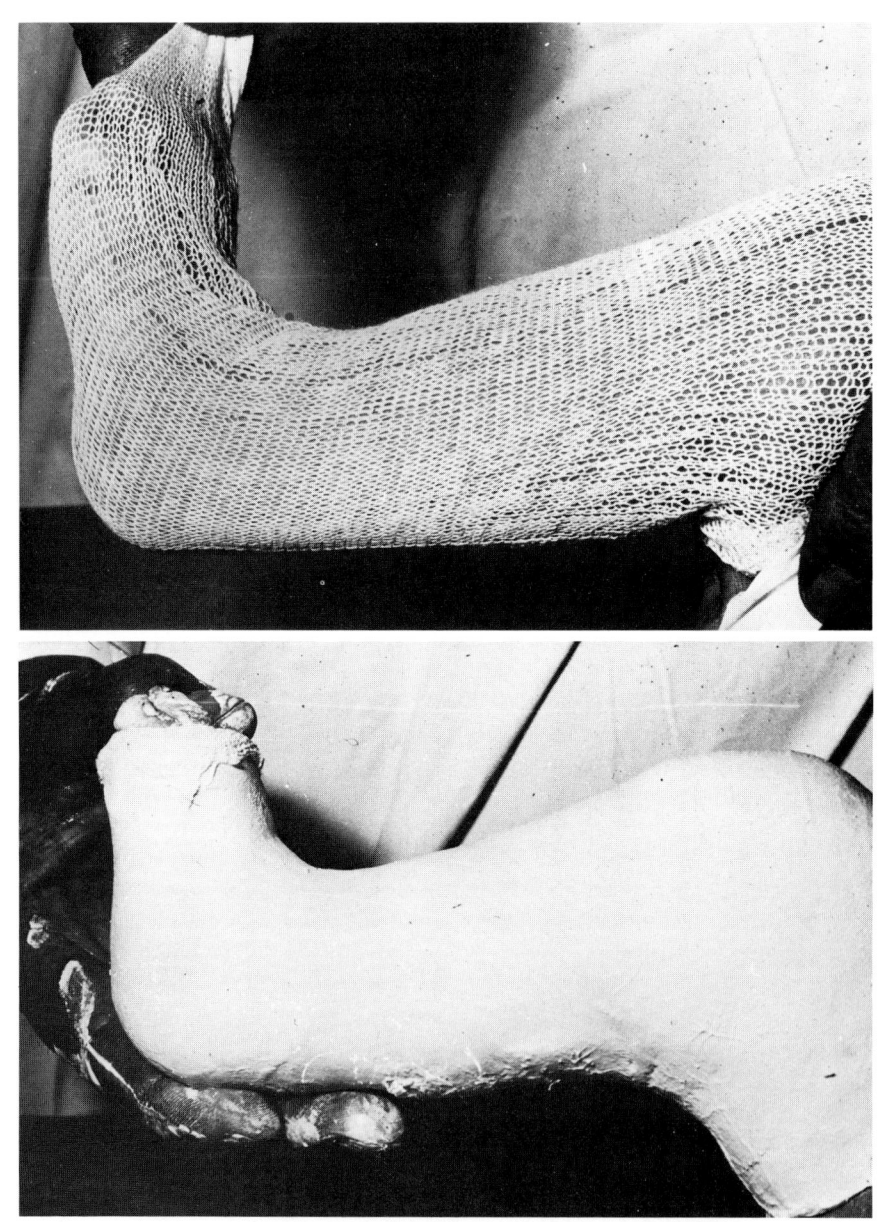

Figs. 2.15 & 2.16 The application of a plaster cast for congenital talipes equinovarus. Tube gauze is applied to the leg as high as the groin. The distal end of the tube is left long so that it can be held between the right thumb and forefinger of the assistant. The assistant holds the thigh in his left hand and pulls the foot—by pulling the end of the tube gauze—in the direction of calcaneo-valgus. There is no force employed in the correction of the deformity. The below-knee portion of the cast is then applied. (*Bottom*) When the below-knee portion has dried, the cast is completed to above the knee.

The resistant or relapsed club foot

Failure to correct in the first few months or relapse after correction indicates that surgical intervention is required. Surgical release can be planned according to the deformity present, as shown in Table 2.2.

Table 2.2   Appropriate surgical release of club foot deformities

Deformity	Release
Equinus	Posterior
Varus	Medial
Cavus	Plantar
T-N dislocation	T-N and plantar

In the neonatal club foot, resistant equinus occurs most frequently but persisting talonavicular subluxation is almost as common. The latter is easily recognised both by a palpable hollow where there would normally be a prominent navicular tubercle and also by a transverse skin crease which is often found in the same region (Fig. 2.17).

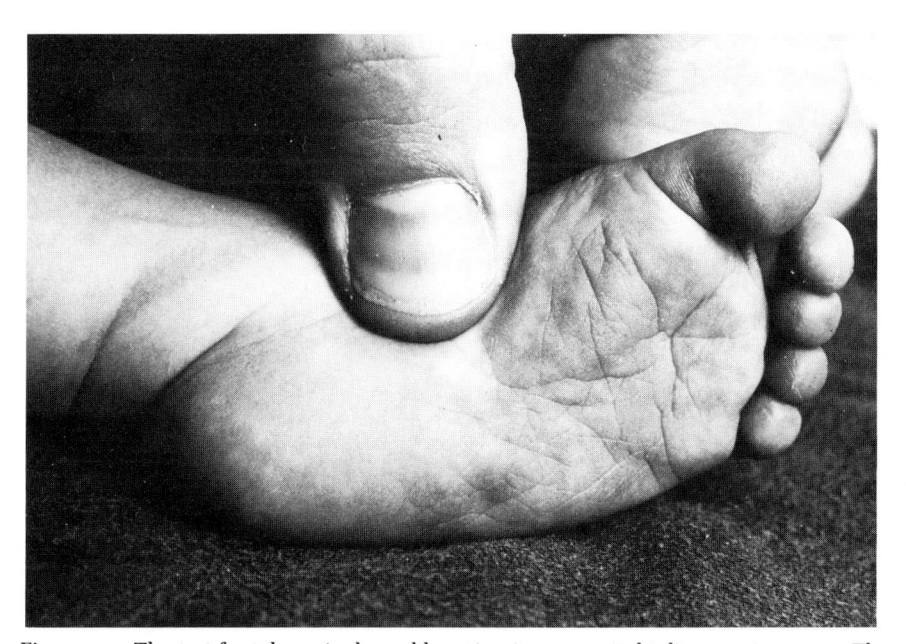

Fig. 2.17 The test for talonavicular subluxation in congenital talipes equinovarus. The clinician's thumb passes into a depression at the site of a skin crease just anterior to the medial malleolus.

OPERATIVE DETAILS

It is not proposed to discuss the surgery in any detail but the important features of each release will be mentioned.

Exposure. A universal incision is needed so that if one part of this is used at any given time it may be extended as the indications arise without fear of producing ischaemia in the flap so produced. A suitable incision is shown in Fig. 2.17a. Note that the vertical limb lies halfway between the tibia and tendo-Achilles for, in this position, the scar will not form a keloid nor rub on the shoe. The horizontal limb is high up on the foot to prevent bowstringing of the scar.

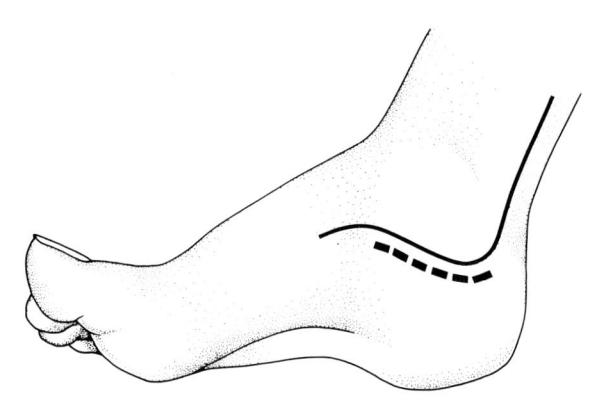

Fig. 2.17a A universal incision suitable for surgical release of club foot. The broken line indicates that part of the incision which may be used for talonavicular release.

Posterior release. The tendo-Achilles is lengthened in the Z manner, and the distal limb is left attached to the lateral half of the os calcis. The posterior capsule of the ankle joint is not usually contracted but the posterior talofibular ligament and the posterior fibres of the deltoid ligament are important structures to release. Using suitable retractors it is possible to divide the posterior structures from the tip of one malleolus to the tip of the other.

Talonavicular release. Using the full horizontal component of the universal incision the neurovascular bundle is isolated and retracted with a tape. The sheath of the tibialis posterior is opened in the line of the tendon and the tendon lengthened in the Z manner making the limbs of the Z as long as possible. The distal limb is retracted downwards and by sharp dissection between the medial malleolus and the navicular the talonavicular joint is opened. This is not always easy as the medial capsule of the joint is greatly thickened by contributions from the deltoid ligament and the sheath of the tibialis posterior. Having divided the medial capsule, the inferior capsule (spring ligament) and the tough dorsal capsule are divided. It may now be possible to reduce the dislocation but if there is any difficulty two further moves may be necessary.

Firstly, on the lateral side of the talar neck the capsule may be adherent so that there is no space into which the navicular may move. In infants this space can be provided by passing a blunt curved dissector into the joint but, in older children, it may be necessary to make a lateral incision to free the capsule adequately. Secondly, if the navicular has been badly subluxated and especially if there is a cavus element to the deformity, plantar release is necessary to allow the forefoot to swing around into the new position.

After satisfactory reduction it is wise to secure this with a fine Kirschner wire which is buried under the skin on the dorsum of the foot and removed two weeks later at the first change of plaster. The tibialis posterior tendon is repaired in the lengthened position and the skin closed with a subcuticular suture.

Medial release. A full medial release is indicated when hindfoot varus is present and, in these circumstances, talonavicular subluxation is usually an accompaniment. The operation therefore consists of talonavicular release together with the following: 1 Tenotomy of flexor hallucis longus and flexor digitorum longus, together with excision of their sheaths. 2 Division of the medial talocalcaneal capsule and the interosseus ligament. 3 Division of the deep fibres of the deltoid to expose the ankle. This should be avoided if possible but may be necessary in older children with severe deformity. 4 Division of the calcaneal branches of the neurovascular bundle. This is necessary to allow the bundle to dislocate forwards as the foot is corrected.

Closure. The dissection will allow the foot to be placed in a position of much overcorrection but this position must be avoided not only because skin closure will be difficult but also because an overcorrected valgus foot may result. It is safer to place the foot in a little valgus and calcaneus and this may be slightly increased if desired at the first plaster change two weeks following surgery when the skin will have healed.

Plantar release. The abductor hallucis has a long origin starting from the os calcis behind and curving along the inner border of the foot (Fig. 2.18). This must all be released together with the plantar fascia and the calcaneal branches of the bundle if the operation is to be effective.

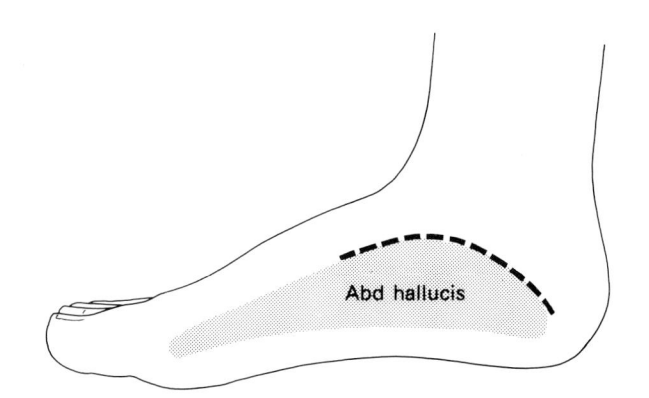

Fig. 2.18 The abductor hallucis muscle has a long origin shown here by a broken line.

Length of immobilisation. After surgery the length of immobilisation will depend on the age of the child and on the amount of previous treatment. This time will vary from six weeks to six months but, as a rule, it can be said that longer immobilisation is always better than shorter. Long periods of post-operative immobilisation are more likely to produce a mobile foot rather than a stiff one.

OTHER OPERATIONS

These may be classified into two groups: those occasionally required and those rarely required. The first group includes *Osteotomy of the os calcis (Dwyer)*. This operation was originally designed for pes cavo-varus and, for this indication, gives excellent results. When used in club feet the results are disappointing, probably due to the small size of the heel and the fact that deformity in the midfoot is usually present as well. *Metatarsal osteotomy*—persistent hooking of the forefoot is occasionally seen in the absence of talonavicular subluxation and causes rapid distortion of footwear. The medial four metatarsals are divided at their bases and the fifth shortened by removal of a small segment. *Triple arthrodesis*—when unacceptable deformity is present at maturity, triple arthrodesis is indicated. The operation should never be performed on immature feet for, while correction may be obtained, there is considerable growth arrest and relapse is the rule. In most children the foot can be considered sufficiently mature for bone surgery at the age of 12 years.

The second group includes *Tendon transfers*—transfer of the tibialis posterior forwards or tibialis anterior laterally have been popular at various times and undoubtedly have a place in paralytic talipes. In congenital talipes they have a regrettable tendency to produce a gross valgus deformity. *Tibial derotation osteotomy*—very occasionally true tibial intorsion exists in the older child and produces an unsightly gait. It is worth repeating here that when the foot is turned in it is more likely to be due to unreduced talonavicular subluxation or to an inset hip posture than to tibial intorsion. When the latter is present, correction is carried out in the lower third of the tibia and maintained by pins embedded in the plaster. Delayed union may occur. *Astragalectomy and amputation* should never be required.

CONGENITAL DYSPLASIA AND DISLOCATION OF THE HIP

The term *dysplasia* describes either an inadequate acetabulum or a deformity of the upper femur, or both of these conditions. In practice, however, use of the term is commonly restricted to a description of the acetabulum. The term *dislocation* is used to describe the condition where there is an alteration in the relationship of the head of the femur to the acetabulum. Dislocation may be subdivided into: subluxation—where the femoral head is displaced laterally but the limbus is still in contact with the head and superior to it. If the hip is examined there is no sensation of dislocation or reduction. Dislocation—where the head is no longer in contact with the acetabulum and the limbus now lies medial to the head. On manipulation there may be a sense of dislocation and reduction if the hip is reducible.

INCIDENCE

The incidence of this condition in Australia, North America and Europe is usually quoted as 4 per 1000 live births. This figure would be much increased if every child who has a 'clunking' hip at birth is diagnosed as having a congenitally dislocated hip. Many of these 'clunking' hips do so for a few days only and it is doubtful if they should be included.

The incidence of the condition is low amongst the Chinese and high in certain North American Indians, Italians, Yugoslavs, Greeks and Japanese. These variations are probably due both to genetic and environmental factors.

SEX RATIO

The sex ratio differs in different countries but is 5–10 times more common in girls.

AETIOLOGY

It is probable that there are two groups of aetiological factors responsible for dysplasia and dislocation of the hip: 1 excessive generalised joint laxity; and 2 defective growth and development of the acetabulum. Either of these factors alone may account for the genetic predisposition to hip dislocation. There appears to be a greater proportion of the joint laxity type in neonatal dislocations and more of the acetabular dysplasia type in dislocations diagnosed at a later age. The pattern of inheritance remains uncertain as both systems are probably acting together in many cases. Generalised joint laxity may be acting by dominant inheritance and acetabular dysplasia by polygenic inheritance.

In addition, there are environmental factors. The condition is more common in breech presentations, in babies who have undergone version late in pregnancy, in the first-born child, in children born in winter, and in those children who are swaddled with their hips in an extended and adducted position during the first months of life.

GENETIC COUNSELLING

With normal parents the risk to subsequent siblings of an index patient is 6% (brothers 1%, sisters 11%). If one parent has congenital dislocation, the risk of a child is 12% (sons 6%, daughters 17%). If one parent and already one child has congenital dislocation of the hip, then the risk to a second child is 36%.

DIAGNOSIS IN THE NEWBORN

Every baby should be examined for hip dislocations during the first day of life and again before discharge from the maternity hospital. The baby is stripped and examined on a large, firm bench. They must be completely relaxed and examination should be gentle. If the baby is crying, try offering a bottle or dummy to suck. With the legs extended, any asymmetry of the legs or adductor creases is noted. A flexion contracture of 30° is normal in the newborn.

The examiner then holds the leg to be examined in his hand (his hand is the opposite hand to the side of the hip to be examined) with the knee flexed, the thumb over the lesser trochanter and the middle finger over the greater trochanter (Figs. 2.19–2.21). The pelvis is steadied by the other hand and the flexed thigh is abducted and adducted and any 'clunk' or jerk is noted. With the hip abducted about 45° the femur is gently rocked backwards and forwards on the pelvis and again any jerk or clunk is noted (Figs. 2.22 & 2.23). The findings on this examination may be of four kinds.

1   A *fine click* in the hip joint not associated with any laxity or abnormal movement between the femur and the pelvis. This is very common and of no significance. It is probably a vacuum phenomenon.

2   A *laxity* in the hip joint not associated with any jerk on abduction of the hip.

The Infant 35

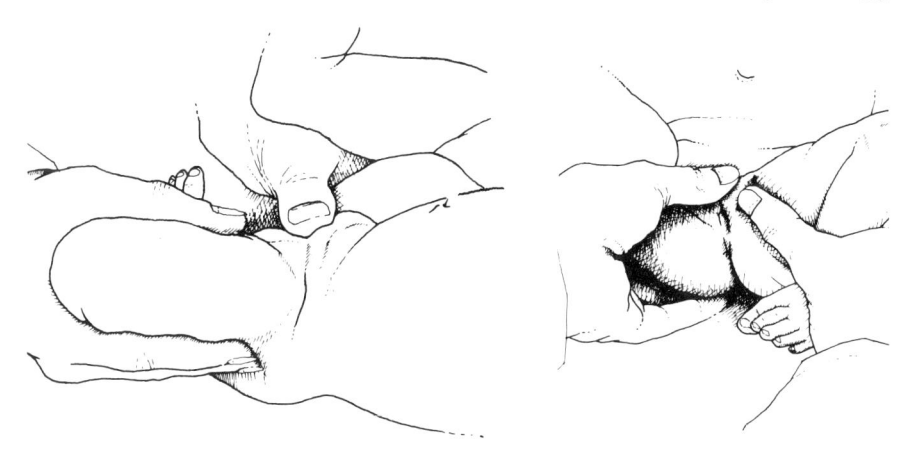

Figs. 2.19 & 2.20 The left hip is grasped gently between the examiner's right thumb and fingers.

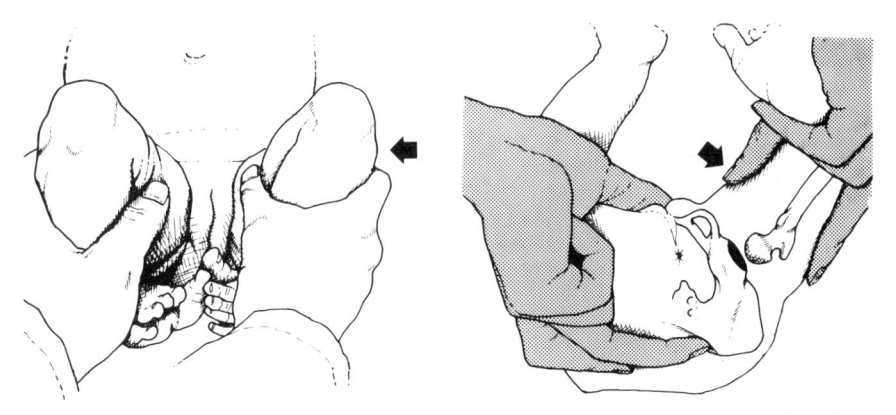

Figs. 2.21 & 2.22 The leg is adducted and the examiner gently presses back with the thumb. The head of the femur can be felt to jerk backwards out of the socket.

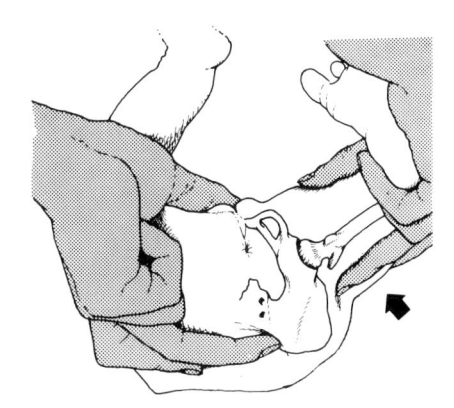

Figs. 2.23 As the leg is abducted, the head of the femur is felt to 'clunk' forwards into the socket.

The hip can be felt to dislocate smoothly without any 'clunk'. This is common in the first two or three days of life, especially in premature and shocked babies. It usually disappears within a week and it is probably of no significance. Persistent laxity is significant and the baby should be regarded as having a potential dislocation of the hip and be treated for this. Those who have temporary laxity (disappearing within a week) should be subjected to re-examination and x-ray at the age of 3 or 4 months.

3   A *palpable and visible jerk forward* of the upper end of the femur when the flexed thigh is abducted to approximately 45° (Ortolani's sign of re-entry). The thigh can then be fully abducted. When the thigh is then adducted to 45°, the upper end of the femur jerks backward. The head of the femur, which is half an inch (12 mm) in diameter at this age, can be moved in and out of the acetabulum over the posterior rim. This distinctive sign is palpable, audible and visible. If untreated, these hips are likely to progress to congenital dislocation as seen in young children.

4   There is *considerable restriction of abduction* in flexion usually on both sides but the Ortolani sign cannot be elicited. This usually means that the hips are dislocated and irreducible—a group referred to as teratological dislocations because the hip has been manufactured in the dislocated position. These hips require operative reduction at a later date. Note that other congenital anomalies may be present in these infants.

Radiography has no place in the diagnosis of congenital dislocation of the hip in the neonatal period. The diagnosis is clinical and treatment is dictated by the clinical findings. All children whose hips were suspect at birth (whether or not signs of dislocation were still present by the time the orthopaedic surgeon saw the child) should have an antero-posterior x-ray of the pelvis (with the legs in neutral position) at the age of 3 or 4 months. All siblings and first degree relatives of children with congenital hip dislocation should also have x-rays at this time to rule out the possibility of symptomless dysplasia.

TREATMENT IN THE NEONATE

If the dislocated hip is held in a flexed and abducted position for three months it will usually develop normally. We have found the Pavlik harness to be a very satisfactory orthosis (Fig. 2.24). It allows a range of motion at the hip joints, but prevents excessive adduction and extension of the hips. If the signs of dislocation of the hip have not disappeared by the tenth day of life, then the harness is applied. The hips should not be excessively abducted nor excessively flexed. Double napkins ensure that the hips do not adduct and the mother is instructed to lie the babe either prone or supine, but not on their side. If the hip is clinically stable after a month, the harness may then be removed daily so that the baby can be bathed.

At the age of 3 months, the harness is discarded and radiographs are taken. In general, the clinical features and x-rays are normal at this stage, however interpretation of the x-rays may still be difficult if the ossific nucleus has not

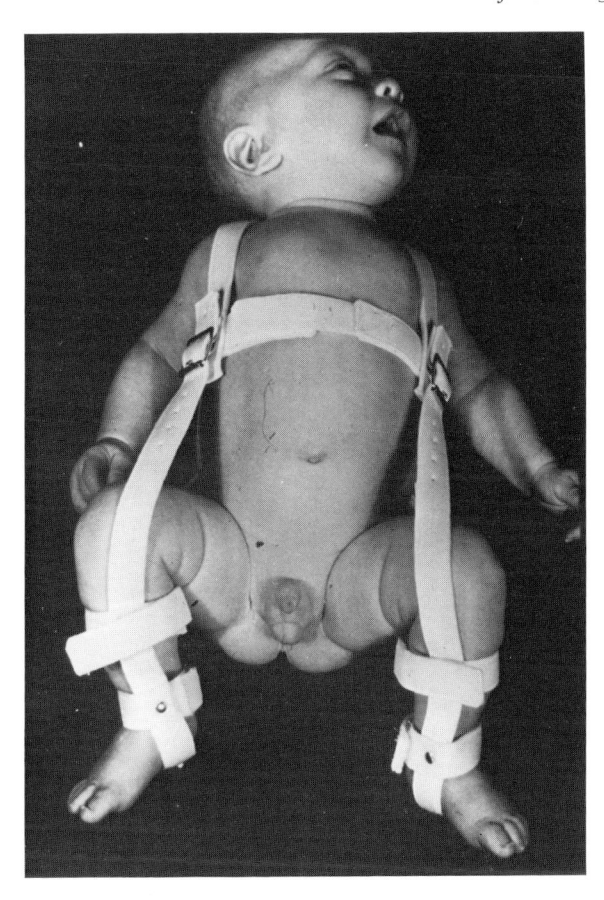

Fig. 2.24 The Pavlik harness.

appeared and, in this case, further x-rays are taken two months later. In all children with neonatal dislocation, x-rays are repeated when the child is walking.

DIAGNOSIS IN THE OLDER INFANT

Palpable dislocation and reduction becomes more difficult to elicit during the first few weeks of life but is sometimes present up to the age of 6 months. As this physical sign disappears, new physical signs appear because the head of the femur is no longer in the acetabulum. There is now limited abduction of the flexed hip. This sign is not diagnostic but should warrant an x-ray where there is asymmetry in the range of abduction of the hip or when the range of abduction of both hips is inappropriate for the age of the child. During the first year of life the range of abduction in flexion should be approximately 60° and this arc lessens with age.

With the hips extended, the relationship of the tip of the greater trochanter to the anterior superior iliac spine should be palpated on both sides simultaneously. Elevation of the tip of the trochanter indicates hip dislocation or coxa vara. There may be difficulty in palpating the pulsations of the femoral artery at the groin, broadening of the perineum, or asymmetry of the gluteal or adductor creases; telescoping may be present; in unilateral cases there is shortening of the affected leg. Over the age of one year, the child may present because of delay in walking or because of an abnormal gait.

SUBLUXATION OF THE HIP

Here the abnormality of gait is much less obvious and hence presentation tends to be later. This group cannot be diagnosed at birth as there is no sense of dislocation and reduction. The physical signs have already been mentioned above but are less obvious.

Radiological diagnosis

Changes are present in the acetabulum, the upper end of the femur, and the relationship between the acetabulum and the femur.

The acetabular roof is less horizontal than normal and there is an absence of the normal outer lip to the acetabulum. There would seem to be little point in measuring the 'acetabular index' as there is a wide range of normality in the first twelve months of life and the angle can be varied by positioning the child during the x-ray examination. The original concept of Putti that 'predislocation' could be diagnosed at birth by measurement of the acetabular angle is no longer tenable.

The upper end of the femur shows a reduction in the femoral neck shaft angle so that the neck of the femur and the shaft of the femur tend towards a straight line. This is due to anteversion of the femur rather than to coxa valga. The femoral neck capital epiphysis is delayed in appearance and, when present, is smaller than normal for that age and, in unilateral cases, smaller than the epiphysis on the non-affected side.

There are varying degrees of dislocation of the hip. The essence of examination of the x-rays in unilateral cases is to compare carefully the two hips. For unilateral or bilateral dislocation, any lateral and upward displacement of the upper end of the femur in relation to the pelvis is noted. Shenton's line and Perkins' line should be estimated and any increase in the medial joint space assessed. Compare also the degree to which the head of the femur is covered by the acetabulum on the two sides.

Management

0–6 MONTHS

Management in the neonatal period has already been considered. The Pavlik harness may be used successfully in most children who present up to the age of 6 months. Even if there is limited abduction-in-flexion and the sign of reduction cannot be demonstrated, the harness may be applied and the hip will often reduce during the next few weeks. That such reduction has occurred should be confirmed clinically and radiologically. Care must be taken to ensure that the harness is not used in such a way as to abduct the hip too rapidly or to place the hip in an extreme position since avascular necrosis of the femoral head may result.

If circumstances do not allow the use of a harness or if the harness is ineffectual, then the child should be admitted to hospital for coronal traction (see below).

6–12 MONTHS

A few children who present in the early part of this period may be managed in a Pavlik harness. However, the majority require admission to hospital for traction. This traction is necessary to stretch the soft tissue so that, after reduction of the hip, it can be placed in a stable position with little risk of avascular necrosis of the femoral head.

The child is placed on gallows traction and the two legs are slowly separated until the angle between them is approximately 60° (Fig. 2.25). This process should occupy at least two weeks. The baby is then taken to the operating theatre and, under general anaesthesia, the hips are examined.

In general, it is found that the dislocated hip will reduce by being placed in a

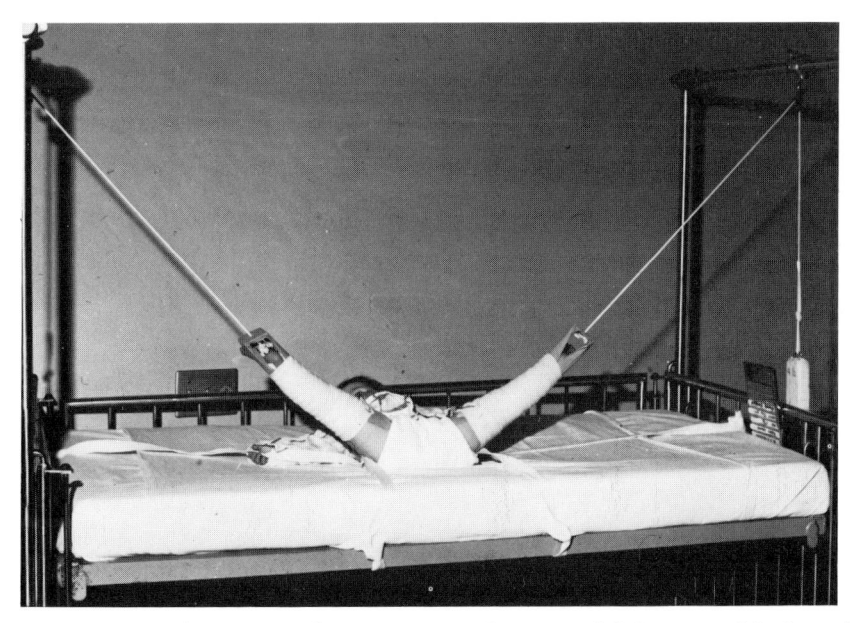

Fig. 2.25 Coronal traction in the managment of congenital dislocation of the hip. The legs should not be further abducted than is shown here.

position of flexion and abduction. The hip is usually very stable if placed in a little more than 90° of flexion and in approximately 70° of abduction. If radiographs confirm this reduction, a double hip spica is applied and the position of abduction selected should be one which is about 10° short of the maximum available. This will ensure that there will not be excessive pressure on the articular cartilage of the joint on the one hand, and that the reduction will be stable and capable of being retained by the cast on the other. Frequently the femoral head stands out somewhat from the acetabulum but, provided there has been a good sense of reduction and this is stable, then the femoral head will sink into the acetabulum over the ensuing two months.

At six weeks following reduction the double hip spica is removed, x-rays are taken to confirm that reduction has been maintained and a Denis Browne CDH splint is applied. This is retained until x-rays show good acetabular development. The total period from reduction of the dislocated hip to discarding the splint will be not less than six months.

If examination under anaesthesia reveals that the hip is irreducible or, although reducible, it dislocates as soon as it is extended or adducted a few degrees, then operative reduction is performed (see page 178). Contrast arthrography is not routinely performed because it does not affect the decision; the investigation is reserved for the patient with complex problems brought about by previous failed treatment.

(See also p. 95 for the management of CDH presenting over the age of 1 year.)

SPINA BIFIDA

Spina bifida belongs to a group of disturbances of development of the vertebral arches. These are often associated with abnormalities of structures derived from the neural tube and the meninges. There may be associated cyst formation.

DEFINITIONS

Myelomeningocele is the form of spina bifida which most commonly requires treatment. There is a fluid-filled cystic swelling formed by dura and arachnoid which protrudes through a defect in the vertebral arches. The spinal cord and nerve roots are carried out into the fundus of the sac. If the neural plate material is spread out on the surface of the cystic swelling (or in a shallow depression on the back itself) the condition is spoken of as a *myelocele*.

Meningocele is a relatively uncommon variety of spina bifida. There is a defect in the vertebral arches and a cystic swelling of the dura and arachnoid without inclusion of the spinal cord which is entirely confined to the vertebral canal. The term spina bifida cystica includes meningocele and myelomeningocele.

Spina bifida occulta is an unfused condition of the vertebral arches without any cystic distension of the meninges. This form occurs in approximately 10% of adult spines and most commonly affects the fifth lumbar and first sacral vertebrae. There may or may not be changes in the overlying skin or abnormal neurological signs of pathology in the spinal cord. The latter occurs in a small number of patients and leads to progressive neurological signs (see page 236).

The various forms of spina bifida are represented diagrammatically in Fig. 2.26.

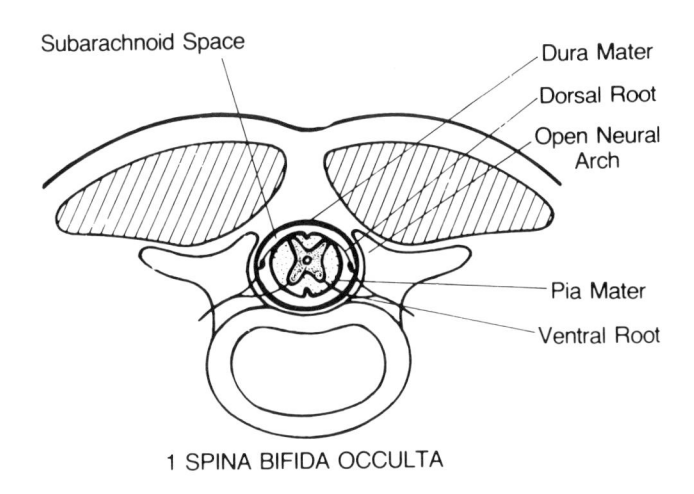

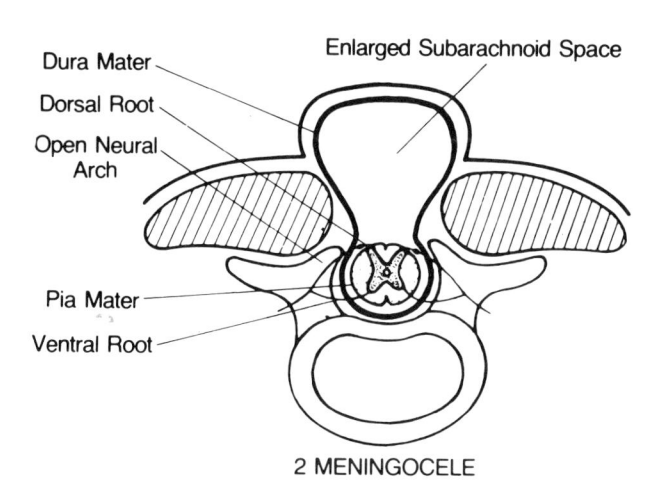

Fig. 2.26a Two types of spina bifida.

42 Chapter 2

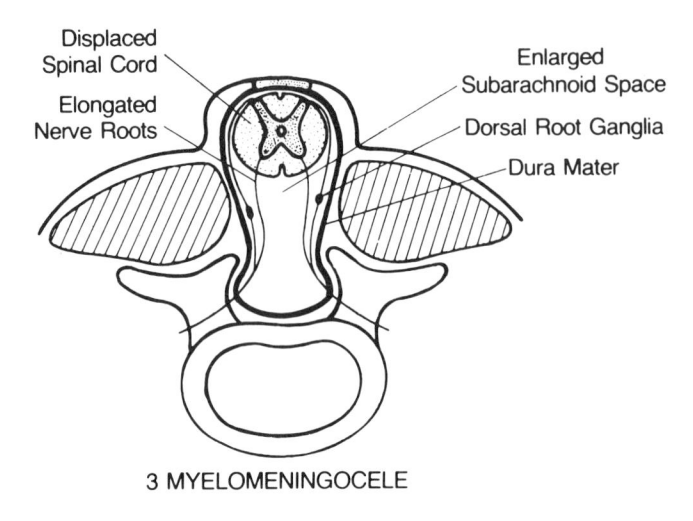

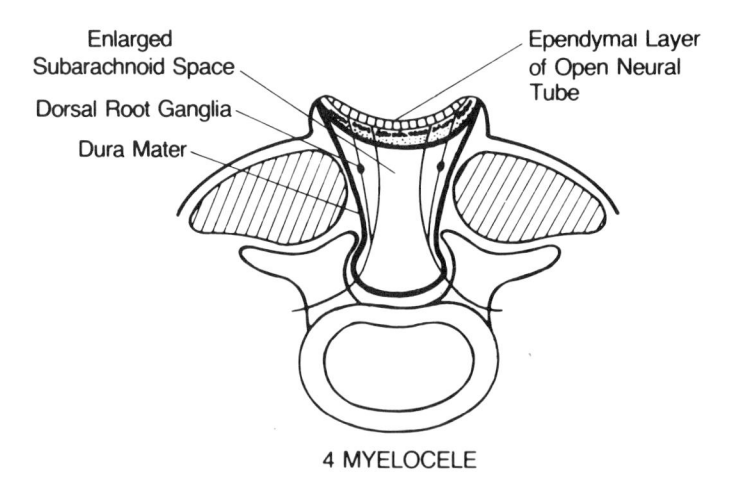

3 MYELOMENINGOCELE

4 MYELOCELE

Fig. 2.26b Two further types of spina bifida.

MULTIPLE SYSTEM INVOLVEMENT

In addition to the gross spinal abnormality other pathology is generally present: the Arnold–Chiari malformation, hydrocephalus, cerebellar hypoplasia, hydromyelia, syringomyelia, diastematomyelia and others. The majority of patients also have upper limb disabilities due to a variety of subtle neurological lesions.

Children with myelomeningocele generally have paralysis of the bladder, bowel incontinence, and a propensity to trophic ulceration in areas of skin anaesthesia. 72% of patients develop significant hydrocephalus. Between one-half and two-thirds of patients have intelligence in the normal range.

Incidence of neural tube defects

The incidence varies in various geographic areas. The overall incidence in Australia is 0.95 per 1000 live births whereas in Western Europe the incidence varies from 1.5 to 4 per 1000 live births. 58% of patients are female.

CAUSES OF DEFORMITY

MUSCLE IMBALANCE DUE TO LOWER MOTOR NEURONE LESIONS

This imbalance is due in large part to the developmental defect. However, further lower motor neurone lesions may be produced by prenatal traction on the abnormally tethered cord, direct pressure and longitudinal shearing forces during delivery, and post-natal drying and infection of the neural plate.

Various patterns of paralysis are seen (see Table 2.3). Children who are paraplegic from T12 down have no deformity, those with activity in L1 (only) tend to lie with their hips flexed and abducted, those with the second lumbar segment spared lie with their hips a little flexed and adducted. Those with the third segment spared tend to have a varus deformity of the foot due to isolated tibialis anterior action. Those with L5 spared have a calcaneus foot, those with S1 spared have an equinus foot and those with the upper two sacral segments spared tend to have claw toes.

Muscle imbalance will cause an abnormal posture of the limb. It is axiomatic also that, in the growing child, it will culminate in fixed deformity in those cases where it persists (Figs. 2.27 & 2.28).

Paralytic dislocation of the hip is generally related to clear cut muscle imbalance (Figs. 2.29–2.31). If the muscles around the hip are either normal or totally paralysed, there is less danger of dislocation. If the muscle imbalance is maximal (namely activity spared in the fourth lumbar segment but no activity below this) dislocation is likely to be present at birth or to develop in the first year of life. With partial imbalance (L2 or L5 lesions) early dislocation is unlikely but increasing flexion adduction contracture and later subluxation can be expected.

MUSCLE IMBALANCE DUE TO UPPER MOTOR NEURONE LESIONS

Two-thirds of infants with myelomeningocele have an additional upper motor neurone lesion. There is an interruption of long spinal tracts with preservation of purely reflex activity in isolated distal segments. Three subtypes can be recognised. In the first, cord function is intact down to a certain level where there

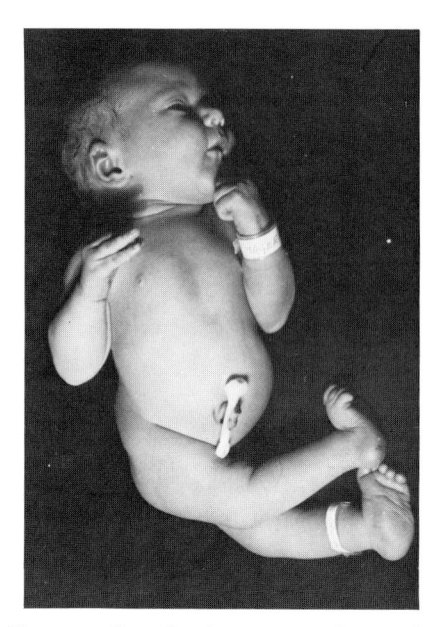

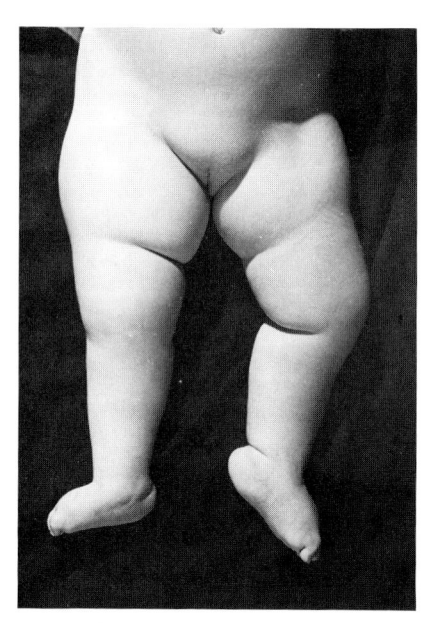

Figs. 2.27 & 2.28 A neonate with a myelomeningocele which was repaired at birth and healed primarily. There is strong activity in the hip flexors, knee extensors and dorsiflexors of the foot where there is the characteristic deformity of vertical talus. (*Right*) The same child at the age of 18 months. None of the previously functioning muscles are now active. The possibility of this train of events should make the clinician wary in assessing the prognosis of lower limb function.

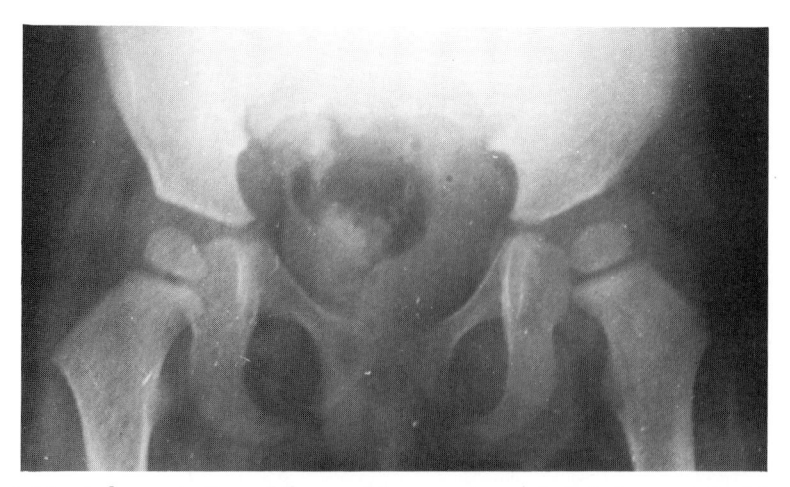

Fig. 2.29 A demonstration of the need to correct muscle imbalance at the hip. The patient had paralysis below the fifth lumbar neurosegmental level on the left and below the first sacral level on the right. She had weak gluteal function on the left, and radiographs at the age of three years show early subluxation of this hip.

The Infant 45

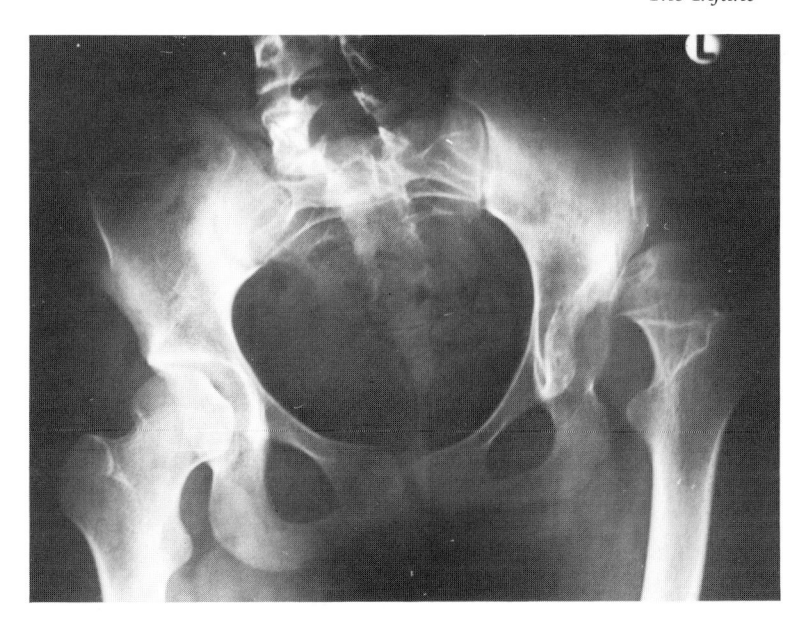

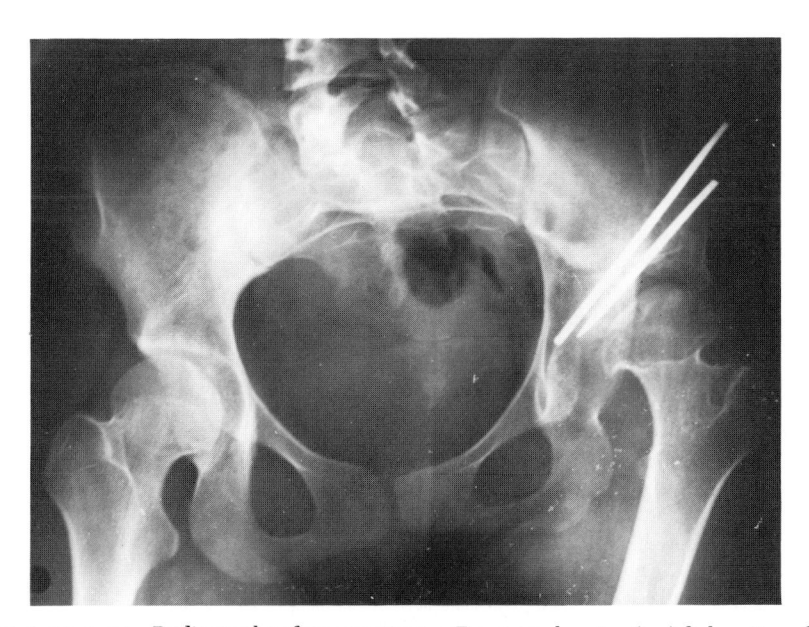

Figs. 2.30–2.31 Radiographs of same patient as Fig. 2.29 showing (*top*) dislocation of the hip due to muscle imbalance abetted by supra-pelvic pelvic obliquity; note the right lumbar scoliosis. There was, in addition, some flexion deformity. (*Bottom*) Following Chiari osteotomy. Heavy threaded wires had been used to maintain the post-operative position. If these or a lag screw is employed, plaster immobilisation is not necessary.

is flaccid paralysis with loss of sensation and reflexes; more distally there is isolated cord function as evident from exaggerated reflex activity. In the second, the 'gap' in cord function is narrow—amounting virtually to a cord transection. There is no movement of the lower limbs when the infant is crying but a wealth of purely reflex activity (including flexion withdrawal) can be elicited by direct stimulation. In the third subtype, where transection of the long tracts is incomplete, the child will have a spastic paraplegia with preservation of some voluntary movement and sensation.

Thus the muscle imbalance producing deformity in spina bifida may be of three types:
- i normal muscle v. flaccid antagonist
- ii spastic muscle v. normal antagonist
- iii spastic muscle v. flaccid antagonist.

The last type produces the worst deformity.

There is evidence that important upper motor neurone lesions occur around the time of birth. Deformities due to spasticity are therefore not present at birth but develop in the early months of life. The effects of such lesions are tabulated at the bottom of Table 2.3.

INTRA-UTERINE POSTURE

Sometimes fixed deformity is present at birth in totally paralysed lower limbs. In some of these cases, deformity may be already fixed which shows that muscle power (and imbalance) has been present in fetal life. In others, the pattern of deformity suggests that it has resulted simply from the pressure of the uterus on paralysed limbs.

HABITUALLY ASSUMED POSTURE AFTER BIRTH

Deformity can develop after birth in flaccid legs which are allowed to lie in one particular posture. Thus the hips may develop a fixed external rotation, flexion, abduction deformity. The knees may develop flexion, and the feet equinus deformity.

CO-EXISTENT CONGENITAL MALFORMATION

This is probably not a common cause of deformity in spina bifida. Syndactyly of the second and third toe is a co-existent congenital malformation, but dislocation of the hip and club foot deformity are due to muscle imbalance.

ARTHROGRYPOSIS

Some of the limb deformities have the same characteristics as those seen in

Table 2.3 Effect of the neurosegmental level of the lesion on muscle activity and limb posture.

Lowest neurosegmental level functioning	Muscles acting	Limb posture
T12	–	Dictated by gravity
L1	Sartorius Ilio psoas (weak function)	Flexion and external rotation at hip
L2	*As above* plus Ilio psoas (strong) Pectineus, Gracilis, Adductors of the hip, Rectus femoris	Flexion and adduction at hip
L3	*As above* plus Quadriceps (power slightly diminished)	*Hip* flexed and adducted *Knee* extended or hyper-extended
L4	*As above* plus Tibialis anterior (and posterior) Medial hamstrings weak	*Hip* flexed, adducted and externally rotated *Knee* extension and hyper-extension *Foot* varus
L5	*As above* plus T.F.L. Gluteus medius and minimus E.D.C. and Peroneus tertius	*Hip* flexion *Knee* some flexion *Feet* in calcaneus
S1	*As above* plus Gluteus maximus Biceps femoris Gastrocnemius Soleus F.D.L. and B F.H.L. and B	Hip and knee in some flexion Flattening of the sole and clawing of the toes
Lower lumbar level with spastic sacral segment.	Spasticity in hamstrings, calf, peronei.	*Knee* flexion deformity. *Foot* equinus or valgus or vertical talus.

arthrogryposis multiplex congenita. There is a rigidity and lack of abnormal flexion creases. Such deformities are very resistant to treatment.

TRACTION ON NERVE ROOTS

Some children who have had a meningocele closed at birth, present later with progressive foot deformity (usually cavus). Myelography generally discloses abnormal tethering of the spinal cord and this should be treated surgically.

PROBLEMS RESULTING FROM SKIN ANAESTHESIA AND BONE FRAGILITY

Pressure sores and chilblains

These result from skin anaesthesia and poor circulation. If serial plasters are necessary to correct deformity they should be very carefully padded as there is no pain to warn the surgeon of pressure on the skin. In most instances, plaster casts should only be used to maintain correction of deformity which has been achieved by soft tissue surgery. The routine use of lambswool-lined boots minimises the incidence of chilblains and pressure sores on the feet during ordinary activities. Hip spicas should include paralysed feet. Varus feet are always unacceptable and pressure sores are inevitable. Parents should be warned to protect the children from extremes of temperature.

Bone fragility

Pathological fractures occur in approximately 20% of those cases with paralysis in the lower limbs. Epiphyseal displacements are common. Hyperplastic callus formation is the rule following any trauma to bone.

An unusual case of pathological fractures in spina bifida is renal rickets and deficiency of vitamin C has also been implicated as a cause of bone changes.

The principle of treatment of pathological fractures is that there should be minimal immobilisation of the child and fractured limb which is compatible with union in good position.

MANAGEMENT

Genetic counselling and antenatal diagnosis

All parents who have a child with myelomeningocele require genetic counselling and this has now become more important because of the development of methods of intra-uterine diagnosis. Myelomeningocele (and other forms of neural tube defect) may be inherited (following a multifactorial pattern) or may be due to some as yet unidentified environmental factor. Once a family has had one child with myelomeningocele there is a recurrence risk which varies from area to area so that counselling should be based on local experience. In Melbourne, as in London, the recurrence risk is about 4%. If the parents have had two affected children, the risk rises to about 10% and after three children to about 25%. The birth of a child with myelomeningocele also predisposes to the birth of a child with an anencephaly, congenital vertebral body anomalies, or with spinal dysraphism.

The logical end stage of intra-uterine diagnosis is abortion of the baby and there is no point in establishing an antenatal diagnosis unless the parents are prepared to consider this. Tests are undertaken between 15 and 17 weeks' gestation using ultrasound followed by amniocentesis. If this sequence is followed, the risk of producing a miscarriage, in experienced hands, is about 1 in 200. The amniotic fluid is submitted for alpha fetoprotein estimation. Between 80 and 90% of those with myelomeningocele can be recognised by these techniques.

A screening programme which measures the level of alpha fetoprotein in maternal serum is employed in certain areas where there is a high incidence of neural tube defects.

Total management

The parents of babies who have little chance of long term survival or who will only survive with very gross handicap should be offered management which involves placing the child on demand feeding where, it should be made clear, there is little chance of survival. This approach is suggested for those children who have an infected sac at presentation, thoracic and high lumbar lesions, hydrocephalus at birth, meningitis and multiple congenital anomalies, or life threatening diseases. Should the baby thrive despite this regime, then the only condition requiring treatment in the neonatal period is talipes equinovarus and even this deformity can be accepted if active neurosurgical treatment is not contemplated. However, the orthopaedic surgeon should examine every spina bifida patient at birth or as soon as possible thereafter, not only to record basic information but to make it possible to monitor progress over the first few months and to plan orthopaedic treatment if survival seems likely. The case mortality is high in infancy but, if the child survives the first year of life (and about 50% do), then long term survival is the rule.

Because of the many disciplines involved, patients with myelomeningocele should only be treated in a special clinic for such children.

The aim of orthopaedic management

The principal aim of orthopaedic management in spina bifida is to establish stable posture (Figs. 2.32–2.34). If affected children are to stand for long periods and to remain on their feet in adult life, they must have their centre of gravity over their feet and minimal flexion deformity at the hips and knees. Indeed it is very desirable that there be some hyperextension at both hips and knees. About 60% of spina bifida children have neurological deficiencies in their upper limbs and often need to use both hands for activities which normally could be managed single handed. It is for this reason also that a posture must be obtained which allows them to stand for long periods without using their hands for support.

Orthopaedic surgery in this condition has differing goals according to the level of the neurosegmental lesion. This level may be ill defined (because of skip lesions

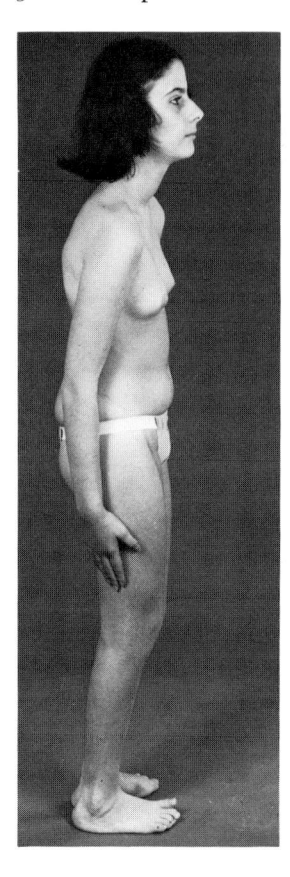

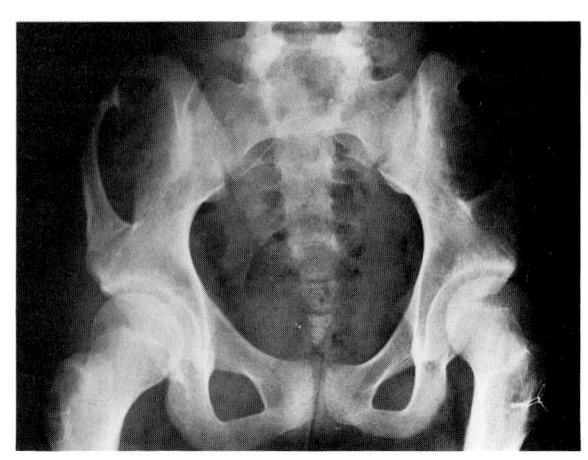

Figs. 2.32 & 2.33 Both hips of this girl with paralysis below the fifth lumbar segment had been subjected to bilateral anterior hip releases and iliopsoas transplantation 14 years previously for increasing flexion deformity and subluxation. She walks with a Trendelenburg gait but without support from a cane or orthosis.

or other neurological or general disabilities). In general, children with *thoracic lesions* will not continue useful walking in adult life (Fig. 2.35). Children with *lumbar lesions* may continue useful walking in adult life if they have strong quadriceps muscles and do not develop significant deformity at their hip joints. Those with strong quadriceps require only below-knee orthoses but may need sticks or crutches in addition. Children with *sacral lesions* can be expected to be useful walkers, without orthoses, into adult life. Those who will not continue walking require simple surgery to provide them with a stable posture in childhood while those who will continue walking require more sophisticated surgery to meet the increased demands of their way of life.

Because the surgery necessary in children with high lesions is relatively minor, it can and should be performed at several levels and in both limbs under one anaesthetic. Muscle imbalance must be corrected in all circumstances so that recurrent deformity does not occur. Radical surgery is necessary to correct rigid, arthrogrypotic-type deformities (notably in the feet) and care must be taken to avoid pressure on anaesthetic skin. For this and other reasons operative correction of deformities is preferable to conservative methods. All management

The Infant 51

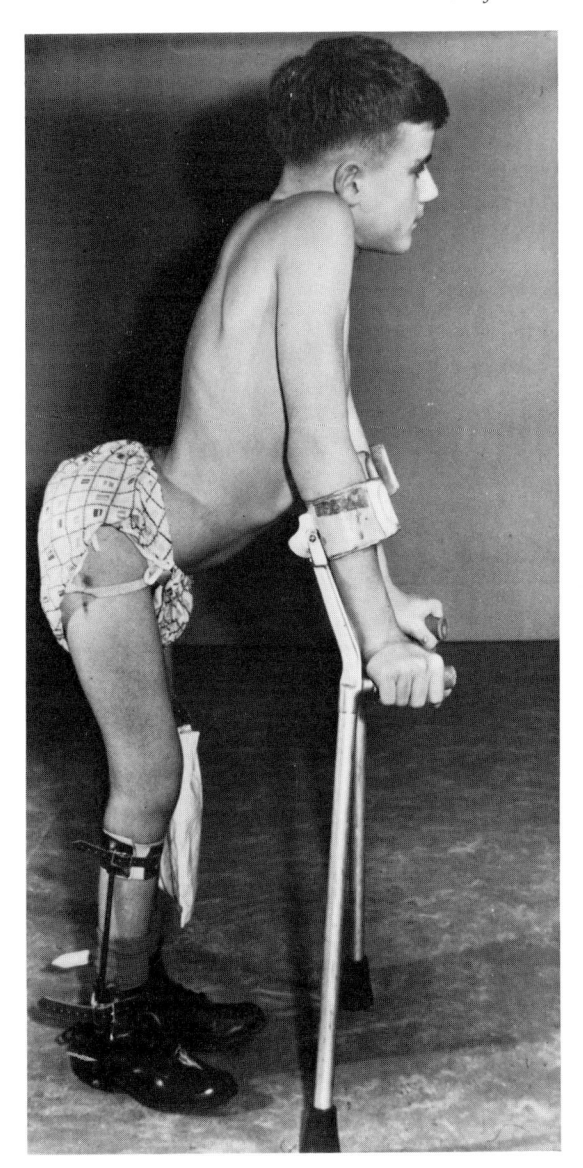

Fig. 2.34 Undesirable flexion posture in a boy with paralysis below the fourth lumbar segment. He has strong psoas muscles and gluteal weakness and has developed fixed flexion deformity of both hips of 60°. Note the gross lumbar lordosis and the fact that his centre of gravity is in front of rather than directly over his feet. He is therefore quite dependent on his crutches.

in spina bifida must involve immobilisation of the child and of the uninvolved limbs for as short a period as possible so that the incidence of pathological fractures is minimised. It can be assumed in the beginning that all these children have the potential to walk, except those who are severely retarded or have gross spasticity. Children should be taught to stand and walk as soon as this becomes feasible. The age at which various orthopaedic procedures are carried out is shown in Table 2.4.

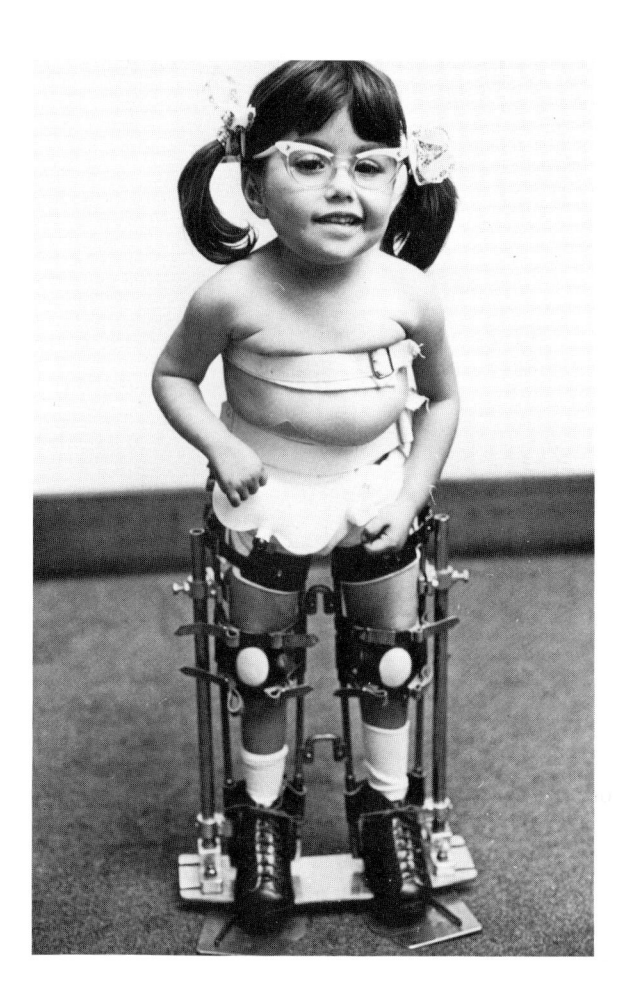

Fig. 2.35
A girl of 4 years with myelomeningocele. She is paraplegic and has gross neurological disturbances in upper limb function so that she cannot use crutches. She uses this swivel walker for progression: by rocking from side to side she progresses forwards.

THE FOOT

Some general observations on the management of foot deformity

Fixed varus deformity invariably requires correction by operation, as complications from weight bearing on a small area of the sole are otherwise inevitable. Undercorrection must never be accepted since further surgery will almost certainly be required.

Valgus feet, while they remain mobile, can usually be controlled with appropriate footwear and orthoses until adolescence. Mobile valgus deformity of the subtalar joint is commonly complicated by torsional and valgus deformity of the ankle mortice; the deformity is difficult to control by bracing and surgery will eventually be necessary to correct this whole complex of deformity.

Table 2.4 Orthopaedic management related to stage of development and age.

Developmental stage	Management
Birth ↓ Head control	Assessment commences with view to determining realistic aims; posturing to correct deformity; correction of equinovarus deformity
Head control	Developmental stimulation
Head control ↓ Sitting	Encourage sitting balance
Sitting	Encourage hand skills and co-ordination
Sitting ↓ Prone mobility	Encourage upper limb strength and co-ordination hand function
Prone mobility	Provide sitting aids
Prone mobility ↓ Upright stance	Continued assessment; increased social stimulation
Upright stance	Provide standing orthosis
Upright stance ↓ Upright mobility	Physiotherapy and bracing appropriate to the neurosegmental level; soft tissue releases for hip deformity; open tenotomy of psoas and adductors; reduction of hip dislocation (in combination with appropriate soft tissue procedure); iliopsoas transfer; Pemberton osteotomy
Upright mobility	Tendon excision of deforming foot tendons
$2\frac{1}{2}$ years ↓ 6 years	Kyphosis surgery; Grice procedure; correction of fixed flexion at knees; quadriceps release
6 years	Chiari procedure
6 years ↓ 10 years	Correction of the early developing scoliosis (surgery for recurrent hip and foot deformity)
10 years ↓ 16 years	Scoliosis and lordosis surgery; osteotomy for fixed hip and knee deformity
16 years	Foot stabilisation

Calcaneus deformity tends to be progressive and should be treated surgically.

Whenever possible, operations on the foot and leg should be performed under the same anaesthetic as other limb surgery, urological surgery or neurosurgery.

Whilst mobile feet are preferable to stiff feet, triple arthrodesis at maturity has a useful place in the management of both varus and valgus deformity in this condition.

Equinovarus deformity

The rigidity of this deformity varies from that seen in the usual form of talipes equinovarus to the extreme rigidity of arthrogryposis. This is the most troublesome foot deformity because of its tendency to recur despite adequate initial correction. Unless survival is unlikely, the deformity should be treated from birth. The feet are placed in well padded plaster casts which are changed frequently whilst the baby is still in hospital and then at intervals of 4–6 weeks. Before treatment, the feet may appear to be purely varus or even calcaneovarus but, as the varus is corrected, it is usually apparent that there is tightness of the tendo-Achilles. In these circumstances closed tenotomy is indicated. Despite this early management, a soft tissue release will generally be necessary between the ages of 4 months and a year. The rigid equinovarus foot will inevitably require postero-medial release and the technique is described on page 30. Since the calf is not functioning, the skin incision need have only a very short vertical component. Portions of the tendons of tendo-Achilles, tibialis anterior, tibialis posterior and the long toe flexors are excised rather than just divided. Only occasionally will the degree of deformity be so mild that conservative treatment will correct the varus and adductus leaving only equinus to be corrected by posterior release.

Tendon transfers have no place in this condition. Should the deformity recur then a repeat soft tissue release is performed. However, if recurrent deformity occurs between the ages of 5 and 14 years, it is generally wise to accept the deformity, provide surgical footwear and perform triple arthrodesis at skeletal maturity. If the child has considerable paralysis, the demands on the feet may be such that pressure effects do not present a problem. Should trophic ulcers appear, then soft tissue releases are preferable to talectomy.

Equinus deformity

This deformity usually responds to closed or open tenotomy of the tendo-Achilles, depending on the severity of the deformity and the age of the child.

Cavus deformity

The management of this condition will depend on the degree of rigidity of the deformity and the age of the child. Minor deformity in a young child may be corrected by open division of the tight plantar structures. If there is heel varus and the child is over the age of 4 years, then osteotomy of the os calcis is appropriate. If the deformity then recurs and the child is too young for triple arthrodesis, then it may be necessary to osteotomise all the metatarsals at their bases. Triple arthrodesis is carried out if there is a combination of cavus and varus deformity in a patient close to skeletal maturity.

Calcaneus deformity

Generally this deformity is left untreated until muscle power can be properly assessed at about 18–24 months. Stiffening the tongue of the boot may control minor degrees of deformity in the young child. If the tibialis anterior is of full strength then this tendon is transferred, through the interosseus membrane to the heel. Any other active ankle dorsiflexors are divided and, if there is fixed calcaneus deformity, an anterior ankle release is combined with this tenotomy. If the anterior muscles are spastic or if they are weak, they are divided and the tendo-Achilles is tenodesed to the fibular metaphysis. The drill hole through the fibula stimulates growth at the lower end of the fibula and this may correct valgus deformity at the ankle mortice—a deformity which commonly occurs in combination with calcaneus deformity. The late-developing calcaneus deformity with a 'pistol grip' heel is best treated by osteotomy of the os calcis removing a wedge posteriorly so that the tuberosity lies less vertically. At the same time restoration of muscle balance is achieved by tenodesis or tendon transfer.

Valgus deformity

This may occur at the ankle mortice, the subtalar joint, or at both these sites. Clinical examination and weight bearing radiographs of the ankle will clarify the site of the deformity. If it is chiefly at the subtalar joint then Grice subtalar extra-articular arthrodesis is appropriate. When there is valgus at the ankle mortice then this is corrected by supramalleolar osteotomy of the tibia. If external tibial torsion is present this can be corrected at the same time; inlay fusion of the subtalar or subtalar and midtarsal joints can also be carried out as part of the same procedure. Subtalar fusion is performed between the ages of 3 and 10 years. Over this age it is preferable to inlay both the subtalar and midtarsal joints and, if possible, to delay this surgery to the age of 14 years. Ankle fusion should be avoided as it has a high failure rate in patients with myelomeningocele.

Paralytic convex pes valgus (vertical talus)

The rigid complex of deformities seen in congenital vertical talus occasionally occurs in children suffering from myelomeningocele or from diastematomyelia. In addition to this rigid deformity there is a less rigid form which develops slowly in the first years of life. The management of this deformity is described on page 59.

THE KNEE

Recurrent flexion deformity is the enemy of extension posture and is the only knee problem to which reference will be made. This condition is frequently due to minor activity or spasm in the hamstring muscles, evident only when the child stands. The result is a slowly progressive flexion deformity and, unless the responsible tendons are divided, the deformity will recur despite supracondylar osteotomy. The knee which is in recurvatum or has limited flexion range will generally require quadriceps lengthening if the muscle is strong or division of the patellar tendon if it is weak.

THE HIP

It has already been indicated that we favour one of two broad approaches depending on the level of the lesion and the likely demands to be made on the hips in adult life. Firstly, those with weak quadriceps require only soft tissue releases and psoas excision to correct fixed deformity at the hip and prevent recurrence (Fig. 2.36). Secondly, those with strong quadriceps require not only soft tissue releases at the hip if fixed deformity is present, but also complex surgery which may include iliopsoas transfer and acetabuloplasty.

The emphasis should be taken away from management of paralytic dislocation of the hip and placed more on correction of fixed deformity. In many spina bifida children a minor degree of hip dysplasia does not lead to subluxation nor subluxation to dislocation. The conventional methods used to correct these conditions carry significant disadvantages in this context. Dislocated hips should be ignored if the dislocation and acetabular dysplasia is bilateral and gross and if

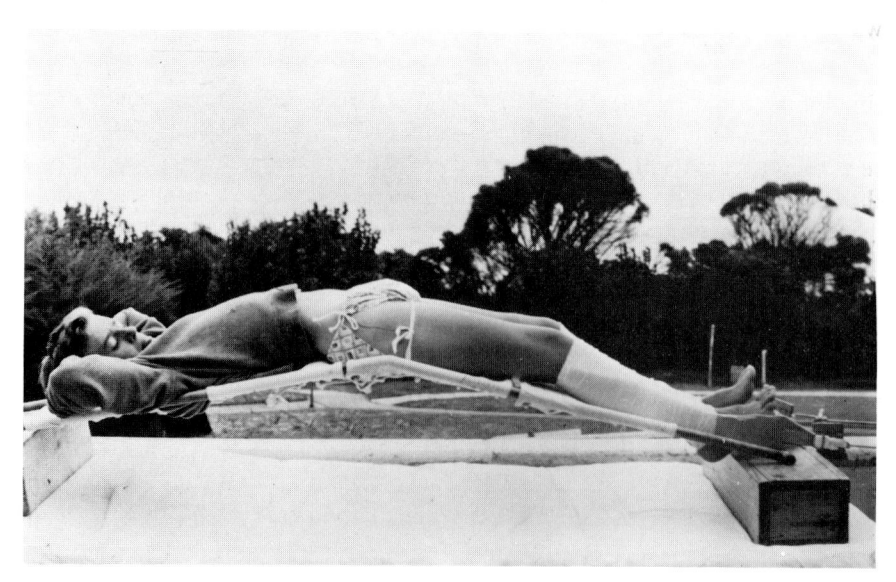

Fig. 2.36 Posture following an anterior hip release, performed for fixed flexion deformity of both hips. The patient is lying on a bent Bradford frame with the angle at the level of the hips. Skin traction is applied to both legs. This posture is alternated with prone lying on a straight frame.

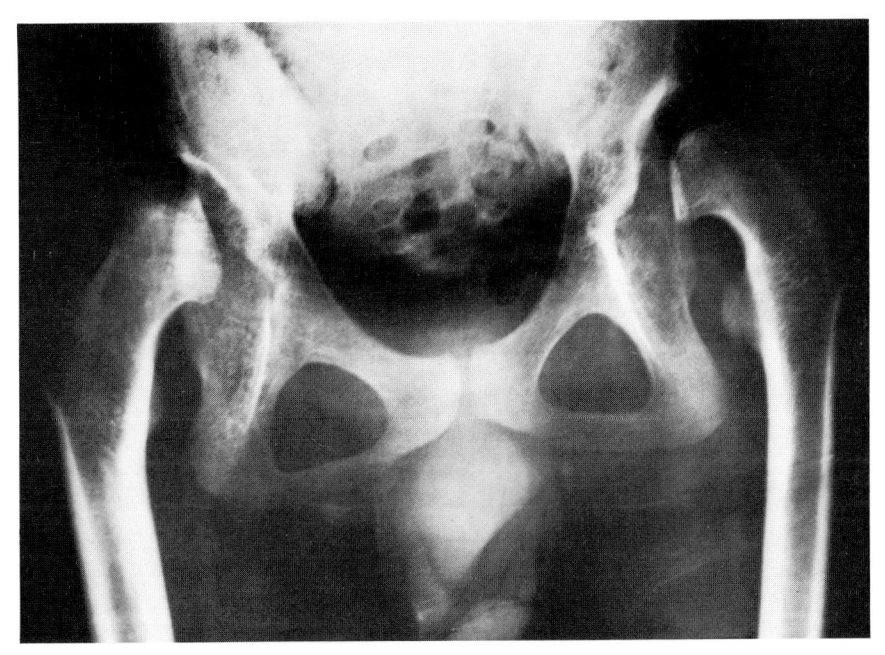

Fig. 2.37 Radiograph of the pelvis of a 17-year-old boy. He is paraplegic but remains on his feet all day and does not yet possess a wheelchair. He has undergone simple soft tissue anterior hip releases for flexion deformity but has had no treatment for hip dislocation, which does not impede his swing-through gait. (*See also* Fig. 2.38)

the child will in any case require long calipers and crutches (Figs. 2.37 & 2.38). In this group there is no difference in the posture and gait between those with hips reduced and those with hips dislocated, but there is a crucial difference between those who do or do not have flexion deformity.

Treatment of dislocated hips will only be indicated if it can be carried out conveniently in combination with the management of fixed deformity and the restoration of muscle balance. It is usually desirable to correct unilateral dislocation as it results in a significant leg length discrepancy (Figs. 2.39–2.41).

SPINAL SURGERY IN SPINA BIFIDA

Although simple surgery is often most appropriate for the legs, it is not so for the spine. The deformities which occur here are often too disabling to be ignored, yet conservative methods of treatment are seldom applicable or effective. A radical approach is therefore necessary; indeed all paralytic spinal deformities which demand treatment need a combination of anterior and posterior fusion. Whilst kyphosis will become a less frequent problem, scoliosis will be with us for a long time to come, since it develops in a high percentage of children with lumbar lesions, and these are likely to survive whatever policy of selection is adopted.

58 Chapter 2

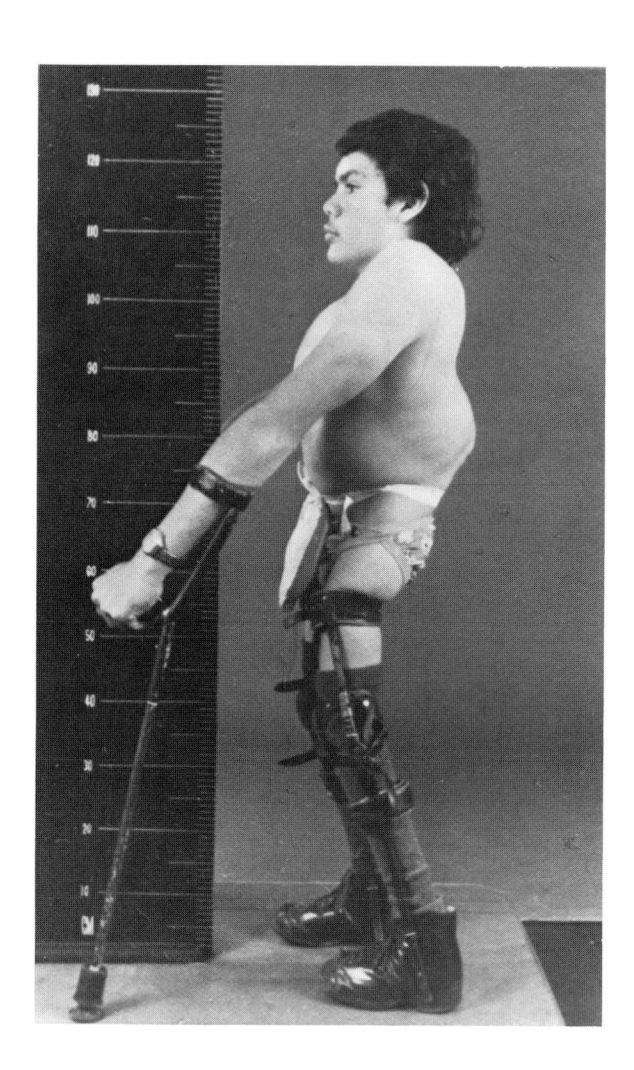

Fig. 2.38 Photograph of the boy whose pelvis is shown in Fig. 2.37.

Scoliosis

All spina bifida patients over the age of 6 years are screened for scoliosis by annual x-rays of the spine (Figs. 2.42–2.44). Management of scoliosis in this condition is surgical and consists of anterior fusion and Dwyer instrumentation, followed two weeks later by a posterior approach and Harrington instrumentation. The anterior instrumentation increases the fusion rate; the posterior instrumentation increases the length of spine that can be fused and enables correction of the pelvic obliquity. Incomplete correction of this obliquity may throw more weight on one ischial tuberosity than was present before surgery. The optimum age for scoliosis surgery is 10–12 years.

The Infant 59

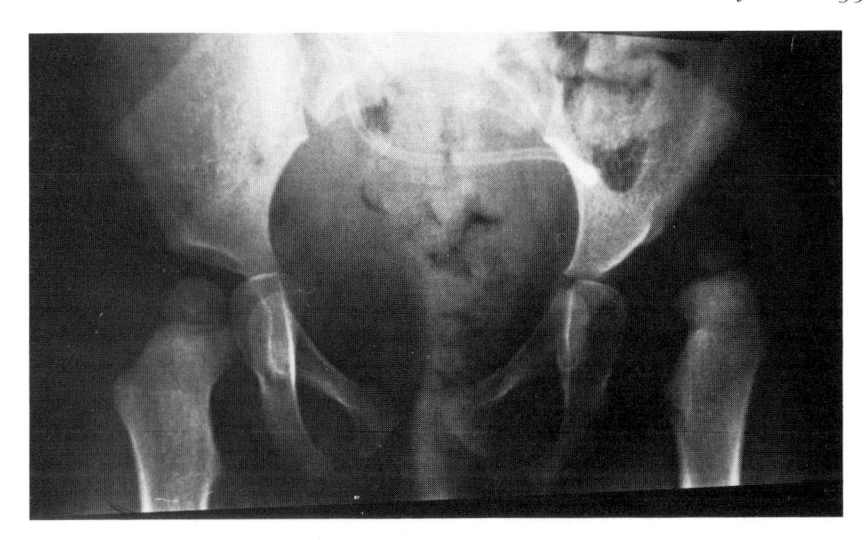

Fig. 2.39 This girl had normal muscle power in the right leg with paralysis below the fifth lumbar neurosegmental level on the left. A radiograph at the age of 2 years shows dislocation of the left hip. Anterior hip release, iliopsoas transplantation, and (unusually) open reduction of the hip were performed.

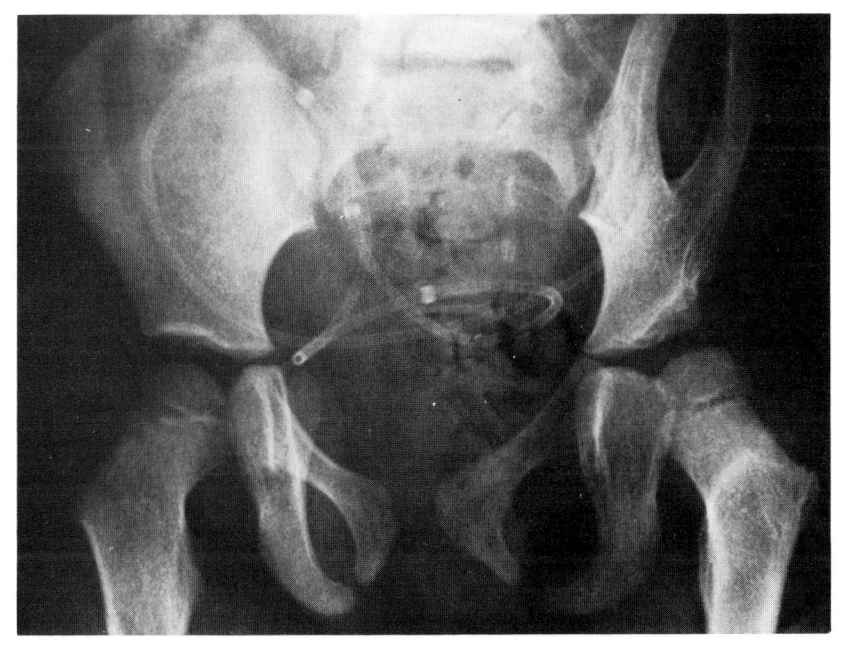

Fig. 2.40 Same patient as Fig. 2.39. Note the improvement two years later in the acetabular dysplasia.

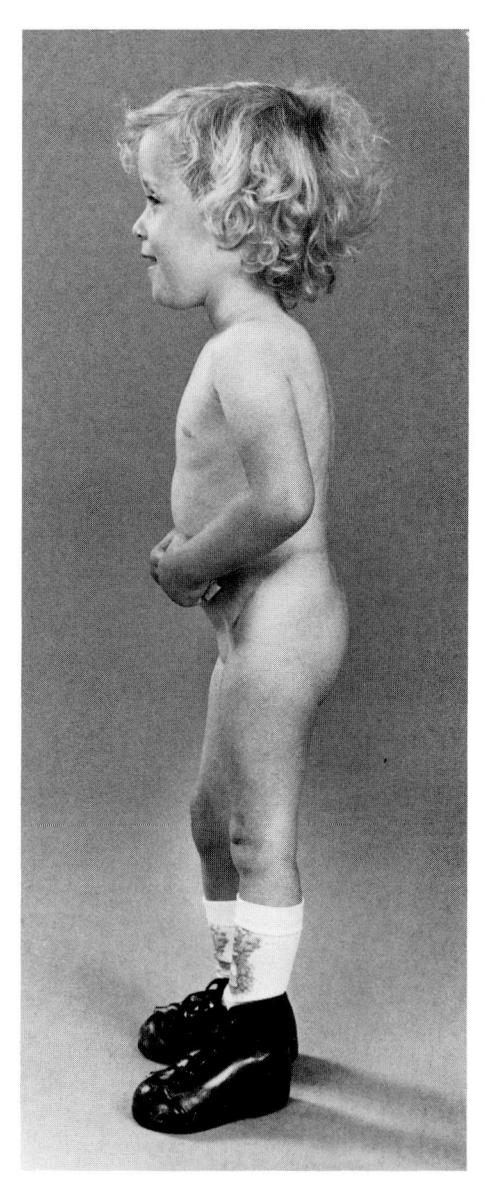

Fig. 2.41 Same patient as Fig. 2.39. Two years later she stands upright without flexion deformity of the hip or lumbar lordosis.

The Infant 61

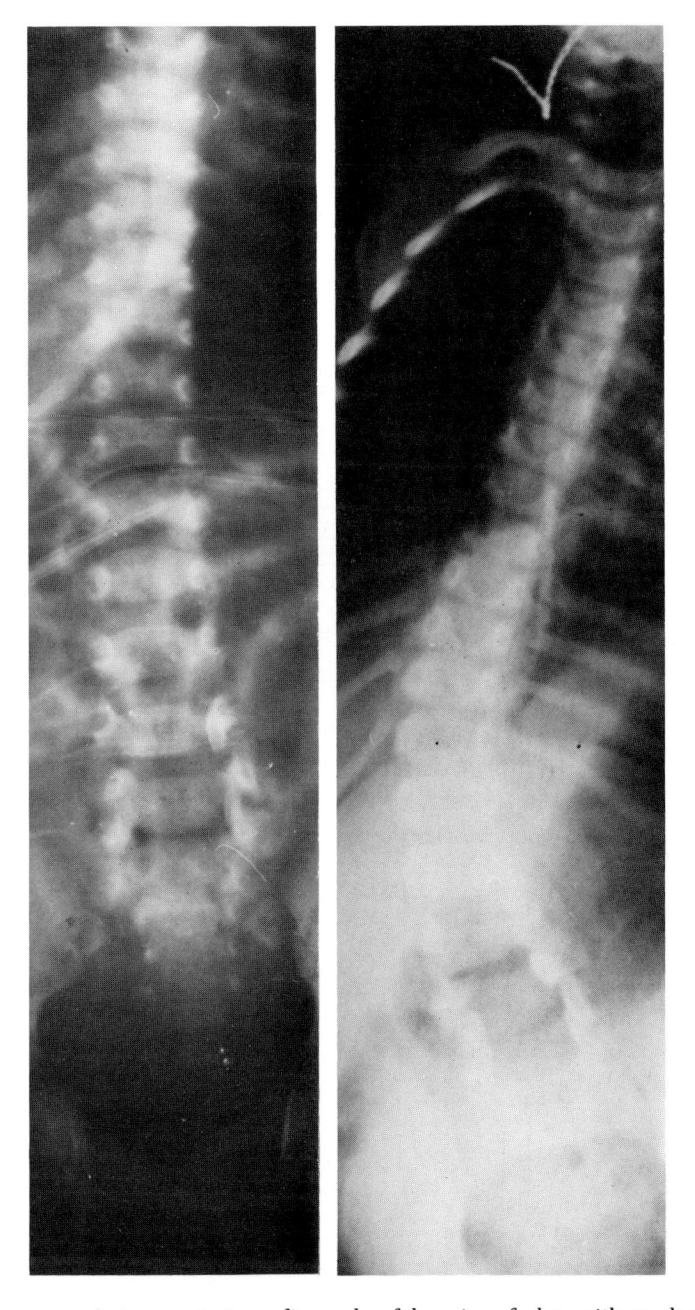

Figs. 2.42–2.43 Antero-posterior radiographs of the spine of a boy with myelomeningocele at the ages of 9 years and 11 years. Note the rapid increase in this characteristic thoraco-lumbar scoliosis, the absence of a minor curve below the major curve and hence the development of pelvic obliquity. The hip on the high side of the pelvis inevitably dislocates in these circumstances.

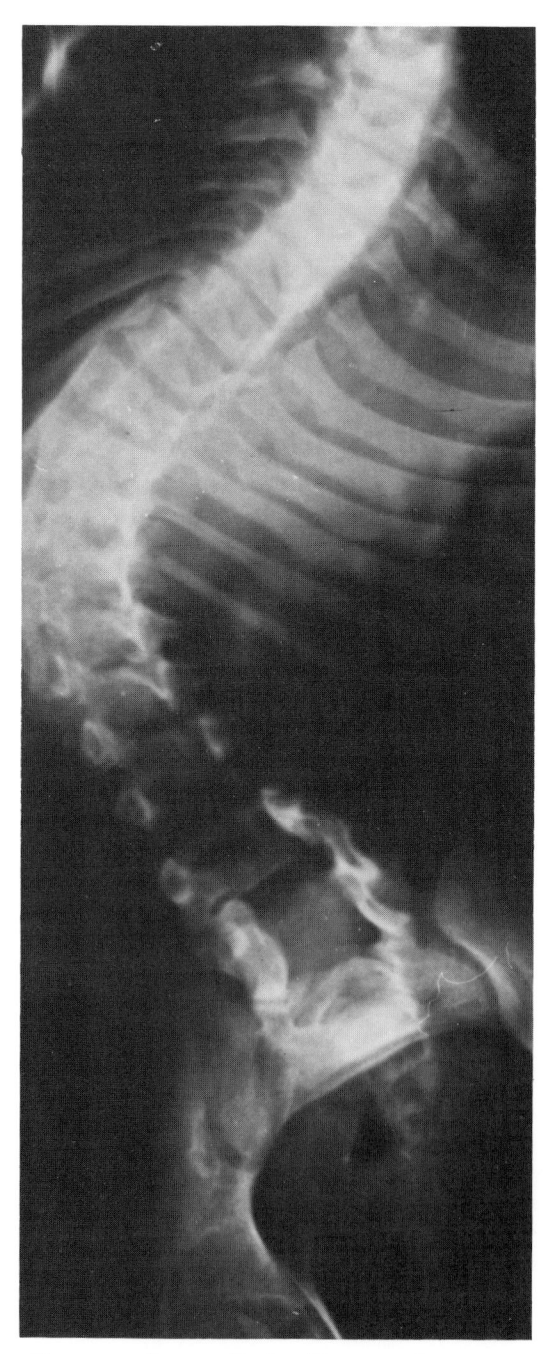

Fig. 2.44 Same patient as Fig. 2.42 at 15 years.

CONGENITAL VERTICAL TALUS
(Congenital flat foot, congenital convex pes cavus)

This is a rare congenital abnormality which may occur either alone or in association with arthrogryposis, spina bifida, or neurofibromatosis.

PATHOLOGICAL ANATOMY

The foot is rigid in a position of calcaneus but the hindfoot is actually in equinus. The midfoot is broken, producing a prominence in the sole, and there is a dislocation of the talonavicular joint. Unlike that seen in club foot, the navicular is displaced dorsally and laterally and the head of the talus points directly to the sole. The talus lies alongside the os calcis rather than on top of it. The extensor tendons are contracted as are the dorsal capsules of the tarsal joints. The disturbed relationship of the various bones are readily visible on x-ray examination.

CLINICAL FEATURES

The deformity is present at birth and is usually readily recognisable. However care must be taken to exclude feet which are mobile and corrigible from the diagnosis as these carry a much better prognosis and require a different approach to treatment. If left untreated, the foot is difficult to shoe and distorts the shoe badly. After some years a large callus appears under the middle of the sole and eventually this area becomes painful.

There are less florid forms in which the foot at birth resembles a severe talipes calcaneovalgus. Instead of correcting itself spontaneously, as does talipes calcaneovalgus, the deformity remains static or worsens to develop increasing rigidity. By the age of 1–2 years it is apparent that the child has a late developing congenital convex pes planus. Another uncommon condition which may be confused with congenital convex planus is reverse club foot. In this condition there is a rigid talipes calcaneovalgus deformity which does not improve spontaneously; it does not develop equinus of the ankle nor dislocation of the talonavicular joint. Two plasters are necessary in the first year of life and generally an antero-lateral soft tissue release of the ankle and subtalar joint is necessary in the second or third year of life.

RADIOLOGICAL APPEARANCE

The talus lies in a vertical or near vertical position (Fig. 2.45). The calcaneus lies in less plantar flexion and the navicular is dorsally displaced relative to the head of the talus. The dislocated position of the navicular cannot be seen radiologically under the age of 2 years as the ossific nucleus is absent. Radiographs in forced plantar flexion will demonstrate that the dislocation of the forefoot does not reduce and views in forced dorsiflexion similarly show that the equinus position of

64   Chapter 2

the heel remains unchanged. These latter features serve to distinguish this condition from severe postural pes plano-valgus.

Treatment

Treatment involves a reduction of the dislocation at the talocalcaneo-navicular joint and correction of the equinus. Although serial casting in infancy may correct some of these feet, surgical reduction has been found more efficient and more likely to produce a permanent result. The operation is best done at 3–6 months when an approach is made on either side of the foot. After division of the extensor tendons, the dislocated joints are opened from both sides. The talus is then replaced onto the top of the os calcis and fixed in position with a fine Kirschner wire passed up through the sole and transfixing the two bones. The

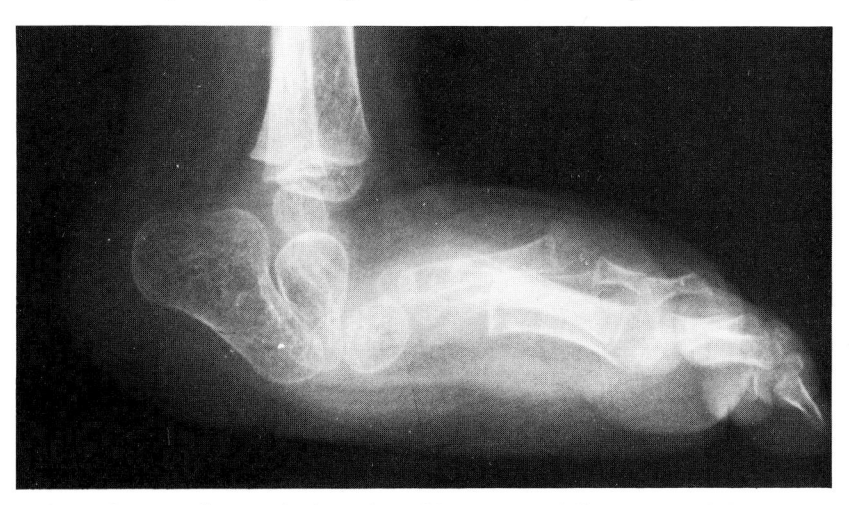

Fig. 2.45 Congenital vertical talus. The ankle joint is in full equinus and there is dorsal dislocation of the talonavicular joint. The head of the talus is not supported by the sustentaculum tali because of valgus deformity of the calcaneum.

talonavicular dislocation is then reduced and this joint is also transfixed with a fine K wire which is buried under the skin on the dorsum of the foot. The foot will now be in considerable equinus so that the tendo-Achilles will need to be lengthened through a separate incision. A plaster cast is used for about three months and followed by night splintage and a day support. After several years it will be found that there is a gradual tendency for the deformity to relapse and as soon as this is in evidence, a Grice extra-articular subtalar fusion should be carried out. This arthrodesis may be carried out at the original open reduction but fusion is difficult to secure in the infant's foot because the tarsal bones are largely cartilaginous.

Many of these feet require secondary procedures at maturity for the relief either of pain or unacceptable deformity.

PROXIMAL FEMORAL FOCAL DEFICIENCY

Proximal femoral focal deficiency is a term first introduced by Aitken to describe a group of anomalies in which the common feature is a deficiency in the proximal femur (Fig. 2.46). The syndrome comprises 1 Deficiencies of the femur which may be short, completely absent, or contain a pseudarthrosis. 2 Anomalies of the hip which may be dislocated or absent. 3 Deficiencies of the femoral neck

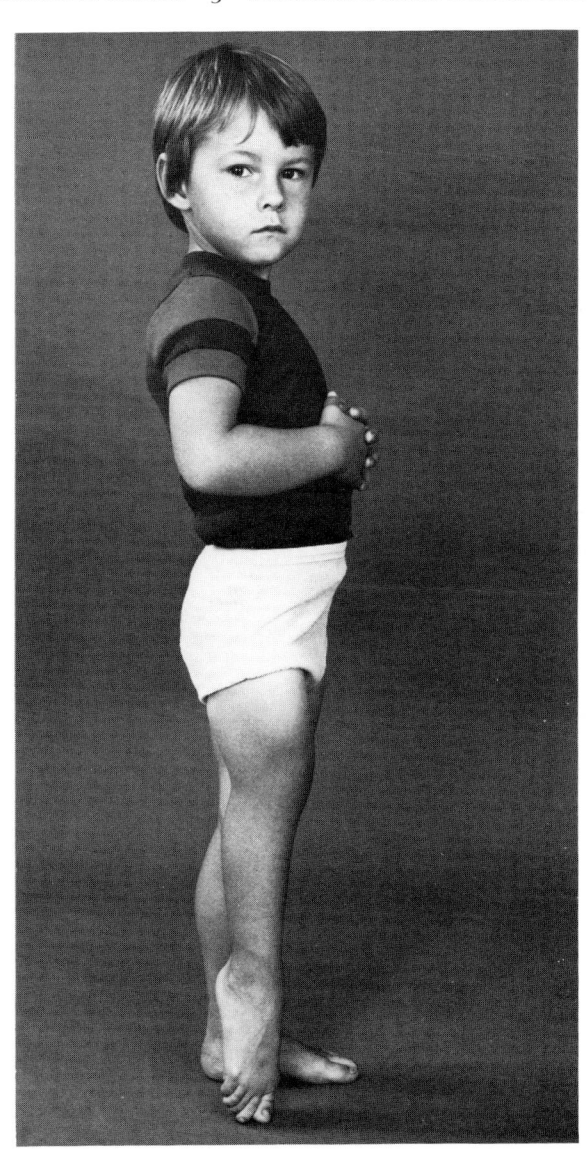

Fig. 2.46 A child showing the typical features of proximal femoral focal deficiency.

66   Chapter 2

such as a coxa vara deformity or a pseudarthrosis. 4 Associated anomalies of the leg, foot and arms.

CLASSIFICATION

The most commonly used classification is that proposed by Amstutz who divided the cases into five separate groups (Fig. 2.47) as follows.

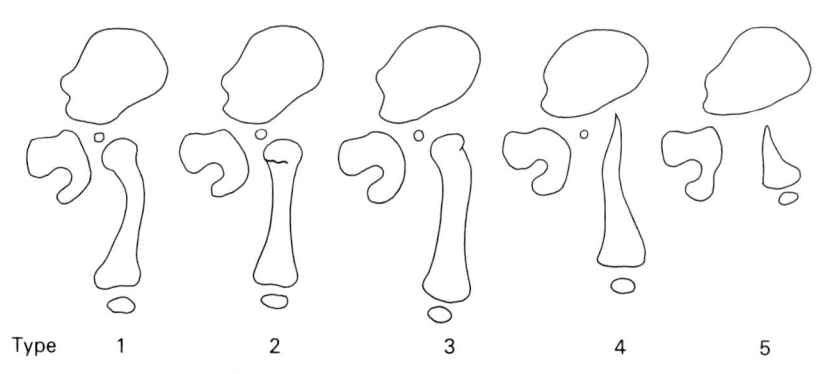

Type   1   2   3   4   5

Fig. 2.47   The five types of proximal femoral focal deficiency.

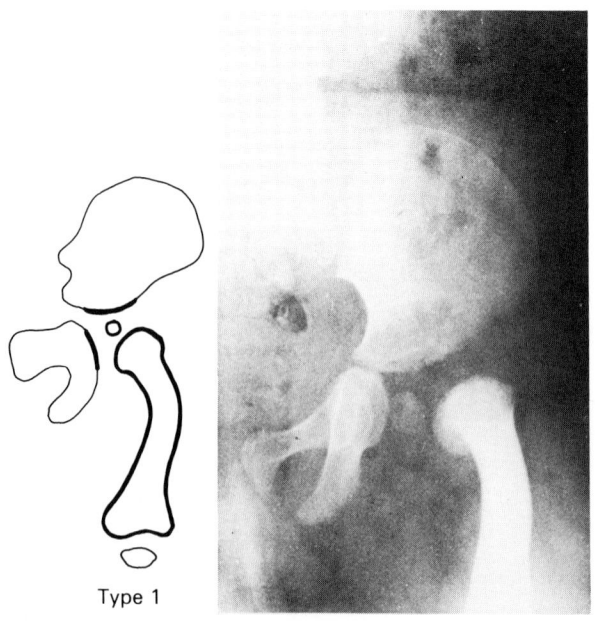

Type 1

Fig. 2.48   The five types of PFFD. (*See* p. 69 for details)

The Infant 67

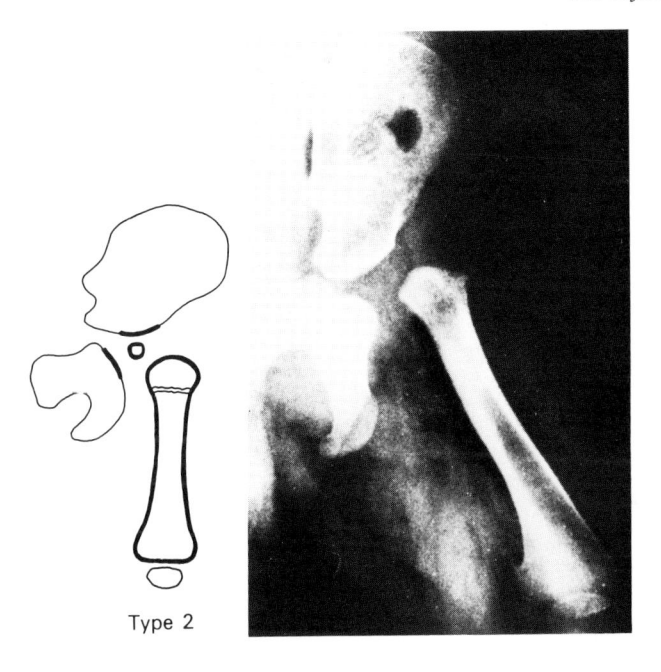

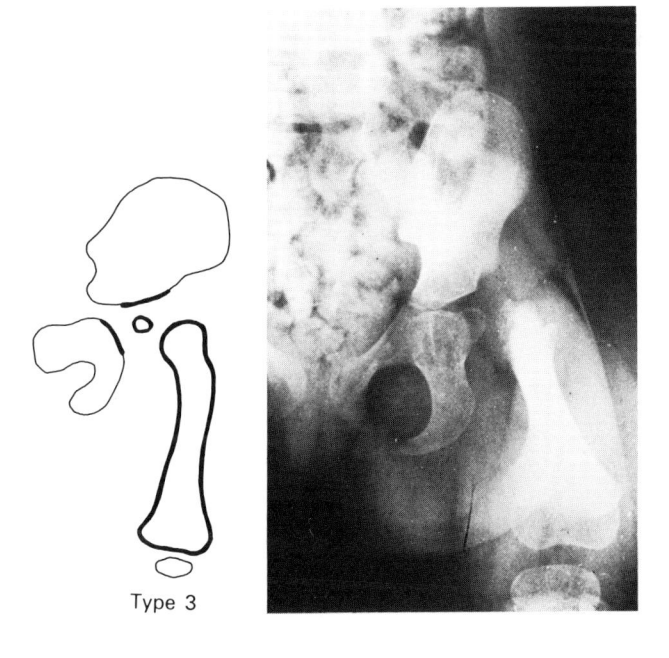

Type 2

Type 3

68 Chapter 2

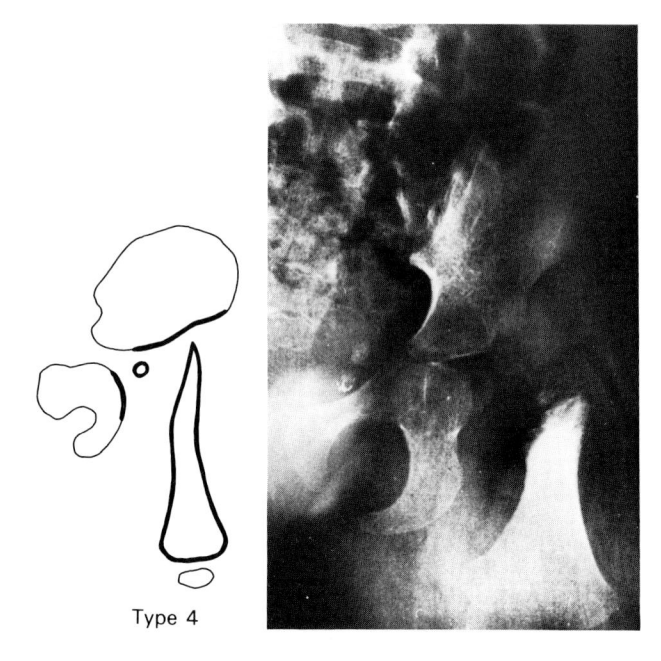

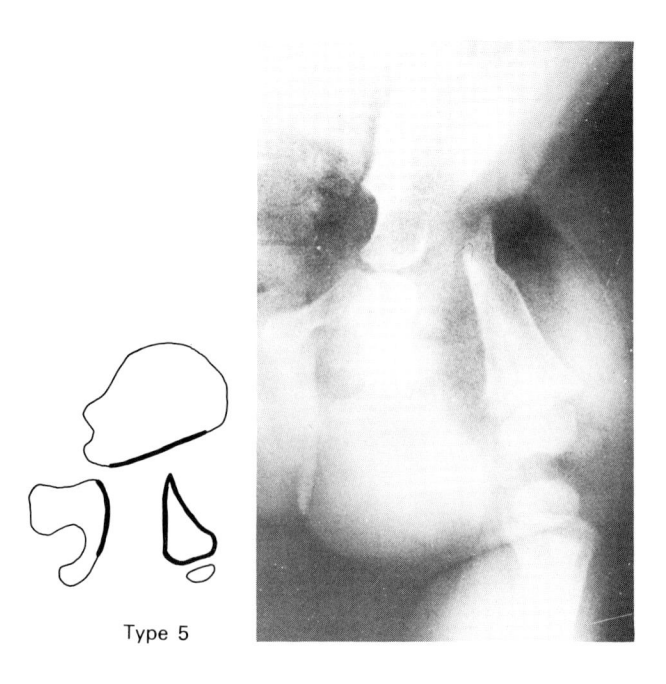

Type 4

Type 5

Type 1—congenital short femur with bowing, coxa vara, and a normal acetabulum. Good hip function ultimately results and shortening is the main problem.

Type 2—short femur with subtrochanteric pseudarthrosis and a normal acetabulum. The pseudarthrosis usually ossifies but significant coxa vara and shortening occur.

Type 3—short femur with a bulbous proximal end. There is a delayed appearance of the femoral capital epiphysis. The neck may ossify or a pseudarthrosis may remain, resulting in extreme coxa vara.

Type 4—complete absence of the proximal femur although the capital epiphysis ultimately appears. The pointed distal fragment of the femur migrates proximally and shortening is extreme.

Type 5—similar to type 4 but no proximal epiphysis appears and the acetabulum is absent.

MANAGEMENT

The birth of a child with a proximal femoral focal deficiency is a tremendous shock to the parents and every effort should be made as early as possible to see that they receive proper advice about the nature of the deformity, the possibilities of treatment, and the likely outcome. As so often happens with birth defects, the parents are assailed by uninformed opinion from nurses, midwives, and others, and this always seems to be far more pessimistic than is justified. In most centres there is usually one orthopaedic surgeon who has a special interest in limb deficiencies and he should be sought out and brought into consultation at the first opportunity. In general there are four basic problems in the management: instability of the hip, malrotation, inadequate proximal musculature, and leg length inequality. These problems will now be discussed in turn.

INSTABILITY OF THE HIP

Instability varies according to the extent of the maldevelopment. However, even in the best varieties with some coxa vara, some instability will be present and this will be greatly exaggerated in the more severe types. Surgery has a limited role to play but the following procedures may be of value. *Valgus osteotomy*—a subtrochanteric osteotomy to correct coxa vara is indicated in types 1 and 2 if the deformity is severe. *Repair of a femoral pseudarthrosis*—this is always worthwhile and usually successful. The adjacent surfaces of the pseudarthrosis may consist of cartilage but this need not necessarily be excised. It is usual to fix the pseudarthrosis with an intramedullary rod and onlay bone grafting can also be used, but is not always necessary (Figs. 2.49 & 2.50). *Reconstruction or repair of the neck*—pseudarthrosis occurring in the region of the neck is a much more difficult problem to manage. In general, while the relationship of the shaft to the

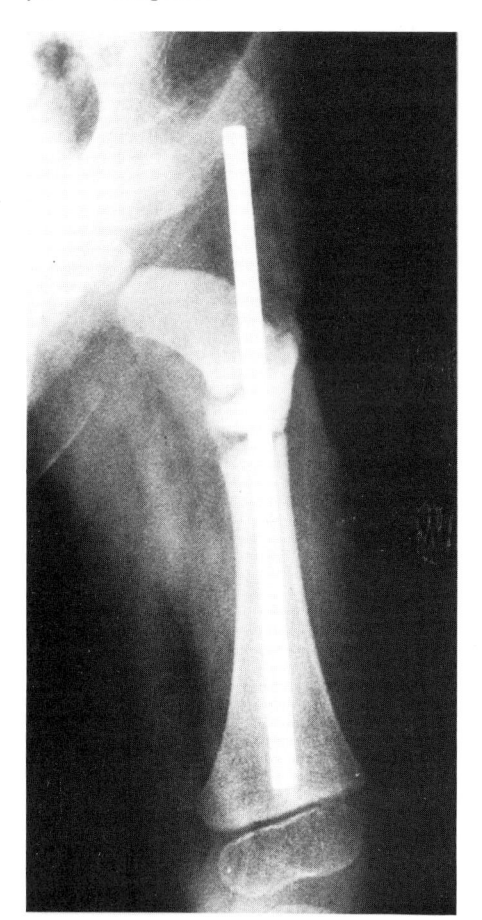

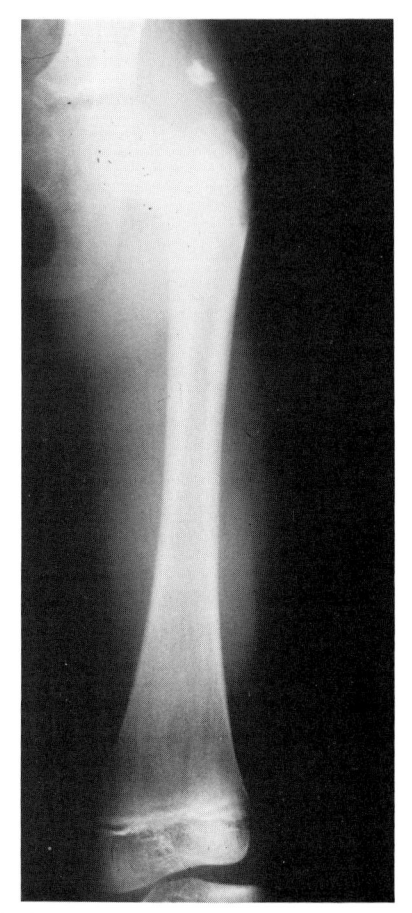

Figs. 2.49 & 2.50 PFFD with a femoral pseudarthrosis. An osteotomy has been done below the pseudarthrosis to correct deformity and an intramedullary rod introduced for fixation. (*Right*) The same case five years after removal of the rod. Union has occurred at both sites without bone grafting.

acetabulum is maintained, it can be assumed that a continuous cartilaginous model is present and it is best to wait for spontaneous ossification to occur. If progressive coxa vara occurs in a few cases, repair can be successful using a small nail and plate and a bone graft supplement. *Arthrodesis of the hip*—although this might appear to be an attractive solution to the instability of the hip, it has been found that mobility is better than stability; arthrodesis should therefore be avoided if possible.

MALROTATION AND INADEQUATE PROXIMAL MUSCULATURE

These two problems are very much inter-related and can be considered together.

The Infant 71

The characteristic posture at the hip is one of flexion, external rotation and abduction. While this looks awkward in the beginning, it should be accepted as the position will improve once the prosthesis is fitted and especially if, at a later date, the knee is fused. There is never any need to carry out release surgery or osteotomy.

LEG LENGTH INEQUALITY

Shortening of the limb provides the greatest challenge and the majority of patients will require some form of orthosis or prosthesis to overcome the problem (Fig. 2.51). The few with a small inequality in length may be managed by leg lengthening procedures or by epiphysiodesis of the normal leg. However in the majority the shortening will be such that, at maturity, the foot of the affected leg will be at approximately the same level as the normal knee. This discrepancy can be handled in the following ways.

A patten—in the young child with a relatively small discrepancy a patten allows good function and this can be used up to about 3 inches (7.5 cm) in height. Over this amount the patten no longer remains functionally or cosmetically acceptable.

Extension prosthesis—by placing the foot in full equinus on a platform it is possible to create a prosthesis of appropriate length. As the discrepancy increases both the knee and the foot may be placed within the socket of a prosthesis with a hinge immediately distal. This type of prosthesis can be regarded as a good interim solution but is cosmetically unacceptable (especially to women) and cannot restore a normal ratio of thigh-to-leg length.

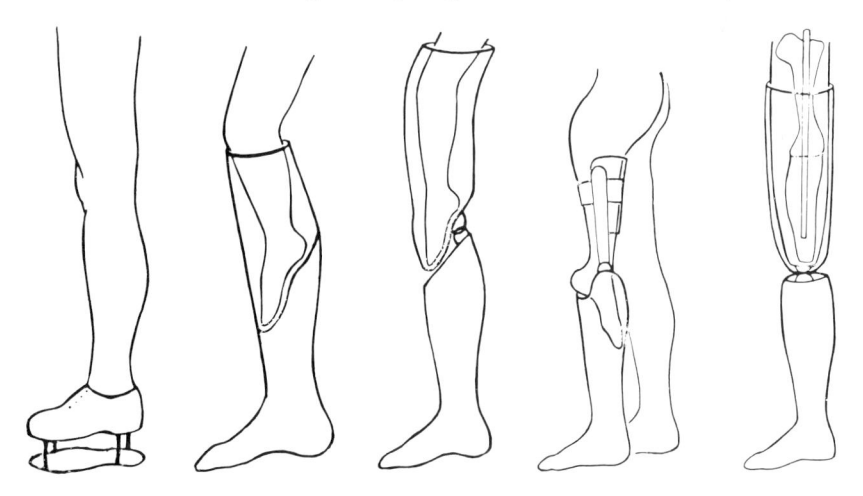

Fig. 2.51 Available methods of overcoming leg length inequality in PFFD. From left to right: patten, extension prosthesis, extension prosthesis with a knee joint, rotation-plasty (Van Nes) allowing the ankle to function at the knee with an extension prosthesis, conventional above-knee prosthesis after a Syme's amputation and fusion of the knee.

Rotation plasty—Van Nes popularised an operation in which the knee was arthrodesed and the distal half of the limb rotated through 180° so that the foot was pointing directly backwards. This brought the ankle into a position where it functioned as a knee with the calf muscles acting as a quadriceps. The operation is difficult to perform and, if done early, derotation occurs with growth. The final appearance of the limb is ugly and our experience has been that it produces an ugly gait and is not well liked by the patient.

Syme's amputation—for the large group of patients with abnormalities of the leg and foot, a decision to amputate the foot through the ankle can readily be made and accepted by the parents; however, where the foot is normal, its loss may be more difficult to accept. In general it can be said that the foot should be retained while the child is still able to put it to the ground and get about without any form of orthosis. Once the shortening is such that it cannot be achieved, there are great prosthetic advantages in removal of the foot and in most cases this will be recommended.

Arthrodesis of the knee—most of the patients with proximal femoral focal deficiency (PFFD) have a knee joint which is close to the pelvis. This increases the instability of the hip region as the available muscles dissipate their effort across two joints. With fixed flexion deformity of the hip, the knee must bend almost to a right angle to allow a vertical posture and this makes it difficult for the prosthetist to provide a satisfactory socket. Arthrodesis of the knee producing a single skeletal lever thus has obvious advantages. Fusion of the knee should be deferred until it is possible to predict the ultimate stump length with some accuracy as it is important that the final stump should not be too long so that the prosthetic knee joint is at too low a level. Sometimes the epiphyses at the knee will require fusion at the time of arthrodesis in order to control the length. There seems to be universal agreement that the best cosmetic and functional results in these cases are obtained by the combination of a Syme amputation and arthrodesis of the knee. While this is true, it is important that this combination should not be regarded as universally applicable and each case should be considered on its merit.

CONGENITAL ABSENCE OF THE FIBULA

Absence of the fibula is more common than absence of any other of the long bones and is twice as common in girls.

CLASSIFICATION

The classification proposed by Coventry and Johnson (Fig. 2.52) is useful.

Type I—the tibia is short but not bowed and the foot is normal. The distal fibula is present to a variable extent. The condition is unilateral and compatible

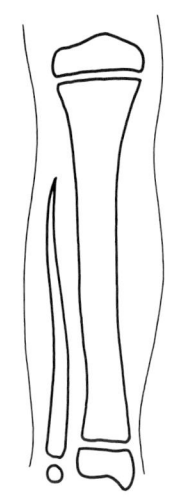

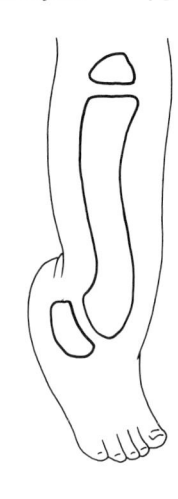

Fig. 2.52 Types of congenital absence of the fibula. On the left type I and on the right type II. type III is similar to type II but is either bilateral or is associated with other defects, e.g. PFFD.

with excellent function, although late deformity at the ankle may occur (Fig. 2.53).

Type II—unilateral but the tibia is much shorter, is bowed anteriorly, and has a skin dimple surmounting it. The foot is in fixed equinovalgus and the outer rays of the foot may be missing (Fig. 2.54).

Type III—similar to type II, but the condition is either bilateral or, if unilateral, is associated with other defects such as proximal femoral focal deficiency.

MANAGEMENT

There is little scope for conservative treatment unless the foot is relatively normal and the tibia long enough to allow the foot to reach the ground. If the foot is in fixed equinovalgus, attempts at closed correction will fail and surgical treatment will be required sooner or later. In unilateral cases, it is usual to make the best of the deformity with special boots while the child is still able to run about barefooted. When the combination of deformity and increased shortening makes this difficult then surgery is advisable. Two procedures are available.

Gruca ankle reconstruction

In bilateral cases or in unilateral cases with acceptable shortening, ankle reconstruction is indicated and will often allow the use of normal footwear for a number of years (Fig. 2.55). This operation is not well known but was described

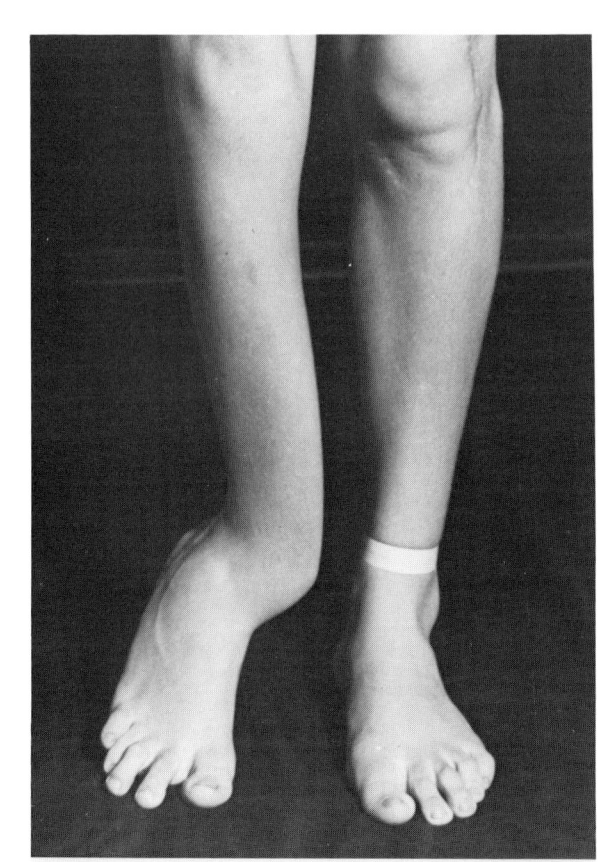

Fig. 2.53 An untreated case of congenital absence of the fibula at the age of 10 years. Surprisingly the ankle remained stable until age 8 years when the talus gradually slipped laterally. It was finally corrected by arthrodesis of the ankle.

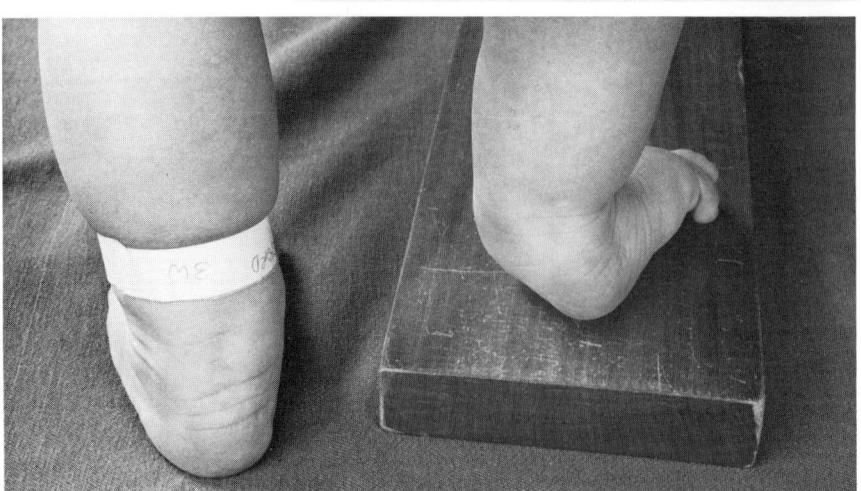

Fig. 2.54 A child with congenital absence of the fibula. The extreme valgus deformity at the ankle is well shown.

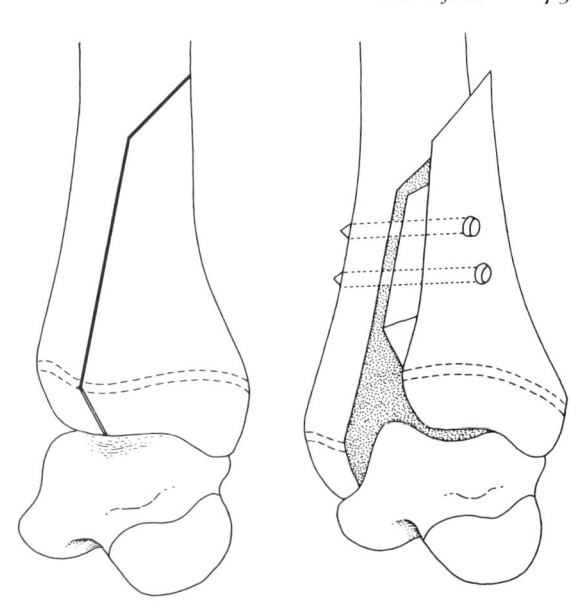

Fig. 2.55 The Gruca procedure showing how a new lateral malleolus is constructed and the growth plate is retained.

by Serafin in the *Journal of Bone and Joint Surgery* in 1967. Briefly, the technique of the operation is as follows:

> From an anterior approach a long oblique osteotomy of the tibia is carried out. When this osteotomy is opened up in front, it is possible to displace the large medial fragment upward and outwards. The talus is now provided with a supporting lateral buttress, consisting of the lateral third of the tibia and with a mortise created, the position can be maintained by two screws and a small cortical graft. The limb is immobilised for 3–4 weeks when union is usually sound and weight-bearing can be allowed.

We have used this procedure on a small number of cases over the last five years but insufficient time has elapsed to demonstrate the long term results. In the short term, all children are walking on the treated foot using normal footwear without bracing. It is felt that, even if deterioration were to occur after a number of years, these children have lost nothing by the procedure.

Syme amputation

Once excessive shortening has developed, it is usual to perform a Syme amputation and this is usually done in the second or third year of life. The surgical procedure is classical but great care is required to position the heel pad over the end of the tibia after scarification of the articular cartilage. Because the subsequent growth tends to retract the pad backwards, a segment of the tendo-Achilles should be removed at the time of amputation. Modern prostheses

76 Chapter 2

fitted to a Syme amputation give excellent function and have a very acceptable appearance even in girls.

ANGULAR DEFORMITIES OF THE TIBIA

Bowing of the tibia arises from both congenital and acquired causes and may be classified on an anatomical basis: anterior, antero-lateral, posterior and lateral.

ANTERIOR TIBIAL BOWING (TIBIAL KYPHOSIS)

The tibia is short, broad and angled forward, the bone being markedly thickened

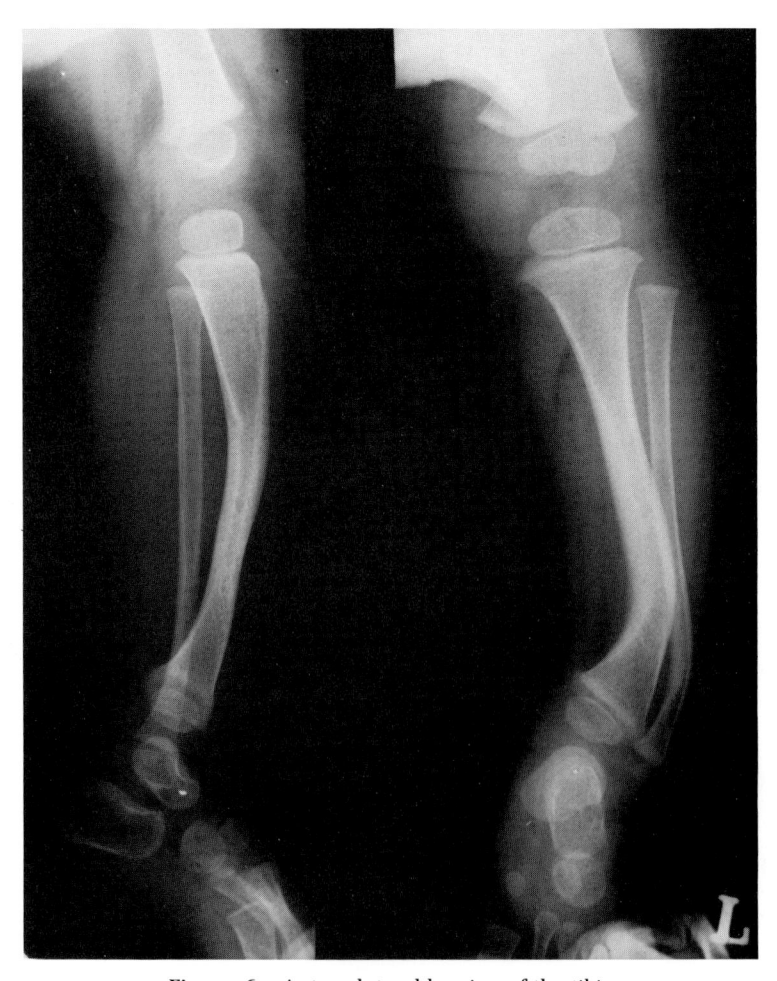

Fig. 2.56 Antero-lateral bowing of the tibia.

on the concave side. Shortening of the calf muscles produces a talipes equinus. Associated anomalies such as absence of the fibula and congenital dislocation of the hip are commonly present. Tibial kyphosis does not lead to pseudarthrosis and treatment is not required unless dictated by any associated anomalies.

ANTERO-LATERAL BOWING (FIG. 2.56)

The tibia is bowed forwards and laterally, the bone being usually small, sclerotic and possibly without a demonstrable medullary cavity at the apex of the deformity. The foot is in calcaneus and there are usually no associated deformities. Fracture eventually occurs and leads to pseudarthrosis.

POSTERO-MEDIAL BOWING (FIG. 2.57)

This deformity is characterised by postero-medial bowing at the junction of the middle and lower third of the tibia and by the presence of talipes calcaneus. A little shortening is usually present in the tibia. Treatment is not indicated as the deformity grows to normality over a period of years.

LATERAL BOWING

This deformity is seen in the physiological bow leg of early childhood, rickets, Blount's disease and epiphyseal injuries.

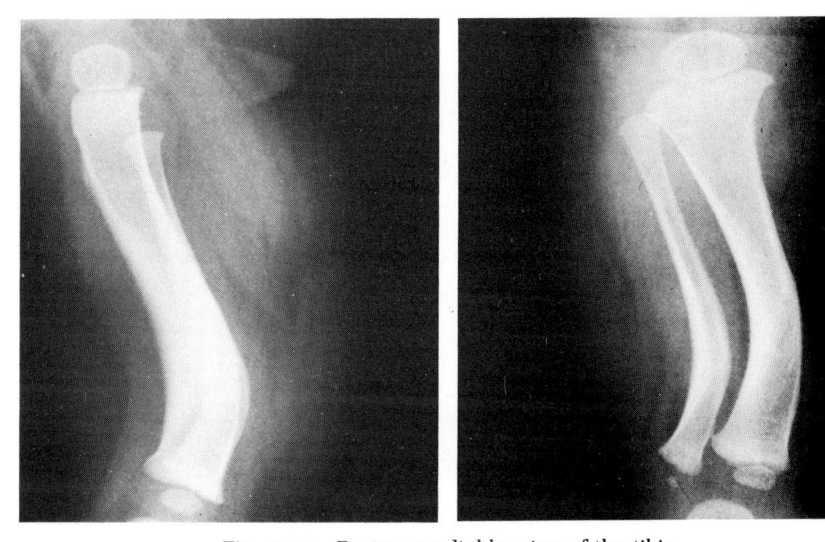

Fig. 2.57 Postero-medial bowing of the tibia.

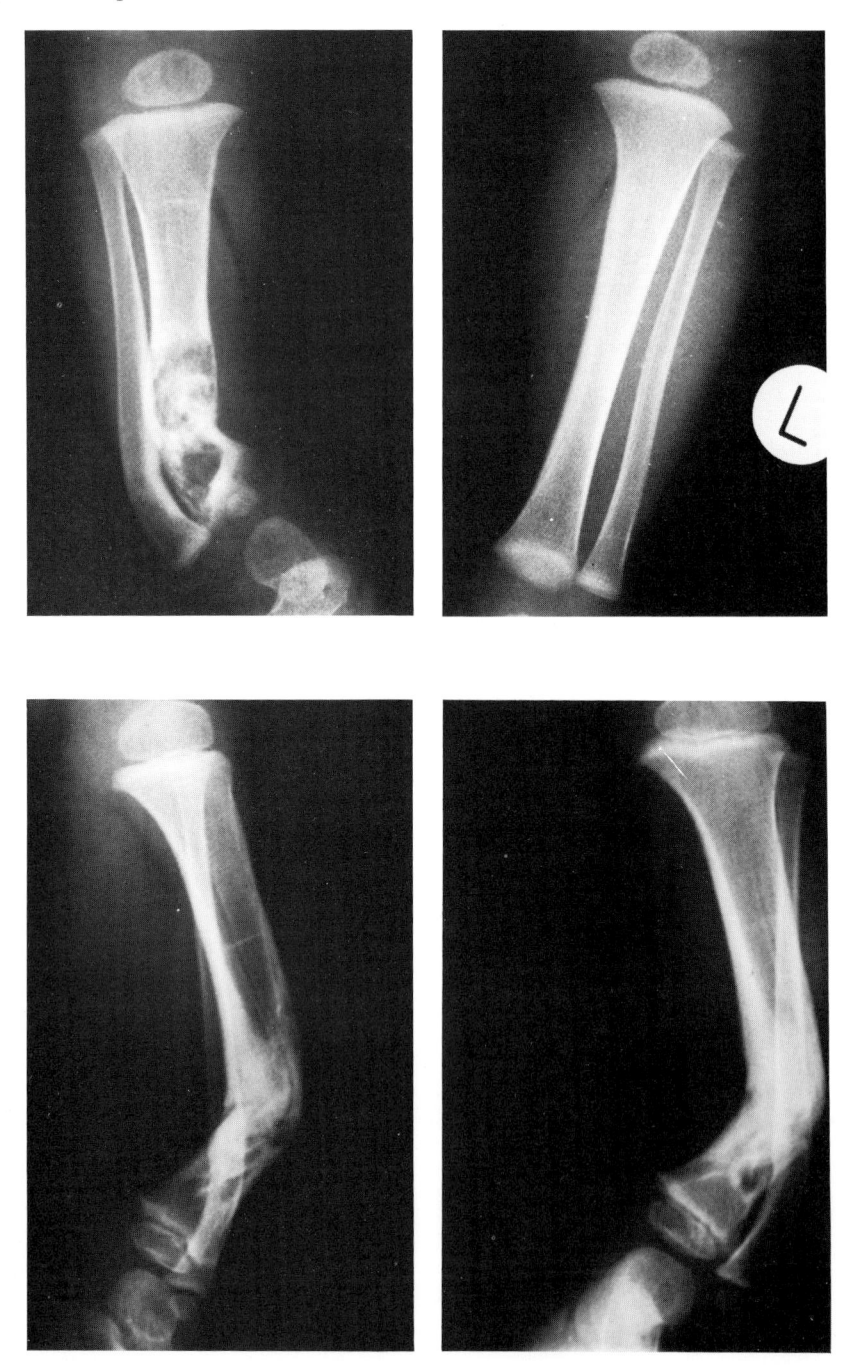

Figs. 2.58 & 2.59 A cystic antero-lateral kyphosis of the right tibia in a child aged 4 months; (*Bottom*) At the age of 2 years.

PSEUDARTHROSIS OF THE TIBIA

Although rarely present at birth, pseudarthrosis of the tibia is related to other forms of tibial angulation and is conveniently discussed in this section. Three clinical types are recognised:
1 Following fracture of a cystic lesion in the tibia (Figs. 2.58–2.61).
2 Following fracture of an anteriorly bowed tibia with a sclerotic segment at the apex of the curve.
3 Present at birth.

The tibia is usually affected at the junction of the middle and lower thirds and the fibula at the same level. Occasionally only the fibula is affected and this leads to progressive valgus at the ankle.

AETIOLOGY

This is unknown but, in some cases, there are clinical associations with

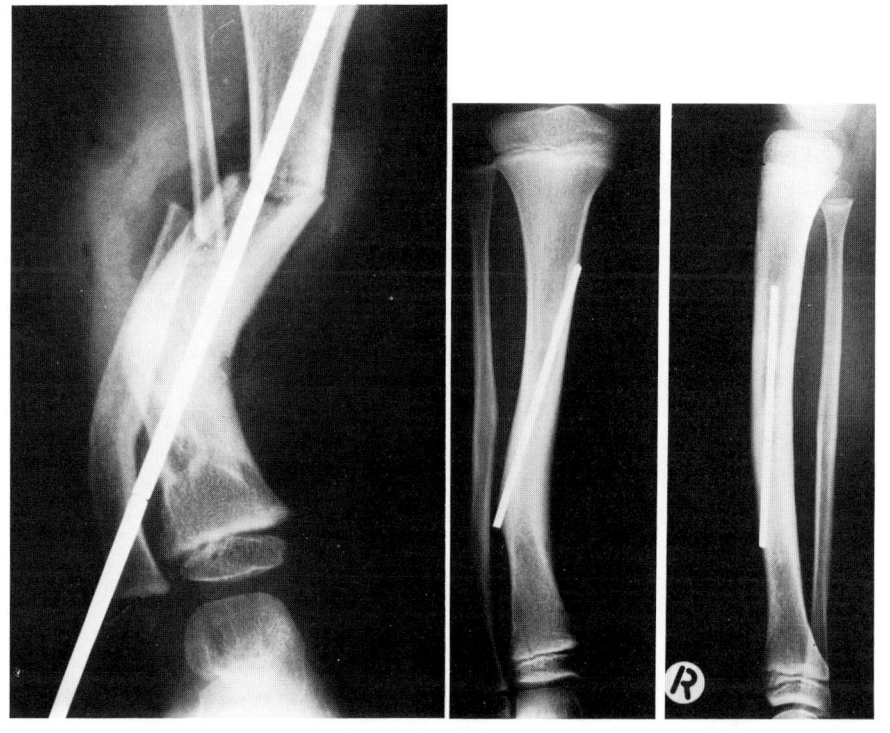

Figs. 2.60 & 2.61 Radiograph taken intra-operatively after an osteotomy had been carried out above the kyphosis. The distal part of the rod was then unscrewed. (See rodding in osteogenesis imperfecta, p. 415.) (*Right*) At the age of 7 years the tibia has moulded to an almost normal shape.

neurofibromatosis and in others the features are identical with monostotic fibrous dysplasia.

TREATMENT

Prophylactic. If the child is seen prior to fracture with one of the two possible precursors, prophylactic treatment is indicated. In the case of a cystic tibia, this should be curetted and the fibrous content removed and replaced with autogenous cancellous bone; for very small infants, maternal or bank bone may be used. It may be necessary to repeat this if the cyst re-forms.

Similarly the anteriorly curved tibia should be reinforced by bone grafts placed in the concavity and this may also need to be repeated until the desired strength is obtained. Following any surgery, external protection from a synthetic mould is required and this should be worn for some years until the medullary cavity is completely reconstituted.

Therapeutic. Once fracture has occurred and pseudarthrosis established, any form of conservative management (however prolonged) is quite useless (Fig. 2.62). Similarly, operative surgery designed to procure union is likely to fail in the young child. It is necessary to avoid repeated bone grafts and prolonged hospitalisation as it is often found that, by the time union is secured, the leg is so short and the foot so small that amputation is indicated.

After many failures of this kind, our present practice is to fix the fracture with an intramedullary rod using the technique described for osteogenesis imperfecta. As soon as the wound is healed, a synthetic orthosis is constructed to encircle the limb and extend from toes to groin. A long leg caliper is worn over this and weight bearing allowed. This regime is continued until the child is 8 years old—the rod and the equipment being changed as required. At this age the bone is re-rodded and formal grafting carried out using a cortical inlay from the opposite tibia and a cancellous supplement. At this age and using this method, success is most likely and sufficient length has usually been preserved. If at any time during the course of treatment it can be seen that shortening is becoming extreme, the advisability of amputation should be discussed.

CONGENITAL ABSENCE OF THE RADIUS (RADIAL CLUB HAND)

This was a very rare deformity until the introduction of the drug Thalidomide when a large number were produced. After withdrawal of this drug, very few cases have been seen.

ANATOMICAL CHANGES

The condition is often bilateral. Usually the entire radius is absent though

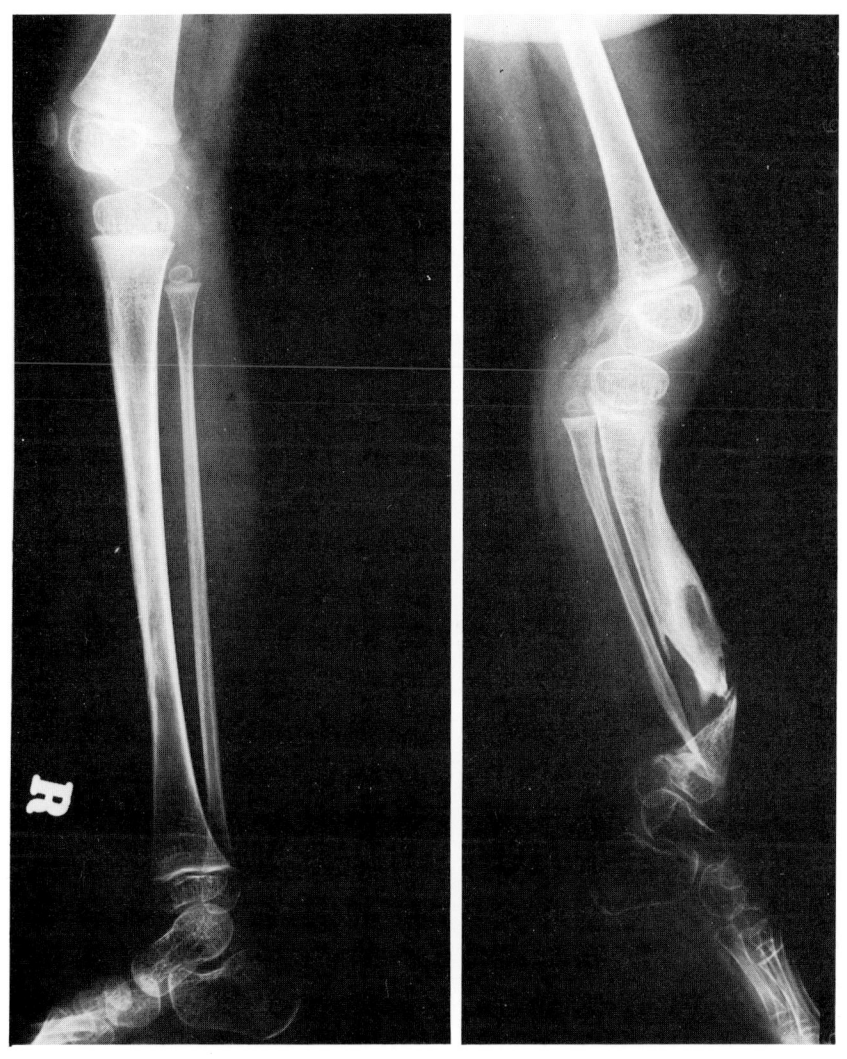

Fig. 2.62 Pseudarthrosis of the tibia persisting despite several attempts at bone grafting. Note the overall shortening of the tibia and the very short distal fragment.

occasionally parts of the bone may be present (Fig. 2.63). The ulna is very short and curved and the hand lies on the side of the arm forming an angle of about 90°. The hand can often be folded up to lie with its radial border opposed to the ulna. The thumb and first metacarpal are usually absent or, if present, will be hypoplastic. Varying degrees of stiffness occur in the metacarpophalangeal and interphalangeal joints and there are many deficiencies in the forearm musculature.

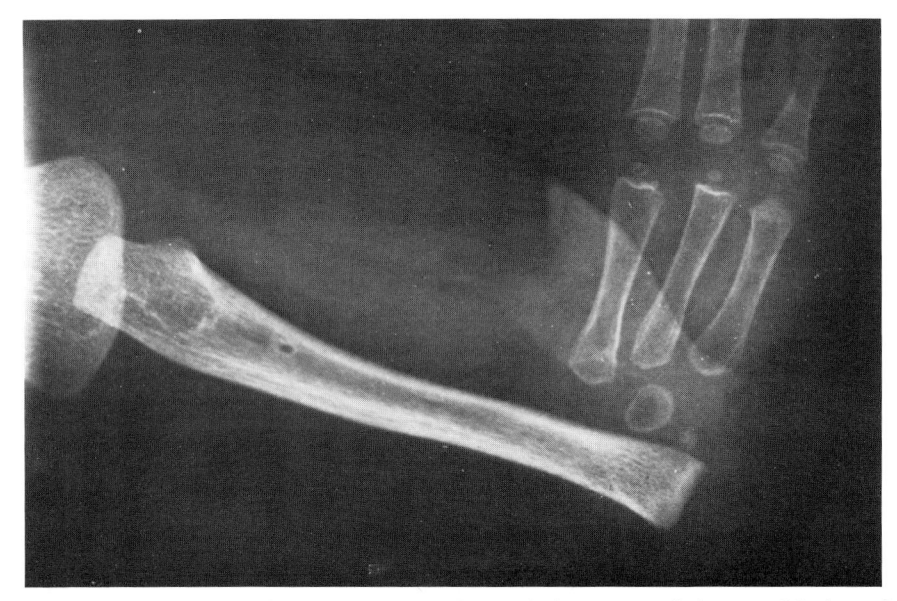

Fig. 2.63 Congenital absence of the right radius with the associated absence of the lateral two rays of the hand.

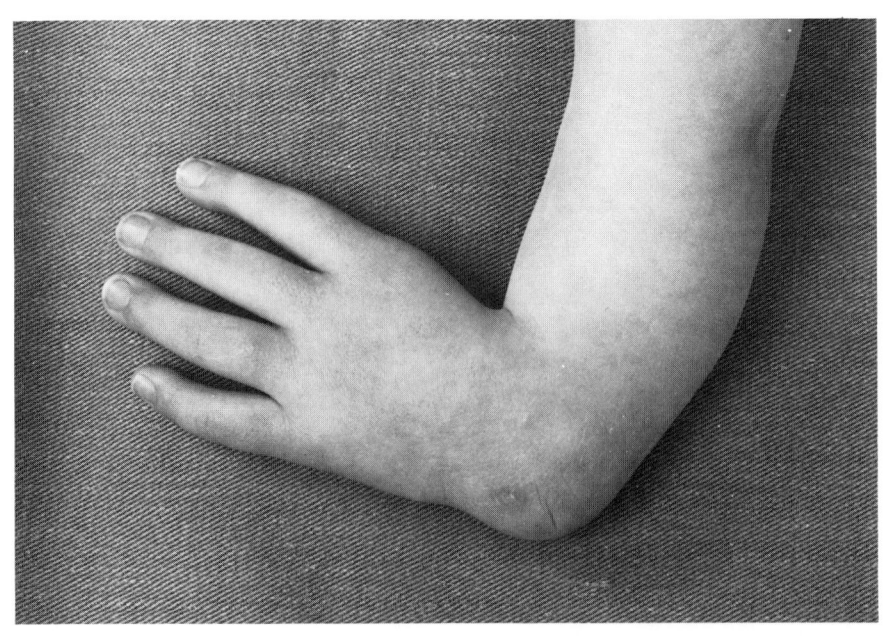

Fig. 2.64 Congenital absence of the radius and thumb with characteristic radial deviation at the wrist.

The Infant

MANAGEMENT

Although remarkable function can be achieved in untreated cases, there are good reasons for attempting correction. After the wrist has been straightened not only is the function improved but the appearance is greatly enhanced.

CONSERVATIVE CORRECTION

In infancy, the smallness of the parts and the lack of subcutaneous fat make it difficult to apply corrective splints or casts, and it is usually more practical to delay treatment until six months of age. The hand can be gradually brought around to the neutral position where it must be held with a removable orthosis until the child is old enough for surgical correction.

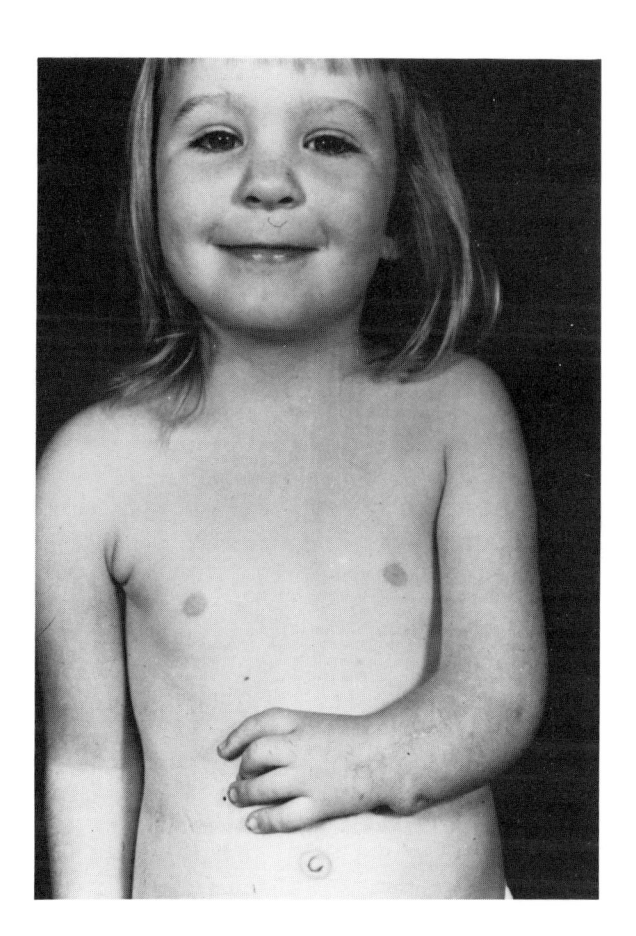

Fig. 2.65 The appearance of the same child two years after centralisation of the ulna into the carpus.

Chapter 2

SURGICAL CORRECTION

Over the years many attempts have been made to reconstitute a new radius but all have failed because it has not been possible to provide a new bone which will grow with the child. The most successful procedure is the centralisation of the ulna in the carpus and this is best done after the second year (although it is still possible up to maturity) (Figs. 2.64 & 2.65)

After careful dissection, the lunate and capitate bones are removed and the lower end of the ulna covered by its capsule is placed into the space so created. A Kirschner wire is usually run up through the metacarpal region across the carpus and into the shaft of the ulna. Fixation is reinforced by a plaster cast and both the cast and the wire can be removed after about two months. Continued night splintage is required for years but, even so, gradual relapse is common and, at maturity, arthrodesis of the wrist may be indicated to retrieve the situation.

CONGENITAL PSEUDARTHROSIS OF THE CLAVICLE

This rare anomaly only affects the right clavicle and is usually not discovered until the child is a year old or more when a painless swelling is noted at the base of the neck. There is marked mobility between the two fragments which become more prominent with growth.

MANAGEMENT

Surgical correction will be indicated in most cases both to improve appearance and to increase the strength of the shoulder girdle. Since intramedully fixation is necessary, the operation should be deferred until at least the age of three years when the bone is big enough to accept a threaded Kirschner wire. The incision should be placed in the neck and not over the clavicle. After freshening the bone end, the threaded wire is introduced into the lateral fragment and wound in until it appears behind the shoulder. The direction can now be reversed and the wire passes the pseudarthrosis to engage the medial fragment. A little bank bone can be added as an onlay and, after closure of the wound, the arm is immobilised in a sling for three weeks. Union is easy to obtain and the wire can be removed after several months.

SUPERNUMERARY TOES (POLYDACTYLY)

There may be one or several supernumerary toes. Most commonly there is a supernumerary hallux or an accessory digit lying lateral to the fifth toe. The accessory digit may be well formed or only partially formed. There may be a

Y-shaped proximal phalanx. In some, there is one or more accessory metatarsals of varying degrees of completeness.

The principle of management is to remove extra toes in such a way as to make the foot of satisfactory cosmetic appearance and the same width as the normal foot. Almost invariably it is best to amputate the digit which lies lateral to a fifth toe, even if that digit is better formed than the more medially placed fifth toe. The same applies to the hallux.

SYNDACTYLY

Syndactyly of the toes are common. It may be partial or complete and does not require treatment.

CONGENITAL HEMIATROPHY AND HEMIHYPERTROPHY

These two conditions may be considered together as they have a similar natural history and indeed it is often difficult to be sure which one is present. Both affect either the whole side of the body, including the face, or in some cases only one limb. All tissues are equally affected and function is usually normal. These conditions are present at birth and are non-progressive, i.e. the discrepancy in length and girth remains constant throughout the growth period.

The leg length discrepancy rarely exceeds one inch (2.5 cm) and, when it does, can be corrected by epiphysiodesis. The difference in girth is often distressing to the child and parents, but usually passes unnoticed by most observers. There is no way of adjusting the discrepancy in girth by any surgical means and orthoses designed for this purpose are hot and cumbersome.

HYPERTROPHY

Enlargement of whole limbs or part of limbs is seen in association with the following conditions: neurofibromatosis (see page 418); gigantism, vascular anomalies, lymphatic anomalies, and muscle hypertrophy in the foot.

Gigantism

Progressive overgrowth of one or more toes or fingers is a rare condition and is sometimes seen in association with neurofibromatosis (Fig. 2.66). Hyperplasia affects all the tissues, particularly the lymphatic and fatty tissues and the enlargement may eventually become grotesque. In the hand the appearance is jeopardised and the function may be impaired due to the clumsy size of the digit.

86 Chapter 2

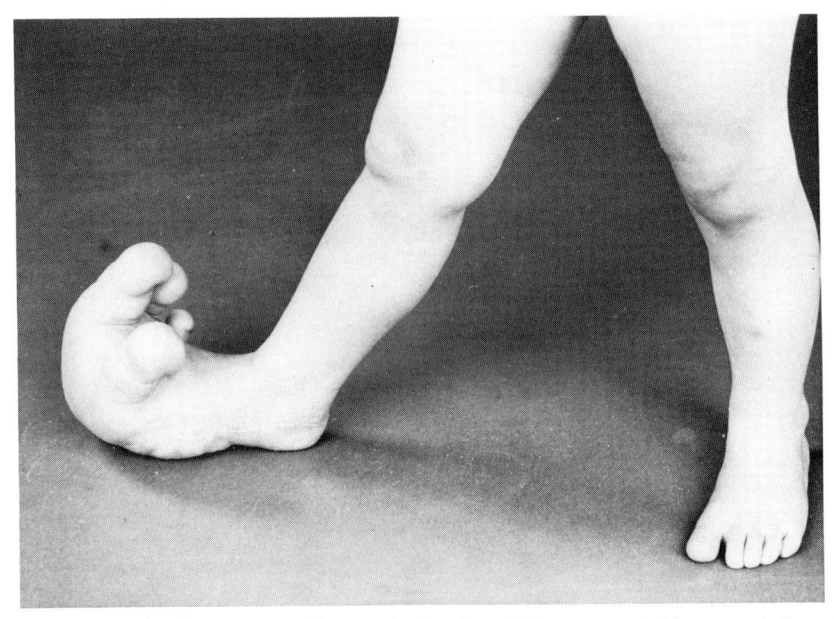

Fig. 2.66 Localised gigantism affecting the forefoot. This was treated by amputation at a tarso-metatarsal level.

In the foot the main problem is the difficulty in shoe fitting and this may become impossible especially if the tissues of the forefoot are involved.

As regards management, many attempts have been made to reduce the size by soft tissue resection, filleting of phalanges and epiphysiodesis, but in most cases these are unsuccessful and amputation becomes necessary. In both the hand and the foot, if only one digit is involved, a better result can be obtained by resection of the whole ray.

Muscle hypertrophy in the foot

Enlargement of one foot is occasionally seen in which there is localised hypertrophy of the abductors of the hallux and the little toe. The cause of this is unknown and there do not appear to be any clinical associations. When shoe fitting problems occur, subtotal excision of the involved muscles will overcome the difficulty.

Vascular anomalies

Congenital vascular anomalies affecting the limbs are rare, especially in the upper limb. All types of involvement are seen. Cavernous angiomatosis may involve part or whole of the limb and be associated with capillary haemangiomas involving the skin or with venous varicosities. The effect is often a bulky unsightly limb which overgrows in length and girth. Spontaneous haemorrhages may occur from the cutaneous involvement and many of the areas of deep involvement are exquisitely tender to touch and the overlying skin sweats profusely. The angiomatous change is best described as a hamartoma and these continue to grow up to the age of about 20 years. During this period incomplete excision is usually followed by recurrence. Lymphatic overgrowth and obstruction is sometimes associated. Arteriography will rarely, if ever, demonstrate any localised arteriovenous connection and by and large the investigation is hardly worth carrying out.

Treatment may be necessary to: *control length*—epiphysiodesis can be safely performed even through areas of involved skin, and *control pain*—excision of large areas of involved muscles, tendons and fat may be necessary on one or more occasions. After repeated surgery, further attempts may be impossible due to involvement of neurovascular bundles by scar and vascular tumour, so that amputation then becomes inevitable.

Even amputation is not without problems as isolated tender patches of haemangiomatous tissue (either in the stump or in the groin and buttock) may make limb fitting extremely difficult. However, with perseverance, local excisions and careful socket construction, a useful prosthesis can usually be obtained.

Lymphatic anomalies

These are virtually confined to the lower limb which becomes oedematous and enlarged due to enormous dilatation of subcutaneous lymphatic channels. This is followed by fibrosis so the limb becomes not only huge but solid. When familial, the condition is known as Milroy's disease.

MANAGEMENT

This is very unsatisfactory. Elastic stockings partly control the oedema but are uncomfortable to wear. Excision of large tracts of involved skin and subcutaneous tissue is possible but the results are unattractive. Amputation may finally be indicated but prosthetic replacement is unsatisfactory.

CHAPTER 3

The Toddler

Principles of child development; The development of locomotion; Sleeping posture

Gait abnormalities, 89
In-toeing, Out-toeing

Other problems in the toddler, 93

Congenital dislocation of the hip, 95
Management

CEREBRAL PALSY, 96
Causes; Classification; The diagnosis of cerebral palsy; Assessment of the child with cerebral palsy; Treatment; The cerebral palsied child in hospital

The changes in postural patterns which occur from birth to maturity occur in a well ordered sequence and a knowledge of this development is required for, if normality cannot be recognised, it is not possible to accurately separate the abnormalities. The following is a brief account of the subject based largely on the works of Gesell, Buhler and Illingworth.

PRINCIPLES OF CHILD DEVELOPMENT

Development is a continuous process. Merely passing a milestone is an insufficient description of progress. It is necessary to observe not only what the child does but how well he does it.

The sequence of development is the same for all children but the timing varies from child to child.

The direction of development is cephalocaudal, e.g. head control precedes sitting balance.

THE DEVELOPMENT OF LOCOMOTION

This occurs in a logical sequence and it is possible to give a fairly accurate average time for the various milestones in the normal child.

Head control—this should be very well developed at 3 months whether tested in ventral suspension, prone or in the sitting position. It should be complete at 5 months.

Sitting unsupported—this will usually be possible at 7 months.

Standing—

5 months—bears some weight on leg if supported.
7 months—able to stand supported with hips and knees fully extended for short periods.
10 months—can pull themselves up to standing position.
11 months—walks sideways along furniture.
12 months—walks with one hand held.

Walking—during the second year the child learns to stand up straight and to balance on a broad base. They walk with feet apart and turned out with a lumbar lordosis and a bulging belly. The average age of independent walking is 15 months and by the age of 2 years the child should be able to run.

SLEEPING POSTURE

In some communities prone sleeping is encouraged in the infant and toddler and there is some evidence that this encourages motor development. In orthopaedic practice the majority of children who present with persisting metatarsus adductus and bowlegs do in fact sleep prone and, while it is not suggested that prone sleeping causes these conditions, nevertheless it does seem that it delays recovery from them. It is common experience that if the sleeping habits are changed there is a rapid resolution of the orthopaedic problems.

GAIT ABNORMALITIES

Minor abnormalities of gait, particularly those associated with in-toeing of one or both feet, constitute one of the commonest worries which assail parents of young children. While it is true that the vast majority of these children do not require treatment, many parents are unwilling to accept reassurance without an adequate explanation and eventually seek an orthopaedic opinion to set their minds at rest.

IN-TOEING

This is the most common presenting complaint in the toddler and is associated with tripping, 'always falling over', and a variety of other side effects. The cause of in-toeing may be at one or more of three anatomical sites—in the foot, in the tibia, or in the hip joint. One, two or all three sites may be implicated in a given patient.

90   Chapter 3

Sometimes a minor degree of deformity may be present at each site; taken singly, each would be unimportant but when the effects of each are summated the functional results can be quite marked.

Causes in the foot

Metatarsus adductus. This posture, which has already been described in the infant, may persist in the toddler (Fig. 3.1). Once the child begins to wear shoes and converts from prone to supine sleeping, resolution usually occurs fairly rapidly. Occasionally a night splint to hold the foot in the overcorrected position will be indicated in more severe cases. Reversal of the day shoes is not recommended since it is uncomfortable for the child and is productive of an awkward gait.

Metatarsus varus. In contrast to the previous deformity, metatarsus varus is extremely uncommon. Although it was fully described by Peabody over 30 years ago the condition has since received only scant attention in the literature and most of the current texts on orthopaedic surgery make little or no mention of it. Nevertheless, it is seen sufficiently frequently and its effects are sufficiently crippling to warrant description here. Metatarsus varus is a true structural

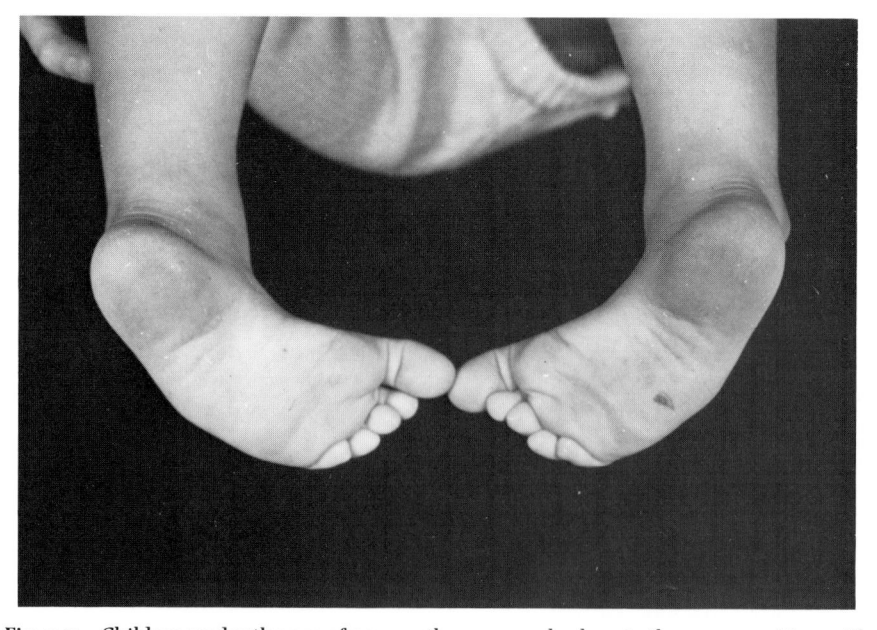

Fig. 3.1 Children under the age of 30 months commonly sleep in the prone position with their feet internally rotated. This posture is not responsible for internal tibial torsion or metatarsus adductus—both of which conditions occur in children who do not adopt this posture. The posture may, however, cause some delay in spontaneous correction of these conditions.

deformity of congenital origin in which the forefoot is not only adducted but twisted into supination, the longitudinal arch is high and the hindfoot is valgoid. Each component of the deformity is rigid. X-ray films show that all the metatarsals are incurved. All this gives the foot a curious sickle shape when viewed from in front and the gait is correspondingly ugly. Small children tend to trip and stumble whilst older ones develop painful calluses on the outer border of the foot and their shoes rapidly lose their shape and wear through. At all times difficulty is experienced in selecting shoes to fit these feet properly. The curious fact is that, although this deformity is classified as congenital, it commonly passes unnoticed at birth and does not usually present until the second year. Untreated, the deformity tends to worsen whereas most children with metatarsus adductus tend to grow towards normality. The deformity of metatarsus varus does not lend itself to conservative treatment and once the diagnosis is established full plantar release should be carried out much in the same manner as is described for the treatment of club foot (see page 19). Continuous splintage will be required for a long period after this and relapse can be anticipated in some cases. In the older child, metatarsal osteotomies and finally even triple arthrodesis may be indicated to produce a satisfactory foot.

Causes in the leg

Tibial bowleg. Causes in the leg operate up to the age of 2 years or at the most $2\frac{1}{2}$ years, for it is during this period that the normal leg (below the knee) enjoys a distinctly bowed appearance. This outward curve of the tibia is always associated to a greater or lesser degree with an inward twist so that, when the patella faces ahead, the feet are directed inwards (Fig. 3.2). Tibial intorsion varies in severity from about 10° almost up to 90° and the degree of in-toeing in the gait is directly proportional to this. It is noted that the outward curve of the tibia presents the foot to the ground on its outer border so that a compensatory pes valgus becomes established. Although the tibial deformity is present from birth, it usually passes unnoticed until the child commences walking and as proficiency in walking is gained persistent tripping and stumbling becomes a feature. Many of these children who exhibit a severe deformity are overweight and nearly all are of sturdy build. It is a curious observation that the child's parents are rarely concerned at this stage with the bandiness, indeed they will often deny its existence, but present for advice on the insistence of relatives or neighbours. Treatment is not often required but, as a guide, it can be said that if the appearance of the child is comical then some help is justified. A Denis Browne bar and boots worn at night is surprisingly effective over a period of about three months. Rarely the deformity is so severe and so persistent that osteoclasis of the tibia will be indicated (Figs. 3.3 & 3.4).

Causes in the hip

The normal mature hip joint has a range of rotation in each direction which is

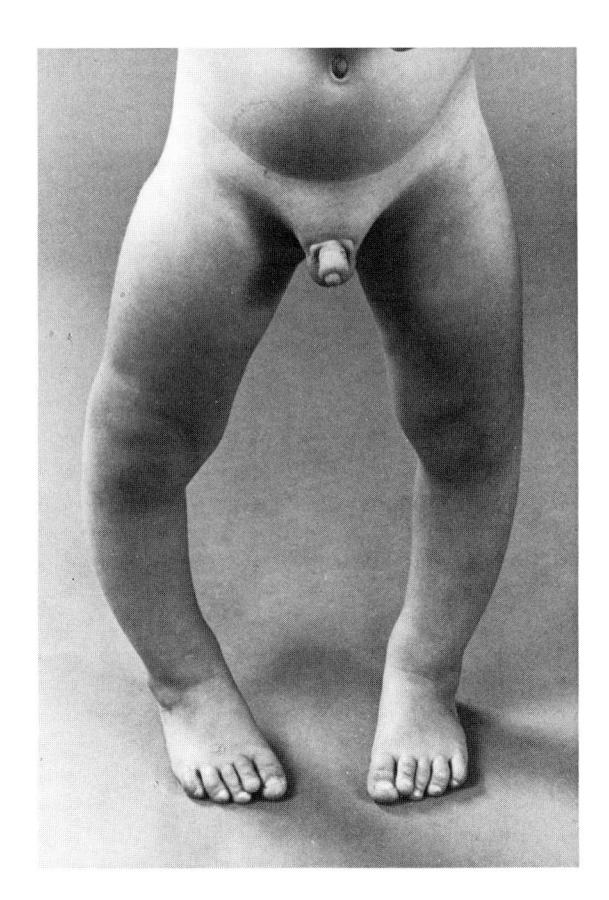

Fig. 3.2 Genu varum and internal tibial torsion (more marked in the right leg) of a boy aged 16 months.

approximately equal. Whilst it is difficult to estimate the incidence at large, in orthopaedic practice children are commonly seen who exhibit an excessive range of internal rotation with a considerably diminished range of external rotation and, in these cases, the history is often so advanced that the children habitually sit as shown in Fig. 4.11, a position which a normal individual finds acutely uncomfortable. Most of the problems associated with an inset hip posture present at a later age, i.e. in the child and in the adolescent and will be further considered in those sections.

OUT-TOEING

An out-toed gait may be assumed by the toddler during his efforts to stand and walk and this is apparently done to increase his sideways stability. Very uncommonly this gait persists in the toddler and will continue through childhood to adult life. In these circumstances examination will reveal that the hips enjoy an

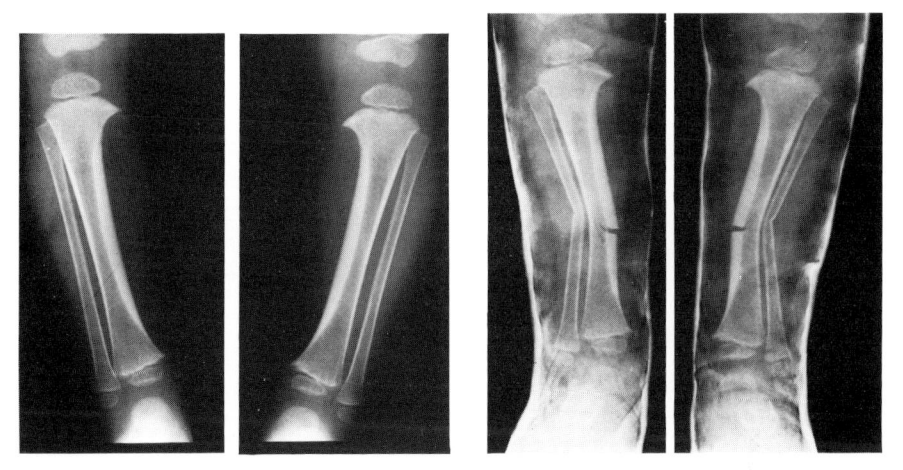

Figs. 3.3 & 3.4 AP view of bow legs of severe degree in a boy aged 2 years and 4 months. (*Right*) The appearance following osteoclasis of both tibiae and fibulae. The osteoclasis usually occurs at a slightly higher level but, even at this low level, the varus and internal torsion is fully corrected.

arc of, say, 90° all of which is in external rotation. The condition is often familial and especially seen in the Jewish race.

Outset hip posture carries certain disadvantages in appearance, in the ability to run fast, and in footwear distortion but is nevertheless acceptable. It is uninfluenced by conservative treatment and surgical correction is not indicated.

It is necessary to re-emphasise that in all the conditions in childhood where in-toeing or out-toeing are a feature, shoe alterations are illogical and useless as a form of treatment. Indeed they may aggravate matters by causing the child to continually trip over on out-of-balance shoes.

OTHER PROBLEMS IN THE TODDLER

Three other orthopaedic problems present in the toddler.

Flat feet

All toddlers have flat feet. This is due to a combination of three factors: 1   the long arch has not fully developed;   2   the hollow in the foot is filled with a large fat pad;   3   the foot rolls into valgus on weight-bearing.

Treatment is unnecessary but since it is expedient for most toddlers to have footwear it is better that they wear boots rather than shoes. Boots have the effect of controlling the valgus and at the same time the real posture of the foot is concealed from the parents' worrying gaze.

Trigger thumb

This is a fairly common abnormality usually presenting in the toddler and often bilateral (Fig. 3.5). The primary lesion is a localised fusiform swelling in the tendon of flexor pollicis longus opposite the metacarpophalangeal joint where it can be easily palpated. There is an associated constriction in the tendon sheath proximal to this. The distal phalanx may trigger for a period as the nodule catches in the constriction until finally the nodule becomes too large to traverse the constriction and the distal phalanx becomes stuck in flexion. The condition is

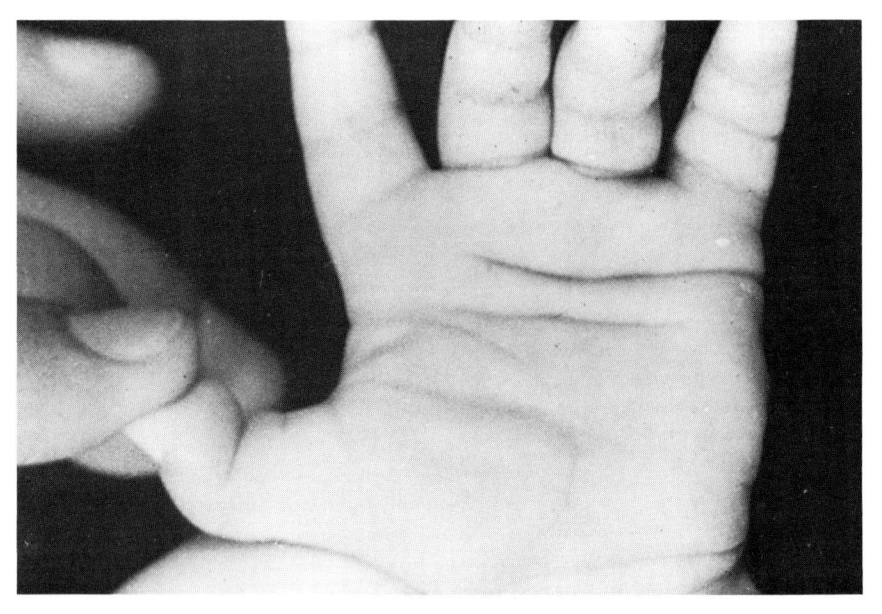

Fig. 3.5 Trigger thumb. There is a fixed flexion deformity of the interphalangeal joint and a palpable hard lump on the volar aspect of the metacarpophalangeal joint.

treated surgically: through a small transverse incision over the nodule the sheath is incised longitudinally to open the stricture. If treatment is delayed into childhood a fixed flexion contracture of the interphalangeal joint develops and may take many months to resolve after operation.

Pulled elbow

A child under the age of 5 years may experience sudden pain and inability to move the elbow following a tug on the arm in play or when being lifted by the hand. The elbow is held fearfully and tearfully in flexion and with the forearm pronated.

The condition is due to a transient subluxation of the radial head causing a tear in the distal attachment of the annular ligament. The proximal part slips into the radio-humeral joint where it becomes trapped. Treatment is simply carried out by holding the elbow in one hand while the other makes a deft supination movement of the forearm. This is accompanied by a palpable click and immediate relief of pain. No after-care is required.

CONGENITAL DISLOCATION OF THE HIP

The aetiology, pathology and management of this condition in the first year of life has been discussed in Chapter 2. Here we are concerned with hip dislocation as it presents over the age of one year. The child may then present because of delay in walking or because of an abnormal gait. All clinical features described in Chapter 2 may be present and, in addition, the child will have a limp. In unilateral cases this is a Trendelenburg gait and in bilateral cases this becomes a waddle. When examined standing, the Trendelenburg sign can be elicited.

Subluxation of the hip

Here the abnormality in gait is much less obvious and hence the children tend to present late. This group cannot be diagnosed at birth as there is no sense of dislocation and reduction. The physical signs have already been mentioned but, like the gait abnormality, they are less obvious.

MANAGEMENT

The child is placed on coronal traction, the hips examined under general anaesthesia and closed or open reduction performed. This management has been described in Chapter 2.

If the hip is reduced by closed means it is placed in a double hip spica in the most stable position, which is generally one of flexion to a little more than 90°, abduction of approximately 70° and neutral rotation. Radiographs confirm concentric reduction and the cast is retained for six weeks. On removal of the cast, under general anaesthesia, the legs are gently moved into a position of flexion (approx. 45°), abduction (approx. 55°) and internal rotation (approx. 15°). Radiographs confirm concentric reduction before a double hip spica is applied with the hips in this position. This spica is maintained for a period of three months and is then removed, under general anaesthesia, and replaced with a Broomstick cast which retains the hips in the same position.

The Broomstick cast is retained until there is satisfactory acetabular development. The total period from reduction to the abandonment of all forms of immobilisation is not less than seven months.

Children who are approaching 2 years of age are more likely to require operative reduction (page 178) than closed reduction. The management of congenital hip dislocation over the age of 2 years is considered on page 176.

CEREBRAL PALSY

Cerebral palsy is a term used to designate those children who are handicapped by motor disorders due to non-progressive disorders of the brain. The motor handicap is usually only one facet of the problem which may include disorders of vision, hearing, and intellectual function.

Cerebral palsy is dealt with in some detail in this section because children with this disorder are not only commonly seen in paediatric practice but often present to the orthopaedist as a gait abnormality when the diagnosis may first be made. The medical student, resident, or physiotherapist who approaches the study of cerebral palsy for the first time soon becomes enmeshed in a confusing, speculative world. Moreover, as every child with cerebral palsy is unique, it is not possible to assemble a series of cases from which to draw conclusions. Whereas the treatment of paralytic disorders (e.g. poliomyelitis) can almost be regarded as a science, the treatment of spastic disorders remains largely an art. It will be the aim of this section to state the few facts that we know, to define the problems, and to state the principles which underlie our management.

CAUSES

Numerous enquiries have been made into the aetiology of cerebral palsy and a great number of causative factors have been identified. However, considerable controversy exists as to which are the major factors, and particularly as to whether the majority of cases may be due to antenatal factors or to unrecognised influences. These questions are unlikely to be resolved for a long time as they must be retrospective and are always likely to be inaccurate. It is important however, to recognise the causative factors and these will be briefly considered below.

Prenatal factors

GENETIC

Several well recognised familial forms of cerebral palsy are known, e.g. spastic paraplegia and tremor, and kernicterus of the type due to haemolytic disease of the newborn. Sporadic cases of cerebral palsy of familial origin also occur and athetosis is seen in this group. Because the facts are not well known, it is difficult to promise the parents of a child with cerebral palsy that another child will not be affected and advice should therefore be tempered with caution.

COMPLICATIONS OF PREGNANCY

Haemorrhage during pregnancy. Premature separation of the placenta leading to bleeding may be responsible for anoxia of the foetus.

Maternal toxaemia. Mothers who develop toxaemia have a slightly increased tendency to produce cerebral palsied children. Similarly, toxaemia due to other causes such as drugs, alcohol, and heavy metals may also have the same effect.

Maternal infection and trauma. Infections of the mother during pregnancy may cross the placenta and infect the foetus so causing prenatal brain damage. These influences mostly cause mental retardation but movement disorders may also occur. The role of trauma to the mother during pregnancy is difficult to determine.

Irradiation. Although therapeutic irradiation of the lower abdomen is always avoided in the first trimester of pregnancy, there is no real evidence to show that this may be a cause of cerebral palsy.

Kernicterus. This term is used to describe permanent damage to the basal ganglia due to improperly treated haemolytic disease of the newborn; it is a preventable condition.

Perinatal factors

ANOXIA

There is little doubt that the commonest cause of cerebral palsy is brain injury in the perinatal period. This injury may be mediated by anoxia or be caused directly by physical pressure. The risk is increased if the delivery is complicated by an abnormal position of the foetus, by disproportion, or by the use of instruments to facilitate delivery. Intracranial bleeding may also occur from similar causes. This bleeding may be subarachnoid, intracerebral or subdural.

PREMATURITY

Children with cerebral palsy are commonly premature. Again anoxia is probably the causative factor, although the fragility of the infant's skull may lead to physical damage.

JAUNDICE

The newborn baby, particularly the premature infant, is at risk in jaundice as the blood–brain barrier to bilirubin is less developed. The bilirubin damages particularly the basal ganglia so that athetosis is more common than the other types.

PURULENT MENINGITIS AND HYDROCEPHALUS

These are two other well known causes of cerebral palsy.

Post-natal factors

Any brain injury occurring after birth during the period of brain development may eventuate into cerebral palsy. This may be caused by trauma, meningitis, encephalitis, and various forms of cerebral haemorrhage. Brain tumours and brain cysts may cause cerebral palsy by causing pressure or a similar condition may follow their removal by surgery. It follows that when cerebral palsy is suspected in a given child, a very detailed history should be obtained in an effort to identify the causative factors.

CLASSIFICATION

The clinical manifestations of cerebral palsy are determined by the site of the brain lesion whether the cause be underdevelopment, ischaemia, or trauma. It is convenient to group these into five main varieties.

Spastic

The lesion is in the pyramidal system of the cerebral motor cortex.

FEATURES

Hypertonus with exaggerated stretch reflexes. The involved limb assumes a typical posture as the increased tone is mostly in the flexors. When the examiner attempts to correct this there is increased resistance until a peak is reached followed by a sudden giving way. The examination of spastic equinus is a good example. *Weakness* of antagonists and a variable loss of voluntary control. This is often seen in the foot where the dorsiflexors of the ankle fail to contract in the swing phase. *Exaggerated deep tendon reflexes* are the rule, clonus may be present at knee or ankle and the plantar response is extensor.

Athetoid

The lesion affects the extrapyramidal system in the basal ganglia.

FEATURES

Involuntary uncontrolled movements of muscle groups in the face and limbs initiated by attempts to stand or move. These may not occur until the child is 3–4 years of age. *Hypertonus* appearing as either rigidity or spasticity in varying degrees. Normal *deep tendon reflexes*. *Speech difficulty* is common but these children are often more intelligent than those in other groups. Contractures and deformities are much less likely to occur compared with the spastic type.

Ataxic

The lesion is in the cerebellum and brain stem.

FEATURES

A rare *disturbance of balance* probably of genetic origin (ataxia is usually a component of the other varieties). *Hypotonia*, involuntary *tremor*, and *nystagmus*.

Rigid

A disturbance of synergistic action due to lesions in both basal ganglia and cortex.

FEATURES

Passive motion in either direction is resisted. This *resistance* may be continuous (lead pipe) or interrupted (cogwheel). *Occurs alone or combined* with other types. May *worsen with age*. Mental retardation is often severe. *Poor response* to any form of treatment.

Floppy (the floppy infant)

In infancy many children who subsequently develop overt signs of cerebral palsy are noted to be hypotonic or floppy. This observation should always be noted with suspicion, although of course many hypotonic babies recover completely.

THE DIAGNOSIS OF CEREBRAL PALSY

Cerebral palsy occurs in all grades of severity and may present at birth if very severe or may be delayed until the child has been walking for several years in mild cases. Diagnosis is rarely easy and the signs are often difficult to elicit; however, if the possibility is kept in mind especially in the first two years of life few mistakes will be made.

HISTORY

The perinatal history may supply information which will alert the physician to the possibility of cerebral palsy, e.g. toxaemia, antepartum haemorrhage, difficult labour, fetal distress, cyanotic attacks and convulsions in the infant, or the development of jaundice.

A developmental history should be sought and failure to pass the various milestones at the correct age will be present in all cases.

EXAMINATION

The infant. Signs of cerebral damage may be present at birth—coma, raised intracranial pressure, fits, involuntary movements, absence of normal reflexes such as blinking to light and sucking or hypotonia. Two special reflexes are important and if present are almost diagnostic of cerebral palsy.

1 *Moro reflex*—the baby is held with the head and trunk supported. The examiner suddenly allows the head to fall backwards and this initiates a mass extensor reflex. The arms are flung out with the fingers opened and the legs may also extend, though this response varies. The reflex is present at birth but usually disappears after 2–3 months. The moro reflex is absent or diminished in hypotonic or severely retarded babies.

2 *Landau reaction*—the examiner holds the baby in ventral suspension. The normal baby from 4–5 months responds by extending head and trunk; by 6–8 months the legs are also included. In hypotonic and severely retarded babies, the reaction is usually absent: they maintain a flexed position in ventral suspension.

The toddler. A history is often obtained of late walking, frequent falls, throwing one leg, turning a foot, or some abnormality in the wear of the shoes. Two main varieties are seen in this age group.

1 *Spastic hemiplegia*—this is recognised by the characteristic posture of the upper limb which is held flexed at the elbow and wrist with pronation of the forearm. In the lower limb the child may merely walk with the foot in a few degrees of equinus so that the heel rises off the floor only when he hurries. This will gradually worsen until by the age of 4 or 5 he walks up on his toe all the time. Examination may reveal that spasticity is confined almost solely to the calf. More severe cases will have involvement of the foot invertors, adductors of the hip, and the hamstrings.

2 *Spastic diplegia*—late walking is the rule and when achieved the gait is jerky and unbalanced. The feet are used in equinus and there will be variable degrees of hip and knee flexion. The upper limbs are relatively normal and these children are often quite intelligent.

Athetosis does not present as such in the toddler, the involuntary movements developing later. Similarly, spastic quadriplegia is not seen in the toddler as these children are usually much more severely affected and will not walk under the age of 5 years, if at all.

ASSESSMENT OF THE CHILD WITH CEREBRAL PALSY

Before treatment can be planned a comprehensive assessment of the child must be made and the data recorded as a base line. Enrolment in a pre-school clinic is a valuable exercise, not only in assessment but also because it allows the mother to be taught important exercises and games, to learn about the home care of her child, and to meet other parents who share similar problems.

Assessment and subsequent planning will depend on the following factors:
Age.
Intelligence—this will vary widely although about two-thirds of cerebral palsied children will have an IQ below 70 and those below this level are likely to respond less well to treatment.

Motivation often cannot be assessed until treatment commences. The success or failure of treatment will depend very much on this factor. Motivation is influenced by emotional difficulties and can be modified to some extent by guidance from therapists, psychologists, and teachers.

Neurological involvement—it is mandatory to define and record the extent and degree of involvement of muscle groups whether by spasticity, weakness, or rigidity. The presence of athetosis is noted.

Associated defects of hearing, vision and speech are determined. These are often found to be present and failure to recognise and treat them will retard the effect of treatment generally.

Orthopaedic assessment—if the child is a non-walker then assessment must be done horizontally although information regarding neck control and sitting balance must be sought. If able to walk or to be walked with assistance, then assessment is done vertically and much more information will be gained from observations than by examination. This is because signs elicited by examination do not necessarily correspond to what happens during walking; for example an apparently severe spastic equinus may be hardly noticeable during walking and the reverse is also true. Likewise it is of little practical value to record ranges of motion available at various joints as these will vary according to the circumstances and the strength of the examiner. Before maturity, fixed deformity beyond that of minor degree is very uncommon in cerebral palsy.

Before commencing any form of treatment it is important to define the objective. This may be: to improve walking, to achieve walking, to be walked (with assistance for transfers etc.), to fix a footwear problem, to facilitate nursing.

The management of cerebral palsied children may be very simple (e.g. a mildly affected hemiplegic) but the more severely affected will require the combined efforts of many disciplines and this can only be effectively carried out in special clinics in the larger hospitals.

TREATMENT

All forms of treatment aim to bring each child up to its full potential and each should be regarded as complementary to the other. For example, surgery to diminish spasticity can facilitate the work of the physiotherapist and may also make bracing unnecessary.

PHYSIOTHERAPY

The physiotherapy of cerebral palsy tends to be surrounded by a considerable mystique and many of the actual techniques used are only understood by the exponents. This has come about because of our ignorance of the processes of learning and motor activity so that it is probably unwise to attempt to justify various physiotherapeutic techniques in terms of neurophysiology. Basically, however, the therapist has a valuable role to play in teaching skills, in evaluation and assessment, and in providing moral support to the parents. The therapist must be sympathetic as well as firm, must try to make the work appear as a game rather than a chore, and, above all, must integrate the parents into the teaching programme. At the same time, it must be recognised that time is likely to be wasted on cerebral palsy of the upper limb, on non-walkers, and on walkers who require surgery.

BRACING

The almost universal use of bracing in the first half of this century has given way to a much more limited application in recent years, largely due to the increased use of surgery. However, bracing is still used, firstly to stabilise the lower limb while the child is learning to walk. A short double iron often with an anterior sandwich strap is usually used for this purpose; secondly, at all times to control weakness, e.g. a long caliper to control quadriceps weakness. Note that bracing should not be used to prevent control or correct deformity.

SURGERY

Surgery is rarely required in the toddler but becomes of increasing importance up to and somewhat beyond maturity. It is used to correct deformity with a view to facilitating physical therapy and the discarding of braces. The aims of surgery are to: weaken the strong by neurectomy, tenotomy, and tendon lengthening; to strengthen the weak by tendon transfer; to fix the joint where no motors are present or in athetosis; and to realign through rotation and angulation in osteotomy.

DRUGS

In cerebral palsy drugs may be used to control or modify the following clinical conditions.

Epilepsy. The most useful drug is undoubtedly phenytoin (Dilantin), but this does have the disadvantage that it causes gross hypertrophy of the gums, acne and coarsening of the facial skin. Sodium valproate has been introduced more recently and, although it does not have the side effects of Dilantin, it can be considerably more toxic and a number of fatal cases of liver failure have occurred.

Spasticity. Although a wide range of drugs have been tried, none has so far proved of any worthwhile value.

Behaviour. Diazepam (Valium) has proved to be a most valuable drug to control hyperactivity and to alloy fear especially before and after surgery.

The surgery of cerebral palsy

In the present state of our knowledge (or ignorance!) the only surgery available to the cerebral palsied child is peripheral, i.e. directed towards the effect of the brain lesion rather than the cause.

Ideally, this surgery should be done early, before secondary changes such as fixed deformity and dislocations have occurred. Early surgery is simple and effective whereas late or salvage surgery is both difficult and much less certain in outcome. Orthopaedic surgery is largely confined to spastic cerebral palsy and has no role in the ataxias or rigidities. In athetosis, surgery is limited to an occasional neurectomy or arthrodesis. When spasticity affects several levels, e.g. the foot, knee and hip, great difficulty is often experienced in deciding which level or levels if any should be released (Fig. 3.6). One school believes that all levels should be corrected at one sitting, but most surgeons agree that there is usually one or perhaps two levels which demand surgery in the first instance and often the other level will improve as a side benefit of this surgery.

It is difficult to lay down any rules as each child is different and must be individually assessed. Generally speaking, however, distal release should precede proximal release. Over the years many attempts have been made to place the whole subject on a more scientific basis but so far gait laboratory studies and other technical investigations have not been able to achieve a better rate than that obtained by careful clinical observation. Whatever surgery is proposed it is paramount to define what benefit is anticipated and ensure that the parents are fully aware of this.

Individual problems and their management

It is not possible to cover all the problems in this discussion but instead it is

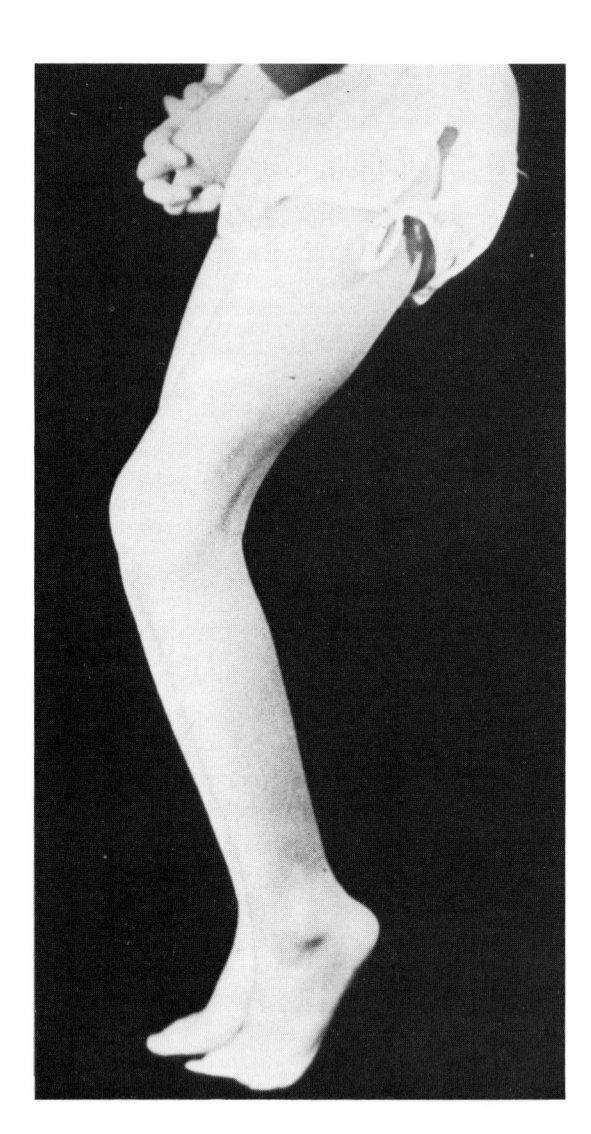

Fig. 3.6 A child with diplegia involving all three levels in the lower limbs. This is the classic dilemma—should all levels be released in the first instance or is it better to do one at a time, and if so which one first?

proposed to select some of the most common and to give an outline of their surgical management.

SPASTIC EQUINUS

Equinus is by far the commonest problem seen. It is usually evident when walking commences and indeed may be the presenting complaint. Untreated it usually progresses and may convert to equinovarus (if tibialis posterior overaction is added) or to equinovalgus (if the tibials collapse and peroneal overaction is added). It is usual to treat spastic equinus conservatively (i.e. by bracing) up till

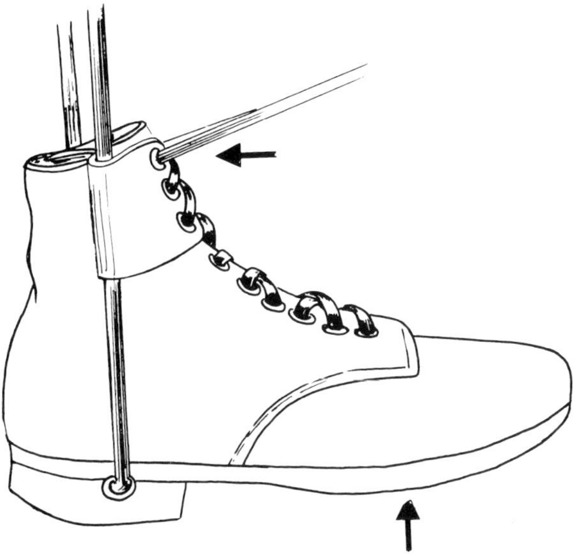

Fig. 3.7 A simple brace to control spastic equinus. The anterior 'sandwich strap' rotates the foot around the ferrule in the heel. This is preferable to the use of a square ferrule which quickly wrecks the boot or a dorsiflexion spring which, by initiating a stretch reflex, increases calf spasticity.

the age of about 5 years (Fig. 3.7). If severe at that time or if the foot is breaking into valgus, surgical release of the calf is indicated. Under the age of 5 years the relapse rate after surgery is very high so that operation should be avoided if possible. The following operative techniques are available:
1 Calf neurectomy (Stöffel).
2 Proximal gastrocnemius release and neurectomy (Silverskiold).
3 Calf recession (Strayer).
4 Aponeurosis lengthening (Baker).
5 Heel cord lengthening.

All have much the same effect as they weaken the calf and reduce the spasticity. The simplest methods should therefore be chosen and we prefer the Baker release up to the age of about 10 years (Figs. 3.8 & 3.9). This technique is simple, gives an excellent midline scar, weight bearing in plaster can be allowed after one week and the plaster can be removed in three weeks. Over 10 years of age the usual Z lengthening of the heel cord is preferred as more length can be obtained. This is followed by six weeks in plaster. Note that the incision for heel cord lengthening should be placed on the medial side half way between the tendo-Achilles and the medial border of the tibia. This will help prevent keloid formation and pressure on the scar from the top of the boot.

SPASTIC EQUINOVALGUS

This deformity is largely preventable by early calf release but even when present in the young child it may still be reversible by surgery (Fig. 3.10). Hallux valgus is another secondary result (Fig. 3.11). As the child grows, the deformity becomes

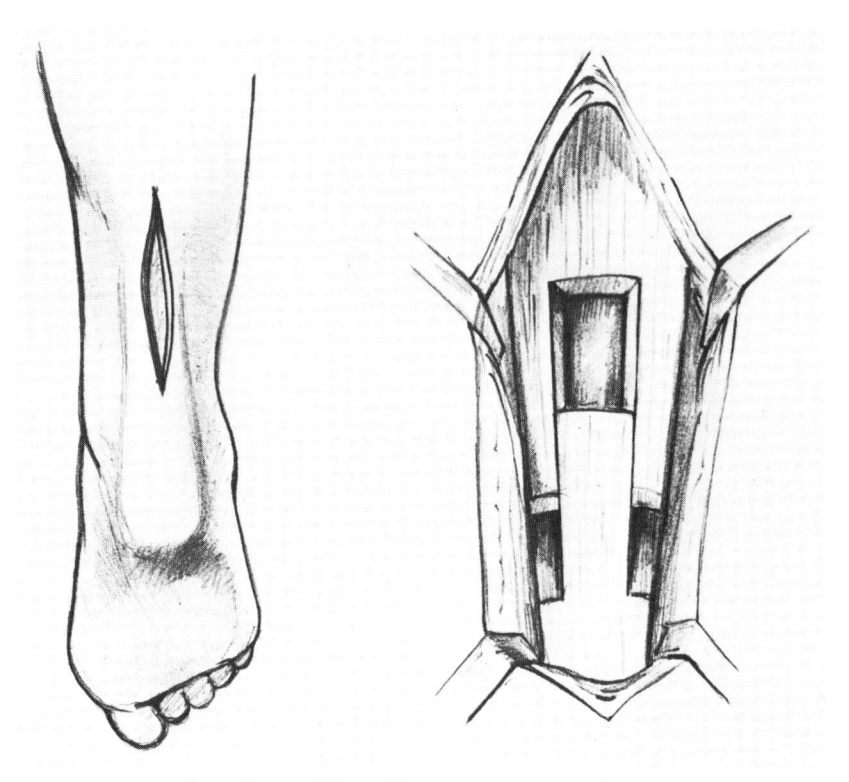

Figs. 3.8 & 3.9 Baker release of the calf aponeurosis. Site of the skin incision. (*Right*) Lengthening of the calf aponeurosis by a tenon and mortice incision followed by extension of the ankle joint.

more and more fixed until by maturity it is irreducible. If presenting at this time, it can often be accepted in those who cover a small mileage but, in others, extreme footwear distortion and finally pain force a surgical reconstruction by heel cord lengthening and triple fusion. This is best done by joint excision using a medial approach.

SPASTIC EQUINOVARUS

This deformity usually presents from the age of 5 onwards and soon becomes impossible to control with bracing. It is a significant disability as it throws the whole leg out of balance and is very destructive of footwear. Early surgical management is indicated and this consists of calf lengthening and transfer of the tibialis posterior forwards to the midline of the dorsum of the foot (Fig. 3.12). This is one of the most rewarding surgical procedures in cerebral palsy and is particularly popular in young girls who can then change their brace and boot for a fashion shoe. If the deformity is neglected it becomes fixed, and can then only be

The Toddler 107

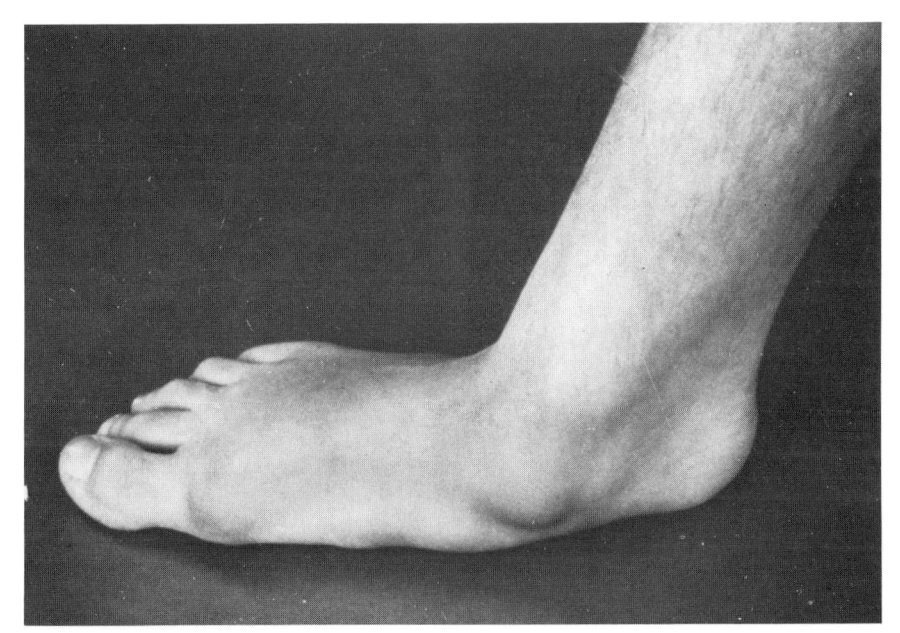

Fig. 3.10 Spastic equinovalgus deformity. Due to unrelieved calf spasticity, the foot is breaking in the middle.

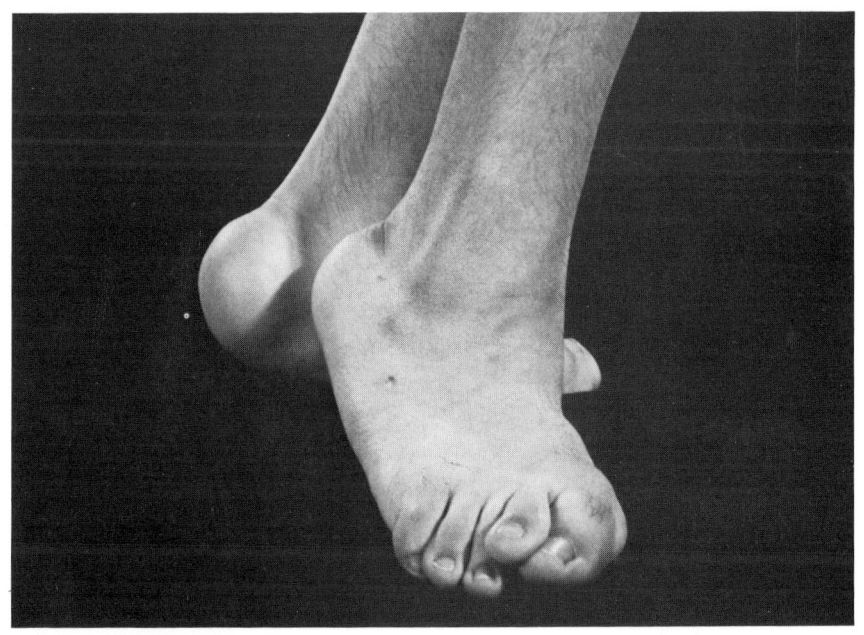

Fig. 3.11 A child with unrelieved spastic equinus showing the secondary development of hallux valgus. This is due partly to the walking posture and partly to spastic contracture of flexor pollicis longus.

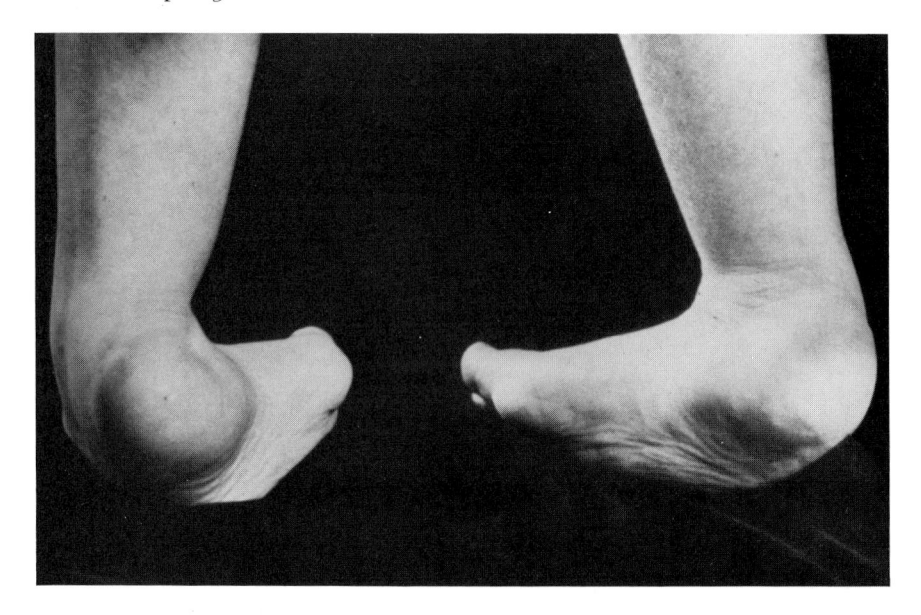

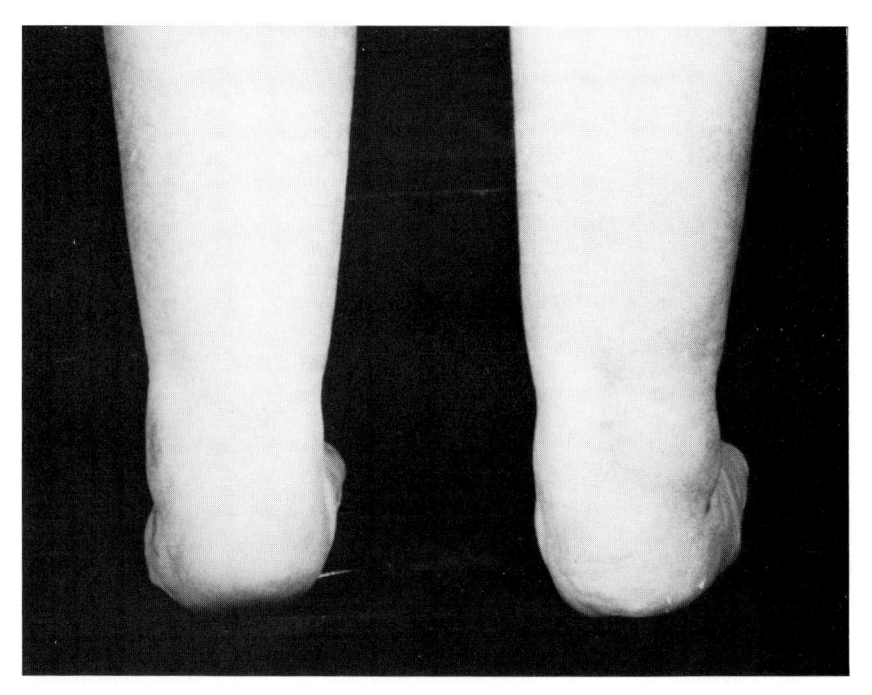

Fig. 3.12 (*Top*) A child with spastic equinovarus of both feet before and (*bottom*) one year following calf lengthening and transfer of the tibialis posterior tendon forwards to the dorsum of each foot.

corrected by triple arthrodesis. At the same time the calf is lengthened and the tendon of tibialis posterior tenotomised.

KNEE FLEXION

Hamstring overaction producing a flexed knee gait is also common; it is often associated with spastic equinus and, to a lesser extent, with spastic hip flexion. The knee joint remains fully mobile for a number of years before flexion deformity appears and the quadriceps tendon stretches. About 15° of knee flexion during gait is acceptable but much more than this is best treated by hamstring release. Transplantation of the hamstrings (Eggers' operation) carries no special advantages. Hamstring release is carried out through a short midline incision above the knee crease. The tendons of semitendinosus and gracilis are cut and the aponeuroses covering semi-membranosis and biceps divided transversely. The knee is then immobilised in a plaster cylinder for ten days. Any residual fixed flexion can be eliminated by wedging the post-operative plaster cast. Proximal hamstring release is not a substitute for distal release and should be reserved for those children whose hamstrings are so shortened that they walk swivelling instead of flexing at the hips. Straight leg raising in these cases is often limited to 10°. If carried out bilaterally for the wrong indications the procedure produces a disastrous degree of pelvic tilt and lumbar lordosis.

Hip involvement in cerebral palsy

There are four common hip problems in cerebral palsy.
1 Spastic hip adduction
2 Subluxation and dislocation
3 Internal rotation
4 Gluteal weakness

SPASTIC ADDUCTION

This is second only to spastic equinus in frequency of occurrence in cerebral palsy. Most often it is a problem in those with diplegic or quadriplegic involvement and in these it is usually associated with spastic involvement at the knee and ankle. The presence of spastic adduction is not in itself an indication for surgical release. If a crossover gait is present, then release is likely to help but care should be taken in assessing those children who use a tripod gait with crutches as they often obtain stability at the hip by pressing the knees tightly together.

Adductor release is carried out as an open procedure through an incision in the line of the adductor longus. The adductor longus, adductor brevis, and gracilis muscles are divided high up together with the anterior branch of the obturator nerve. The neurectomy is desirable to further weaken the muscles and to minimise the risk of recurrence. Broomstick plaster fixation post-operatively is

110 Chapter 3

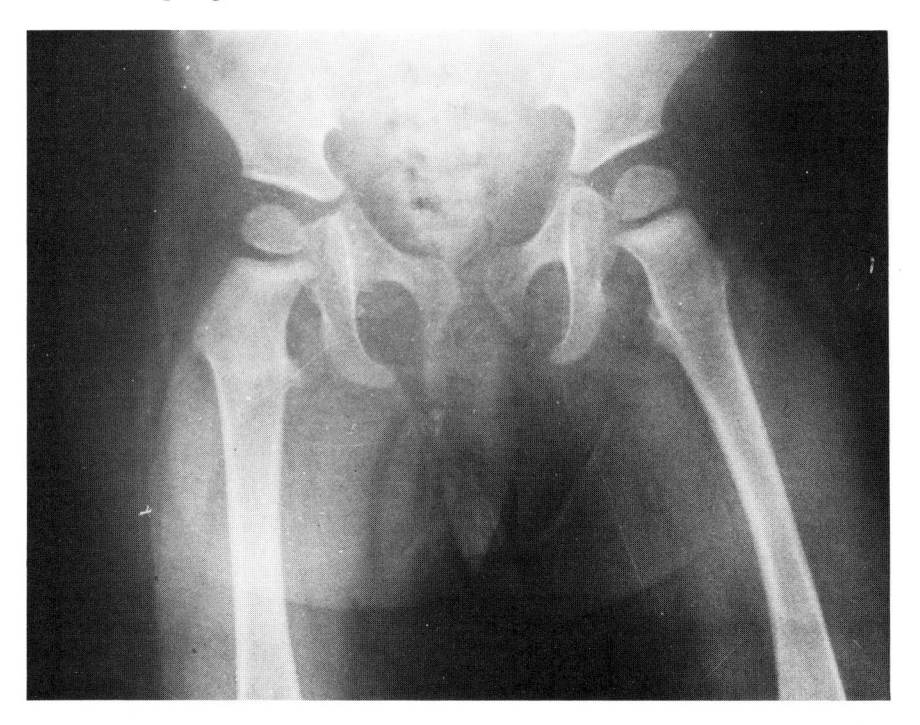

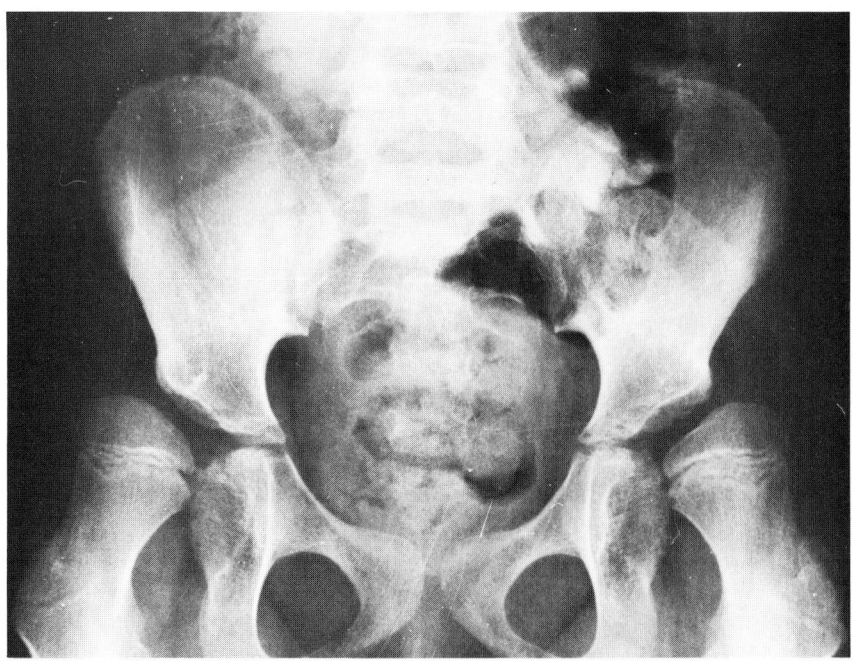

Figs. 3.13 & 3.14 *(See caption opposite.)*

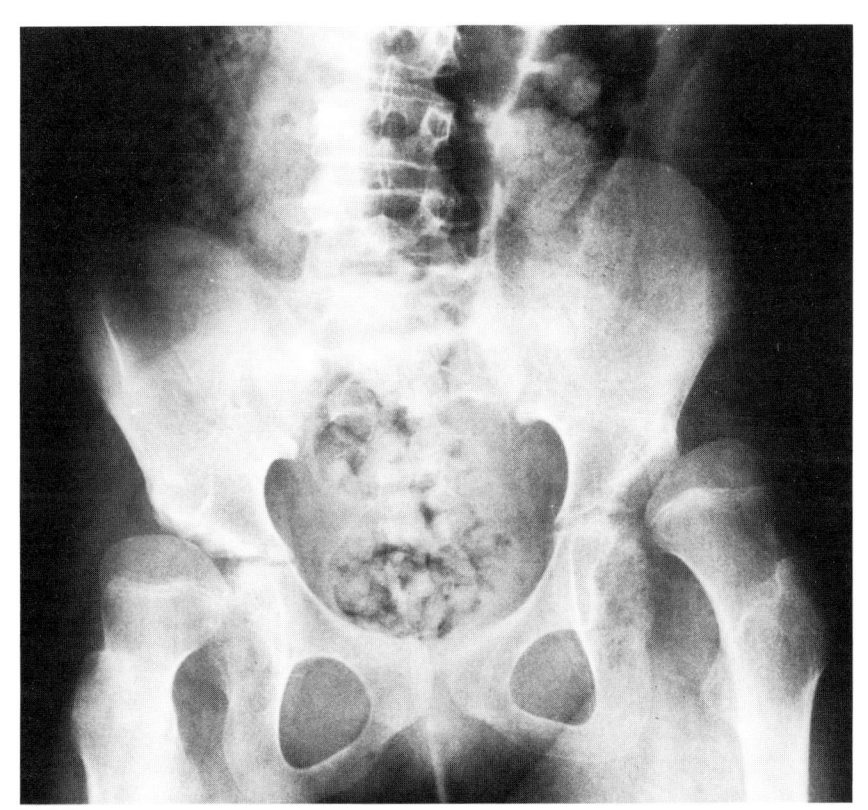

Figs. 3.13–3.15 Cerebral diplegia in a child. (*Opposite top*) Aged 18 months—the hips appear normal. (*Opposite, bottom*) Aged 6 years—dysplasia and subluxation are now present. Adductor release and neurectomy was done at this stage. (*Above*) Aged 10 years—the right hip has improved but the left is about to dislocate. It is still reducible, however, with the limb in abduction and internal rotation. The dysplasia can be controlled by Chiari osteotomy and the anteversion may also require correction by osteotomy.

traditional but is very unpopular with both the child and his parents. A similar effect can be obtained using pillows in bed for about a week.

SUBLUXATION AND DISLOCATION

The hip is at risk in from 10 to 20% of children with spastic cerebral palsy and the possibility of subluxation should be constantly borne in mine (Figs. 3.13–3.15). Each cerebral palsy child should have the hips x-rayed every twelve months until maturity. Untreated subluxation tends gradually to change to dislocation—a disaster for the walker and a great inconvenience to the non-walker. Non-walkers are the most at risk and many of these develop hip dislocation. Marginal walkers commonly develop subluxation and this may proceed to dislocation. Good walkers usually have normal hips, especially those who walk with spastic in-toeing. The formula for dislocation contains three ingredients: 1 Spastic adductors and flexors of the hip (with weak abductors). 2 Coxa valga and anteverta (late weight-bearing). 3 Dysplastic acetabulum (secondary to habitual adduction and pressure of the roof).

Early subluxation. This is an indication for adductor and flexor release almost regardless of other factors. Even those without walking potential should not be allowed to dislocate. The adductors, gracilis and psoas and anterior branch of the obturator nerve are all divided. Subsequently standing is encouraged—if necessary in a frame or box—and some form of soft night splintage is instituted to maintain the hip in abduction. Providing the subluxation is recognised early and treated it should be possible at least to prevent deterioration and in many cases to correct the subluxation.

Late subluxation. When subluxation is discovered late but acetabular dysplasia is minimal, salvage may be possible by carrying out subtrochanteric varo-rotation osteotomy in addition to adductor myotomy, neurectomy, and psoas tenotomy. The osteotomy is fixed with a plate and four screws or a small blade plate may be used.

Imminent dislocation. When subluxation has advanced to the point where dislocation is imminent there is always significant acetabular dysplasia present. In these circumstances a combination of adductor release and Chiari osteotomy has been found to be remarkably effective. Internal fixation is used as well as an external plaster cast for about three weeks.

Actual dislocation. Once dislocation has occurred attempts to salvage the hip joint usually fail. It is better to accept the dislocation—although, in exceptional cases of unilateral dislocation, arthrodesis may be warranted. If the dislocation is painful, as it sometimes is in non-walkers, adductor release can be tried; however, failing this, it is necessary to resect the head and neck of the femur. In very high dislocations, resection of the upper end below the lesser trochanter may be the only way to relieve pain and facilitate nursing care.

INTERNAL ROTATION

Internal rotation at the hip is an important disability in cerebral palsy as it produces a gait which is not only very unattractive but also is very energy consuming, destroys footwear rapidly, and virtually prevents the ability to run (Fig. 3.16). Although much research on this subject has been carried out, there is still no agreement as to which muscles are responsible and it is therefore not surprising that operations directed towards redressing muscle imbalance nearly always fail. The psoas, adductors and medial hamstrings are usually involved in

The Toddler 113

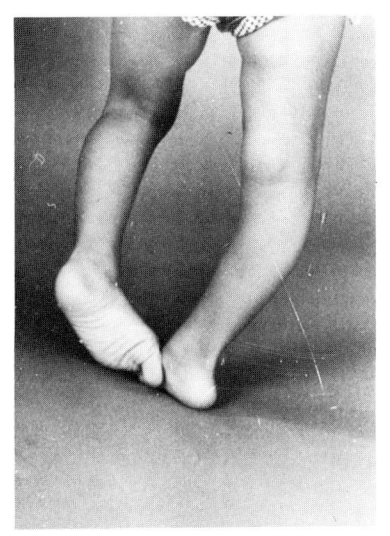

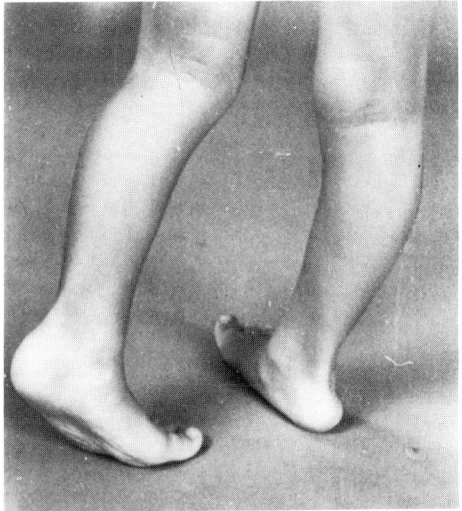

Fig. 3.16 Spastic diplegia with in-toeing as the major problem.

varying degrees and, if these are released for other indications, some slight benefit to hip internal rotation may be noticed.

Real correction can only be obtained by de-rotation osteotomy of the femur. This is best done in the upper third of the femur and the osteotomy fixed with a heavy compression plate so that walking can recommence after a few weeks. The operation should not be performed on children under 8 years of age as experience has shown that the recurrence rate is high in the younger group. It is important to remember that, if the spastic hip when examined pre-operatively has an arc of 0–90° all in internal rotation, then the amount of correction at operation must be 90° in order to achieve a reasonable gait. In non-spastics only 45° correction should be necessary to achieve the same result (Fig. 3.17).

Femoral osteotomy does not usually increase speed, agility or distance capability, but will invariably improve appearance, overcome footwear problems, and conserve energy. Although not often indicated, in selected cases the result can be very rewarding.

GLUTEAL WEAKNESS

Hip instability due to gluteal weakness is a common feature of diplegia and necessitates the permanent use of crutches or sticks. No form of bracing or surgery is available to overcome this problem.

The upper limb in cerebral palsy

The upper limb is often severely disabled in cerebral palsy and the components of

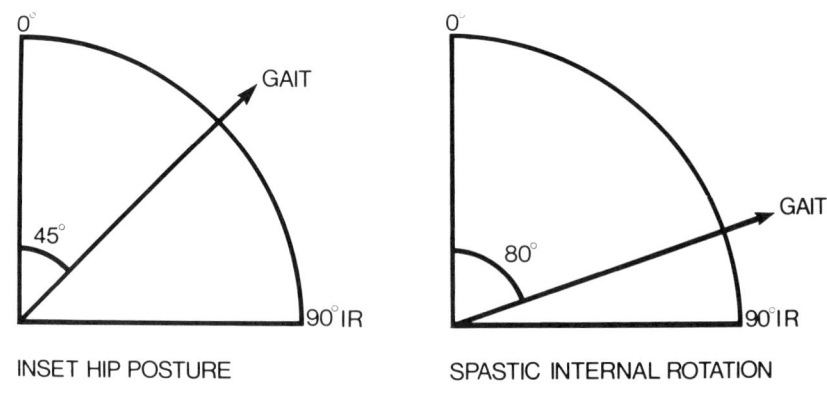

Fig. 3.17 A diagram illustrating the difference between an internal rotation gait occurring in children with inset hip posture (femoral anteversion) and those with cerebral palsy. The implication is that, if correction is to be obtained by femoral osteotomy, twice as much correction is required in the spastic cases.

this disability may include spasticity, athetosis, weakness, loss of sensation, astereognosis, and finally fixed deformity.

Very little improvement can be gained by physiotherapy and it is doubtful whether the time and effort expended is worthwhile. Surgery too has a very small role to play and this is confined almost exclusively to spastic hemiplegia. In selected cases, improvement in both function and appearance can be obtained, and the latter is particularly valuable in the adolescent.

Assessment is difficult and time consuming but it is essential to a good result, not only to know the available function of the hand and its sensibility, but also the intelligence and motivation of the child. Largely because of the sensory deficit and the fact that the other hand is usually normal, increased function obtained by surgery is not often used to capacity—it is easier to do the job with the good hand. However, advantage will be taken of the improvement in situations where two hands are required. Again it is essential to have the parents understand what is likely to be achieved by any proposed surgery.

The surgery of the hand is very specialised and cannot be detailed here. Instead there is set out below a useful summary of the methods available.

THE USELESS HAND

This hand is often held clenched in the fingers and flexed at the wrist. There is no voluntary control and it is used mainly as a paperweight. The elbow is commonly held in a flexed position. Function cannot be improved but the appearance can, and this should be offered to those adolescents who are disturbed by this aspect of their disability. This improvement in appearance can be achieved in the following ways.

Wrist fusion—wrist flexors should be divided to prevent later loss of position.

Internal fixation with removable Kirschner wires is desirable and the position for fusion is neutral. Techniques which employ an inlay iliac graft are the most successful.

Elbow release can be done at the same time. The biceps tendon, lacertus fibrosis, and the brachialis are divided. In the adolescent it may occasionally be necessary to perform an anterior capsulotomy of the elbow to overcome a fixed deformity. The brachioradialis should be left intact to preserve some active elbow flexion.

Finger and thumb release—following successful arthrodesis of the wrist, the finger and thumb flexors often relax sufficiently to produce an acceptable hand. If the fingers remain clenched, all sublimis tendons can be divided at the wrist and the profundis tendons lengthened by the required amount. The thumb is best released by the technique of Matev (1963).

THE USEFUL HAND

This hand will usually have fair grasp and release, fair sensation, a flexed wrist and clenched thumb. Innumerable combinations are possible but, broadly speaking, improvement may be possible by tendon transfer, tendon lengthening and very occasionally, by arthrodesis.

The following three procedures are considered to be the most reliable:
1 Transfer of flexor carpi ulnaris to extensor carpi radialis brevis around the ulnar border of the wrist. This will often provide active dorsiflexion of the wrist. The transfer should not be made through the interosseus membrane as experience has shown that adhesions form later and prevent the transfer acting. 2 Transfer of flexor carpi radialis to abductor pollicis longus and extensor pollicis brevis. The metacarpophalangeal joint of the thumb is fused at the same time. It is a useful transfer to overcome the thumb in palm deformity, but rarely provides full active abduction of the thumb. 3 Thumb release is useful if there is fixed adduction of the thumb.

Surgery in athetosis

The range of operations described for spastic cerebral palsy is not applicable in athetosis where muscle imbalance is not present. Similarly braces to control unwanted movements are usually discarded as being both uncomfortable and ineffective. Occasionally, foot and wrist arthrodesis are useful at maturity and selective neurectomy can be employed to control unwanted movements. Neurectomy should always be preceded by injection of alcohol or nerve crushing so that the effect can be seen before it is made irreversible.

Other orthopaedic problems

Leg inequality. In hemiplegic children, shortening may occur up to one inch (2.5

cm) and this can usually be accepted as it is of some advantage for the affected leg to be somewhat shorter.

Spinal deformity. Kyphosis is common in those who spend their lives in a wheelchair and it is usually best to accept this as conventional methods of treatment cannot be used. Severe thoracic kyphoscoliosis occurs but fortunately is rare. Bracing is not tolerated and surgical correction with instrumentation is so hazardous due to difficulties in nursing, lack of co-operation, and poor hygiene, that it should rarely be attempted.

THE CEREBRAL PALSIED CHILD IN HOSPITAL

The orthopaedic surgeon should realise that hospitalisation of cerebral palsied children often causes considerable emotional disturbance which may last for many months after discharge and interfere with rehabilitation. Every effort should therefore be made to prepare the child and the parents for this episode and to ensure that the nursing staff appreciate that many mothers devote their lives to the care of their afflicted child and become overprotective and even resentful of others trying to care for them. Because the pain threshold in cerebral palsy is diminished these children require more analgesics than might be expected. Valium is a most useful drug to control both fear and spasticity and should be given almost routinely before and for a week or so after surgery. Plaster fixation is not always tolerated—especially hip spicas and broomstick plasters—and their use should be avoided if an alternative exists.

CHAPTER 4

The Child

Normal and abnormal gait (limp) in childhood, 118
Limp

Posture and gait, 123
Flat feet; Knock knees—genu valgum; In-toed gait; Obesity; Footwear and the foot

INFECTIONS OF BONE AND JOINT

Acute osteomyelitis, 138
Methods of spread of infection; Chronicity of infection; Management; Complications of acute osteomyelitis

Chronic osteomyelitis, 142
Chronic osteomyelitis as a sequel to acute infection; Chronic osteomyelitis in which the onset is insidious

Septic arthritis, 149
Management

Leg length inequality and management, 153
Calculation of matured discrepancy and time of arrest; Specific management

The foot, 162
Pes cavus; Metatarsus varus; Sore heels; Deformities of the lesser toes

The knee, 172
Osteochondritis dissecans and abnormalities of ossification of the lower femoral epiphysis; Quadriceps contracture; Discoid meniscus; Popliteal cyst

The hip, 176
The late-presenting congenitally dislocated hip; The surgical management of congenital hip dislocation; Perthes' disease; Irritable hip; Coxa vara

The spine, 200
Classification of spinal deformities; Scoliosis

Spinal dysraphism, 236
Investigations; Indications for surgery; Surgical management

Torticollis, 240

The shoulder, 245
Dislocation of the shoulder

Head injuries in childhood, 246
Management

The period of childhood is from about the age of 2 years to the onset of puberty at 10–12 years. During this period there is a gradual reduction in the rate of growth each year to be followed by a rapid increase at the onset of puberty. Ligamentous laxity is a feature of childhood and tends to decrease as maturity is approached. It accounts for the generous range of joint motion of children and for some elements of posture in this age group.

Posture varies throughout childhood; at the age of 2 years the child frequently has some residual bowing of the legs and internal tibial torsion but this soon corrects spontaneously. Then the opposite deformity of knock knee often appears: this also is a temporary posture and will correct by the age of 6–7 years. In early childhood, flat feet are the rule and children generally stand with more marked lumbar lordosis than is commonly seen in adulthood. The commonest reasons for the child to be brought to the orthopaedist are minor abnormalities of gait and posture so that it is appropriate to consider these topics at this point, before moving on to discuss infections of bone and joints.

NORMAL AND ABNORMAL GAIT (LIMP) IN CHILDHOOD

Gait is a term used to describe the style of walking (ambulation, locomotion). This rhythmic and effortless performance is dependent not only on normal muscles and joints but also upon an intact central and peripheral nervous system and normal labyrinthine function. The ability to analyse normal and abnormal gait is of fundamental importance to the orthopaedic surgeon. In childhood, when a satisfactory history is often unobtainable, observation of the gait will often suggest both the site and the nature of the disability.

Walking is divided into two phases (Fig. 4.1): *the stance phase* in which the foot is on the ground. This is further subdivided into heel-strike, mid-stance, and push-off. *Swing phase* in which the foot is not in contact with the ground. This is further subdivided into acceleration, swing-through, and deceleration.

In normal gait, the pathway followed by the centre of gravity of the body (which lies just in front of the second sacral vertebra) follows a smooth regular curve. By the time maturity is reached, this motion fluctuates, in a vertical plane, with an average rise and fall of approximately 1.8 inches (47 mm), and in a side-to-side plane of 1.75 inches (45 mm).

In normal walking, the pelvis rotates forward on the side in the swing phase. This rotation is accompanied by alternate internal and then external rotation of the hip joint in the stance phase. As the pelvis rotates forward it also tilts downwards a little.

At heel-strike, the knee is in extension. It then flexes until the mid-stance phase. Soon after this it extends briefly and then flexes once more as the limb passes into the swing phase. At heel-strike, the ankle is dorsiflexed. It then plantar flexes and the foot lies flat on the ground until the heel rises before push-off. As the ankle is rising (both at push-off and heel-strike), the knee is flexing and this

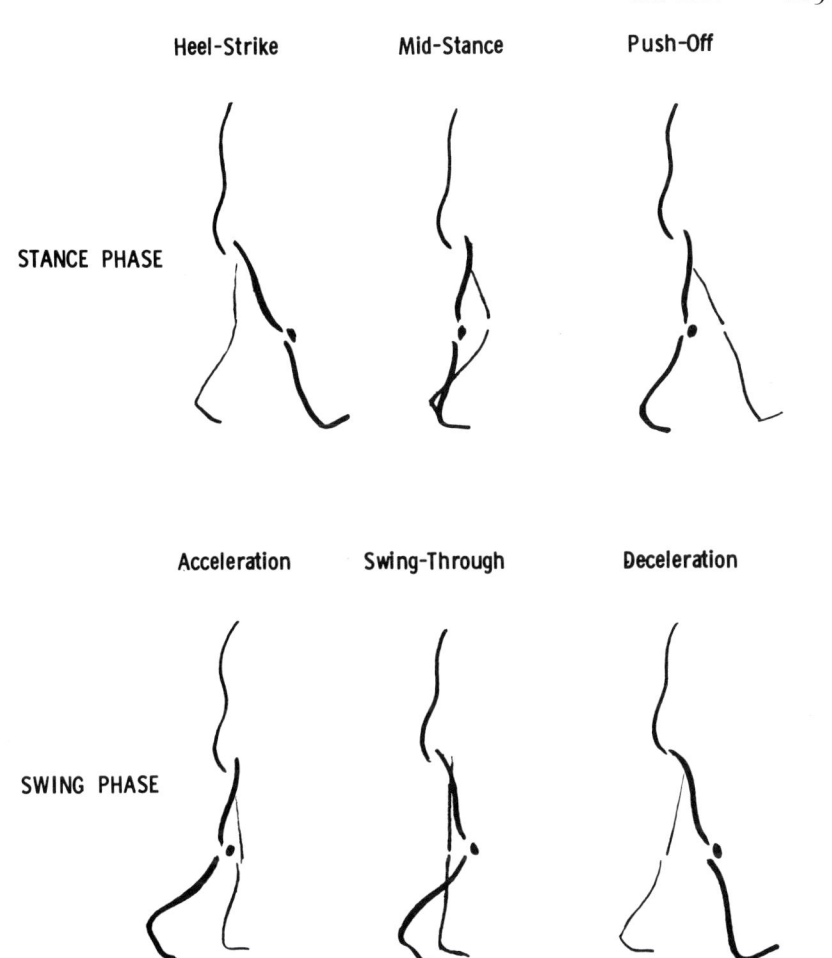

Fig. 4.1 The terms employed to describe the phases of normal gait. The terms apply to the heavily drawn right leg. During the stance phase the foot is in contact with the floor and the body weight is born through the leg. During the swing phase the foot does not touch the floor and the opposite leg bears the body weight.

reciprocal motion prevents wide fluctuation in the height of the centre of gravity of the body.

During walking, muscles act over a very short period. For long periods, the extremity is propelled forward by its own momentum. Muscles are used to stabilise, accelerate or decelerate the moving leg. Major muscle activity commences in the deceleration segment of the swing phase. The following muscles then act in sequence: the hamstrings, the erector spinae, the anterior tibial muscles, the adductors and abductors of the hip, the extensors of the hip, and the quadriceps. This activity is already subsiding at heel-strike. The calf muscles act at mid-stance through to push-off, there being little other muscle activity at this stage. During the last 10% of the stance phase, there is activity in the erector spinae muscles, the hip adductors and to a lesser extent in the quadriceps and gluteus maximus.

60% of the cycle is stance and the remainder is swing phase since there is a period when both feet are on the ground.

LIMP

The term limp implies a pathological gait pattern. Limp may be due to muscle weakness, shortness of the leg, stiffness of the joints, pain, instability of joints, inco-ordinated muscle action, spasticity of muscle, proprioceptive disturbances, or hysteria. These are discussed below.

SHORT LEG LIMP

The head and pelvis fall as the body weight is taken on the short leg. This is difficult to discern at maturity if the discrepancy is less than one inch. The limp is disguised by pelvic tilt, by holding the ankle of the short leg in equinus and the hip and knee of the long leg in flexion.

ANTALGIC LIMP

The stance phase is shortened. In addition, the patient places the foot of the painful limb more gently onto the ground at heel-strike.

UNSTABLE HIP LIMP

In order to understand the various ways in which an unstable hip limp may occur, it is necessary to appreciate the biomechanics of the hip joint. Around the hip there is a simple lever system consisting of a fulcrum, lever, and motor (Fig. 4.2). Instability may occur due to some derangement of any of these three components (see below), the result being a positive Trendelenburg sign and a gait with similar characteristics. When body weight is taken on the affected leg, the opposite side of the pelvis drops. At each stance phase of walking the patient swings his trunk over towards the affected side to bring the centre of gravity over and then beyond the hip joint. The result is a gait which sways from side to side and, if both hips are unstable, this is accentuated to form a gait which is usually described as a waddle. Instability may result from changes in fulcrum (congenital hip dislocation), lever (short neck, coxa vara—Perthes' disease), or motor (gluteus medius weakness—poliomyelitis, cerebral palsy).

Fig. 4.2 Diagrammatic representation of the factors responsible for the normal relationship of the pelvis to the femur when the patient stands on one leg. The body weight is indicated by the central arrow. The motors (A) are the gluteal muscles. The fulcrum (B) is the hip joint and the lever (C) is the femoral neck. If each of these are intact and the patient stands on one leg the opposite side of the pelvis will rise.

Trendelenburg's sign is positive—that is the opposite side of the pelvis will fall—if the motors are weak or ineffective because their origin is approximated to their insertion; if the fulcrum is unstable because the hip is dislocated or destroyed; or if the lever is inefficient because the femoral neck is short, varus, or fractured.

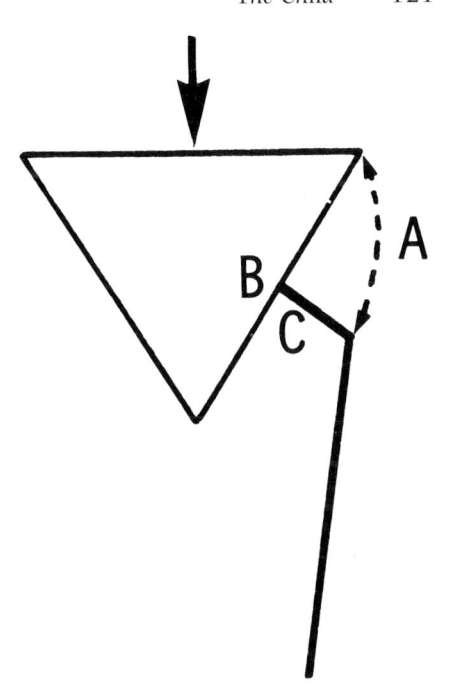

GLUTEUS MAXIMUS WEAKNESS

The patient walks with his hip in hyperextension so that his centre of gravity is behind the hip joint.

THE GAIT IN QUADRICEPS WEAKNESS

There may be little or no limp as the knee can be locked by hyperextension. The patient is unable to climb stairs normally. If there is associated flexion deformity at the knee, then the patient will either place his hand on his thigh or bring his centre of gravity forward with a lurch to lock the knee in the stance phase of gait. These mechanisms are even more necessary if there is weakness of the gluteus maximus.

CALCANEUS GAIT

This is due to calf weakness. There is no push-off. The tibia moves posteriorly over the talus at the end of the stance phase which gives a 'hitch' at each step.

DROP FOOT GAIT

In the swing phase the foot drops so that, to clear the ground, the patient flexes the knee and flexes and externally rotates the hip. This gait is due to weakness of the pre-tibial muscles.

STIFF HIP GAIT

During the swing phase there is increased motion of the pelvis on the lumbar spine. The limp should be minimal if the joint is fused in 25° of flexion and in neutral position in other respects.

STIFF KNEE GAIT

The pelvis is raised during the swing phase of the affected hip so that the heel will clear the floor.

THE GAIT IN CEREBRAL PALSY

A wide variety of patterns may be seen. In hemiplegia of mild degree, the gait abnormality may be subtle indeed: the patient may merely walk without swinging the arm on the affected side. More commonly the child will walk holding the elbow on the affected side in a flexed position. Such arm abnormalities may not be obvious as the child walks but become obvious on running. With more severe involvement, the arm on the affected side is characteristically held flexed at the elbow, adducted and internally rotated at the shoulder; the forearm is pronated, the wrist flexed, the thumb adducted and the fingers flexed.

Abnormalities of posture and gait in the legs will vary from barely discernible toe-walking to severe bilateral 'scissors gait'. The latter term implies that the hips are held in adduction and internal rotation; the knees may be pressed hard to each other or crossed one in front of the other. There may be an associated gluteus medius limp. Frequently there is a flexion deformity at the knees throughout all phases of walking.

ATAXIC GAIT

Spinal ataxia. The child may walk with his feet well apart to give him stability. The feet are brought to the ground with a characteristic 'double tap' as the heel and then the sole flap down. The child walks with his eyes held to the ground and, if asked to close their eyes, will become unsteady or fall. It is characteristically due to brain stem lesions which result in loss of appreciation of the position and motion of the various parts of the body.

Cerebellar ataxia. Again the gait is with the legs well apart and unsteady; there may also be tremors or persistent deviation towards one side. The gait is not affected if the child closes the eyes.

In Friedreich's ataxia, both forms of ataxia are present.

Hysterical gait

Conversion hysteria is far from rare in childhood and is mostly seen in girls in early adolescence. The gait is usually bizarre and unlike anything seen before. It is usually possible by diverting the child's attention to show that the gait is inconsistent and does not fit with the available physical signs. There is usually a history of emotional turmoil in the family home, at school, or in both areas.

POSTURE AND GAIT

There is a wide range in what may be regarded as normal posture and gait during childhood. While this is commonly recognised in cases of knock knees and pigeon toes, it is less commonly appreciated in regard to foot posture. Thus unnecessary treatment continues to be ordered for flat footed children. The conditions considered in the following paragraphs require, as the chief form of therapy, parental reassurance based on an accurate knowledge of the natural history of the condition.

FLAT FEET

There are four propositions on which a logical attitude to this condition is based. First that foot posture varies with age. Second that, whilst the majority of the population develop a medial longitudinal arch, there are others who (for reasons that are presumably genetically determined) do not. Third that it is very doubtful whether we can alter the ultimate shape of the foot any more than we can alter the colour of our patient's hair or any other genetically determined feature. And last that those who remain flat footed seldom have trouble resulting from the planus shape of the feet. Persisting valgus however may cause footwear problems.

With regard to the natural history of foot posture, when any child begins walking, they do so on feet that appear flat, partly because of true flatness of the medial arch and partly because of a fat pad which occupies the arch (Fig. 4.3). The fat pad inevitably disappears and over the next four or five years the majority of children develop a medial longitudinal arch. In Australia, there are approximately 15% of Caucasians who remain flat footed throughout life, though this figure will differ with different races and different communities. Clearly, the results of any form of treatment for flat feet are going to be excellent if 85% will improve without treatment.

It is important to make a distinction between planus of the longitudinal arch and valgus of the subtalar joint. Many children go through a phase where they have planus with very little heel valgus. These children tend to push down the medial half of the upper of their shoe. This is a slow process and they have generally grown out of their shoes before they distort them sufficiently to become

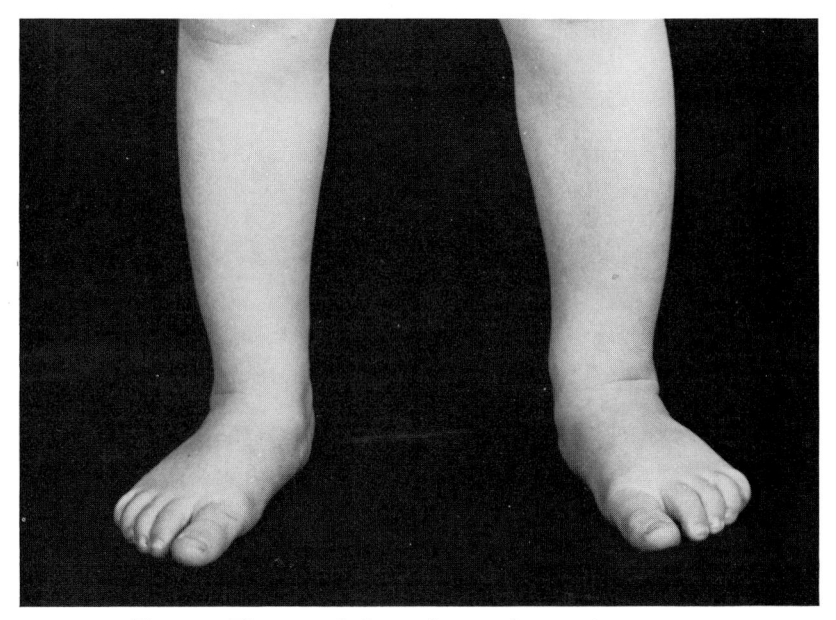

Fig. 4.3 The normal planus feet in a boy aged 18 months.

unserviceable. Some go through a phase, commonly between the ages of 8 and 12 years, when they have both planus and valgus. During this period they are likely to distort their shoes very quickly indeed and the orthopaedic surgeon can give helpful advice about how to preserve the footwear. Any footwear modifications or orthoses that he recommends are unlikely to affect the ultimate shape of the feet.

History and examination

It is important to establish the reason for the child's presentation to the orthopaedic surgeon. Most commonly it is because the parents wonder whether treatment should be instituted in order to prevent some problem in adult life. Less commonly it is because there is a footwear problem at the time of presentation and details of this should be sought and the footwear examined.

A family history of the foot shape should be taken and is often rewarding as flat feet are commonly familial. It is convenient to be able to point out to the flat footed parents of flat footed children that there is no reason why the children should be any more symptomatic than are their parents.

Examination of the child's feet should be carried out, standing and walking, walking on the toes and walking on the heels. This examination may give an indication of the rigidity of any deformity, of tightness of the tendo-Achilles, and of muscle weakness. With the child lying on the couch the feet are inspected for evidence of pressure over the navicular bones and the shape of the weight bearing skin of the sole of the foot is observed. The passive range of movement at the ankle, subtalar and midtarsal joints is examined. When assessing the range of extension at the ankle joint it is important to hold the heel in the neutral position so that the tendo-Achilles does not 'bowstring' laterally as this will mask a tight tendo-Achilles.

Treatment

If the child presents because the parents wonder whether some treatment should be carried out to prevent a future problem, then the parents are reassured. They are told the facts which have been outlined above and are generally satisfied by this explanation and the offer of a further consultation should a problem occur in the future.

If the shoes have become deformed sufficiently to make them wear out before the child grows out of them then arch supports will generally solve the problem. Certain brands of children's footwear are strengthened along the medial side and these can be recommended. In selecting footwear, preference should always be given to those brands which have a very stiff counter. Regrettably much modern footwear lacks this stiffening and the resultant sloppy counter soon allows the shoe to lose its shape. If these measures are not enough, boots may be necessary for a short period. Very rarely indeed do otherwise normal children require an ankle–foot orthosis or iron and T-strap. However, such orthoses may be necessary to control the gross plano-valgus deformity which occurs in some mentally defective children (Figs. 4.4 & 4.5) and in some neuromuscular disorders.

There are a very few children (perhaps 1 per 1000 of those brought to us with flat feet) who have persistent flat feet of such a degree that, in the latter part of the first decade, they develop symptoms. Some of these children have a tight tendo-Achilles which forces the foot to break into plano-valgus. Lengthening of the tendo-Achilles is then appropriate. The lengthening should be such as to allow a range of approximately 15° of dorsiflexion at the ankle joint.

A few children present between the ages of 8 and 12 years with symptomatic plano-valgus deformity of a degree which precludes sporting activity and normal enjoyment of life. Some of these will have peroneal spasm and radiographic evidence of a tarsal coalition but the majority have mobile feet and normal articulation. A weight bearing lateral radiograph is needed to plan further treatment. If these demonstrate a break at the naviculo-cuneiform joint, we have found the procedure described by Miller to be very satisfactory. Here the heel cord is lengthened, the tibialis posterior advanced distally and the naviculo-cuneiform joint fused. If radiographs show that the break is at the talonavicular joint, then some form of triple fusion is indicated preferably using an inlay technique (see Williams & Menelaus (1977) *J. Bone Joint Surg.* **59 B,** 333–6.).

It is to be noted that physiotherapy and exercises have no place in the management of mobile flat feet.

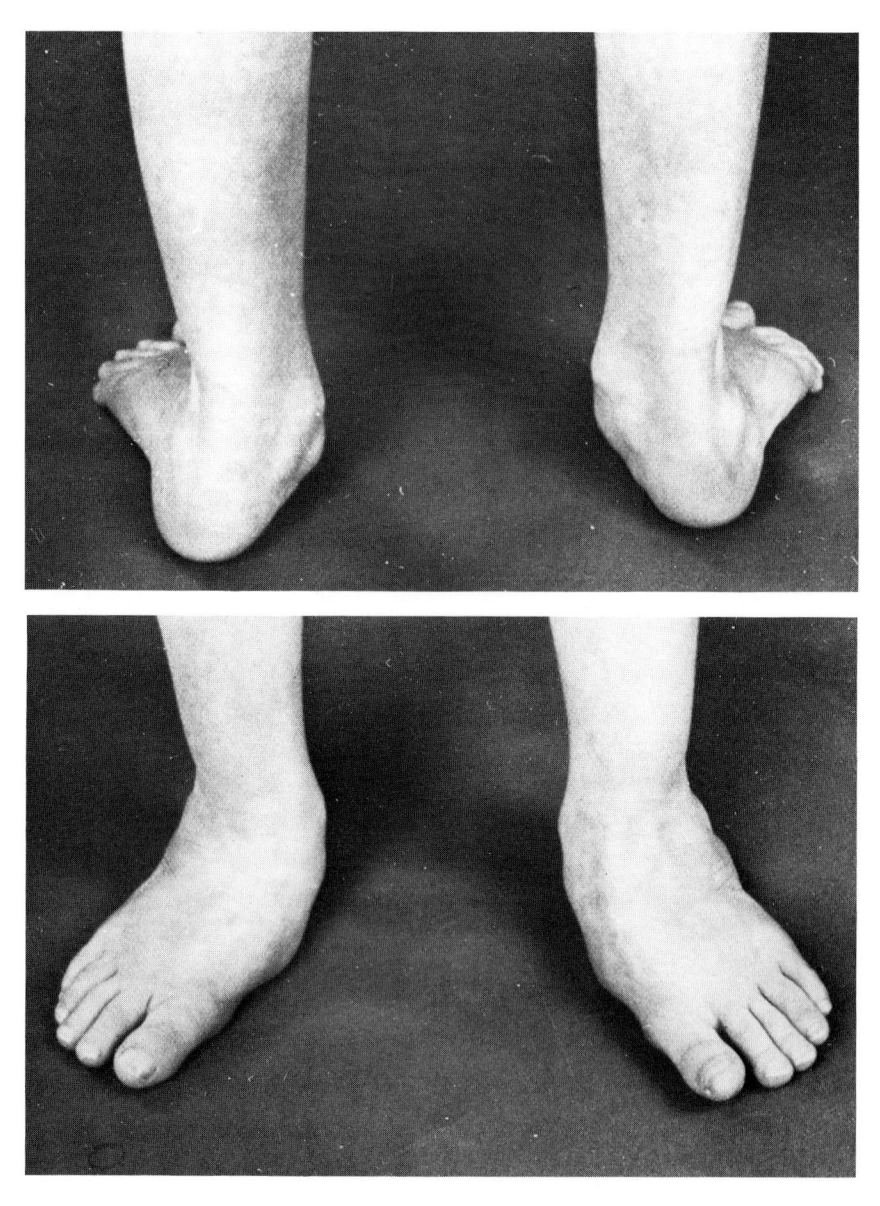

Figs. 4.4 & 4.5 Severe plano-abducto-valgus deformity of the feet in a mentally defective boy aged 8 years.

The Child 127

KNOCK KNEES—GENU VALGUM

A high proportion of the population between the ages of $2\frac{1}{2}$ and 7 years have knock knee deformities (Fig. 4.6). While we see knock kneed adults, this is very seldom of sufficient degree to make their appearance bizarre. Knock kneed men are well disguised by their trousers and it is seldom that we are critical of the shape of womens' legs because of their knock knees.

The advocates of inside wedges to the heels will have a very high percentage of successes but there is no evidence that this measure is of any value. Night splintage will also be successful in a high percentage of cases but this is very seldom justified. If a child aged between 6 and 7 years has a bizarre appearance owing to knock knee deformity then it is reasonable to order a night splint. It is surprising how seldom this is necessary and, even then, it is probable that these children are merely late developers and that the condition would have improved

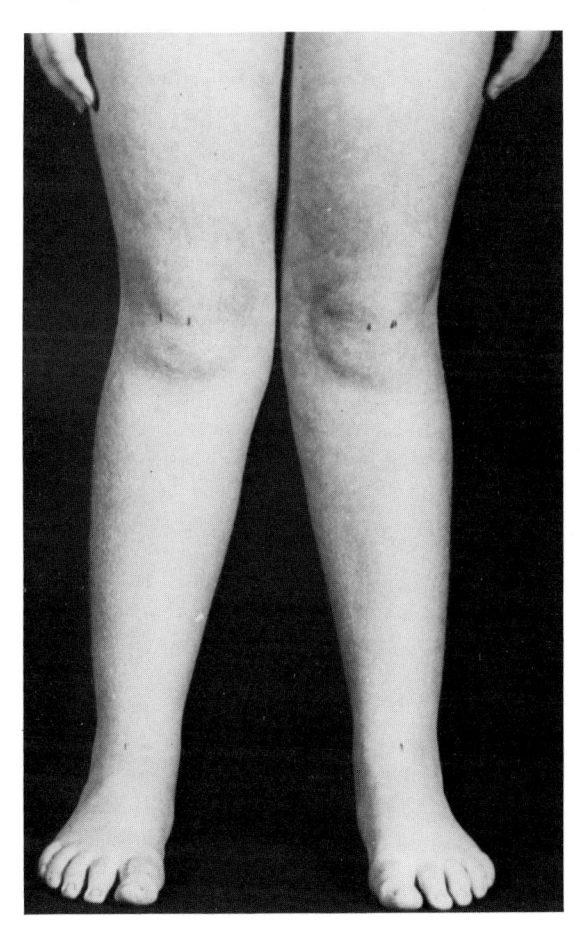

Fig. 4.6 Knock knee at the age of 4 years. There are 4 inches (10 cm) of separation of the medial malleoli. Appropriate management is to reassure the parents that spontaneous correction will occur by about the age of 7 years.

whether or not a night splint had been ordered. In general, parental reassurance is the only treatment necessary. Children presenting with excessive knock knee are commonly obese and here the treatment is in the kitchen rather than in the brace shop.

IN-TOED GAIT

In-toed gait in children may have one or more of the following three anatomical causes:

Inset hips—hips which have internal rotation in excess of the range of external rotation. This is common between the ages of 3 and 8 years.

Internal torsion of the tibia—this is commonly present from the age of walking to $2\frac{1}{2}$ years (page 91).

Metatarsus adductus—commonly present from birth to 4 years (page 132).

These three conditions are present at certain ages and all have a very strong tendency to improve. As for bowlegs and knock knees, these conditions do not require local treatment unless they are present at an unexpected age. Parental reassurance, based on a knowledge of the normal age range for each of these conditions, is the major form of therapy necessary.

Inset hips

EXAMINATION

The child is examined lying with the hips extended. The surgeon stands at the end of the couch and rotates the legs by grasping the feet. The position of the patellae rather than the feet is used to calculate the arc (Figs. 4.7–4.11). It can be demonstrated clinically that those children who have an in-toed gait due to inset hips have excessive anteversion on the neck of their femora. If the examiner palpates the greater trochanter as he internally rotates the leg he will find that the trochanter is most laterally situated when the hips is in full internal rotation and this finding confirms excessive anteversion. The range of internal rotation in these children commonly approaches 90° and the range of external rotation approximates to 20° or less. This allows these children to sit on the floor in the manner illustrated in Fig. 4.11.

CLINICAL FEATURES

Children with an inset hip posture present in a variety of ways.

In-toed gait. This is the commonest presentation.

Awkward children. The parents complain that the child is always falling over

The Child 129

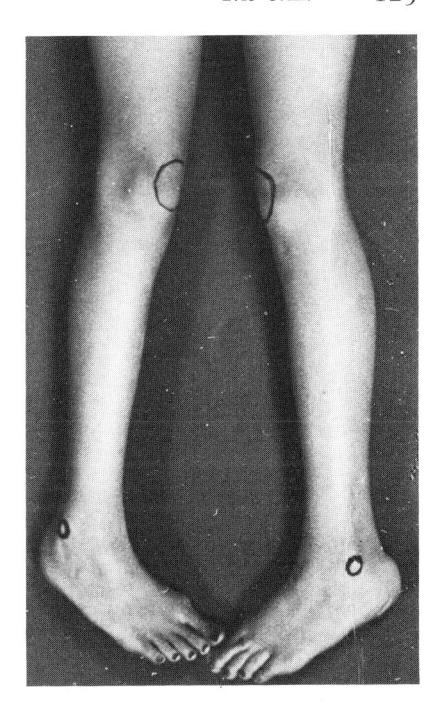

Fig. 4.7 The range of internal rotation of the hips is demonstrated to be approximately 80°. (The patellae and malleoli are ringed with a skin pencil.)

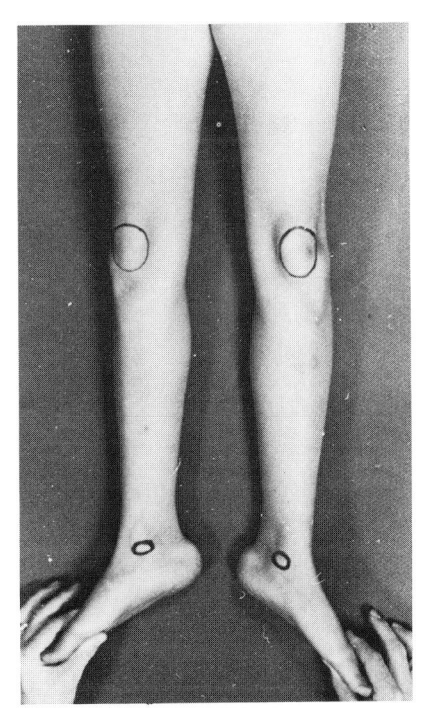

Fig. 4.8 Same patient as Fig. 4.7. The range of external rotation at the hips is 10° only. Note that with the hips in full external rotation the patellae are directed forwards. The ankles and feet are pointing laterally because of the associated external tibial torsion.

130 *Chapter 4*

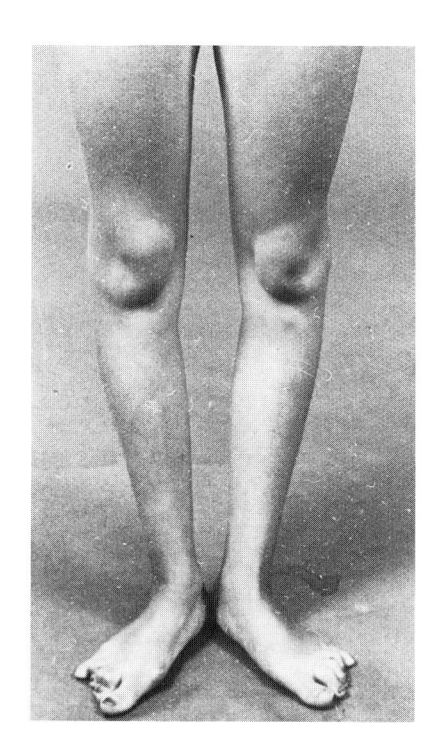

Fig. 4.9 Same patient as Fig. 4.7. The patient standing with the patellae directed forwards (and the feet outwards) gives an appearance of bow legs.

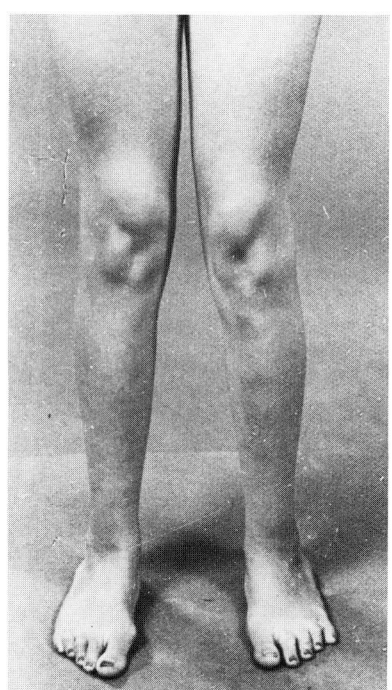

Fig. 4.10 Same patient as Fig. 4.7. With the feet pointing forwards (and the knees inwards) there is an appearance of knock knee.

The Child 131

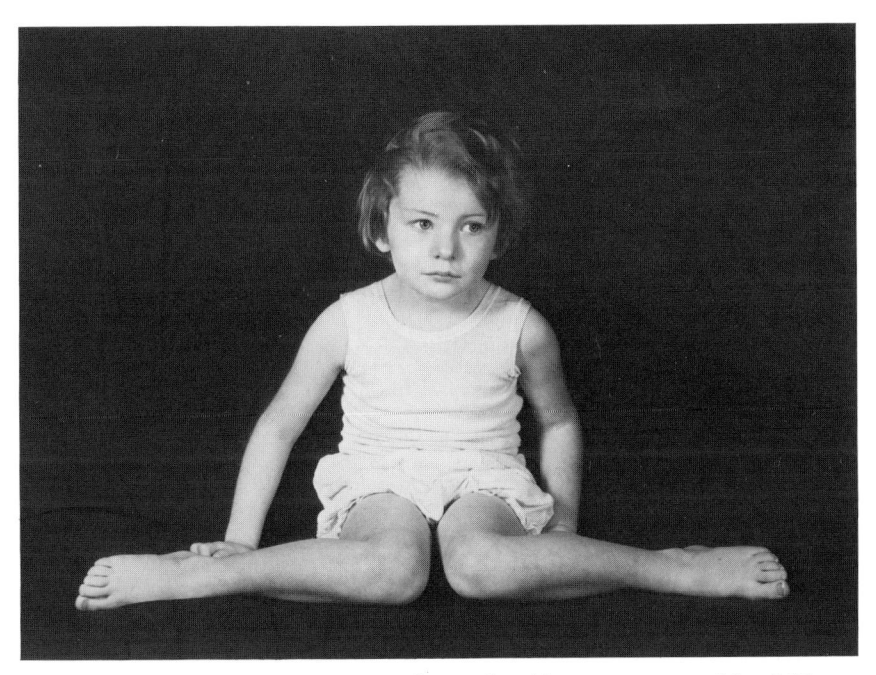

Fig. 4.11 Same patient as Fig. 4.7. The comfortable sitting posture of the child.

himself and that he can't run efficiently. This is because when walking or running, the feet do not swing backwards but outwards.

Knock knees or bowlegs (Figs. 4.9 & 4.10). Such children are frequently described by the parents as being knock kneed. Careful examination reveals that they do not have knock knees but appear to be so because they stand and walk with their knees pointing towards one another, and if they do this with their knees a little flexed, then apparent knock knee results. There may be apparent bowlegs owing to slightly recurved knees facing each other.

Flat feet. In an effort to overcome the in-toeing, the child may roll the feet into valgus so that shoe distortion or flat feet become the presenting symptoms.

NATURAL HISTORY OF INSET HIPS AND THEIR MANAGEMENT

Inset hip posture is present in variable degree in the majority of young children. During growth there is a very strong tendency for the degree of femoral anteversion to gradually diminish and this process continues up to the age of approximately 8 years. When children present under this age, the parents can be told that the vast majority (i.e., about 95%) correct spontaneously by the age of 8 years and that treatment is unnecessary. This is just as well because there is no evidence that the condition is influenced by any form of treatment. Various expensive and uncomfortable night splints have been proposed but should not be used. Of the few who do not correct, some will develop compensatory external tibial torsion which is cosmetically unattractive in a girl but must be accepted. Theoretically, correction is possible by a combination of femoral and tibial osteotomies, but it would be hard to justify this on cosmesis alone. Those who remain inset into adult life seldom have gross deformity and it is almost unknown for an adult to present with a complaint of in-toeing.

Metatarsus adductus

It is important to differentiate this condition from metatarsus varus (see page 167). The term metatarsus adductus implies that there is a deformity at the tarso-metatarsal joints, such that the metatarsals are adducted towards the midline of the body, with the metatarsal heads in the same plane as each other and in the same plane as the hindfoot. The deformity is generally mobile and does not usually become rigid. The condition has a strong tendency to correct itself spontaneously and it may be that all patients with this condition would correct spontaneously without treatment.

Metatarsus adductus (Fig. 4.12) may be present at birth but commonly presents at a later age and frequently after the child has begun walking. An in-toe gait is then noted. There may be difficulty in shoe fitting or the shoes may readily become deformed but these are not commonly presenting features.

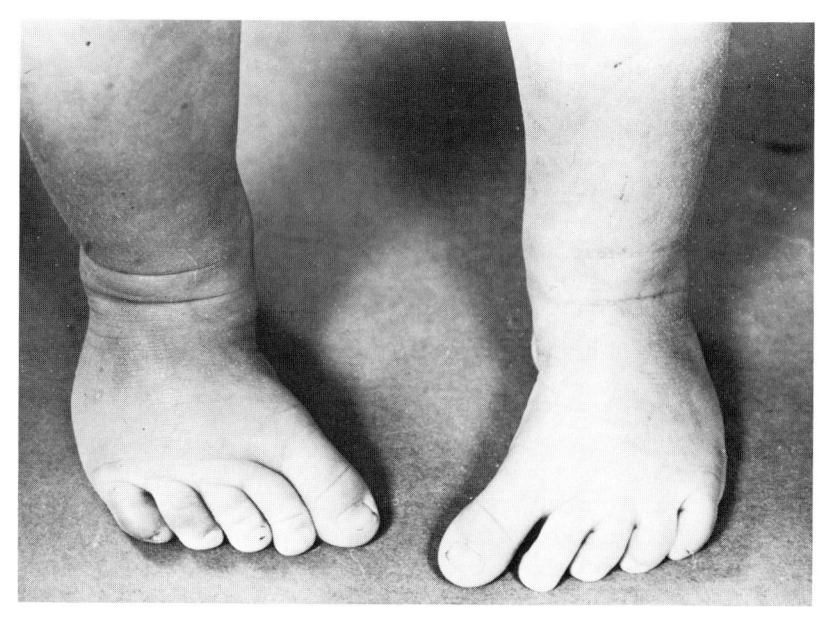

Fig. 4.12 Bilateral metatarsus adductus in a child aged 14 months.

On examination there is the deformity which has been described above. By manual pressure the adduction deformity of the metatarsals can be corrected. If the child has reached the age of standing and is examined standing, then it is noted that there is the adduction deformity, an obvious medial arch to the foot, some convexity of the lateral border of the foot, and frequently the hallux is markedly abducted from the midline of the foot so that it is widely separated from the second toe. The heel is in neutral or valgus.

DIFFERENTIAL DIAGNOSIS

Metatarsus varus. This can be differentiated from metatarsus adductus because, in the former condition, the child presents at a later age and there is rigidity of the deformity, cavus deformity, supination of the forefoot, and valgus deformity of the heel. The deformity is progressive.

Congenital talipes equinovarus. Metatarsus adductus can be differentiated from this condition by the ease with which the deformities can be corrected in metatarsus adductus and by the absence of any deformity of the hindfoot.

MANAGEMENT

Most children who present with metatarsus adductus do not require any active treatment for the foot deformity. The parents must be reassured by an explanation of the natural history of the condition. It should be pointed out that metatarsus adductus is extremely common in childhood and that, even if it is not treated, the condition is very rarely seen in adults. In addition the parents should be brought to see that metatarsus adductus improves slowly over a variable period of time up to the age of 5 or 6 years, although most have corrected spontaneously before that age.

Because the condition takes some time to spontaneously correct itself it may be necessary to see the child and the parents on a number of occasions. Very occasionally indeed does one see a patient with metatarsus adductus which shows no tendency to improve. There may even be slight worsening deformity and the foot may take on the features of metatarsus varus (page 167). In these circumstances, the foot requires management appropriate to that condition.

Although serial plasters and night splints have been popular in the management of metatarsus adductus, we do not find them necessary.

OBESITY

Obesity, in childhood and adolescence, has orthopaedic implications and requires management. This requires sensitivity on the part of the orthopaedic surgeon as many children are particularly embarrassed about their appearance. It is generally wise to discuss the problem initially with the parents alone and then later in the presence of the child. If the parents are also obese then there is little possibility of helping the child unless the parents are prepared to diet.

Obese children are more likely to have poor general posture with a tendency to flat feet, knock knees, excessive lumbar lordosis, and excessive thoracic kyphosis. They are also more likely to complain of foot strain, recurrent giving way of the ankle, and even discomfort from their knees knocking together, particularly in the winter time. In addition, slipped upper femoral epiphysis is more common in obese subjects. Not only does obesity have specific complications of an orthopaedic nature but, should an orthopaedic condition occur in an obese subject, then the obesity as well as the orthopaedic condition requires management, with the aid of an experienced dietitian. Frequently obesity should be treated prior to the joint disorder; for example, a fat boy who requires arthrodesis of the hip should lose weight before surgery is undertaken.

FOOTWEAR AND THE FOOT

In clinical practice more parents present with footwear problems in their children than with foot problems. Parents have great difficulty in knowing what they should buy and in distinguishing the good from the bad. The whole subject is confused by folklore, old wives' tales, and conflicting advice given by doctors, chiropodists, and shoe fitters. This section is an attempt to present the subject in a logical manner so that parents may be given firm guidelines regarding the selection, alteration, and maintenance of footwear in children.

Normal development of the foot

In the first 6–9 months, foot shape is largely dependent on distribution of fat in the foot. Many appear so chubby that no arches are apparent and when the infant starts to find his feet, he stands on a wide base with everted feet—a stance which is often aggravated by the tibial bowleg commonly present. As the tibia straightens, the foot posture recovers by about the age of 2 years only to receive another setback as the knock knee posture develops. Finally, by the age of about 6 years, the legs have become straight and the definitive posture of the leg and foot becomes established. In the vast majority, the end result is a normal foot without treatment of any sort, but several other factors also influence the shape of the foot.

Hereditary—a foot may be long and thin or short and broad; it may be planus or cavus and it may be big or small. The characteristics which a child may have in its feet are largely determined by the type of feet possessed by the parents. If one or both parents have very flat feet, one should not be surprised if their children follow suit. Attempts to change this state of affairs will be about as successful as trying to change the colour of a child's eyes.

Footwear—if no shoes are worn, the foot tends to be broad and flat but very mobile, and this is perhaps what a normal foot should be. When shoes are constantly worn, however, the foot becomes narrower and develops a more fixed longitudinal arch. Shoes that are too small, especially in the forefoot, may cause deformities of the toes but it is equally true that deformities such as hallux valgus and clawing of the toes are common in some races though shoes are never worn. Tight shoes and tight socks which crowd the toes should obviously be avoided.

Ill health—has a marked effect on foot pressure. Prolonged recumbency associated with illness causes softening of ligaments and bones and, when weight bearing is resumed, the foot tends to sag and will require protection until health is restored.

Definition of the normal foot

What constitutes a normal foot is rather difficult to define as the foot can have different shapes and different postures at different ages. Under the age of 6 years, a planus and valgus posture can be accepted and even after this age there is considerable variation. It can be said that a normal foot is one that fulfils the following three criteria: 1 it can be taken to a shoe shop and easily fitted; 2 the shoe wears evenly on the heel and sole and the upper is not distorted; 3 it is painless.

Definition of a good shoe

In the first instance, shoes were designed to protect the feet from rough surfaces and the weather. Later they were given the added duty of adornment, and in more recent times they have been seen as necessary to normal growth and development of the foot. While shoes may undoubtedly enhance appearance, there is no doubt that a foot can develop normally without them. There is also considerable doubt that corrective shoes have any influence at all on development.

SHAPE

The basic prerequisite for a shoe is that it should be the same shape as the foot with a straight inner border, sufficient toe room, and a well fitting instep and heel. The fit over the instep is important because it not only holds the shoe on, but when walking downhill, it prevents the foot sliding forwards and cramping the toes. Pointed toes come into fashion from time to time and this shape is compatible with a good fit provided the shoe is long enough. In general however, a rounded toe is always preferable for children.

SIZE

Most children's shoes are available in fractional fittings and it is therefore quite easy to select the right shoe once the length, width and height have been measured with the aid of a foot measuring device. In children, always select the size which is one longer than the foot, i.e. one-third of an inch.

CONSTRUCTION

The nomenclature used in shoe construction is illustrated in Fig. 4.13. Traditionally, shoes have been made from leather with the sole sewn to the upper. However, with increasing labour costs, this method of construction has been largely replaced by the use of adhesives. The modern children's shoe is usually made of leather with a stuck-on rubber or synthetic sole and heel; while these are adequate they are a poor substitute for the traditionally made shoe. Because the shoe is much more flexible and the stiffening in the counter is less strong, the shoes deform readily. Parents often present with the problem of a distorted shoe believing that their child has a foot problem—in fact, the feet are normal and the

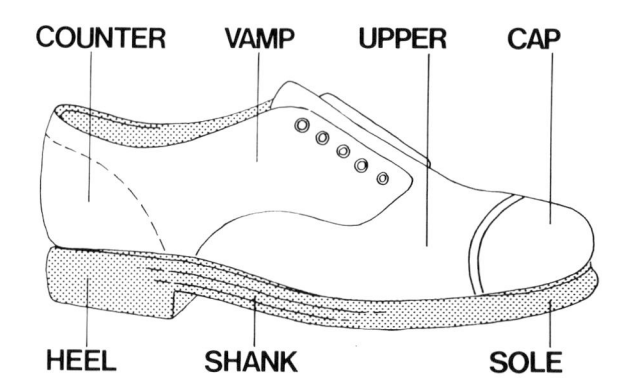

Fig. 4.13 The terminology used to describe the various parts of a shoe.

shoes inadequate. Supplied with stronger and more rigid shoes, the difficulty is overcome.

COST

Although in most instances the most expensive shoes are the best constructed, it does not follow that all cheap shoes are bad. They may not last as long but they are certainly not harmful if fitted with the same skill as an expensive shoe. Shoe retailers tend to create a climate which prevents mothers seeking cheaper footwear for fear of doing harm.

Thongs, runners, sandals

This type of footwear is commonly available in supermarkets, discount stores and the like, and is therefore frowned upon by the legitimate shoe retailers. They are

The Child

all said to be harmful and, in not offering support for the foot, somehow to interfere with proper development. This of course is nonsense. Thongs are worn by about half of the world's population and are probably the only really effective corrective footwear known. Having no sides they do not restrict the foot and may only be held on by proper contraction of the intrinsic muscles at each step. Corns and callouses do not occur in thong wearers.

Runners or sandshoes made of moulded rubber and canvas are favourites with children rather than their parents. Again they are not harmful and their only real disadvantage is that they soon become dirty looking and rather malodorous. Sandals have obvious advantages in hot weather and their use should be encouraged.

Having attempted to define the advantages and shortcomings of the various types of footwear, it only remains to provide answers to the following questions which are commonly asked by parents in orthopaedic practice.

Q Is footwear necessary?
A Shoes are only necessary for protection. They are not necessary to promote normal foot growth and development.

Q Are boots better than shoes?
A In toddlers, boots are preferable because they are less likely to fall off or be taken off. They retain their shape better and are usually more strongly constructed. In older children and adolescents, boots are only preferable for special purposes, for example, hiking and skiing.

Q Is it harmful to use worn shoes (hand down) from other children?
A No. Provided they are big enough.

Q How should I choose socks and stockings?
A Natural materials such as cotton and wool are preferable. Nylon socks become very smelly. Avoid stretch socks at all costs as they crowd the toes.

Q What is the place of building up shoes?
A Very little. The Thomas heel designed for juvenile flat foot is of no value. It is ugly, expensive to maintain and produces an awkward gait. A metatarsal bar is useful for metatarsalgia but an insole with a button is preferable. An outside float is useful for recurrent instability of the ankle. All other alterations should be regarded as historic.

Q What can I do to overcome excessive wear?
A This is most often seen in children with cerebral palsy. Assuming spastic equinus and other aggravating factors have been attended to, the bootmaker can assist by providing metal toe pieces or nylon soles. Rollers may be fitted to the front of the shoe. The problem diminishes after maturity when the patient usually does a smaller mileage at a slower rate.

Q How do I cope with unequal foot sizes?
A When the discrepancy is roughly less than three sizes it is usually possible to

fill up the shoe of the small foot with an inner sole and a plug of paper or cotton wool in the toe cap. Over three sizes, the problem is best managed by the construction of a slipper which converts the small foot to full size and allows a pair of shoes to be worn in comfort.

INFECTIONS OF BONE AND JOINT

Osteomyelitis and septic arthritis may be acute or chronic although, in developed countries, they generally present as acute illnesses. Either should be suspected in any child who presents with an acute illness characterised by pain, swelling or tenderness in any portion of the limbs. With early and vigorous treatment, complete cure can be effected with a minimum of morbidity. Osteomyelitis is now frequently treated and cured without any radiological changes appearing in the affected bones.

ACUTE OSTEOMYELITIS

There may be a history of minor trauma to the affected limb within 14 days of the onset of osteomyelitis. Presumably there has been bruising of tissue and then a bacteraemia has allowed organisms to settle in the haematoma. A responsible focus of infection is only rarely found.

Generally, one bone alone is involved and the commonest sites are the lower femur, the upper tibia, the upper femur, pelvis, and upper humerus. However no site is exempt. Occasionally, multiple sites are involved and the child is then likely to be severely ill with marked systemic features.

It has been suggested that the metaphysis of long bones is involved because there are large sinusoids here in which the blood flows slowly. Furthermore, there are thin-walled blood vessels at the junction of the metaphysis and the epiphysis and it is thought that bacteria might readily leak through these. A local inflammatory response is produced, characterised by infiltration with polymorphonuclear leucocytes and by hyperaemia. Tissue destruction results from the release of proteolytic enzymes and, if sufficient leucocytes are destroyed, then suppuration will result.

METHODS OF SPREAD OF INFECTION (see Fig. 4.14)

The infection may spread to the subperiosteal region with elevation of the periosteum. Spread also occurs into the venous and lymphatic channels of the bone and may pass by this route to the diaphysis. If the infection spreads throughout the shaft of the bone, there is likely to be thrombosis of the peripheral branches of the nutrient artery, or of the nutrient artery itself. Furthermore, the elevation of the periosteum, if allowed to spread, will result in avascularity of the cortex of the bone. If the metaphysis is intra-articular (as in the hip joint) then the infection may involve the joint.

The growth plate acts as a barrier preventing infection spreading to the epiphysis unless the child is under 1 year old, when terminal branches of the nutrient artery may perforate the epiphyseal plate and allow infection to cross the plate.

In general, osteomyelitis is vigorously treated at an early stage and suppuration does not occur, nor does the infection have an opportunity to spread as described above. However in the late-presenting case, these more gross changes may occur and may be followed by chronic infection of the bone.

CHRONICITY OF INFECTION (see Fig. 4.15)

The periosteum ultimately lays down new bone as an involucrum surrounding the dead bone (sequestrum). A small sequestrum may be absorbed or discharged spontaneously through a sinus. If a large sequestrum remains, then there are likely to be recurrent flares of infection and possibly recurrent sinus formation. Pus-filled cavities may occur in the bone and these may contain small sequestra. If

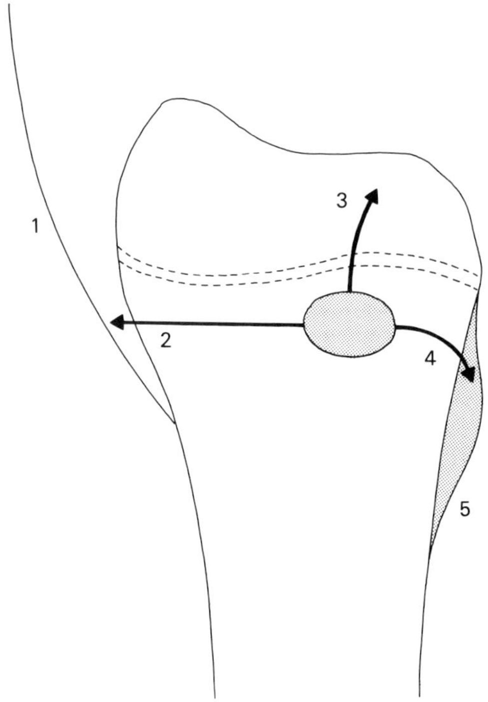

Fig. 4.14 The directions in which a focus of acute osteomyelitis may spread.
1 Joint capsule.
2 Spread of infection into the joint which may occur if the growth plate is intra-articular.
3 Spread of infection through the growth plate into the epiphysis.
4 Spread of infection through the cortex to form a subperiosteal abscess. 5 Stripping up of the periosteum in a distal direction.

there has been damage to the epiphyseal plate then this will not recover and permanent leg length discrepancy or deformity may result. The younger the child, the more likely are metaphyseal and diaphyseal changes to revert to normal. Overgrowth of the affected bone may occur, particularly if the infection has been adjacent to an epiphyseal plate without there having been any destruction of the plate.

Bacteriology

The organism most commonly responsible for this infection is *Staphylococcus aureus*. This organism is responsible for approximately 95% of cases in our community, but the incidence varies throughout the world. The remainder of patients have infection due to a Streptococcus, Pneumococcus, *Escherichia coli*, *Salmonella typhi* and *Haemophilus influenzae*. The latter organism is seldom a cause of oestomyelitis in this community but is responsible for the condition in other parts of Australia and elsewhere in the world.

Clinical features

Generally there is a short history of pain in the affected limb. If it is the lower limb that is involved then the child is soon reluctant to walk. The pain becomes severe and is throbbing in quality. The child becomes generally unwell and is feverish.

There is acute tenderness in the region of the pain. Later there may be swelling and redness, though these changes are seldom seen in developed countries as patients tend to present early in the course of the disease and early treatment prevents the appearance of such features. Rarely, there is swelling of a related joint.

Infants may present with gross systemic features due to septicaemia and, in these circumstances, localisation of the bony element of the infection may be difficult. These children may be extremely sick with gross systemic features. This is the case in neonatal osteomyelitis which may be due to a source of infection in the umbilicus and the organism be a Streptococcus or Staphylococcus. Infection may occur in several bones at the same time.

Investigations

The diagnosis is made on clinical grounds and antibiotic therapy should not await the results of any special investigation. In general the erythrocyte sedimentation rate is raised at an early stage. The white cell count may be normal initially but soon rises to as high as 20 000 cells per cubic millimetre. There is a polymorphonuclear leucocytosis.

Blood should be taken for culturing before an antibiotic is commenced and this investigation should be repeated if the patient continues to show a high temperature. X-rays will be normal for approximately ten days following the onset of the condition. Rarely distortion of the soft tissue shadows will indicate the site of a subperiosteal abscess.

A bone scan using technetium-99 pyrophosphate will almost invariably show a hot spot at the site of the lesion. This investigation is useful if there is doubt as to the diagnosis as may occur if the spine or pelvis are affected.

Differential diagnosis

Cellulitis and erysipelas may be difficult to distinguish from osteomyelitis in the early stages and, if there is doubt, then the patient will be treated for osteomyelitis. The lesion will rapidly subside.

Septic arthritis, particularly in the infant, may also be difficult to distinguish from osteomyelitis, indeed the infection may have arisen in the bone and spread to the joint.

Rheumatoid arthritis and rheumatic fever may occasionally be confused with osteomyelitis. However they can generally be distinguished by their characteristic systemic features.

Ewing's tumour may sometimes give rise to pyrexia in addition to pain and tenderness in the affected bone. The radiological features may also be difficult to distinguish from subacute or chronic osteomyelitis.

MANAGEMENT

The successful management of the child with osteomyelitis depends upon early diagnosis and hence a high index of suspicion on the part of the treating doctor. It behoves orthopaedic surgeons to impart this high index of suspicion to general practitioners and paediatricians.

Any patient with pyrexia and a short history of pain in the limbs, the limb girdles or the spine should be admitted to hospital and investigated as outlined above. Even if these investigations do not show any other abnormality, then appropriate antibiotics should be given unless an alternative diagnosis has been confidently established.

The proper management of acute osteomyelitis in childhood depends upon adequate immobilisation, appropriate antibiotics in high dosage, and the occasional need to release pus.

Adequate immobilisation

The child should be rested in bed and the whole of the affected limb immobilised in a plaster backslab with the limb elevated. Once the child is afebrile a complete cast is applied and retained for a period of six weeks.

Antibiotic management

Adequate blood levels can only be obtained by intravenous administration. In this community the administration of flucloxacillin alone gives the most appropriate cover for the organisms encountered. The drug is administered in a dose of 50–100 mg per kilogram per day until the child has been afebrile for 24 hours. Flucloxacillin suspension is then administered orally half an hour before meals. This suspension is unstable and has to be prepared every ten days. The antibiotic is continued for a period of six weeks.

If, in any community, *Haemophilus influenzae* is cultured from a significant number of children with osteomyelitis then ampicillin is administered (in the dosage employed in the management of septic arthritis, p. 153) in addition to flucloxacillin. In the rare case where a Streptococcus is cultured, penicillin is the antibiotic of choice.

Surgery

If antibiotics are given in adequate dose and early enough then surgery will not be needed because there will have been no abscess formation. If a patient with osteomyelitis has a persistent swinging temperature and develops an extremely well localised tender spot then it is likely that a subperiosteal abscess has formed and this requires immediate surgical drainage.

If the site of the infection is distally situated in a limb then the operation is performed under a bloodless field but without having used preliminary exsanguinating tourniquet. Whether or not a tourniquet has been employed, an incision is made at the site of tenderness and the dissection carried down to bone where the abscess may be disclosed. Once the periosteum has been opened, the pus drains quite freely and there is no need to make any drill holes into the bone itself. If operation is performed and a subperiosteal abscess is not disclosed then the operation has been performed unnecessarily. There is no point in making multiple drill holes and this practice may indeed be harmful and lead to sequestrum formation.

COMPLICATIONS OF ACUTE OSTEOMYELITIS

These include septicaemia, metastatic infection, suppurative arthritis of the related joint, destruction of an epiphyseal plate with retardation of growth of that bone, overgrowth of the affected bone (due to hyperaemia of the metaphysis) and chronic osteomyelitis.

CHRONIC OSTEOMYELITIS

Chronic osteomyelitis may occur either as a sequel to acute osteomyelitis or may have an insidious onset.

CHRONIC OSTEOMYELITIS AS A SEQUEL TO ACUTE INFECTION
(pathology, see p. 139)

If bacteria persist in the bone following acute osteomyelitis they may remain dormant there for very long periods. Commonly there is a flare of infection from time to time. If, in addition, the initial infection has been complicated by bone destruction plus sequestrum formation then recurrent flares of infection are more likely. Cavities may be present which are surrounded by dense sclerotic bone, in which case antibiotics are less likely to be effective. Recurrent abscess formation may occur and be complicated by sinus formation with secondary infection.

Patients with a flare of infection are commonly feverish but not extremely ill or toxic. There is local pain, tenderness, and sometimes redness. If an abscess forms then the pain increases and becomes throbbing in nature. The abscess may discharge spontaneously or require surgical drainage. Sequestra may be extruded. Following the discharge, a persistent sinus may form which suggests that there are one or more sequestra present. The lining of such sinuses is frequently of dense fibrous tissue.

RADIOLOGICAL APPEARANCES AND BONE SCAN

The affected bone generally shows patchy areas of rarefaction surrounded by dense sclerosis. Sequestra may be seen, either in cavities in the bone or lying adjacent to the cortex of the bone. If there is a persistent sinus then a sinugram may be helpful in demonstrating its extent and its relationship to any sequestra that may be present (Fig. 4.15). Bone scanning may supplement radiographs in disclosing the extent of the lesion.

Management

The management of chronic osteomyelitis in childhood is generally conservative. One can never guarantee a cure with either conservative or operative management.

NON-OPERATIVE MANAGEMENT

Children with a flare of infection are rested in bed and the affected limb immobilised in a plaster shell. Antibiotics are of doubtful value but they are given in order to prevent infection spreading.

If a sinus should form then in general it is intially treated conservatively. The patient is discouraged from weight bearing and the affected part is immobilised.

The clinician's attitude to antibiotic therapy in chronic osteomyelitis is influenced to some extent by his past experience with the affected child. If the child has not had previous courses of high dosage antibiotics for long periods then

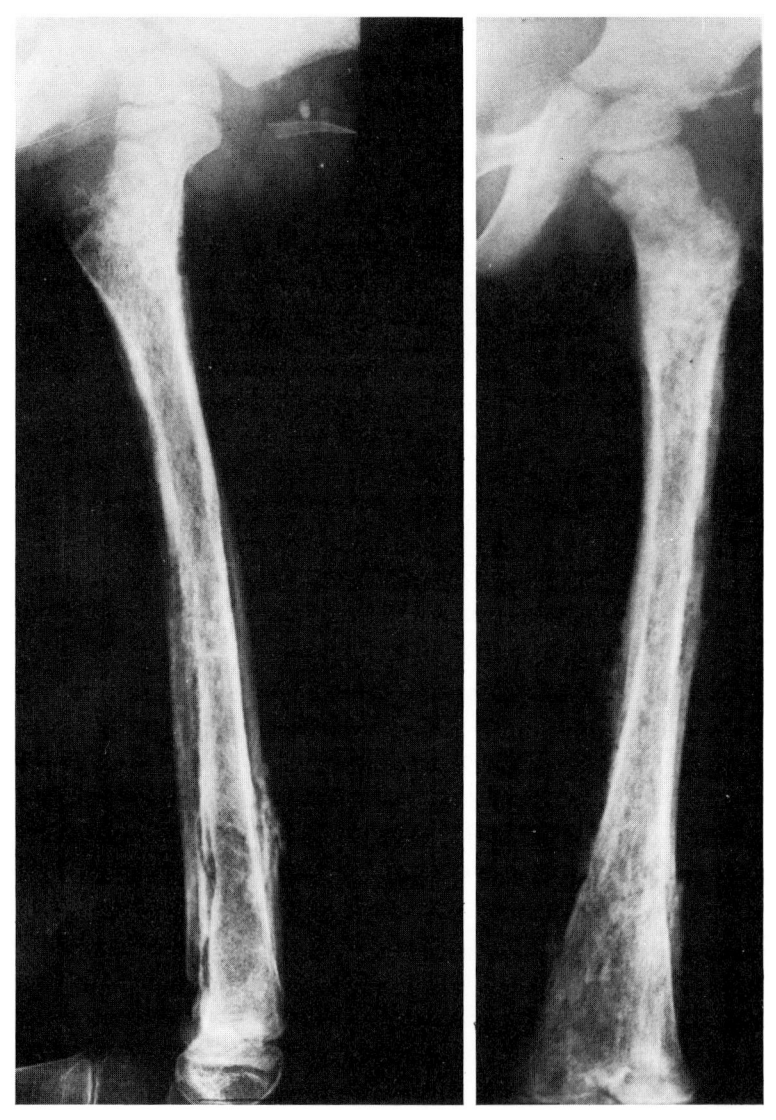

Fig. 4.15 Osteomyelitis involving the entire femoral shaft. The dense outline of the old femoral shaft (sequestrum) can be seen inside the new sub-periosteal bone which encircles it (the involucrum).

such a course is instituted. If the appropriate antibiotic is unknown then the child is admitted to hospital and given intravenous flucloxacillin (100 mg per kilogram) for six days (or until the patient is afebrile for 24 hours) and then a three month course of oral flucloxacillin (100 mg per kilogram).

If the patient has had previous courses of flucloxacillin then some other broad spectrum antibiotic will be employed. At the time of writing and in our community the most appropriate is cephazolin sodium (Kefzol). Estimations of the blood level of the appropriate antibiotic ensure adequate dosage.

If the patient has had previous adequate courses of appropriate antibiotics and continues to have flares of infection or chronic sinus formation, or both, then antibiotics play little part other than to minimise the risk of spreading infection should surgical management be undertaken.

OPERATIVE MANAGEMENT

Indications for surgery. An abscess cavity and/or a sequestrum with repeated flares, persistent pain, or chronic sinus formation.

Nature of surgery in chronic osteomyelitis
1. Sequestrectomy.
2. Cavity drainage with primary skin closure.
3. Cavity saucerisation.

The wound is generally packed open with moist saline packs to encourage the formation of granulation tissue and the wound repacked as necessary until closure has occurred. Split skin grafts may be employed to accelerate closure. Rarely it is possible, following saucerisation of a cavity, to place a muscle belly in the defect and proceed to primary closure of the wound.

If surgery is undertaken in the presence of a chronic sinus then a tourniquet is employed if possible and methylene blue is injected along the course of the sinus to enable the surgeon to identify the sinus in the depths of the wound. In general, the sinus tract is cored out together with the dense fibrous tissue which surrounds it and the wound is laid open so that there are no pockets. All avascular tissue is excised down to bleeding bone. Sequestra are removed as is any dead cortical bone. It is usually safest to pack the wound though, if the surgeon is confident that he has excised all dead and infected tissue, he may perform primary or secondary closure of the wound.

CHRONIC OSTEOMYELITIS IN WHICH THE ONSET IS INSIDIOUS

BRODIE'S ABSCESS

This term refers to an abscess which is usually situated in the metaphysis of a long bone; however, it may occur at any site in the bone. Patients who present with a Brodie's abscess are usually over the age of 8 years and present with local pain. If the affected bone is subcutaneous it will be tender and there may be some overlying swelling. X-rays show an oval lucency in the bone with surrounding sclerosis.

If the patient presents in the manner described above then the condition is treated as for a flare of chronic osteomyelitis. The symptoms and signs rapidly settle following immobilisation and a course of antibiotics. If recurrent flares occur then the treatment is operative: the cavity is opened; generally it contains sterile fluid and there may be a sequestrum present. The cavity is unroofed and the sclerotic abscess wall is removed. The wound is primarily closed and the limb is immobilised for a period of six weeks during which time antibiotics are continued.

TUBERCULOSIS OSTEOMYELITIS

This is a chronic infection which is seldom seen in developed countries. X-rays show bone destruction with ill-defined margins and surrounding bone atrophy rather than the sclerosis which is seen in chronic osteomyelitis of other causes.

Discitis

This term is applied to a form of subacute osteomyelitis which affects two adjacent vertebral bodies. An organism is occasionally cultured. The characteristic early radiological feature is narrowing of one intervertebral disc. A technetium-99 bone scan will show two hot spots in the vertebral bodies adjacent to the affected disc and the diagnosis may be made in this way before there are any radiological changes.

CLINICAL FEATURES

Children present with this condition between the ages of 10 months and 12 years. On occasion more than one intervertebral disc is affected but the most common is that between the fourth and fifth lumbar vertebrae. The lumbar spine is involved in 74% of affected children and, in our experience, the cervical spine has been affected in only one instance.

The commonest symptoms are vague pains in the buttock, thigh, or knee, or simple refusal to walk. Only approximately half of the patients have symptoms relating to the back.

The patients may present with headache and vomiting, painful stiff neck, abdominal pain or a painless limp.

Frequently the children have been extensively investigated before a diagnosis has been made.

The commonest physical sign in lumbar discitis is a stiff back. There may also be a loss of lumbar lordosis or an increased lordosis. There may be tenderness at the site of the lesion or a prominent spinous process. There may be no abnormal physical signs. Most affected children have a pyrexia at an early stage of the illness but generally the temperature is not above 37.5°C and the children do not appear to be sick.

RADIOGRAPHIC APPEARANCES

At the onset, radiographs may be normal. The earliest change is narrowing of a single disc (Fig. 4.16) and this may become evident within three weeks of the onset of symptoms. Further narrowing of the disc takes place over a period of months. There may then be erosion of the adjacent vertebrae with fluffy ill-defined margins to these erosions. Later the erosions develop sclerosed margins (Fig. 4.17). Tomographs may reveal much more bony involvement than is shown

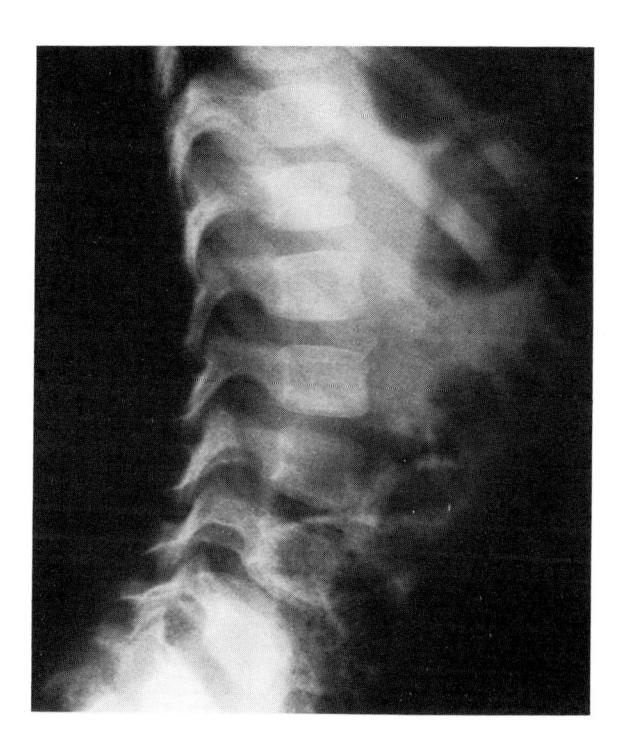

Fig. 4.16 Lateral x-ray of the lumbar spine of a child aged 2 years who presented because she refused to walk. Note that the disc space between the first and second lumbar vertebrae is narrower than the space above and the space below.

in plain radiographs. Generally there is progressive narrowing of the disc, though, on occasions, the disc space may widen after initial narrowing (Fig. 4.18).

There is no related soft tissue abscess visible radiographically.

OTHER SPECIAL INVESTIGATIONS

The blood sedimentation rate is raised in approximately half of the affected children but it seldom exceeds 60 mm in the first hour.

Technetium-99 bone scan will generally show hot spots in the adjacent borders of the two affected vertebrae. Very rarely indeed is the patient seen at such an early stage that the bone scan is normal.

A Mantoux test is performed and is generally negative. Brucella and

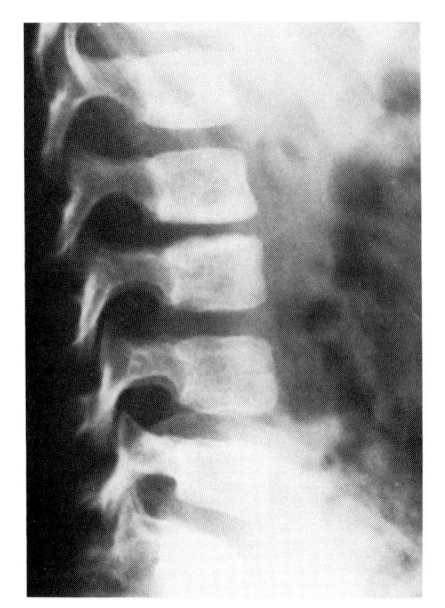

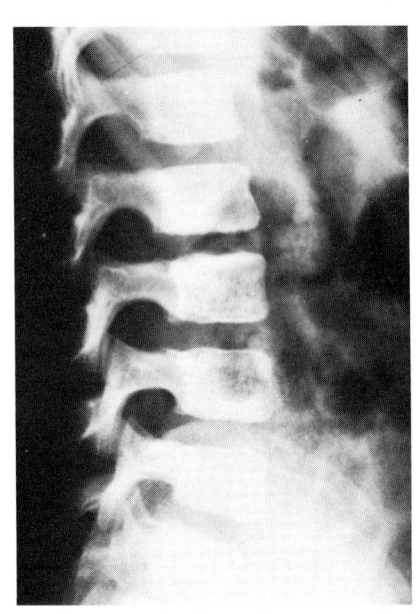

Figs. 4.17 & 4.18 Same patient as Fig. 4.16. Three months later there is marked narrowing of the affected disc space and some sclerosis of the adjacent vertebral margins. (*Right*) Six months later there is some reconstitution of the disc space.

Salmonella agglutination tests should also be carried out to eliminate the possibility of these infections.

DIFFERENTIAL DIAGNOSIS

The bone scan is quite diagnostic. A differential diagnosis only arises if the clinician has not thought of the diagnosis and has neglected to carry out a scan. Symptoms and signs similar to discitis may occur in the Guillain–Barré syndrome. Such patients may be distinguished clinically from those suffering from discitis if the lower limb deep reflexes are reduced.

Frank osteomyelitis of the spine is a much more severe infection than discitis and there will be marked systemic features.

Tuberculosis of the spine runs a much slower course and the child is generally unwell as distinct from the healthy appearance of those with discitis.

Rarely a patient is seen with a single narrow disc and the clinical features of discitis. At four weeks a further x-ray shows gross flattening of the vertebral body above the narrowed disc and this will be caused by eosinophilic granuloma of that bone—Calvé's disease.

MANAGEMENT

The principles of management are to rest the spine in recumbency until there is no pain or limitation of movement, the blood sedimentation rate is normal and radiographs indicate that bony erosion is not progressing.

Affected children are generally rested in a short double hip spica or on a Bradford frame until these criteria have been satisfied. Others report satisfactory results from ambulant treatment but our experience has shown that prolonged recumbency is the surest method of treatment. Antibiotics are reserved for those children with persistent pyrexia.

SEPTIC ARTHRITIS (see also p. 14)

Septic arthritis in childhood generally has many features in common with osteomyelitis: there is an acute onset of pain and reluctance to use the limb together with marked systemic features. In infancy however there may be few local signs related to the affected joint and the constitutional symptoms are then relatively slight.

Staphylococcus pyogenes is most commonly the responsible organism, though infections with *Haemophilus influenzae* are not uncommon. Infection reaches the joint from the blood stream or by secondary spread from local osteomyelitis, the latter being more likely to occur if the metaphysis is intra-articular. Penetrating wounds, sometimes complicated by retention of foreign material in the joint, may lead to septic arthritis. This most commonly occurs in the knee.

Acute septic arthritis may occur, particularly in infancy and in children with a nutritional disturbance, as part of a fulminating acute infective disease with severe systemic features; in these circumstances, management is first concentrated on maintaining life.

Pathology

The synovial membrane becomes hyperaemic at an early stage of the infection and this can be readily confirmed at operation. Oedema of the synovial membrane shortly follows and then it becomes infiltrated with polymorphonuclear leucocytes. There is excessive production of synovial fluid which contains numerous polymorphs and the breakdown of these cells releases proteolytic enzymes which rapidly destroy articular cartilage. Furthermore, streptokinase and staphylokinase from the responsible organism may activate plasminogen to produce a protease which breaks down the protein–chondroitin sulphate complex of the cartilage matrix. If the process continues, granulation tissue may spread over the articular surface resulting in further chondrolysis and irreversible joint damage. Fibrosis may occur later with a resultant fibrous or bony ankylosis. Avascular necrosis of bone may occur—notably of the femoral head in septic arthritis of the hip (Figs 4.19 & 4.20). In this condition the hip may dislocate (see p. 15).

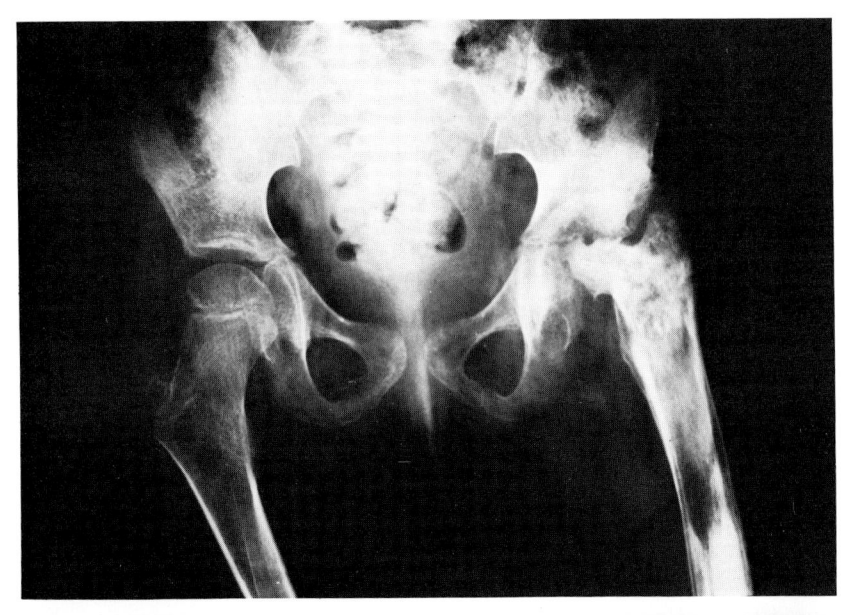

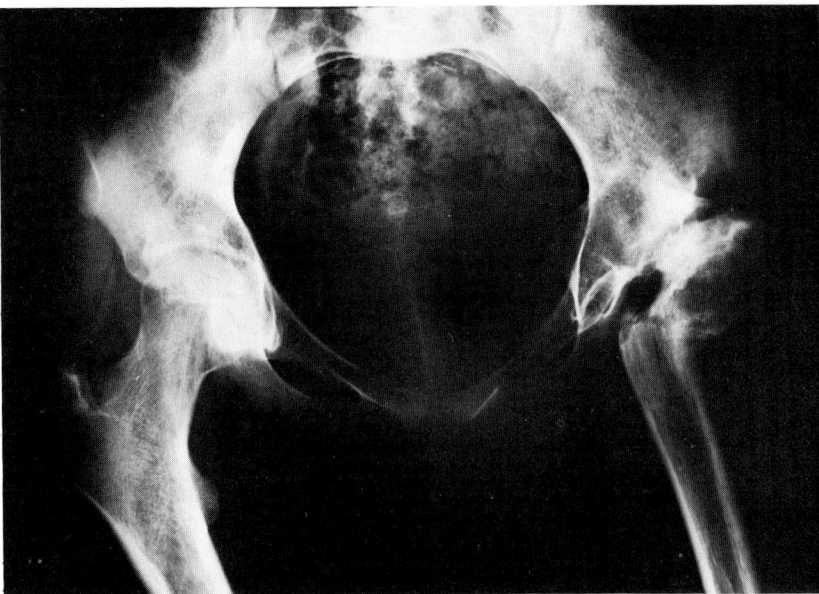

Figs. 4.19 & 4.20 Antero-posterior x-ray of the pelvis of a girl aged 5 who had presented late with osteomyelitis of the left femur and septic arthritis of the left hip. Note partial destruction of the femoral head with avascular necrosis of the remainder of the head, absence of the growth plate, and shortness of the femoral neck. (*Bottom*) At the age of 15 years the left hip had developed 40° of fixed flexion deformity (note the contour of the pelvic inlet which is an index of this deformity) and 40° of fixed adduction deformity. An intertrochanteric osteotomy has been performed to rid the patient of these deformities.

Clinical features

Generally there is an acute onset and the symptoms are similar to those of acute osteomyelitis: pain, pyrexia, and reluctance to move or use the affected limb. In general there is soon a marked limitation of movement of the affected joint with severe muscle spasm and pain on attempted movement.

Radiological appearances

The soft tissue outline of the joint may be seen to be increased at an early stage for the more peripheral joints. At the hip there may be an alteration in the normal soft tissue shadows but such alterations are not a reliable method of diagnosing the condition. After about six days, porosis may develop in the bone adjacent to the affected joint. Much later there will be narrowing of the joint space if the condition has progressed to a stage where there is destruction of articular cartilage.

Special investigations

In general the erythrocyte sedimentation rate and white cell count show changes suggesting an acute infection. Blood is taken for culture.

The most satisfactory investigations are carried out on material obtained by arthrotomy of the affected joint or by aspiration. An immediate smear may demonstrate the responsible organism. The joint fluid generally contains approximately 100 000 cells which are chiefly polymorphonuclear leucocytes with a reduction in sugar content and an elevation in protein.

Culture of the synovial fluid reveals the responsible organism only in approximately 50% of patients with septic arthritis. Of those with a positive culture a *Staphylococcus aureus* is grown in approximately half and *Haemophilus influenzae* type D in approximately a third of cases. *Haemophilus influenzae* is only isolated in children between the ages of 4 months and 4 years. Streptococci, Pneumococci, or Meningococci are sometimes the responsible organisms. Candida albicans may be responsible for multiple joint involvement in children with gross immunological deficiency.

Differential diagnosis

Initially, particularly in the neonatal period and in infancy, there may be difficulty in distinguishing acute osteomyelitis from acute septic arthritis and the child then requires treatment which is appropriate for both conditions.

Rarely, the patient presenting with rheumatic fever may be thought to have septic arthritis of the first joint affected. However, further joints are soon involved and the diagnosis becomes apparent because of the characteristic clinical features of rheumatic fever.

Rheumatoid arthritis is seldom confused with septic arthritis but on occasions septic arthritis may be wrongly diagnosed as juvenile chronic arthritis especially if it has a subacute rather than an acute onset. Any child with a painful and irritable joint should be assumed to have a septic arthritis until proved otherwise.

MANAGEMENT

The essence of management of septic arthritis in infancy and childhood is firstly, to try and obtain the responsible organism by aspiration of the joint. This distinguishes the management from that of osteomyelitis where it is seldom appropriate to employ local aspiration. Secondly, to begin antibiotic treatment at an early stage before the joint is distended with pus. Thirdly, to remove pus from the distended joint as early as possible in order to prevent damage to the articular cartilage.

Management then consists of arthrotomy or aspiration, the administration of appropriate antibiotics in adequate dosage, and immobilisation.

Arthrotomy or aspiration

Since pus in the joint damages the articular cartilage, it is important to remove this as soon as possible. The most certain way of achieving this is by performing arthrotomy rather than simple joint aspiration. Once it has been established that there is turbid fluid in a joint, then the safest management is to perform arthrotomy (though in the case of a knee joint aspiration alone may prove adequate provided the orthopaedist carefully observes the local and general response to therapy and is prepared to repeat aspiration).

As soon as the special investigations have been performed, the patient is taken to the operating theatre and a general anaesthetic administered. An intravenous infusion is set up as this will provide the route for subsequent antibiotic therapy.

A needle is inserted into the joint and aspiration is performed. One of three courses of action is then dictated by the findings: 1 If turbid fluid or pus is obtained, then arthrotomy is performed. 2 If clear fluid is obtained, there is no need for arthrotomy. 3 If no fluid is obtained then arthrotomy is performed; this is the only way one can be certain that pus is not present because the needle may not have been in the joint or may have been blocked by the oedematous synovium filling up the joint.

Should arthrotomy be performed then, once the synovial membrane has been opened, the fluid in the joint is collected for microscopy, Gram staining, culture and antibiotic sensitivity studies. The synovial membrane, which is generally swollen, red and oedematous is biopsied and similarly examined. A wide opening is made in the synovial membrane and capsule and the joint is washed out with saline. The wound is loosely sutured and the joint immobilised in a plaster cast.

In the case of a hip joint this procedure is carried out through a limited

Smith–Petersen approach (performed through an anterior oblique incision which is the lower part of the Salter incision). A one and a half hip spica is applied for immobilisation.

Antibiotics

The antibiotics employed must be effective against Staphylococci and *Haemophilus influenzae*. They should be begun once the joint has been aspirated.

The current antibiotic regime employed is flucloxacillin and ampicillin—100 mg per kilogram per day of each intravenously, until the patient has been afebrile for 24 hours, then flucloxacillin 50–100 mg per kilogram orally plus amoxycillin in the same dosage. Antibiotics are continued for at least four weeks from the onset of the condition.

Flucloxacillin forms an unstable suspension and has to be prepared freshly every ten days. It also has an unattractive flavour which children are more likely to tolerate if it is mixed with a fruit flavoured elixir of amoxycillin. If a Streptococcus is the responsible organism then penicillin is the antibiotic of choice.

Immobilisation

Rest in recumbency is continued until the child has been afebrile for at least 24 hours. The affected limb is immobilised in a plaster cast for 3–4 weeks. At the conclusion of this period the joint should not have any residual swelling and will rapidly mobilise without physiotherapy.

LEG LENGTH INEQUALITY AND ITS MANAGEMENT

The causes of leg length inequality are listed below.

CONGENITAL

Coxa vara
Various forms of underdevelopment of the femur and leg bones with or without absence of the whole or part of these bones
Tibial kyphosis
Congenital dislocation of the hip
Congenital leg atrophy or hypertrophy
Vascular abnormalities
Congenital talipes equinovarus

TRAUMATIC

Traumatic injury to the epiphysis of the femur or tibia with suppression of growth. Total suppression of growth leading to shortening; partial suppression of growth leading to deformity and shortening

Fracture of the shaft of one or more long bones with union in excessive shortening

Fractures of the metaphysis or shaft of long bones with growth stimulation

Severe burns

INFLAMMATORY

Diaphyseal osteomyelitis with growth stimulation

Diaphyseal osteomyelitis complicated by epiphyseal plate destruction with premature fusion of the epiphyseal line

Septic arthritis with joint destruction and or dislocation

NEUROLOGICAL CONDITIONS

Poliomyelitis
Cerebral palsy

TUMOURS

Neurofibromatosis
Fibrous dysplasia

MISCELLANEOUS

Old Perthes' disease
Old slipped epiphysis
Prolonged immobilisation of one limb
Radiation of one or more growth plates

Leg length inequality requiring active treatment is most commonly due to 1 trauma—malunion of fractures with shortening or epiphyseal damage leading to premature fusion. These conditions are increasing in number due to high speed motor vehicle injuries. 2 Congenital short femur in its various forms. 3 Congenital atrophy and hypertrophy of the whole of one leg. 4 Hypertrophy due to a vascular anomaly. 5 Poliomyelitis—Although uncommon in developed countries, this remains the commonest cause of significant leg length inequality in underdeveloped areas. 6 Septic arthritis of the hip in infancy with or without destruction of the head or dislocation.

Examination and management

A full general history is taken. Examination includes inspection for evidence of those conditions (listed above) which have generalised manifestations. Radiographs of both legs are taken to exclude multiple anomalies.

Measurement of leg length discrepancy

IN THE FIRST YEAR OF LIFE

Accurate measurement is impossible and generally unnecessary. Minor discrepancies are best discerned by careful palpation of the anterior superior iliac spine and greater trochanters and the inspection of the relative levels of the medial malleoli when the infant lies supine with both legs at right-angles to a line joining the anterior superior iliac spines. A useful method is to mark the tip of each malleolus with a ball point pen and, while the ink is still wet, apply equal traction to each foot and press the two ankles together. If the legs are equal in length the two marks will coincide and if not, a gap will show the discrepancy.

MEASUREMENTS BY TAPE

Real and apparent shortening are measured by this means. Accurate location of the anterior superior iliac spine is best achieved by the examiner's thumb creeping upwards to meet the point of the spine. Location of equivalent points on both medial malleoli is difficult and this method does not take into account discrepancy in the height of the heel (from the skin of the heel to the tip of the medial malleolus). Nor does this method take into account discrepancies which may be brought about by weight bearing (commonly valgus deformity at the subtalar joint).

MEASUREMENTS USING BLOCKS (FIG. 4.21)

This is the most accurate form of measurement as it eliminates the shortcomings of tape measurement. Measurements should be taken to both the anterior and posterior iliac spines.

RADIOLOGICAL MEASUREMENT

This investigation is appropriate only if very accurate measurement of the individual long bones is necessary. It is less accurate in determining the overall shortness of a limb than clinical assessment with blocks as it is difficult to measure the weight-bearing limbs or the distance from the ankle mortice to the skin of the heel. Orthoroentgenography is as accurate as scanography or teleradiography.

Serial examinations

Appropriate management depends largely on an annual examination with accurate recording of standard measurement. Clinical examination alone is generally adequate. For children over the age of 2 years, measurement using blocks provides adequate records of total leg length discrepancy. Tape measure-

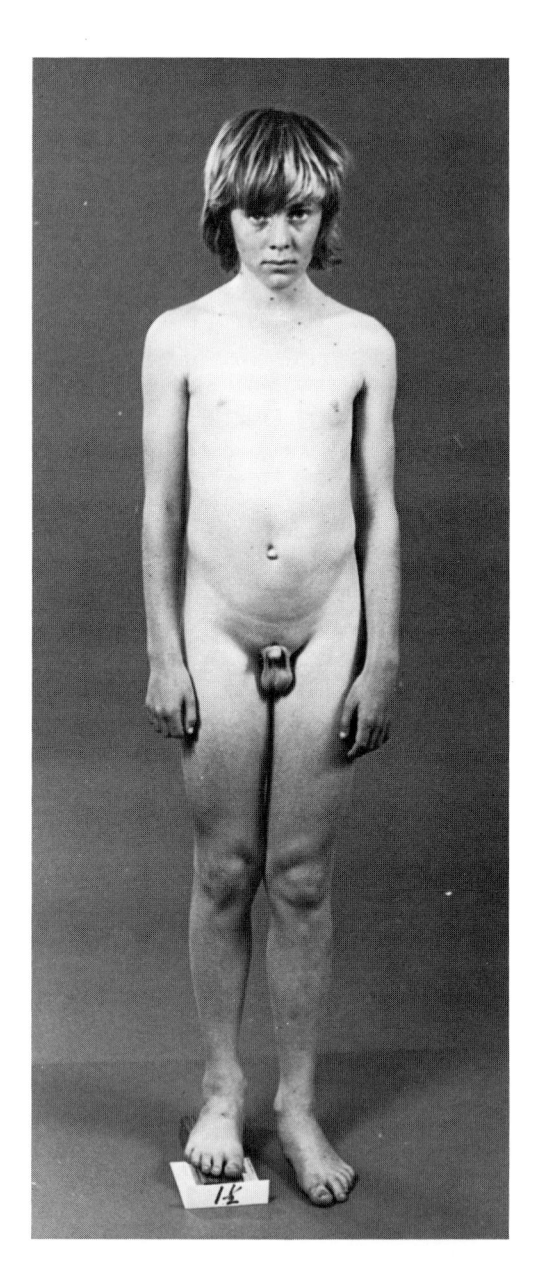

Fig. 4.21 Right hemiatrophy. Note that the whole of the right half of the body is affected. The use of blocks, as shown here, to bring the anterior superior iliac spine level, provides the most accurate estimation of leg length discrepancy.

ments are generally adequate for differential measurements of the femur and tibia. Radiographic examination has its greatest application in children who have undergone epiphyseal injury with partial or complete suppression of growth. Patients with partial suppression of epiphyseal growth also require accurate measurement of the deformity.

The Child 157

Patients are photographed at presentation and every two years thereafter. Skeletal age estimation is made over the age of 6 years and repeated at an appropriate age if an epiphyseal arrest is contemplated. Skeletal age estimations are also used to enable estimation of mature height.

CALCULATION OF MATURED DISCREPANCY AND TIME OF ARREST

Mature discrepancy

In order to forecast with accuracy the length of discrepancy at maturity, it is necessary to know the annual increment—that is the amount of length lost or gained each year. This can be obtained by annual measurements of the child's leg length. It may be found that the rate of loss is not constant year by year but it is usually possible to strike a mean after about four years of observation. If the cause of the discrepancy is premature fusion of one of the growth plates, then the loss of length can be predicted fairly accurately (see below).

TIMING OF ARREST

Of the various methods of calculation available we have found a modification of that described by Warren White the most convenient in use and as accurate as any other method (Fig. 4.22). Although it involves accepting inaccuracies, these are not significant provided the skeletal age does not differ from the chronological age by more than 18 months. The method is based on two assumptions. Firstly, that fusion of the lower femoral and upper tibial epiphyses occurs in boys at

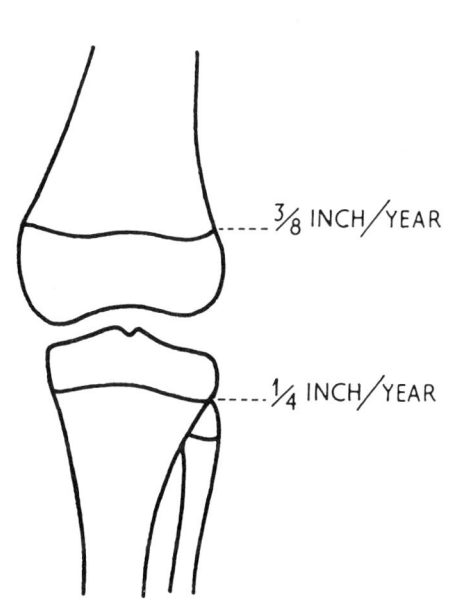

Fig. 4.22 The assumptions which are made in timing lower femoral and upper tibial growth plate arrest.

chronological age 16 years and girls at chronological age 14 years. Secondly, that the lower femoral epiphysis provides $\frac{3}{8}$ inch of longitudinal growth per year, while the upper tibial epiphysis provides $\frac{2}{8}$ inch of longitudinal growth per year.

For example, a girl aged 11 years has a leg length discrepancy of $1\frac{1}{2}$ inches. The annual increment in discrepancy is $\frac{1}{8}$ inch (this is obtained by examination of the annual records). The estimated mature discrepancy then equals $1\frac{1}{2}$ inches plus $\frac{1}{8}$ inch multiplied by 3, i.e. $1\frac{7}{8}$ inches.

If it were desired to completely correct the leg length discrepancy by epiphyseal arrest then lower femoral and upper tibial arrest should be performed at the age of 11 years ($\frac{5}{8}$ inches × 3 = $1\frac{7}{8}$ inches). Arrest of these epiphyses at the age of 12 years would retard growth by $1\frac{1}{4}$ inches ($\frac{5}{8}$ inches × 2)—leaving a discrepancy of $\frac{5}{8}$ inches. Complete correction of a leg length discrepancy is not usually the aim. Calculation may be performed to allow a residual discrepancy of up to one inch as this amount carries no disability and minimises loss in stature. The patient's records should read:
1. Chronological age (CA) = 11 years
2. Skeletal age (SA) = 11.5 years
3. Leg length discrepancy (LLD) = $1\frac{1}{2}$ inches
4. Annual increment (AI) = $\frac{1}{8}$ inch
5. Expected mature discrepancy (EMD) = $1\frac{7}{8}$ inches
Arrest of femur and tibia now = $1\frac{7}{8}$ inches
Arrest of femur and tibia Aet. 12 = $1\frac{1}{4}$ inches

In making the calculation for patients with considerable difference between skeletal age and chronological age, the surgeon should veer on the side of undercorrection, perhaps fusing one epiphysis initially and later fusing the second epiphysis if unacceptable undercorrection is seen to be occurring. Leg shortening can always be performed at maturity if there is doubt as to the appropriate age for epiphyseal arrest.

SPECIFIC MANAGEMENT

The various methods considered below may be used alone, or in varying combinations for severe discrepancy.

DISCREPANCIES IGNORED

If the estimated mature discrepancy is less than one inch it can generally be ignored. Such patients do not have an increased incidence of backache in adult life and need not wear raised shoes.

CONSERVATIVE MANAGEMENT OF LEG LENGTH DISCREPANCY

Modifications to footwear are available to accommodate discrepancies of almost any degree. The following is a rough guide to the various devices.

$\frac{1}{2}$ inch—raise heel only.
$\frac{1}{2}$–2 inches—raise heel and sole using outside cork or synthetic material. The latter is now cheaper, lighter and more durable than cork. As an example, a prescription might read $2''-1\frac{1}{2}''-1\frac{1}{4}''$ being the height of the heel, tread and toe respectively.
2–5 inches—patten and boot.
5–9 inches—patten plus double short irons with a ferrule in the patten. This is to control instability at the ankle.
9–14 inches—extension prosthesis (O'Connor boot).

EPIPHYSEAL ARREST (EPIPHYSIODESIS)

This is appropriate when the estimated mature discrepancy varies between 1 and $2\frac{1}{4}$ inches. The estimated mature height is discussed with the child and parents. Very short stature may preclude the procedure but, in general, those children who are estimated to have a short mature height come from small stock in whom short stature is regarded as normal.

Phemister's technique is employed when performing epiphyseal arrest. The growth plate is exposed through two incisions, one on its medial and one on its lateral aspect. The incisions to expose the medial aspect of the lower femoral and upper tibial epiphyses should be directed vertically and be placed on the medial aspect of the leg so that the subsequent scars (which are frequently broad and unsightly) will not be visible from in front or behind when the child is standing in the neutral position. The lateral femoral incision should be obliquely placed and passed laterally as it passes distally; the lateral tibial incision should pass obliquely, distally and medially. Starting over the metaphysis, the periosteum is raised and stripped towards the growth plate. Periosteum becomes adherent at the plate which is thus identified. A one inch square of bone, consisting of one-half epiphysis and one-half diaphysis, is removed and the growth plate is thoroughly curetted out using a small Volkmann spoon or mastoid gouge. The white line of cartilaginous growth plate can be followed to the centre of the bone and only the peripheral rim of plate is left undisturbed. The curettings are then returned to the narrow, deep crevasse and punched in tightly. The cortical square is returned into place but is rotated through 90° from its original alignment. The procedure is then repeated on the opposite aspect of the plate to be arrested.

Complications of the procedure are few; the most serious complication being the cosmetic appearance of the scars. This is best minimised by directing the incision as has been described above. Staples should not be employed for growth plate arrest as they have a high complication rate.

BONE SHORTENING

This is indicated in children who present when they are too old for epiphyseal arrest or when the timing of an arrest will be inaccurate due to poor records,

160 Chapter 4

erratic increments or when there is a gross difference between skeletal and chronological age.

Femoral shortening. This is performed at the subtrochanteric level (Figs. 4.23 & 4.24). The patient lies on the side opposite to that being shortened. Through a lateral approach, a Trifin nail is passed up the neck of the femur. Using an end-cutting power saw a segment of femur is removed at a subtrochanteric level. The cut ends of the femur are then brought together and secured using a plate attached to the nail.

Up to $2\frac{1}{2}$ inches of femur may be removed without causing permanent disability in limb function or appearance. There is generally some weakness of the quadriceps muscle for up to twelve months following this procedure.

Tibial shortening. This procedure is carried out at a diaphyseal level. Using an end-cutting saw, a Z cut is made in the tibia with the longitudinal limb of the Z 4–6 inches in length (Fig. 4.25). Two segments of tibia are then removed, at the upper end of the lower fragment and at the lower end of the upper fragment. The length of each segment removed is at the length of tibia to be resected which should be not more than two inches. Once the tibia has been shortened two screws are passed across the osteotomy from the medial to the lateral aspect of the tibia and the leg is immobilised in plaster until union is sound.

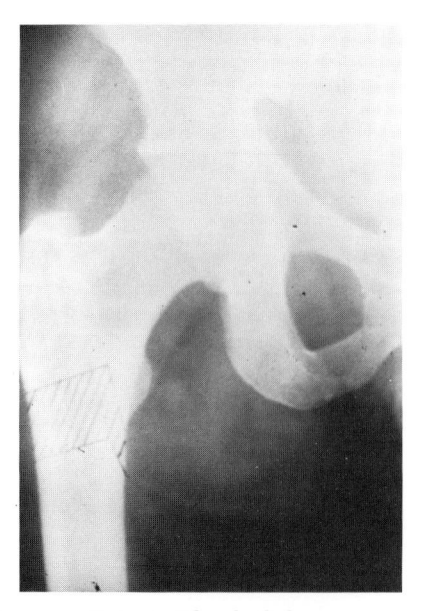

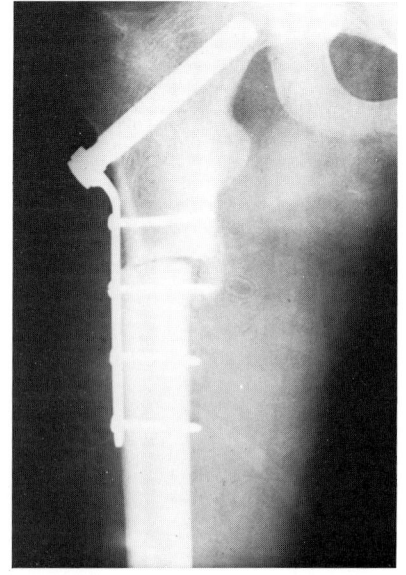

Figs. 4.23 & 4.24 The shaded area represents the segment to be excised. It is high and hence likely to unite readily, stable and does not interfere with the insertion of iliopsoas. (*Right*) The post-operative appearance. The upper osteotomy is a little lower than is ideal. It has been internally fixed with a Thomas King nail and plate.

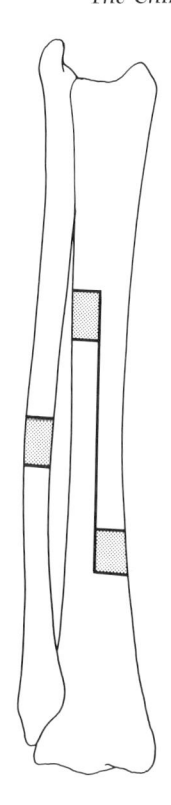

Fig. 4.25 Shortening of tibia and fibula in the management of leg length discrepancy. A step cut is made in the tibia and a segment (hatched) is excised from either fragment. A segment of the same length is excised from the fibula. The shortened tibia is internally fixed by two transverse screws.

The calf is generally weak for up to twelve months following this procedure. There is some increased bulk in the calf and as this procedure is generally performed on the side of the bigger leg this does constitute a disadvantage.

RESECTION OF BONE BRIDGE AND IMPLANTATION OF FAT AT THE GROWTH PLATE (LANGENSKIÖLD)

Partial closure of a growth plate will result in shortening of the affected bone and there may be angular deformities due to asymmetrical growth. Langenskiöld has shown that the bony bridge may be excised allowing the undamaged portion of the growth plate to continue its growth (Fig. 4.26). A free fat graft is packed into the defect produced by the bone bridge resection. Not only may further growth occur following this procedure but also angular deformity may correct with growth.

A bone bridge occupying up to three-quarters of the area of the growth plate may be excised with resumption of growth. Such resumption may occur up to two years after cessation of epiphyseal growth. The procedure is performed using the operating microscope to allow a good light source and accurate identification of the physis.

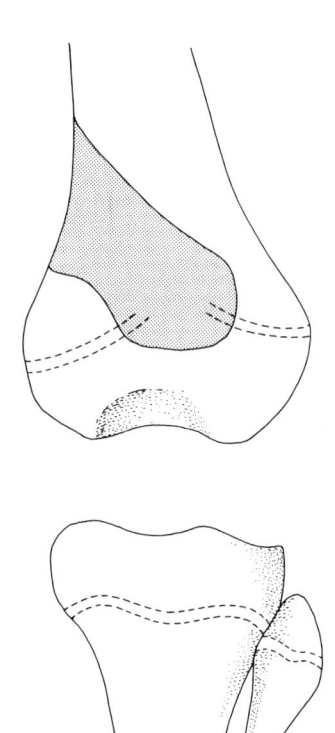

Fig. 4.26 Excision of central bone bridge crossing the lower femoral growth plate. The hatched area of bone is excised to leave a tongue of growth plate protruding into the cavity.

LEG LENGTHENING

This is a major procedure with a high complication rate and a high morbidity over a period of up to twelve months. It is only appropriate for children with major leg length discrepancy (more than $2\frac{1}{2}$ inches) which cannot be managed by simple means. Lengthening may be used in combination with other techniques. Tibial lengthening is performed by the Anderson technique but using Wagner apparatus, and two inches should be the maximum lengthening. It is doubtful whether femoral lengthening should be performed as the complication rate is unacceptably high.

AMPUTATION

This is appropriate if there is gross shortening and deformity and the circumstances are such that a prosthesis will give better function and better cosmesis.

THE FOOT

PES CAVUS

The term 'pes cavus' describes the foot which has an excessively high medial longitudinal arch. A well marked lateral longitudinal arch may also be present and there may or may not be associated clawing of the toes.

Aetiology

The modern view is that most cases are caused by some form of neuromuscular disease although the presence of this is often difficult to establish. The following classification is suggested.

Congenital—many families and some races have a tendency towards development of pes cavus.

Idiopathic—when a specific cause cannot be demonstrated. This category is becoming smaller as our knowledge of the causation increases.

Neuromuscular disease—the defect may be in *muscle* (muscular dystrophy, especially the pseudohypertrophic type) when it often develops before ambulation ceases and is aggravated by recumbency; *peripheral nerve* (e.g. sciatic nerve injury, Charcot-Marie-Tooth, polyneuritis); *anterior horn cell* (e.g. poliomyelitis, spinal dysraphism, myelomeningocele and diastematomyelia); *cord tracts* (e.g. Friedreich's ataxia produces one of the most severe forms of cavus); and the *brain* (e.g. cerebral palsy).

Physical insults—burns and irradiation. No account of the cavus foot would be complete without reference to the worst type of claw foot produced by the ancient art of foot binding in China. The practice started in the 9th century and spread to all levels of society, even to the Imperial Household. The treatment started at about the age of 6 years and was continued throughout the life of the individual. The result was accomplished by kneading and binding and in unskilful hands was painful and often led to ischaemia. Its aim was undoubtedly to enhance the sexual attractiveness of the woman. Also the exaggerated motion of the hip brought about by walking with this deformity was apparently much appreciated by the male of the day. The practice of foot binding was outlawed in mainland China early this century but persisted for a number of years in Chinese communities elsewhere.

Pathogenesis

Very little is known about the pathogenesis of pes cavus. A number of theories have been proposed such as intrinsic muscle failure, intrinsic overaction and muscle imbalance.

Investigation

Most cases of pes cavus when presenting should be investigated further especially if the deformity is unilateral.

FAMILY HISTORY

If there is a strong family history towards pes cavus further investigation is probably unnecessary.

NEUROLOGICAL EXAMINATION

A full neurological examination is required to detect evidence of generalised neurological disease or spinal disease.

SPINAL X-RAY

This may show laminal defects ranging from a simple split in a spinous process to partial absence of the lamina; such findings are highly suggestive of the presence of spinal dysraphism. Diastematomyelia may also be suspected. If there are any suspicious areas at all in the plain x-ray, myelography is indicated. Air myelography will often yield almost as much information as contrast media. If a myelogram illustrates a space-occupying lesion or a low conus, a good case can be made out for exploratory laminectomy, especially in cases of unilateral pes cavus.

However it should be noted that any surgical treatment on the back is unlikely to improve the orthopaedic condition present at that time although it may prevent progression. Since the progressive changes only occur during growth it may be wise to accept the presence of spinal dysraphism in a child near maturity and to treat the orthopaedic manifestations on their merit. On the other hand if there is urinary incontinence in addition to pes cavus, neurosurgical exploration will be mandatory.

Clinical features and management

There are various associated deformities which may be present with the cavus deformity and these will often determine the symptoms and the treatment required. These include varus of the hindfoot; equinus (there may be true equinus deformity at the ankle or a midfoot equinus due to dropping of the forefoot); adductus; and clawing of the toes. With time, secondary changes occur—the tread becomes thin and calloused and corns develop over the rigid claw toes. The presenting problem can be considered under four headings.

Footwear. Because the foot is usually short, broad, and tall it is difficult to obtain properly fitting footwear. Even when this is found wear of the sole and heel is often uneven and there is distortion of the upper due to the varus deformity of the hindfoot. In mild cases, simply fitting oversized shoes is acceptable whereas at other times specially made surgical shoes will be required. Sometimes boots are more serviceable than shoes.

Forefoot problems. The main problem in the forefoot is metatarsalgia due to the steep angle of the metatarsals which soon cause thinning and callusing of the tread. An outside metatarsal bar may give relief in mild cases although, in general, a well made metatarsal insole with a firm central dome is more likely to be helpful. The calluses require regular chiropody so that they do not become too hard and thick.

Toes. If the toes are rigidly clawed it is difficult to obtain shoes with sufficient room in the toecap and corns are the inevitable result. The only conservative measure of any value is the provision of shoes with sufficient room to accommodate the toes.

Ankle. Many adolescents present with recurrent sprains of the ankle. The varus and the adductus components of the deformity are responsible for initiating inversion strains and these may be helped by the provision of boots or by prescribing an outside float on the heel.

Surgery of pes cavus

It is difficult to lay down the indications for surgery as these will vary with the cause, the severity of the deformity, and the age of the patient. The important thing is to define the problem and to select a procedure which is likely to solve that problem. A wide variety of procedures exist but most are designed to correct one or other aspect rather than restore the foot to normal. In general a number of soft tissue procedures are available in childhood before the deformities are fixed and most bone operations are reserved until maturity. A difficult decision arises when the child presents not because he has any symptoms but simply because his parents are unable to find footwear to fit him. Since this is likely to be a lifelong problem, a good case can often be made out for restoring the shape of the foot. The following operations can be used in selected cases.

PLANTAR RELEASE

This procedure is useful before the age of 8 years, especially if adductus is an associated feature. The operation is identical to that done in cases of club foot and should be done as an open procedure. The incision is placed high up on the medial side of the foot well away from the arch. The neurovascular bundle is isolated and the calcaneal branches divided. The operation sets out to release abductor hallucis, the plantar aponeurosis and ligaments. Occasionally it is necessary to lengthen the tibialis posterior tendon as well. A plaster cast is applied with the foot in the corrected position and retained for at least two months.

DWYER OSTEOTOMY OF THE OS CALCIS (FIGS. 4.27 & 4.28)

This operation is designed to convert a varus heel into one which is slightly valgus

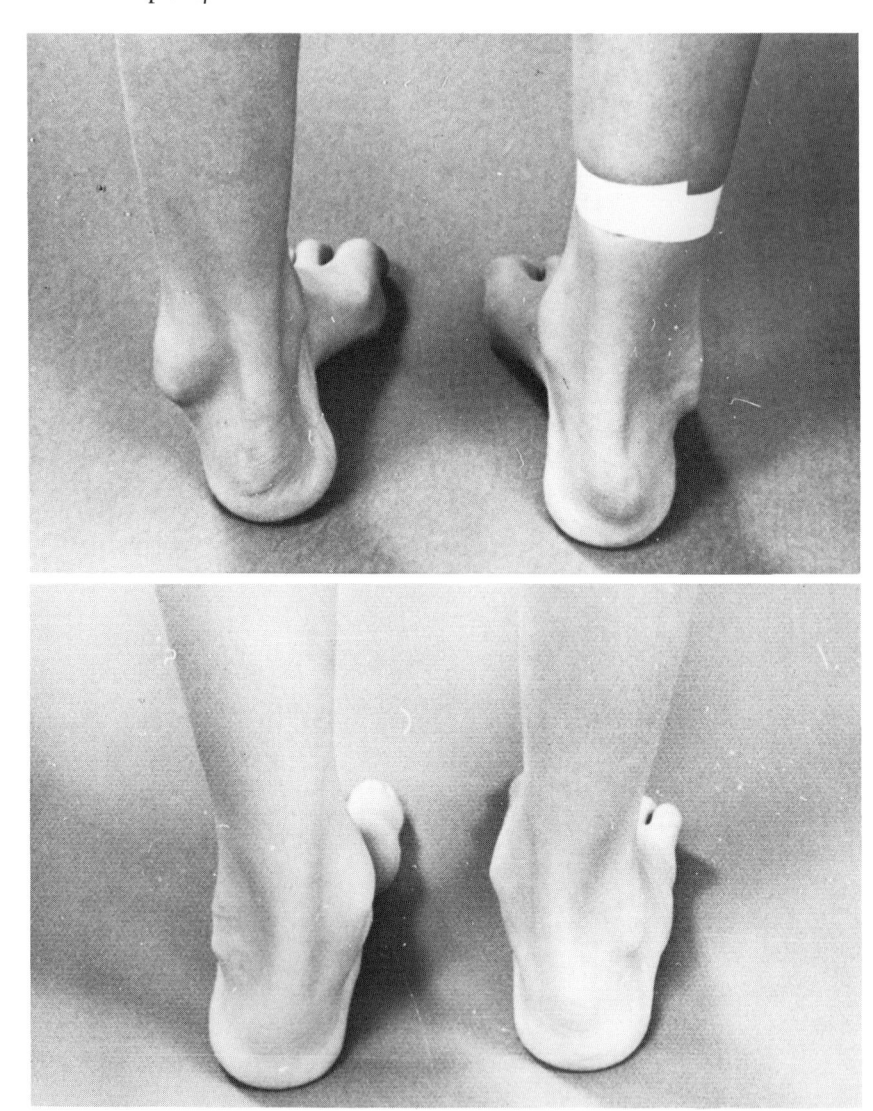

Figs. 4.27 & 4.28 Pre-operative view of a boy aged 7 years who presented with idiopathic cavo-varus deformity of the left foot. (*Bottom*) Two years following a Dwyer osteotomy of the os calcis.

and is very useful up until the age of 10 years in those who have mild cavus deformity but severe varus. Experience has shown that the foot tends to grow towards normality following operation. It is worthwhile noting however that the varus deformity must be fixed for, if it is not, the operation will produce a cavo-valgus deformity which is as bad, if not worse, than the cavo-varus it replaced.

TRANSFER OF THE TOE EXTENSORS

All the extensor tendons can be transferred to the necks of the metatarsals. This operation is useful in paralytic pes cavus. In the case of the hallux the interphalangeal joint is fused at the same time (the Robert Jones procedure).

TRIPLE ARTHRODESIS

After the age of 12 years, triple arthrodesis may be indicated for severe cavo-varus causing insuperable footwear problems. The results of triple arthrodesis are better than those obtained by midtarsal wedge resection but even so recovery after operation is often protracted. Meticulous attention to detail is required to obtain a satisfactorily shaped foot.

SURGERY OF THE TOES

Surgery designed to straighten the toes may be indicated when the deformity is severe and painful corns are present. If the toes are mobile open flexor tenotomy will often provide sufficient correction to relieve symptoms. Flexor to extensor tendon transfer is a laborious operation which produces a row of stiff toes and cannot be recommended. If the toes are already rigid, interphalangeal arthrodesis as described by Lambrinudi should be considered. Because the toes are usually fixed with intramedullary Kirschner wires, they tend to be too straight; this not only makes them look unattractive but also renders them functionless. An attempt should always be made to leave the toes slightly curved and if successfully carried out, the result will be most rewarding. Phalangeal filleting of the toes to relieve corn problems is not recommended in adolescents.

METATARSUS VARUS

Metatarsus varus is an uncommon condition which is to be distinguished from metatarsus adductus (see p. 132). Metatarsus varus is characterised by the following deformities all of which soon become fixed: forefoot adduction, forefoot supination, heel valgus, and cavus deformity of the foot. The affected child generally presents between the ages of 3 and 6 years because he distorts and destroys his shoes very rapidly (Fig. 4.29).

If recognised early, when the deformity is relatively corrigible, considerable improvement can be obtained by the operation of plantar release as described for club foot. However once the deformity becomes fixed bony operations become necessary. Before maturity osteotomy of all the metatarsals will often give sufficient correction but after maturity, triple arthrodesis is usually indicated.

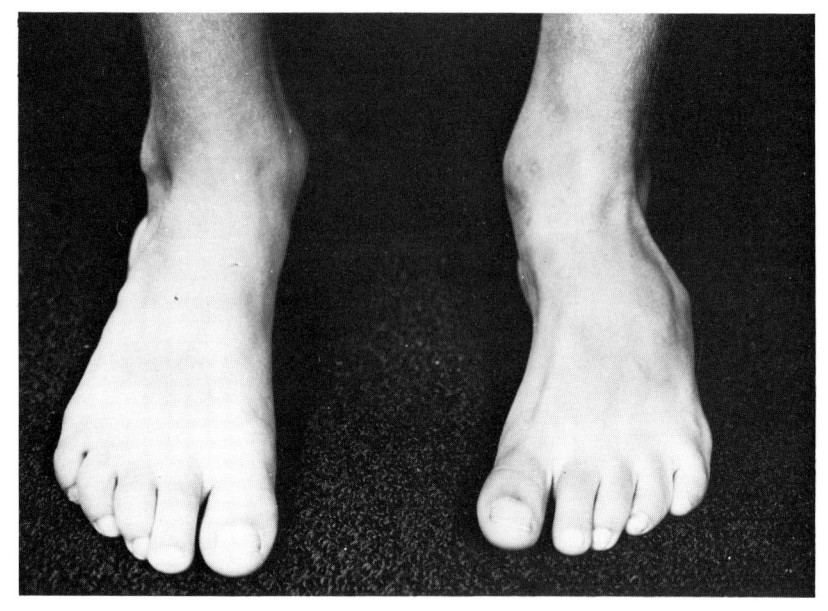

Fig. 4.29 Metatarsus varus of the left foot in a boy aged 6 years. He presented because his left shoe was worn out in a period of six weeks. Note the hooked appearance of the forefoot due to a combination of cavus and adductus.

SORE HEELS

Children commonly present between the ages of 9 and 12 years with soreness of the heels. Although it is the heel that is sore, the child often refers to the soreness being in 'the ankle'. There is generally no abnormality on examination and the child merely points to the posterior or to the plantar aspect of the heel as the site of discomfort. There may be tenderness here or in the lower inch of the tendo-Achilles.

The cause of this condition is uncertain. In the past it had been considered to be due to osteochondritis of the apophysis of the calcaneus. X-rays may show fragmentation of this apophysis but such an appearance is a common normal feature, present also in children who have no complaints of heel soreness. Thus, radiographs do not definitely establish the diagnosis even if a degree of osteochondritis is the responsible pathology. It may be that the condition is due to inflammation in a bursa adjacent to the tendo-Achilles.

In general it is sufficient to reassure the child and parents that this condition will get better with the passage of time. The higher the heel of the shoe the more comfortable are affected children and some are prepared to choose higher heels or have a heel raise whilst they await recovery.

DEFORMITIES OF THE LESSER TOES

Mallet toe, hammer toe, claw toe and curly toe

DEFINITIONS (FIGS. 4.30 & 4.31)

Mallet toes have flexion deformity of the terminal interphalangeal joint. Hammer toes have flexion deformity of the proximal interphalangeal joint. Claw toes have hyperextension at the metatarsophalangeal joint and flexion deformity at the proximal and frequently the distal interphalangeal joints. The term curly toe implies that the affected digit has a varus deformity so that it comes to lie beneath its medial neighbour (Figs. 4.32 & 4.33). Some patients present because the second toes tend to lie higher on the dorsum of the foot than do the other digits. In these circumstances the third toe will be found to be curly and responsible for the deformity of the second toe.

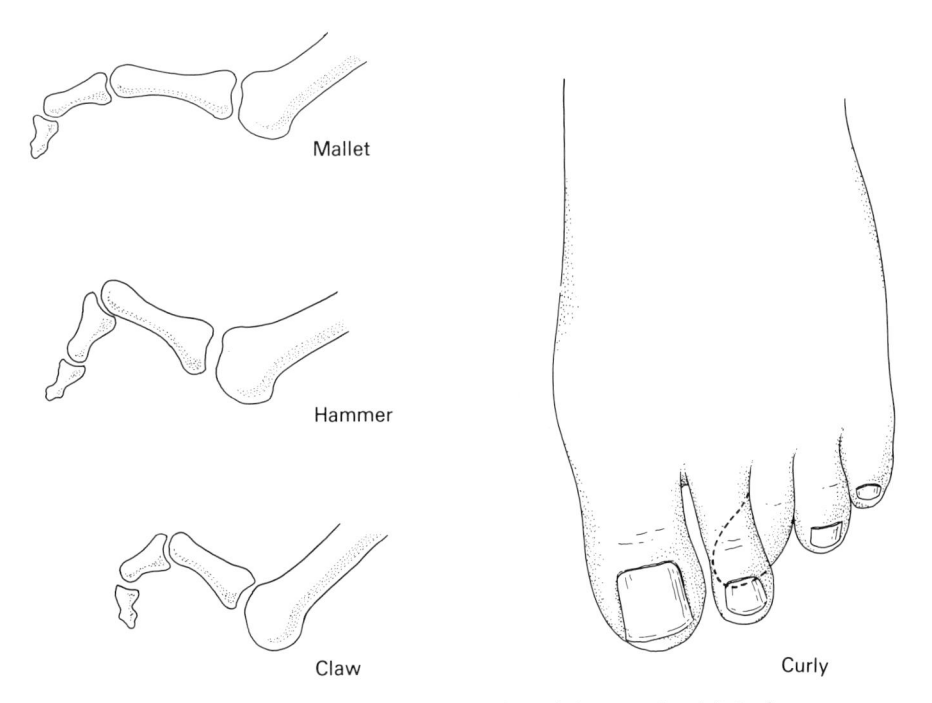

Mallet

Hammer

Claw

Curly

Figs. 4.30 & 4.31 The nomenclature of toe deformity. (*Right*) Curly toe.

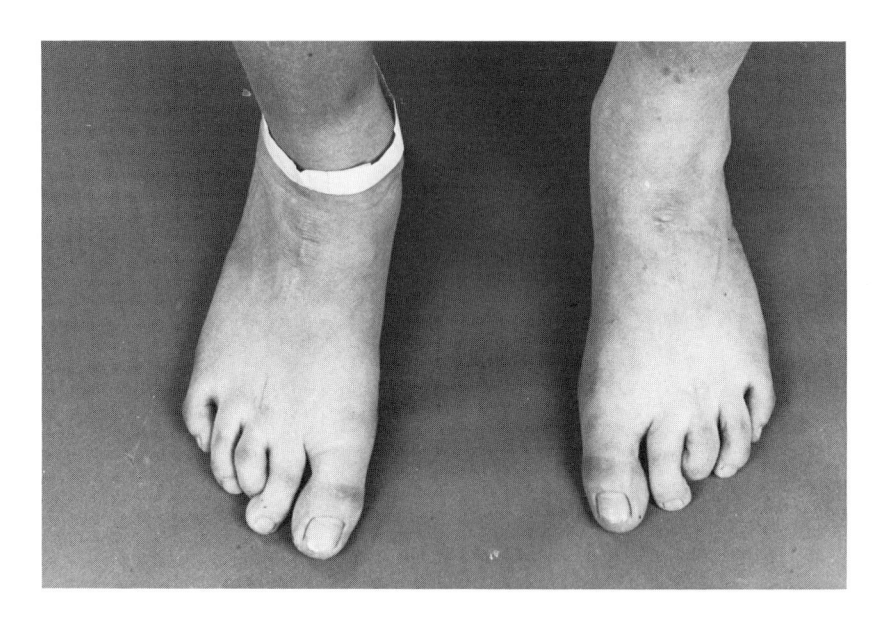

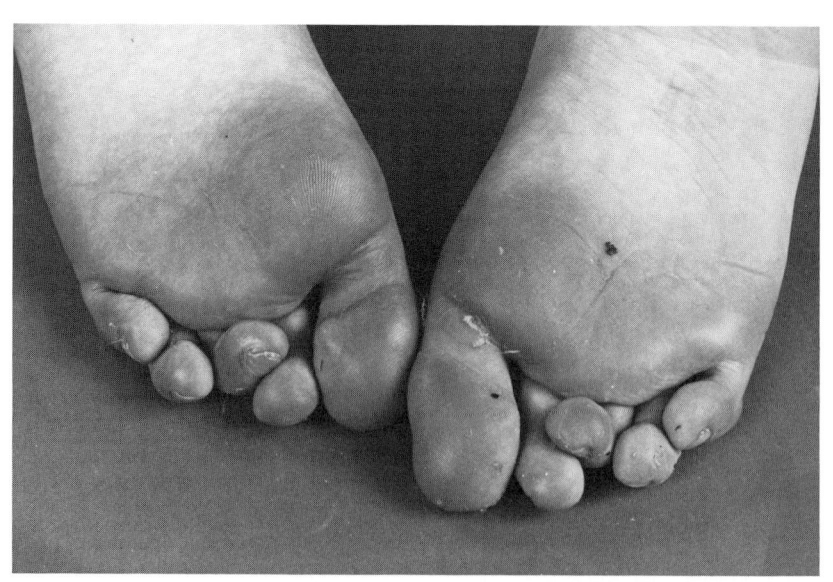

Figs. 4.32 & 4.33 The third (and fourth) toes are curly and underlie the digit lying medial to them. Flexor tenotomy of each third toe is the appropriate management. (*Bottom*) View from underside.

MANAGEMENT

Hammer and curly toes are best ignored until the patient is at least 3 years old. This allows for spontaneous correction of minor degrees of deformity. Over the age of 3 years a decision can usually be made as to whether the deformity is likely to be troublesome later in life. Minor degrees of hammer toe deformity may be ignored, particularly in boys. Curly toes are likely to cause symptoms and embarrassment and should always be corrected surgically.

Division of the long flexor tendons will generally correct the deformity of hammer and curly toes. That this surgery will be effective in correcting hammer deformity should be confirmed clinically by flexing the metatarsophalangeal joint and observing that the interphalangeal joints will then fully extend.

The surgery is performed under general anaesthesia. Through a longitudinal incision in the midline of the plantar aspect of the proximal phalanx of the affected toe, the long and short flexor tendons are exposed and divided. Usually the deformity is then fully corrected. If there is some residual flexion deformity at the proximal interphalangeal joint or varus deformity at this joint then plantar capsulotomy of the joint will correct any residual deformity. Two interrupted sutures of plain catgut close the skin.

Overlapping or cocked up fifth toe

There is a common group of congenital anomalies in which the fifth toe is hyperextended at the metatarsophalangeal joint so that it lies on a more dorsal plane than the other digits. In addition the toe is smaller than is normal for the fifth toe and may have a varus deformity so that it lies on the dorsum of the fourth toe.

Symptoms do not invariably follow such a deformity (particularly in men), but it is generally best to correct this deformity in childhood because of the cosmetic impairment and the possibility of symptoms. Although this deformity looks as if it would be readily susceptible to correction there is an incidence of failure following all forms of surgical correction, and this should therefore be carefully planned and precisely executed. Either the Butler or the Holdsworth procedures are preferred.

BUTLER PROCEDURE

A racket-shaped incision is made to encircle the base of the toe with the racket handle on the plantar aspect in the long axis of the foot. All the ligaments of the metatarsophalangeal joint of the toe are then divided, as is the extensor tendon. The toe is then displaced in a plantar direction so that it occupies the position of the racket handle. The wound is then closed in such a way that it becomes the shape of a racket but with the handle on the dorsum of the foot.

HOLDSWORTH PROCEDURE

This procedure is an advancement flap. The little toe forms the apex of the flap to be advanced onto the plantar aspect of the foot and the plantar flap is swung onto the dorsum of the foot to replace it. The extensor tendon and medial and lateral collateral ligaments are divided.

Whether the Butler or the Holdsworth procedure is performed it is wise to place a suture through the pulp of the little toe suturing it to the plantar aspect of the foot in the region of the fourth metatarsal head. One is not then dependent on post-operative bandaging for the maintenance of an appropriate posture for the toe.

THE KNEE

OSTEOCHONDRITIS DISSECANS AND ABNORMALITIES OF OSSIFICATION OF THE LOWER FEMORAL EPIPHYSIS

Osteochondritis dissecans most commonly presents in adolescence and young adult life and is therefore discussed in greater detail in Chapter 5. The condition rarely presents under the age of 10 years. Children in this younger age group commonly injure their knees and this leads to an x-ray which shows irregularity of ossification which resembles osteochondritis dissecans. Such abnormalities may take varying forms. There may be some roughening of the margin of the lower femoral epiphysis with small foci of calcification immediately beyond the roughened edge. There may be large localised marginal indentations, best seen in an intercondylar view and generally situated at the point of greatest convexity of either femoral condyle rather than in relationship to the intercondylar notch. An independent island of calcification or ossification may lie within the indentation (Fig. 4.34). Such abnormalities are more common in the lateral condyle and in boys; indeed the majority of boys between the ages of 3 and 13 years show such irregularities. It is assumed that these radiological appearances are due to irregularity in the process of cartilage proliferation and that provisional calcification is appearing outside the main mass of calcified cartilage. As ossification continues these irregularities disappear spontaneously. If there is doubt as to whether a lesion represents true osteochondritis dissecans then serial radiographs will clarify the diagnosis.

QUADRICEPS CONTRACTURE

Quadriceps contracture is not infrequently seen in orthopaedic practice and patients present in a variety of ways. At birth, they may present with a stiff extended knee, congenital recurvatum, or congenital dislocations. In the first few

The Child 173

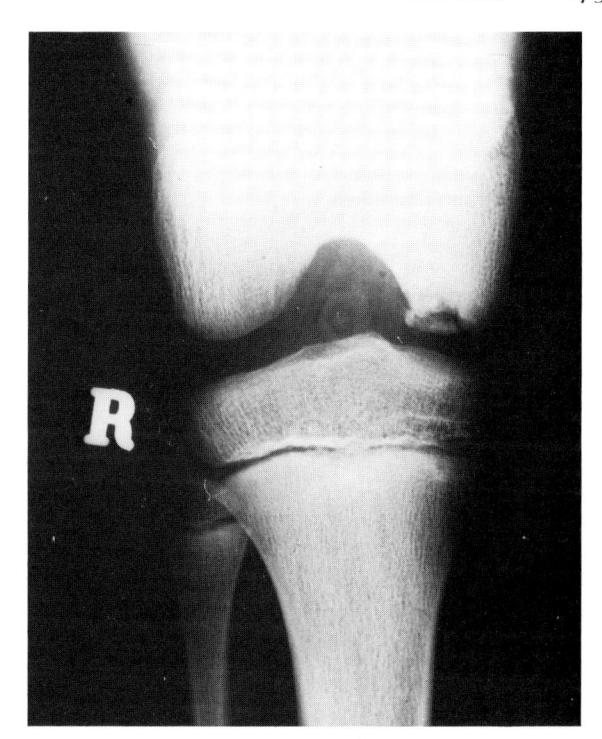

Fig. 4.34 Irregular ossification simulating osteochondritis dissecans in a boy aged 8 years. There is a notch on the convexity of the medial femoral condyle best seen in this intercondylar view. It contains an independent area of ossification.

years after birth they may present as progressive loss of knee motion and in later childhood with habitual dislocation of the patella.

Aetiology

No single cause has yet been found and it seems likely that there is more than one factor. In those seen at birth, the lesion may be similar to the contractures seen in sternomastoid torticollis, in club foot, or a form of localised arthrogryposis. The contractures which appear in later years are difficult to explain on a congenital basis and some of these have been shown to be due to repeated intramuscular injections of antibiotics. However, in some of the cases in this group, there are abnormal bands and connections in the tendinous insertion of the quadriceps which seem to be undoubtedly of congenital origin. Late presentation in these cases may be caused by unequal growth of muscle and bone, so that the effect on the knee is not apparent for a number of years. The three groups can now be considered.

STIFF KNEES

These children present with a limited range of knee flexion which, if it is observed over a period, is found to be progressive. Different parts of the quadriceps may be implicated in different cases. Hnevkovsky described involvement of the vastus intermedius in most of his cases but this has not been our experience. The type of quadricepsplasty carried out in these cases is similar to that used in the next group.

HABITUAL DISLOCATION OF THE PATELLA

This condition is described in more detail in Chapter 5. Suffice it to say that these children present at a later age than the previous group and although it is tempting to postulate that the untreated stiff knee may eventually move by dislocation of the patella, we have not been able to observe this transition in clinical practice.

ARTHROGRYPOTIC QUADRICEPS CONTRACTURE

Involvement of the knee is common in arthrogryposis and those which are stiff in extension have a combination of fibrous adherence of the patella to the front of the femur and contracture of the rectus femoris. A quadricepsplasty consists of dissecting the patella away from the femur and lengthening the rectus such that the joint can be bent to a right angle. The quadriceps is repaired in this position. It is important that these cases be treated in the first year of life and preferably in the first six months, for secondary changes occur in the otherwise unaffected structures.

DISCOID MENISCUS

This term is employed to describe an abnormality of the lateral (and sometimes of the medial) meniscus (Fig. 4.35).

The abnormal meniscus is generally much thicker than normal, it covers the whole tibial plateau, and may have an abnormal posterior attachment to the medial femoral condyle. It is not attached to the tibia posteriorly. There is no satisfactory embryological explanation for this condition as at no stage in development does the meniscus resemble a discoid meniscus.

Clinical Features

The child generally presents over the age of 5 years because of a loud snap arising in the knee or because of instability or pain on the outside of the knee. Adolescents and young adults may present with an effusion in the knee and locking episodes secondary to a tear in the discoid cartilage.

As the knee is actively or passively extended, the examiner may feel a sudden movement of the edge of the lateral cartilage or of the tibia in relationship to the femur. This movement may also be seen and may be accompanied by an audible

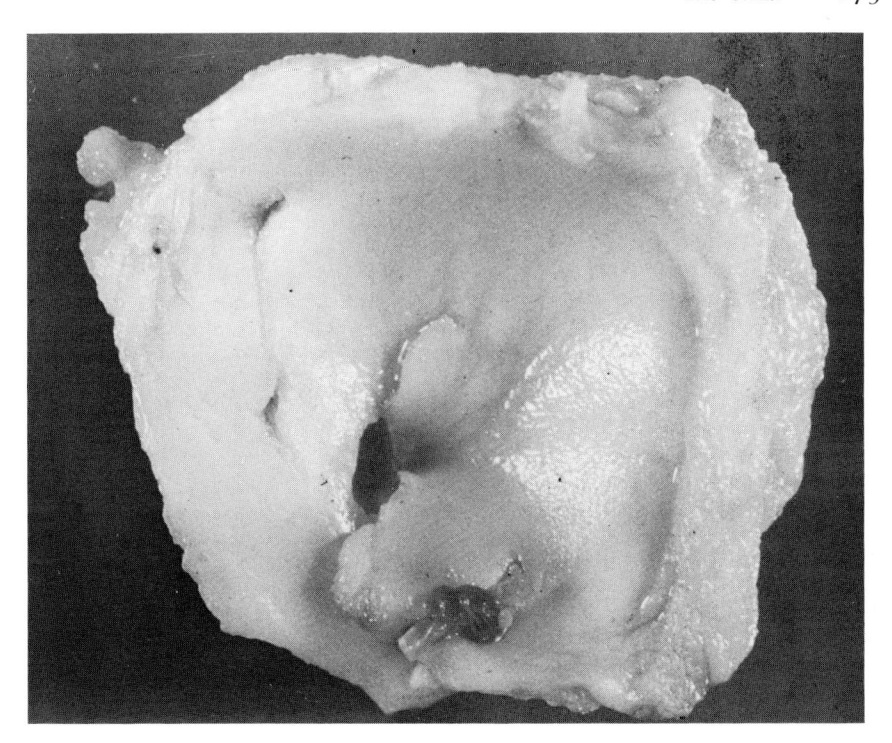

Fig. 4.35 Torn discoid lateral meniscus which had been removed from a child aged 5 years. There is a central perforation from which a tear extends for one-third of the distance to the mid-lateral periphery of the meniscus (upwards on this illustration). A second tear is seen to the left of the central tear. Discoid menisci are frequently thicker than this example.

'snap'. There may be tenderness on the lateral joint line and an effusion in the joint. X-rays may show a slight increase in the lateral joint space.

Management

In the typical case, with a visible, audible and palpable snap, the diagnosis can be readily made. Some children present with less characteristic symptoms and may require examination on a number of occasions. Arthroscopy can be used if the diagnosis is in doubt.

The discoid cartilage is removed through an antero-lateral approach. Care is taken to divide the posterior femoral attachment of the cartilage.

Children withstand meniscectomy very well indeed. There is little postoperative pain and swelling and the quadriceps muscles rapidly regain their function and bulk. Thus physiotherapy is not necessary. The child can be discharged home on crutches on the fourth post-operative day and commences knee flexion exercises at 7–10 days.

POPLITEAL CYST (Synonyms: Baker's cyst, semimembranosus bursa)

Children frequently develop a cystic swelling in the popliteal fossa. It is most common under the age of 8 years and boys are more frequently affected than girls. The majority of these cysts are filled with synovial fluid and are lined by synovial tissue. They are generally assumed to represent a bursa which communicates with the joint. However a few of these cysts are filled with clear jelly and resemble ganglia.

The patient presents because the swelling has been noted. Usually the condition is unilateral. On examination there is a cystic translucent swelling in the popliteal fossa lying just below the flexion crease of the knee.

Popliteal cysts will invariably resorb spontaneously. The patient and parents are told that the lump will be there for up to two years and during this period it will vary in size. It may be necessary to see the child from time to time to reassure the parents that there is no indication for surgery. An added indication for such a conservative approach is that operative removal of such cysts is associated with a high recurrence rate.

On the rare occasion when a popliteal cyst progressively enlarges, then biopsy should be performed to exclude tumour.

THE HIP

THE LATE-PRESENTING CONGENITALLY DISLOCATED HIP

The early management of this condition has been discussed in Chapters 2 and 3. Over the age of 2 years open reduction is preferred as it is the least traumatic means by which reduction can be achieved. A small percentage of children may be treated by closed means; that is those hips which, when examined under anaesthesia prior to surgery, readily reduce and are stable.

Operative reduction need not be preceded by preliminary traction. If, at operation, it is found that the femoral head does not fall readily into the socket, then femoral shortening is performed in addition.

Those children who present towards the age of 5 years will almost certainly require femoral shortening and some will require the Klisic procedure which is described in the following paragraphs.

Management between the ages of five years and the onset of puberty

In this age group it is generally necessary to perform the Klisic procedure (Figs. 4.36 & 4.37). This involves open reduction, femoral shortening and Chiari osteotomy. If, at operation, the acetabulum is found to be adequate and the

The Child 177

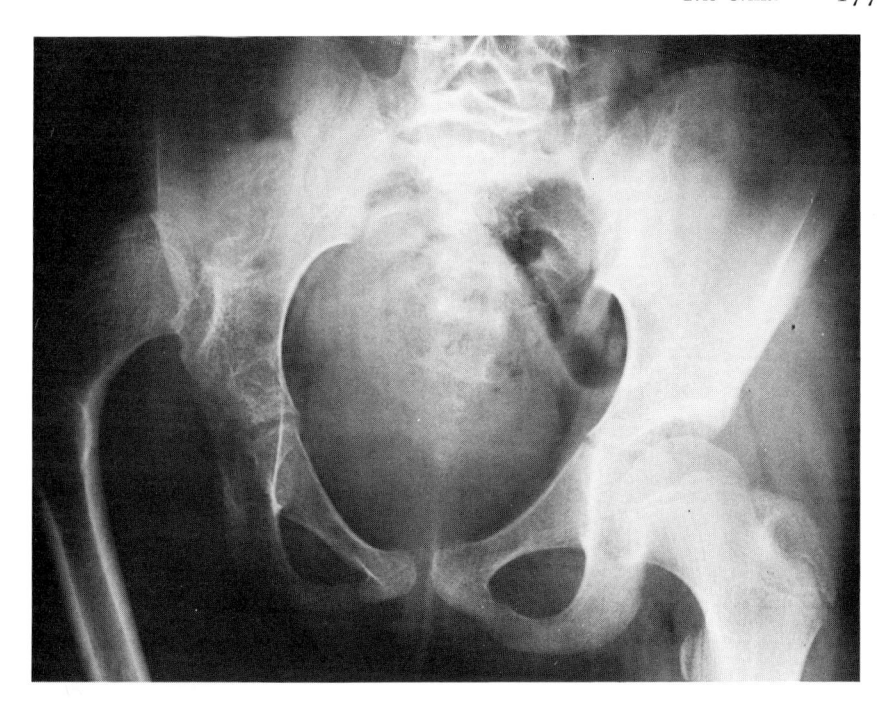

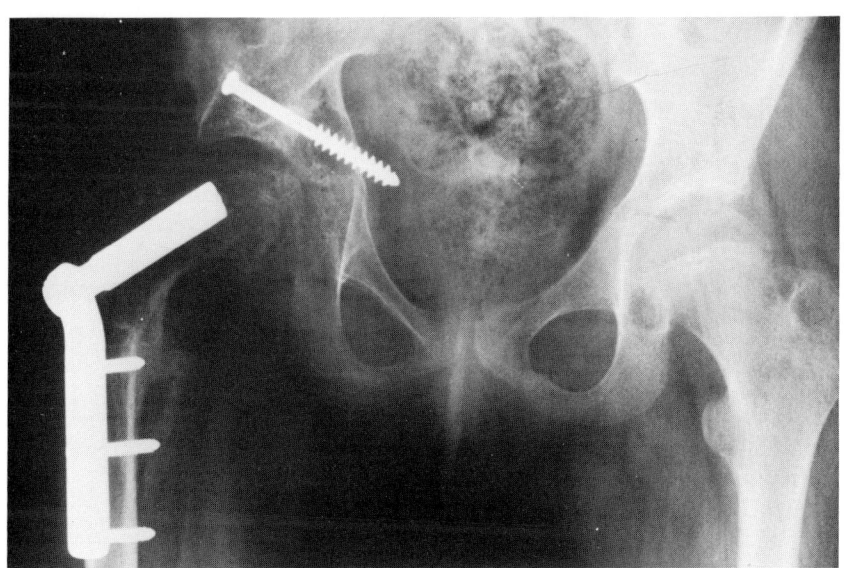

Figs. 4.36 & 4.37 A–P x-ray of the pelvis of a 9-year-old Turkish child who presented with an untreated right CDH. (*Bottom*) The appearances one year following one-stage open reduction, femoral shortening plus de-rotation and Chiari osteotomy. She now has a nearly full range of motion. There is a residual length discrepancy of $1\frac{1}{2}$ inches (4 cm) to be managed by left lower femoral growth plate arrest.

reduction is stable, then Chiari osteotomy is deferred; it can always be performed later.

In this age group, unilateral dislocation is invariably treated as the limp resulting from hip instability and leg length inequality is unacceptable. Bilateral dislocations will be treated in the younger children of this age group—the decision here is difficult and depends on the degree of femoral and acetabular dysplasia, the upward displacement of the femoral heads, the degree of limp present, the maturity of the child, and the attitude of the child and the parents to surgery.

THE SURGICAL MANAGEMENT OF CONGENITAL HIP DISLOCATION

Primary surgery—operative reduction of the dislocated hip

The *indications* for this procedure have been considered in the preceding paragraphs and on p. 40. They may be summarised as, firstly, failure to achieve stable reduction—assessed by examination under anaesthesia after a period of coronal traction. Secondly, children, generally older than 2 years of age, with high-lying femoral heads. In these circumstances closed reduction will either fail or will be accompanied by undue pressure on the femoral head. Primary open reduction without preliminary traction, is performed and, if reduction does not readily occur, then femoral shortening is carried out. Thirdly, children with arthrogrypotic and teratological hip dislocation.

TECHNIQUE OF OPERATIVE REDUCTION

The procedure is performed through an anterior Smith–Petersen approach but using a straight oblique skin incision (as described by Salter for innominate osteotomy). The capsule is opened transversely and the interior of the joint is inspected to visualise the obstacles to reduction of the hip. Each of these obstacles is removed in turn.

OBSTACLES TO REDUCTION

Ligamentum teres—this is the first thing seen on opening the joint. It is long, wide and thick and is excised completely. The ligament, if followed medially, provides a valuable guide to the true acetabulum.

Pulvinar—the fat pad is often enlarged and fills the floor of the true acetabulum.

Transverse ligament—it is important to excise or divide this ligament to allow the femoral head to descend under the limbus.

Limbus—this is rarely an obstacle to reduction after the other barriers have been removed. There is never need to excise the limbus, indeed excision is detrimental to the stability of reduction and to the future development of the acetabular margin.

After each of the obstacles has been removed, if easy reduction is still not possible, open adductor tenotomy can be performed; however, if reduction remains difficult, then femoral shortening is indicated.

Closure—reduction is usually most stable in some flexion, abduction and internal rotation. Stability can be increased if the supero-lateral part of the capsule is sutured to the limbus using a heavy silk mattress stitch. This obliterates the false acetabulum. The skin is closed with an absorbable subcuticular suture and a double hip spica applied.

After-care—following open reduction the period of immobilisation is the same as for closed reduction.

Secondary procedures

SALTER INNOMINATE OSTEOTOMY (FIGS. 4.38 & 4.39)

Indications. The procedure is performed for acetabular dysplasia which is not improving. This osteotomy should not be performed at the same time as open reduction and there are several reasons for this. Experience has shown that there is a much higher incidence of complications if the two procedures are performed together. Moreover, since the acetabulum has a tremendous potential for development, early osteotomy may well be unnecessary in most cases.

Prerequisites for the procedure are that the child is between 3 years and 10 years old, and that radiographs (both in the neutral position and in full abduction of the hip) demonstrate that the hip is concentrically reduced in the acetabulum.

Following the final removal of the cast, after closed or open reduction of the hip, the child is allowed to mobilise and radiographs are taken, initially at four-monthly and later at six-monthly intervals. The acetabular dysplasia, whatever its degree, generally improves once the dislocation has been reduced. Even gross degree of acetabular dysplasia may slowly revert to near normal and whilst the dysplasia is improving there is no need for surgical intervention; if improvement ceases and the acetabulum does not look normal then the osteotomy is performed. If the hips start to subluxate and acetabular dysplasia is present then osteotomy is performed.

FEMORAL DEROTATION OSTEOTOMY

This procedure is used as primary treatment of subluxation of the hip over the age of one year, and for late subluxation after reduction of a dislocated hip.

Before this operation is performed for either of the above indications it must be demonstrated that concentric reduction of the hip is obtained by placing the leg in a position of internal rotation. If there is doubt as to whether this reduction is

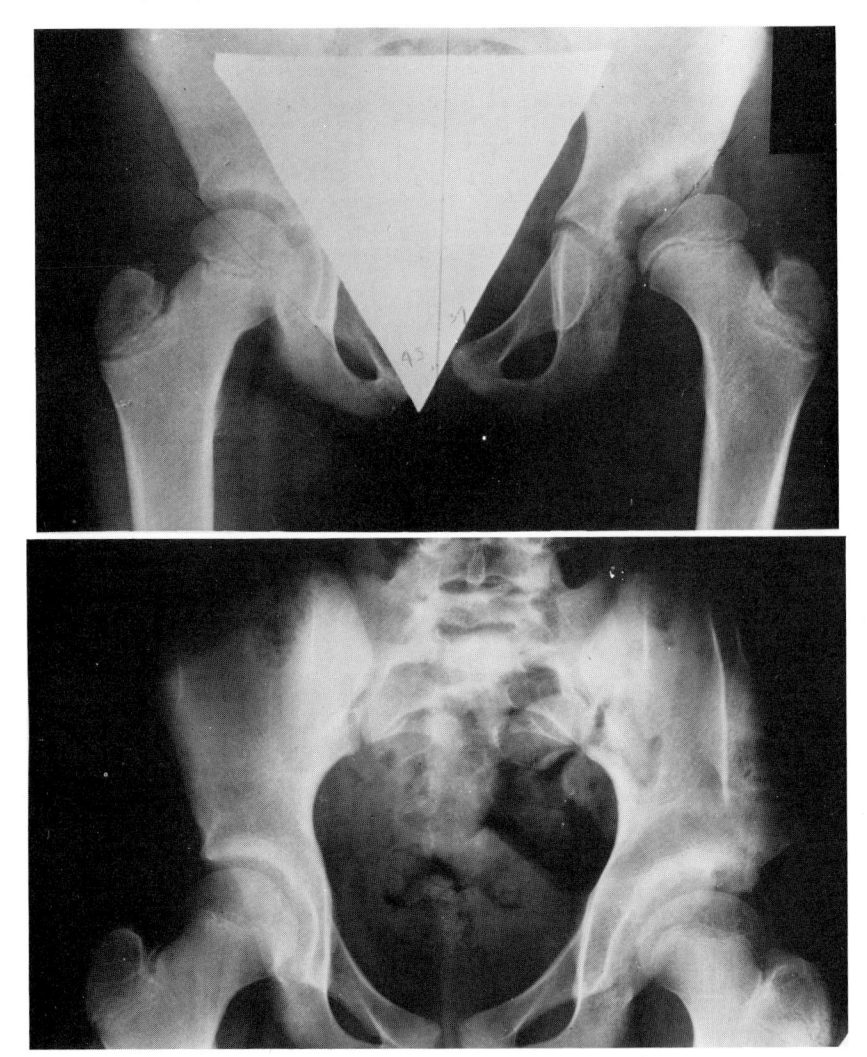

Figs. 4.38 & 4.39 Antero-posterior x-ray of the pelvis of a girl aged 5 years who had been treated, at the age of 18 months for a left CDH. The acetabulum has not developed into the normal cup shape and is rather saucer shaped. There is upward and lateral displacement of the femoral head. (*Bottom*) The radiological appearance three years after left Salter innominate osteotomy.

concentric then arthrography is performed. There must be a range of internal rotation of at least 45° and frequently the range approaches 90°.

The subluxated hip which has these prerequisites and indications for femoral osteotomy may also have a dysplastic acetabulum. In these circumstances, innominate osteotomy plus capsular reefing is a preferable alternative to femoral osteotomy, as this will attend to both problems at the same time.

It is to be noted in the above description that varus is not imparted at the osteotomy site as this displacement leads to prominence of the greater trochanter, widening of the perineum and, in unilateral dislocation, to shortening of the leg.

Salvage procedures

SHELF ARTHROPLASTY (FIG. 4.40)

This procedure is indicated for the correction of acetabular dysplasia between the ages of 12 and 20 years. Slight subluxation of the hip is not a contraindication. Shelf arthroplasty is not performed if x-rays show that there are arthritic changes.

Most of the children requiring this procedure complain of aching about the hip joint after activity; physical examination discloses that pain can be produced by stressing the joint.

Technique. An anterior Smith–Petersen exposure is made. A full thickness iliac graft is taken in such a way that the iliac crest is left intact. This graft is approximately $1\frac{1}{4}$ inches in width along the edge which is to be driven into the pelvis, fans out to approximately $1\frac{1}{2}$ inches in width and is over $1\frac{1}{2}$ inches in length. The outer lip of the acetabulum is carefully identified and a slot constructed to receive the graft. This slot must be positioned so that the graft lies immediately against the capsule overlying the uncovered portion of the femoral head and between the capsule and the reflected head of rectus femoris. The concave pelvic surface of the graft is directed distally and the graft hammered into the prepared slot. Partial fracturing of the outer table of the ilium enables the slot

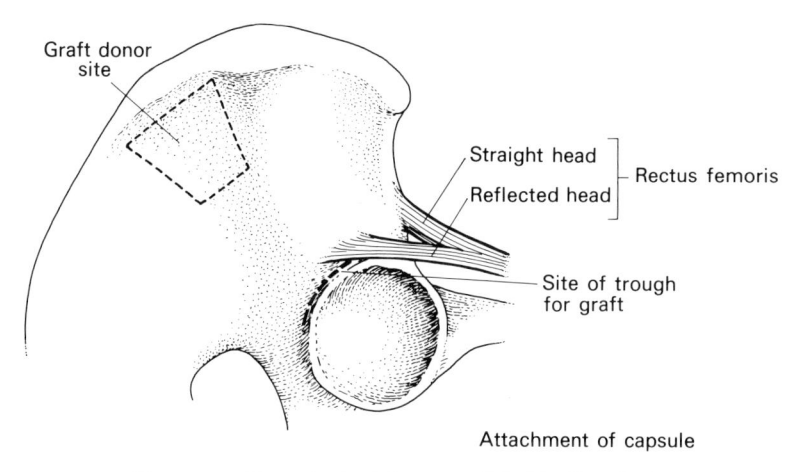

Fig. 4.40 The principal features of shelf arthroplasty.

to be sprung open to receive the graft which is thus securely fixed to the pelvis so that internal and external fixation are unnecessary. Skin traction is applied for ten days when the patient is allowed up on crutches; weight-bearing on the affected leg is not allowed for eight weeks.

CHIARI PELVIC OSTEOTOMY (FIGS. 4.41 & 4.42)

In childhood and adolescence the Chiari osteotomy should be regarded as a salvage procedure when other types of operation are contraindicated. The operation is most useful when a hip has already been subjected to other procedures which have failed to give stability. It is therefore used in the group under 10 years of age for this purpose. Over the age of 10 years there is a small group where the hip is eccentric and dysplastic and may even be arthritic. In these circumstances the Chiari osteotomy will often produce a useful hip which will last for many years.

The femoral head must lie lower than the level of the sacro-iliac joint so that an oblique osteotomy can be performed which passes medially through the pelvis and enters the inner table of the ilium below the level of the sacro-iliac joint. If Shelf arthroplasty can be performed then it is to be preferred to the Chiari procedure as the latter generally produces gluteal weakness and an aggravated limp.

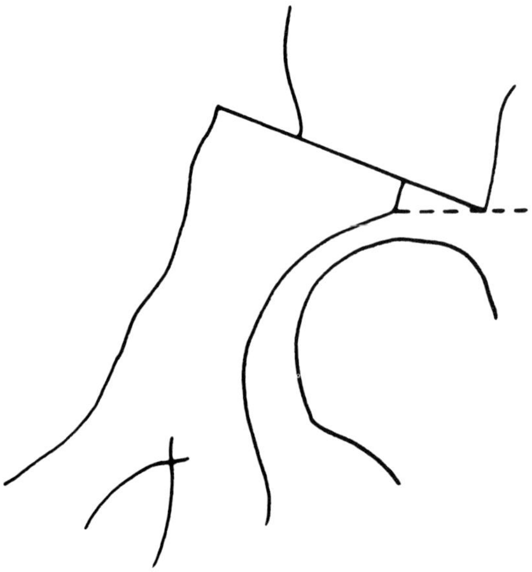

Fig. 4.41 The Chiari osteotomy. Note that the line of the osteotomy must slope gently upwards to emerge just below the sacro-iliac joint. If the hip is too high to allow this, the osteotomy is not indicated.

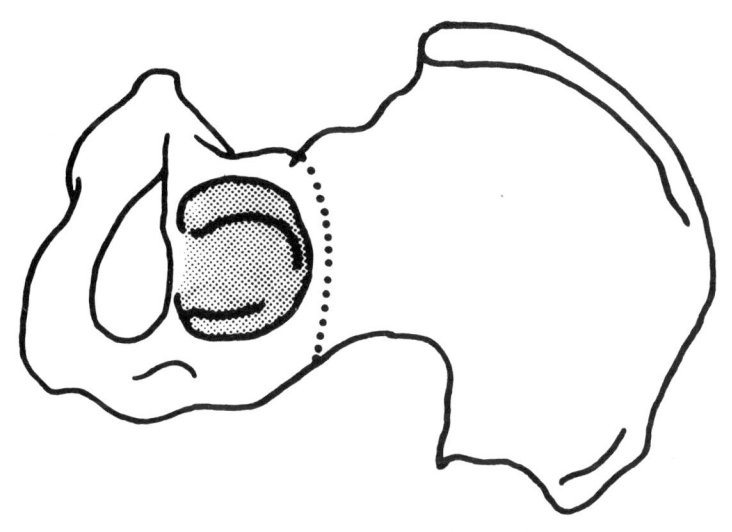

Fig. 4.42 Seen from the side, the osteotomy should have a slight curve concave distally.

ARTHRODESIS OF THE HIP JOINT

Arthrodesis may be indicated when there is painful unilateral hip disease, particularly when the patient is a boy. Precise indications cannot be given, but in general there will be one or more of the following features present: gross degenerative changes in the hip joint; a femoral head which lies high on wing of the ilium; or gross deformation of the upper end of the femur. These abnormalities may force the surgeon to perform arthrodesis on the worst hip in painful bilateral hip dislocation knowing that an arthroplasty will eventually be needed on the opposite side. Arthrodesis is still the only operation of the hip which carries a life long guarantee of pain relief and stability.

TOTAL HIP REPLACEMENT

This procedure should rarely be performed in the second decade of life. The stresses which young people place on their hip joints are in general too great to be withstood for long by any form of hip replacement and loosening of one or both components of the prosthesis is almost inevitable. Furthermore, the situation is difficult to salvage should infection or other complications occur. These considerations should lead the surgeon to consider continued conservative management or more conservative surgery rather than perform hip replacement. Precise indications for hip replacement cannot be given here as they depend on a number of factors which cannot be quantitated—the degree of pain, the degree of femoral and acetabular dysplasia, and the attitude of the child and parents to surgery. If replacement surgery is undertaken then it may be necessary to affix the excised femoral head to the pelvis to provide adequate bone stock.

JOINT RE-SURFACING

This procedure offers the advantages of total hip replacement but enables the surgeon to perform a second procedure (total hip replacement) should late complications ensue. It is too early to give precise indications for this operation.

PERTHES' DISEASE

Perthes' disease is a condition characterised by idiopathic avascular necrosis of the whole or portion of the femoral head followed by re-vascularisation. It is one of a group of conditions loosely grouped together under the name 'osteochondritis juvenilis'. These conditions are characterised by similar avascular changes with a specific age and sex incidence. Perthes' disease is most common in boys between the ages of 4 and 10 years.

Aetiology

The fundamental cause of this condition remains uncertain. Whatever it is it mediates its effect by interfering with the circulation to the head of the femur. It is likely that several episodes of circulatory impairment produce the condition. Between the ages of 4 and 8 years (with individual variations) the femoral head is supplied almost exclusively by the lateral epiphyseal vessels. These vessels might be thrombosed or obliterated by trauma, or increased intrasynovial pressure due to an effusion or other insult. Children with a low birthweight are more likely to suffer from the condition and hence Perthes' disease is more common in the children of mothers who smoked in pregnancy. Delayed bone age is commonly found in association with the condition.

Incidence

The condition occurs once in 740 boys under the age of 15 years. It is five times more common in boys than in girls and is rarely seen in Negroes, Indians or Polynesians. Male infants weighing $5\frac{1}{2}$ pounds (12 kg) or less at birth are five times more likely to have Perthes' disease than male infants with a birth weight more than $8\frac{1}{2}$ pounds (18.7 kg). 17% of cases are bilateral.

Pathology

From an early stage the synovial membrane is thickened and more vascular. In particular there is an increased size of the pulvinar. Microscopy reveals that there are villi on the surface of the synovial membrane. The articular cartilage remains normal.

There is bone death followed by bone repair. *Bone death* is evidenced by death of osteocytes and coagulation of the bone marrow. The trabecula pattern and mineral content remain unaltered at this stage and therefore there is as yet no radiological change in density or trabecular structure. *Bone repair* is characterised by three factors. 1 Re-vascularisation by granulation tissue which leads to absorption of dead bone. 2 Re-ossification of increased trabecula width and bulk as a result of new bone being laid down on dead bone. This results in increased bone density. Different areas are affected at different times. 3 Absorption of dead bone which may take place over a period of years. As bone re-vascularises some dead trabeculae may be absorbed, but most act as a framework for appositional bone growth. If dead trabeculae become completely ensheathed, they present no free surface for absorption and never absorb. The new bone which forms early is woven bone which is more mouldable or plastic.

The condition affects varying portions of the head of the femur but, if only part is affected, it will be the anterior part. The physis may be affected and this may lead to premature fusion of part or whole of the epiphyseal line with resultant broadening and shortening of the femoral neck.

In more severe forms of the condition the femoral head is not well covered by the acetabulum (Fig. 4.43), either as a result of lateral extrusion of the femoral head with increased head–tear-drop distance (Fig. 4.44) or of broadening of the neck and head of the femur. There is increased vascularity of the metaphysis adjacent to the afflicted portion of the femoral head.

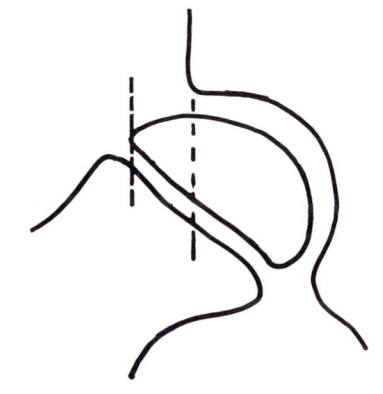

Fig. 4.43 Diagrammatic representation of the relationship of the femoral head and the acetabulum in severe forms of Perthes' disease.

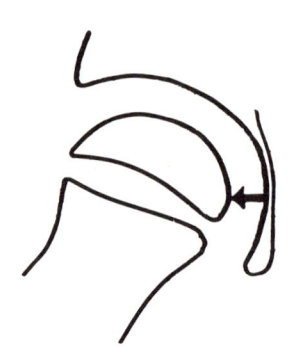

Fig. 4.44 Diagrammatic representation of lateral extrusion of the femoral head leading to increased head–tear-drop distance.

Types of Perthes' disease

It is generally recognised that the more extensive the degree of involvement of the femoral head the more likely it is that deformity will occur, in which case the radiological course will be different from that of cases with minor involvement of the femoral head. The clinical course may be the same regardless of the degree of involvement, but persistent limitation of joint motion is more commonly seen in children with extensive involvement of the femoral head.

Clinical features

The patient most commonly presents with a painless intermittent limp. Sometimes the child is reluctant to walk on rising in the morning and may limp in the earlier part of the day or after prolonged walking. Ill-defined leg aches may be described but there is seldom pain. The condition may be diagnosed during the radiological investigation of the urinary tract and is then often asymptomatic and frequently remains so. This raises the question as to whether this condition may be much more common than the incidence quoted above and these asymptomatic cases may be responsible for some cases of 'idiopathic' osteoarthritis of the hip in adults.

Physical examination in the early stages generally reveals limitation of all movements at the hip joint, flexion being the least affected. At a late stage the most characteristic findings are restriction of abduction in-flexion, adduction in-flexion, and internal rotation. The degree of limp parallels the degree to which hip motion is restricted.

Radiological features

Epiphyseal changes. Initial x-rays may be normal. The earliest change is concentric widening of a joint space. Initially this may be due to an effusion in the hip joint; later it is due to failure of ossification of the cartilaginous portion of the head, commonly the medial joint space will widen more than the superior joint space. An early sign that is occasionally seen is subchondral radiotranslucency. This occurs as a lucent line which may be seen in the lateral x-ray and indicates the extent of the involvement of the head. The translucency may be so marked as to suggest a fracture line. As diffuse atrophy occurs, the head becomes relatively increased in density. As revascularisation occurs, a true increase in density (relative to the opposite hip) occurs due to the laying down of appositional bone. When revascularisation is complete the head eventually returns to normal density. If less than half of the head is involved, normal head height is maintained and there is usually little increase in either the width of the neck or the tendency of the head to extend beyond the confines of the acetabulum (Figs. 4.45 & 4.46). If more than half of the head is involved, there is generally loss in epiphyseal height, increased width of the head and neck, and reduced covering of the head with loss of sphericity (Fig. 4.47 & 4.48).

Metaphyseal changes. There is irregularity and rarefaction of the metaphysis and the degree of this change (which is assumed to be due to increased vascularity) varies with the degree of involvement of the head and underlies the involved

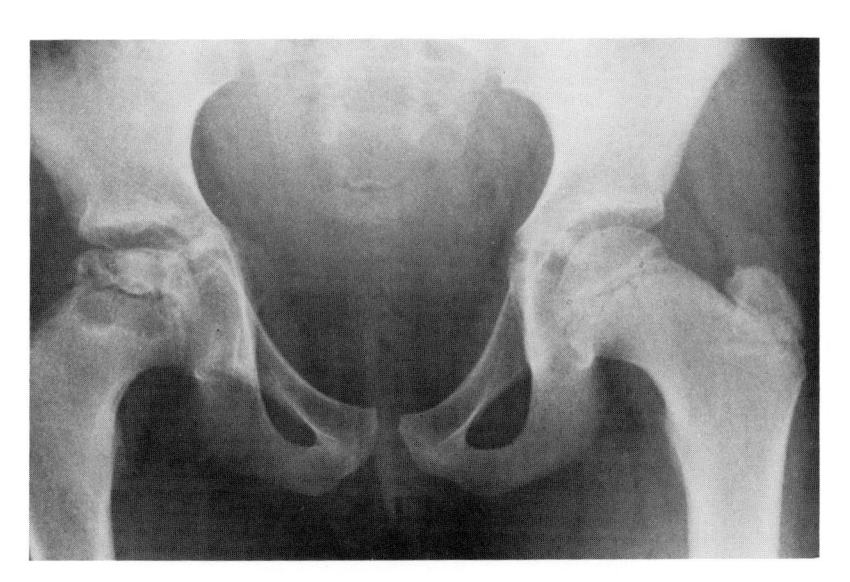

Fig. 4.45 Perthes' disease. Antero-posterior x-ray of the pelvis of a boy aged 7 who presented with a painless intermittent limp. Note the increased head–tear-drop distance and the well marked metaphyseal changes. The femoral head is only slightly more uncovered on the affected than on the unaffected hip.

188   Chapter 4

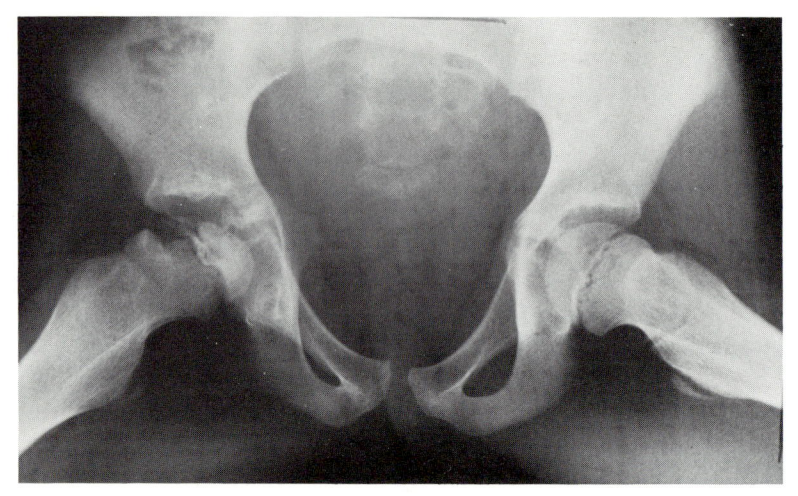

Fig. 4.46 Same patient as Fig. 4.45. The posterior half of the femoral head is unaffected by the disease which accounts for the well maintained epiphyseal height and absence of extension of the head beyond the limits of the acetabulum.

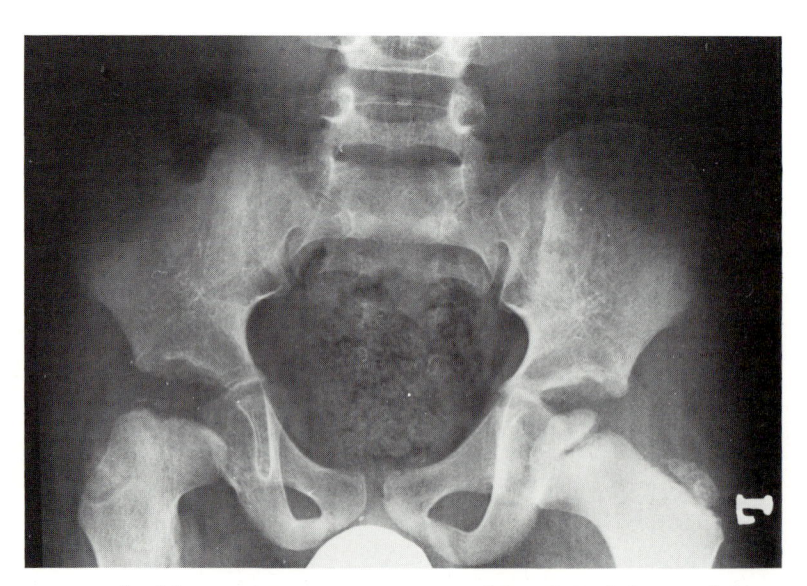

Fig. 4.47 Perthes' disease. Antero-posterior x-ray of the pelvis of a boy aged 6 years who presented with a painless intermittent limp of 10 months' duration. Note the gross resorption of bone which has occurred in the femoral head, the broad short femoral neck, and the slightly less contained head from that on the unaffected side.

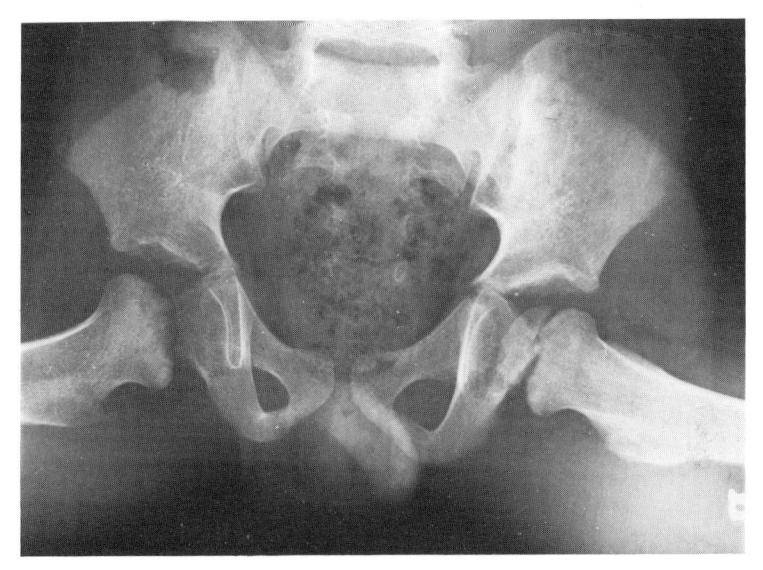

Fig. 4.48 Same patient as Fig. 4.47.

portion of the femoral head. If there is premature closure of the epiphyseal line (which occurs in the more severe forms of the condition), then shortening and widening of the femoral neck occurs.

Bone scan

Bone scanning is capable of confirming the diagnosis and indicating the extent of the avascular bone in Perthes' disease.

Differential diagnosis

The irritable hip or observation hip. This is the principal differential diagnosis in a small group of children who present before there is any radiological change. If bone scans are performed on these children, some will show avascularity of the head and yet these children may not subsequently develop Perthes' disease.

Multiple epiphyseal dysplasia. This is to be suspected in bilateral cases and a skeletal survey should be performed.

Other causes of avascular necrosis of the femoral head. Avascular necrosis may also occur in association with steroid therapy, infection, juvenile chronic arthritis, or in renal disease.

Tuberculosis of the hip. This remains the principal differential diagnosis in those countries where this condition still occurs. In tuberculosis there is narrowing rather than widening of the joint space and widespread osteoporosis.

The natural course of the disease

Long term studies of Perthes' disease show that most children who have suffered the disease lead an active life throughout their later childhood and have no symptoms in early adult life. During this period there is commonly some persistent restriction of hip motion.

At 30 years after the onset of the condition about one-third of patients have no symptoms and few physical signs, one-third have discomfort or intermittent pain in the hip, and one-third have frank osteoarthritis of the hip which requires treatment. Those patients who, at the conclusion of the pathological process, do not have a spherical head (as measured with Mose's rings on antero-posterior and lateral radiographs of the femoral head) and those who then have poorly covered heads are more likely to suffer osteoarthritis later in life. If the disease begins under 5 years of age, then a spherical head and a good long term prognosis are more likely to ensue.

Factors indicating prognosis

CLINICAL FACTORS

It has been indicated in the preceding paragraphs that those who present at a chronological age of less than 5 years have a better prognosis than those who present at a late age; those who present over the age of 10 years have a particularly poor prognosis. Children who have persisting restriction of joint motion despite adequate treatment also have a poor prognosis and, in general, girls have a worse prognosis than boys.

RADIOLOGICAL FACTORS

Uncovering of the femoral head at presentation (Fig 4.43). This uncovering is measured as the horizontal distance between a vertical line with the outer lip of the acetabulum and a second line, parallel to this, through the lateral edge of the femoral capital epiphysis. The measurement should be compared on the two sides. The greater the degree of uncovering at the onset of the condition the poorer will be the radiological result at the conclusion of the pathological process. More than about 3 mm of uncovering (in excess of that on the normal side) indicates a poor prognosis.

Catterall's assessment. Catterall has grouped patients with Perthes' disease into four groups depending upon the amount of the femoral head involvement as assessed in radiographs (Table 4.1). Those in which only the anterior half of the

Table 4.1 Catterall classification.

	Grade I	Grade II	Grade III	Grade IV
Percentage of head involved in disease process	Up to 25%	Up to 50%	Up to 75%	100%
Collapse of head	None	None or slight	Moderate	Severe
Sequestrum formation	None	Present	Present	Present
Metaphyseal change	Seldom and, if present, mild	Anterior only	Extensive	Extensive

head is involved (groups I and II) have a good prognosis; those in which the greater part of the head is involved (groups III and IV) have a poorer prognosis in that there is more likely to be permanent deformation of the hip joint. He has also drawn attention to various factors which worsen the prognosis whatever group the patient belongs to. These include lateral displacement of the head, calcification in the head lying lateral to the acetabulum, Gauge's sign, a horizontal epiphyseal line, and gross metaphyseal changes.

Catterall's assessment is of reliable prognostic value but it may not be possible to determine the grouping of some patients for a period of up to eight months after presentation.

Management

It is possible, and should always be the aim, to carry out management which causes the least interference with the patient's home and school life. Only those children who are likely to have arthritis later in life require vigorous treatment. It is therefore necessary to define those features which suggest a poor prognosis and merely to treat the symptoms in the remainder. The child with a poor prognosis presents after the age of 5 years, has uncovering of the femoral head of more than about 3 mm in excess of the uncovering on the unaffected hip, and has Catterall grade III or IV disease.

MANAGEMENT IF THE PROGNOSIS IS GOOD

It has been shown that many children who have Perthes' disease recover with an excellent radiological and clinical result when the condition has only been treated symptomatically. Symptomatic treatment involves periods of restricted activity if the child limps badly or complains of pain. At other times, a way of life is designed to avoid throwing excessive strain on the hip. The child is taken to or from the school by car and is not pressed into walking. Regular sporting activities are curtailed, although swimming is encouraged. The hip is observed clinically and radiologically at four-monthly intervals. If, despite rest at home, the child continues to limp badly or complain of pain then he is admitted to hospital and the affected leg is suspended from a frame by two springs each attached to a sling; one sling supports the thigh, the other the calf. Should the child be reluctant to keep his leg in the slings then skin traction is added. A period of ten days' treatment is usually adequate for these periods of irritability.

MANAGEMENT IF THE PROGNOSIS IS POOR

If the prognosis is considered to be poor at the onset or if features suggesting a poor prognosis develop, then treatment designed to contain the femoral head within the acetabulum is carried out. The only exception is the child who presents late and in whom it is assessed that treatment will not improve the result. In this case the patient receives only symptomatic treatment for the phases of irritability.

There is no evidence to suggest that any one method of containment gives superior results nor does logic suggest that this should be the case. Prolonged conservative methods of containment are not employed as they disturb the child's life unnecessarily at an age when activity is desirable for normal physical and emotional development.

CONSERVATIVE CONTAINMENT

Many forms of orthoses and casts have been employed to achieve containment by non-operative means; however usually these must be used for a long period and also prevent a normal active life. Broomstick casts are employed for those children who have a poor prognosis yet lack the hip mobility which is necessary for surgical containment. If the affected hip will not abduct sufficiently to allow the cast to be applied with the head properly covered, then a period on slings and springs may achieve this. Adductor tenotomy is rarely necessary. Once containment has been achieved, broomstick casts may be used as the definitive form of management but more commonly operative containment is then performed.

OPERATIVE CONTAINMENT

This approach is favoured as the child can generally resume a normal life with no further interruptions for treatment. Both innominate osteotomy and femoral osteotomy can give the same results, though the former procedure has been favoured (Figs. 4.49–4.53). It is performed only if, firstly, radiographs suggest that the condition is not of longstanding and, preferably, the symptoms have been present for less than 6 months; secondly, there is a nearly full range of motion at the hip, though it is acceptable for the hip to lack 10° of internal rotation or

The Child   193

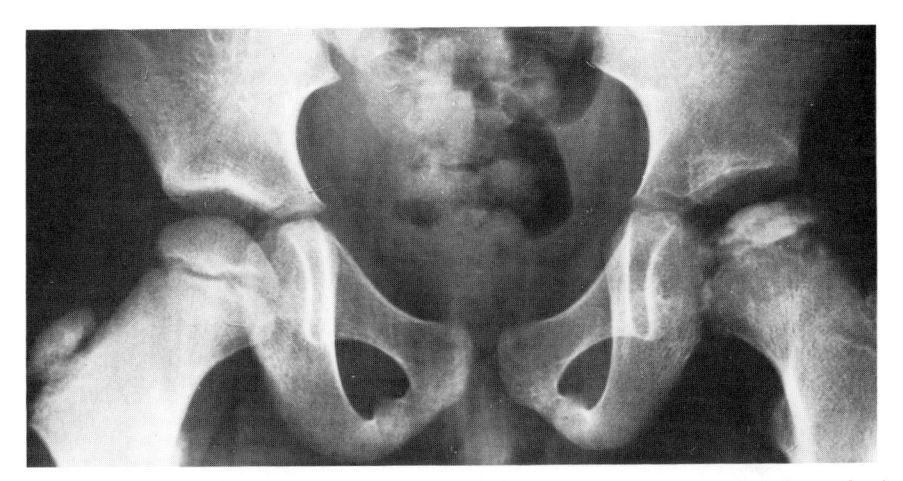

Fig. 4.49 Antero-posterior x-ray of the pelvis of a boy who presented with Perthes' disease of the left hip at the age of 7 years. In the antero-posterior view note the uncovering of the femoral head. As the prerequisites for Salter innominate osteotomy were fulfilled, it was elected to perform this procedure (Figs. 4.51–4.53).

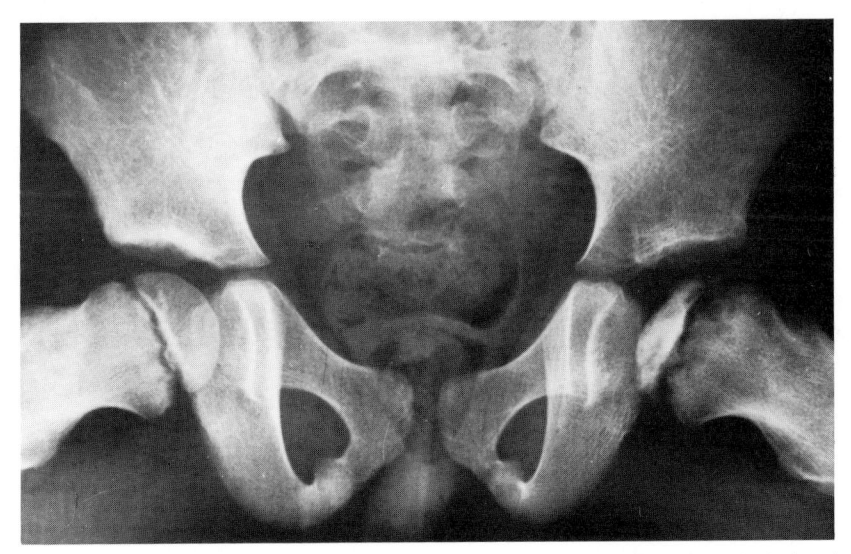

Fig. 4.50 Same patient as Fig. 4.49. Lateral view showing that the whole head is involved.

abduction or adduction in flexion (when compared with the unaffected hip); and lastly, x-rays in full abduction demonstrate that the femoral head can be covered by the acetabulum. Arthrography to demonstrate that the cartilaginous head is spherical is not necessary if surgery is performed only on patients with early disease. The head is then invariably spherical.

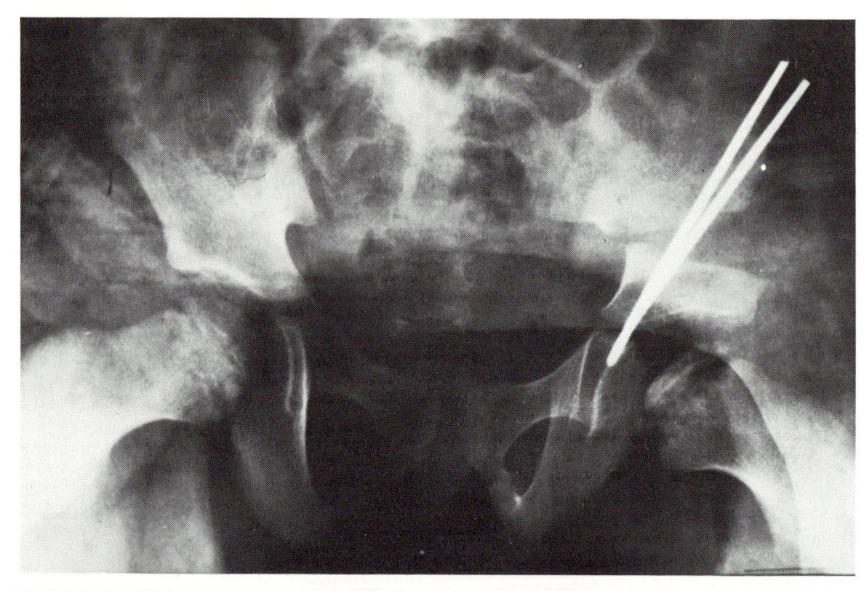

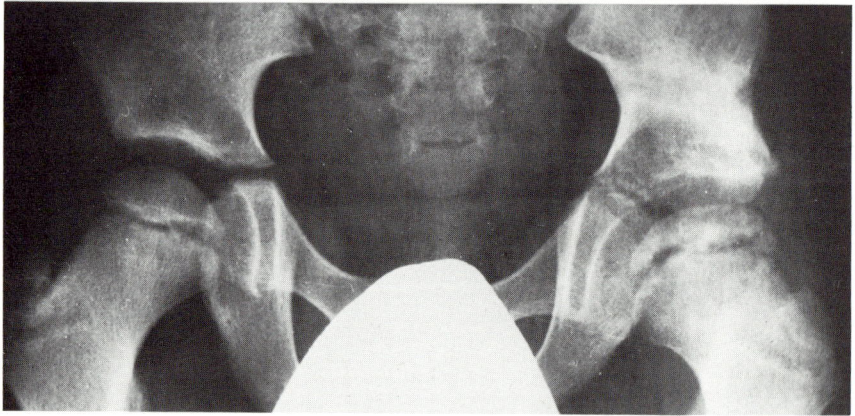

Figs. 4.51 & 4.52 (*See caption opposite.*)

IRRITABLE HIP (Synonyms: transient synovitis, observation hip)

This is a benign condition affecting children between the ages of 2 and 12 years. The condition is usually characterised by a limp and limited hip motion.

AETIOLOGY

This is uncertain. The condition does tend to occur most commonly in spring and autumn. Sometimes there may be a preceding throat infection. The higher incidence in boys has been used as evidence of a traumatic aetiology.

The Child 195

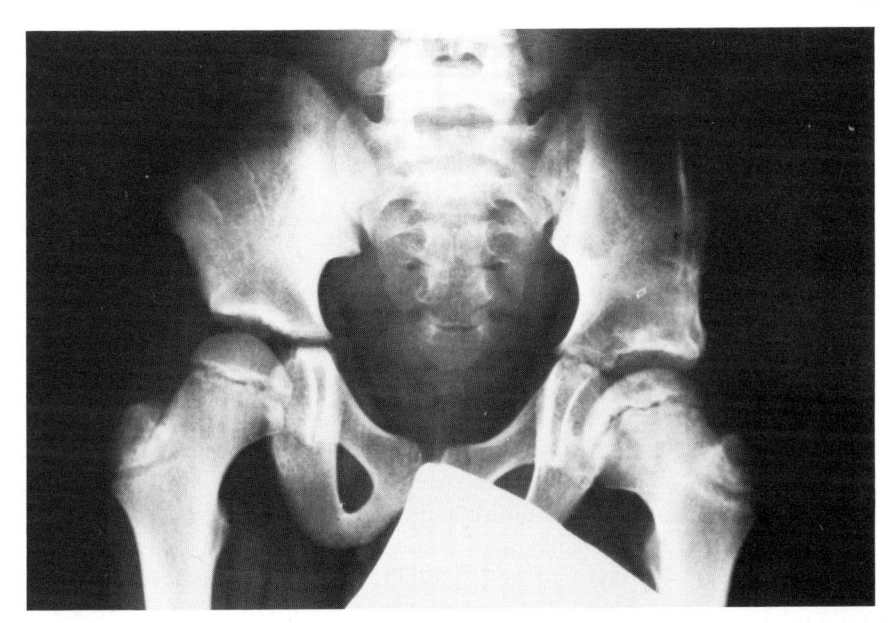

Figs. 4.51–4.53 Same patient as Fig. 4.49. Salter innominate osteotomy was performed two weeks after presentation. (*Opposite top*) This radiograph in the post-operative hip spica shows proper displacement at the osteotomy site. Displacement is maintained by two heavy threaded Steinmann pins. (*Opposite bottom*) The appearance five months after surgery. There was a full range of motion and the boy had returned to full sporting activity. (*Above*) The radiological appearance at the age of 10 years.

CLINICAL FEATURES

A child between the ages of 2 and 12 years (and most commonly between the age of 3 and 6 years) presents with pain in the thigh or knee, reluctance to walk, and limitation of hip motion. The onset is generally acute. All movements of the hip are restricted and there is generally tenderness about the anterior aspect of the hip. There may be a slight pyrexia.

RADIOLOGICAL FEATURES

Usually the x-rays are normal throughout. There may be slight widening of the joint space and such widening may displace the femoral head laterally.

OTHER SPECIAL INVESTIGATIONS

In general the erythrocyte sedimentation rate is normal, though it may be slightly elevated. If the joint is aspirated, then the fluid obtained is clear. If the synovial membrane is biopsied, the histology shows small round cell infiltration which is quite non-specific.

DIFFERENTIAL DIAGNOSIS

Perthes' disease. Some children present with Perthes' disease without radiological change. This is uncommon but the possibility of the diagnosis of Perthes' disease must always be entertained and, if the symptoms do not settle rapidly or recur, then further X-rays should be taken.

Septic arthritis. Some children present with a painful irritable hip and with marked limitation of hip motion. Septic arthritis can then only be excluded by aspiration of the joint.

TREATMENT

The treatment is general and local rest. If the signs are not marked then this rest can be carried out by resting the child in bed at home. If the local features are more marked then the child is admitted to hospital and Pugh's traction applied for up to ten days. Generally the condition settles with 4–5 days of skin traction.

Once the irritability is settled then the child is allowed to resume full activities. It is of the utmost importance to differentiate the irritable hip from the septic hip and, if there is doubt, the joint should be aspirated.

COXA VARA

The normal neck shaft angle in childhood lies in the range of 135–145° and any decrease in this angle is referred to as coxa vara.

CAUSES

Coxa vara may be classified as follows:
1 Infantile
2 Idiopathic—slipped upper femoral epiphysis
3 Traumatic—fracture of the neck or trochanteric region
4 Local bone disease—osteomyelitis, tuberculosis, Perthes' disease
5 General bone disease—rickets, steroid osteopathy, osteogenesis imperfecta

Infantile coxa vara

This condition is sometimes described as congenital coxa vara but since it cannot be recognised at birth when x-rays are normal, it is best referred to as infantile (Figs. 4.54–4.57).

A characteristic feature is the presence of a separated triangular fragment of metaphysis in the lower part of the femoral neck (Fig. 4.58). This triangular fragment has its base on the neck of the femur, the epiphyseal line forms the

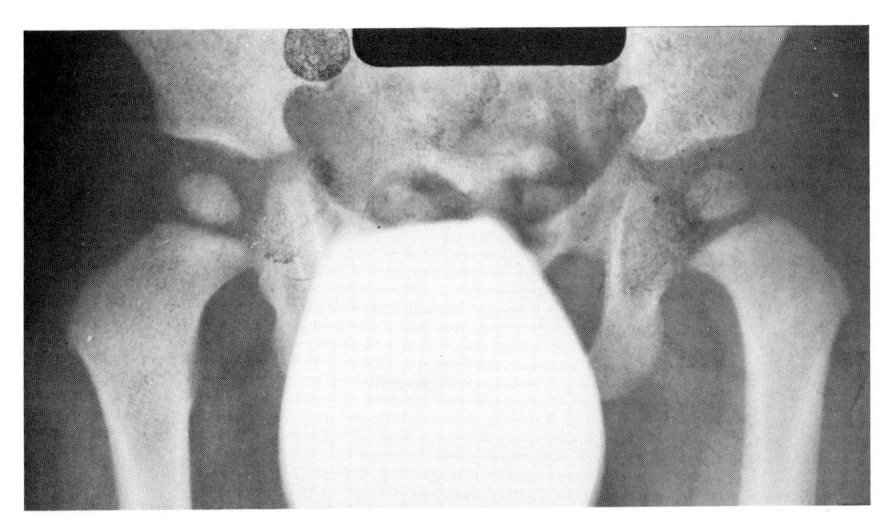

Fig. 4.54 Infantile coxa vara. Normal radiological appearance at the age of 1 year. This badly stained radiograph was part of an abdominal film.

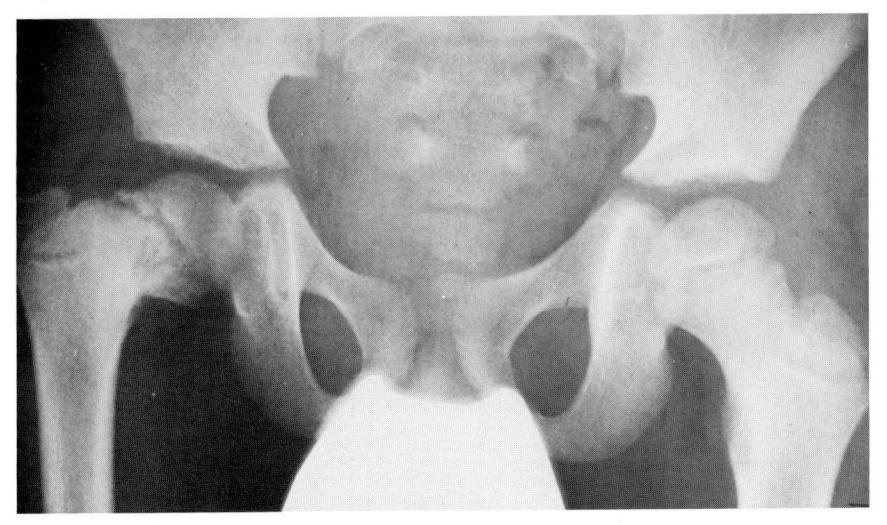

Fig. 4.55 Coxa vara has developed by the age of 6 years.

medial side and there is a fissure on the lateral side of the triangle. It is postulated that the condition is due either to severe trauma in normal bone or, more frequently, to shearing stress on an abnormal femoral neck. The nature of the abnormality is unknown. One patient in four is affected bilaterally. The child usually presents after the age of 2 years with a limp, if unilateral, or a waddle if bilateral. Although there will be limitation of abduction at the hip, the Ortolani sign is negative and shortening is minimal. During growth, the degree of coxa

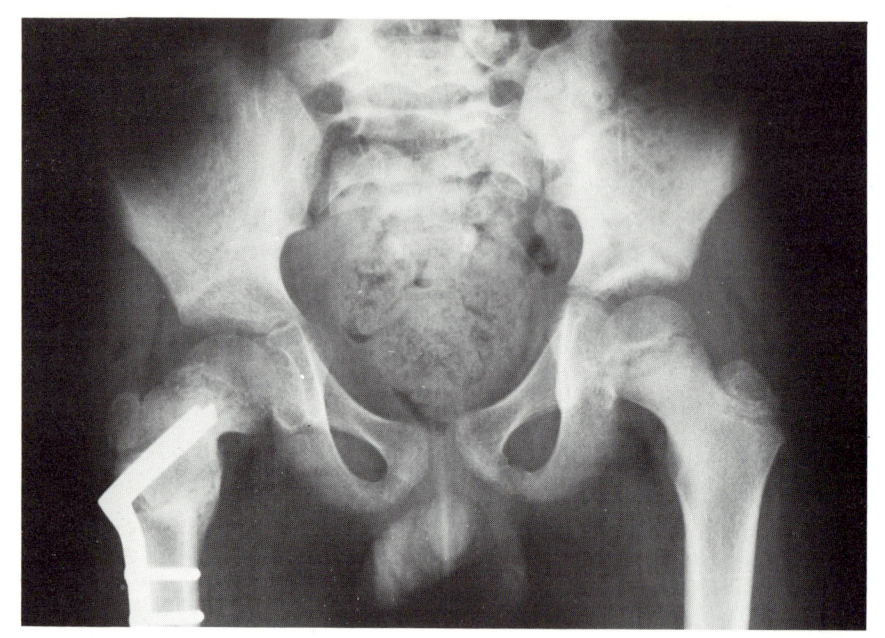

Fig. 4.56 Appearance following sub-trochanteric valgus osteotomy.

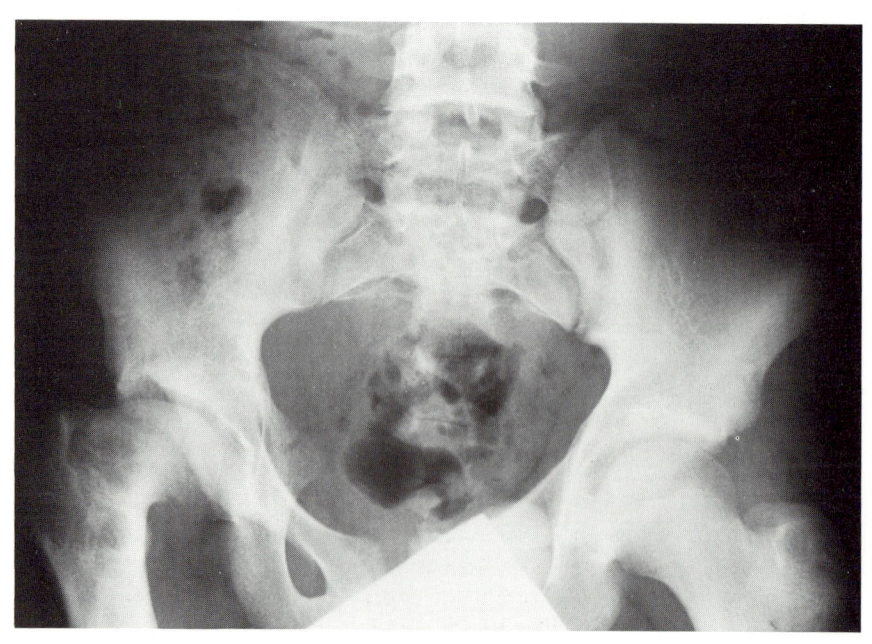

Fig. 4.57 Recurrence of deformity at the age of 17 years.

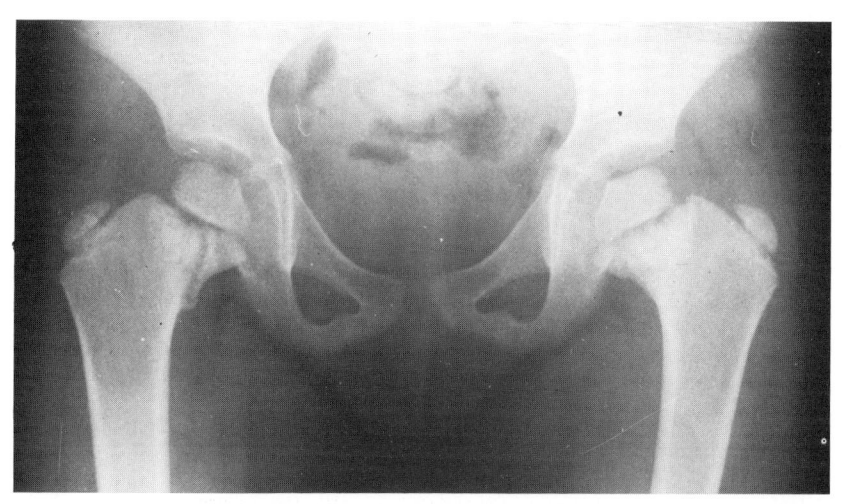

Fig. 4.58 Bilateral infantile coxa vara in a girl of 4 years who presented with a painless limp. Note the characteristic triangular fragment in the inferior part of the metaphysis.

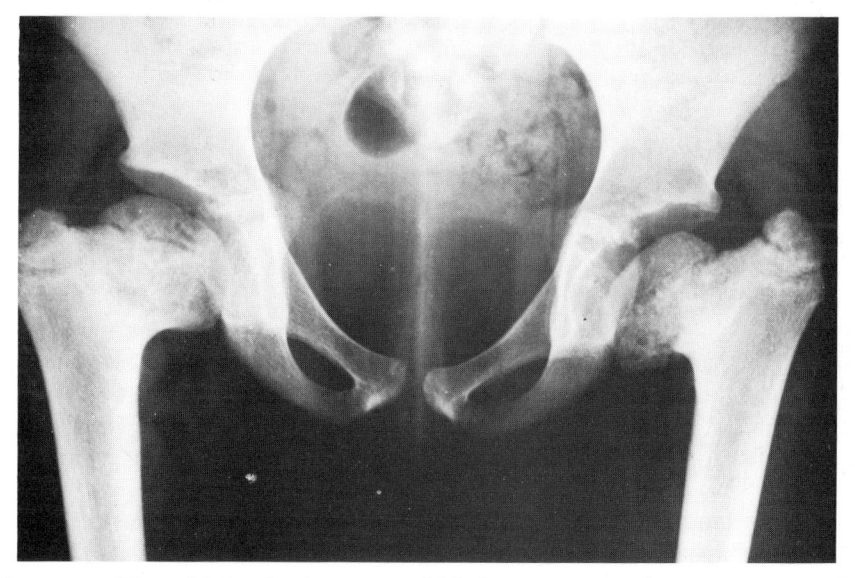

Fig. 4.59 Bilateral infantile coxa vara which has not received treatment. Note the shortness of the femoral neck and high trochanter, more marked in the left hip.

vara increases, the neck becomes relatively short while the trochanter overgrows (Fig. 4.59). When both growth plates eventually fuse a classical Shepherd's crook deformity of the upper femur is established. Although cases are occasionally seen where the deformity is mild and does not progress, the majority grow progressively worse. If serial x-rays show progression, treatment is indicated. Any

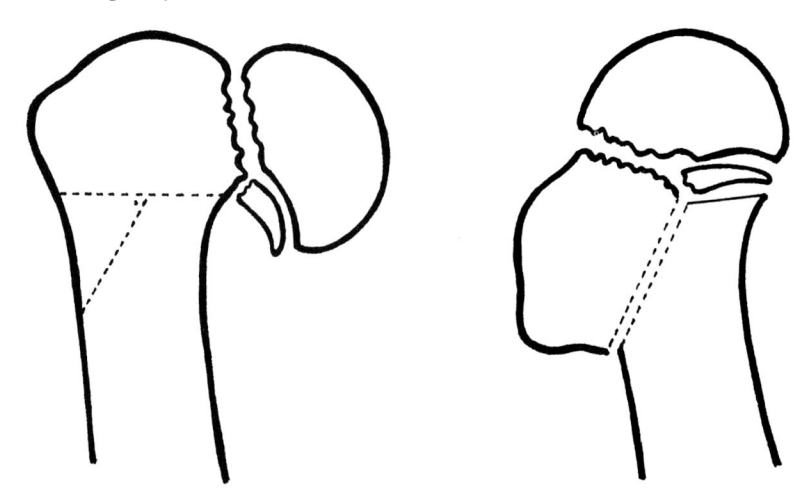

Figs. 4.60 & 4.61 Pauwels' osteotomy for infantile coxa vara. The biomechanical weakness of the neck is overcome by angulation plus displacement of the osteotomy. Osteotomies are performed along the two dotted lines and the triangle between them is excised. (*Right*) The upper fragment has been adducted and the lower fragment displaced medially and abducted. Pauwels holds the displacement using a wire suture; we prefer the temporary insertion of a heavy pin. (For further details see Pauwels, F. (1976) *Biomechanics of the normal and diseased hip*. Springer-Verlag, Berlin.)

form of conservative treatment, such as weight-relieving calipers, has no effect and subtrochanteric osteotomy is generally accepted as the treatment of choice. There has been considerable variation of opinion as to when this should be done because recurrence is so common.

Pauwels, however, has shown with a 40 year follow-up that his Y-shaped intertrochanteric osteotomy (Figs. 4.60 & 4.61) designed on biomechanical principles will not only correct the deformity, but will prevent recurrence. Althought this osteotomy is demanding technically, the extra effort is worthwhile. The lines of the osteotomy are drawn on a tracing of the pre-operative radiograph and at operation these are reproduced with the help of two Kirschner wires drilled into the bone under x-ray control. The displacement is maintained by a circular wire loop and a plaster hip spica with the leg in abduction. Using this method the end result should be a normal functioning hip with an acceptable degree of shortening.

THE SPINE

CLASSIFICATION OF SPINAL DEFORMITIES

The classification outlined in Table 4.2 is that recommended by the Scoliosis Research Society.

Table 4.2 Classification of spinal deformities.

Structural scoliosis	*Kyphosis*
Idiopathic	Postural
infantile	Scheuermann's disease
juvenile	Congenital
adolescent	Neuromuscular
Neuromuscular	Myelomeningocele
neuropathic	Traumatic
myopathic	Post-surgical
Congenital	Post-irradiation
Neurofibromatosis	Metabolic
Mesenchymal disorder	Skeletal dysplasias
Rheumatoid disease	Collagen disease
Trauma	Tumour
Extraspinal contractures	Inflammatory
Osteochondrodystrophies	
Infection of bone	*Lordosis*
Metabolic disorders	Postural
Related to lumbosacral joint	Congenital
Tumours	Neuromuscular
	Post-laminectomy
Non-structural scoliosis	Secondary to hip
Postural scoliosis	flexion contracture
Hysterical scoliosis	Other
Nerve root irritation	
Inflammatory	
Related to leg length discrepancy	
Related to contractures about the hip	

Embryology and early development

It is essential to understand the development of the vertebral column and spinal cord in order to discuss the problems of congenital spinal abnormalities. More details of this can be obtained from standard texts, but a short review follows.

The development of the spine and spinal cord has close associations with other systems such as the heart and great vessels and the genitourinary system, and therefore associations of congenital deformities involving all these structures are frequently seen.

There are two centres of chondrification for the vertebral body and failure of development of one of these accounts for the formation of a hemivertebra. Hypoplasia in development produces a lateral wedge vertebra. The neural arches are also chondrified from two centres which originate in the pedicle region and extend forwards and backwards fusing with one another.

Ossification occurs from three centres, one for the body and two for the posterior elements. Secondary centres of ossification develop for the upper and lower surfaces of the body and these do not completely incorporate into the body until skeletal maturity.

SCOLIOSIS

Scoliosis (curvature of the spine) was recognised in ancient times and medical literature referred to techniques of treatment consisting of traction and crude casts. It is only in recent times that adequate techniques of bracing and surgery have been available to satisfactorily manage the condition.

The formation of the Scoliosis Research Society has resulted in a more scientific approach to the problem and it is possible, with the techniques now available, to manage even the most difficult of spinal curvatures.

Terminology

In December 1978 the Scoliosis Research Society provided a revised glossary of the terminology to be used in discussing scoliosis. This terminology has, where possible, been adhered to in the following pages.

Natural history of childhood scoliosis

In recent times with the introduction of school screening programmes and with the more satisfactory prospective longitudinal studies of the condition, our knowledge of the natural history of scoliosis has been considerably improved. Without this knowledge it is impossible to treat the condition logically.

The prevalence of scoliosis in the community has been extensively studied by a number of workers; recent school screening programmes suggest that the incidence is approximately 4% and that only 13.6% of those found to have scoliosis demonstrate progression. Progression is more likely to occur in the female. The other interesting finding in these surveys has been that the sex incidence for minor curves is equal, and that curve progression is more likely in the female and more commonly requires treatment.

The natural history of untreated scoliosis is still subject to debate. Clarisse reviewed 110 patients with curves between 10 and 29° and followed them without treatment until such time as they progressed to 30°. If they presented at a very young age with these degrees of curvature they were more likely to progress than if they presented after the onset of menarche.

The time of progression of these curves corresponded to the growth spurts. Ponseti and Friedman reviewed 394 untreated patients and followed them to skeletal maturity. They found also that the earlier the presentation the more likely progression was to occur.

Natural history of adult scoliosis

Progression of scoliosis in adults is also an area under investigation. The studies of Nilsonne and Lundgren and of Nachemson suggest that in adult life the curves produce significant problems with an increase in mortality rate and a reduced capacity for work with an associated high incidence of back pain.

Ponseti and Weinstein presented the follow-up of the original cases studied by Ponseti and Friedman and their findings did not suggest nearly as gloomy a prognosis as those of the previous authors. They were able to compare current with original films in a number of patients and found that the average deterioration of the curve was 3° per decade. They did note that, the more severe the curve at the time of skeletal maturity, the more likely it was for progression to occur; in thoracic curves progression was seen to average 12.5° per decade if the curves were between 50 and 80° at skeletal maturity.

Clinical assessment

HISTORICAL EVALUATION

An adequate history is of vital importance in determining the aetiology. It must take into consideration the deformity itself, when it was first noted, and if it has increased while under observation.

The history of complications from the deformity is also important, in particular the pain produced by effect of the deformity on the spine, the difficulties in breathing produced by effect of the deformity on the respiratory system, and changes peripheral to or at the level of deformity produced by the effect on the neurological system.

A family history must be carefully taken to determine if there are other members of the family who have spinal deformities, or if there are other conditions such as neurological disorders which may be of a familial nature to explain a secondary cause for the curve.

A full history of the patient's general condition is of importance in planning future treatment. Past history including the neonatal stage may be of significance in certain patients. The developmental milestones are another important pointer to neurological problems, as is the schooling record.

An estimate of growth potential and skeletal maturity is relevant and a history directed at determining if growth is still occurring will be helpful in assessing the likelihood of progression. Such things as the onset of menarche and the occurrence of a rapid growth spurt would indicate the likely proximity of early growth cessation.

PHYSICAL EXAMINATION

Physical examination must also include full general examination as there are frequently findings on a general examination which may make one suspicious of a secondary cause for the scoliosis. The general shape of the body, height (both sitting and standing), arm span and the presence of features such as webbing of the neck in relation to the scapula, flexibility of the joints, presence or absence of café-au-lait spots and many other cutaneous findings may well suggest an abnormality which is the cause of the scoliosis. Full neurological examination is an essential component of this thorough general examination.

The spine is inspected with the patient standing erect (Fig. 4.62). An assessment can be made as to the degree of compensation manifest by the level position of the shoulders and pelvis, and as to the absence or presence of deviation to either side by using a plumb line dropped from the occipit (Fig. 4.63). The measurement of any leg length discrepancy is carried out at this stage using blocks to level the pelvis (Fig. 4.64).

The flexibility of the spine can be determined by assessing the range of movements. Flexibility of the deformity can be assessed by suspension or lateral flexion and observation of the apex of the deformity during these manoeuvres. The curvature is more obvious in forward flexion since the rotary element is revealed more clearly in this position. This vertebral rotation produces elevation of the ribs on the convexity of the curve and depression of the ribs in the concavity (Figs. 4.65 & 4.66). On the anterior aspect of the chest this deformity of the

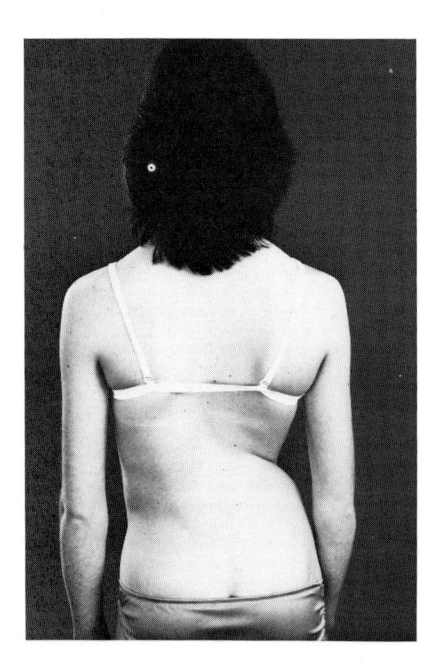

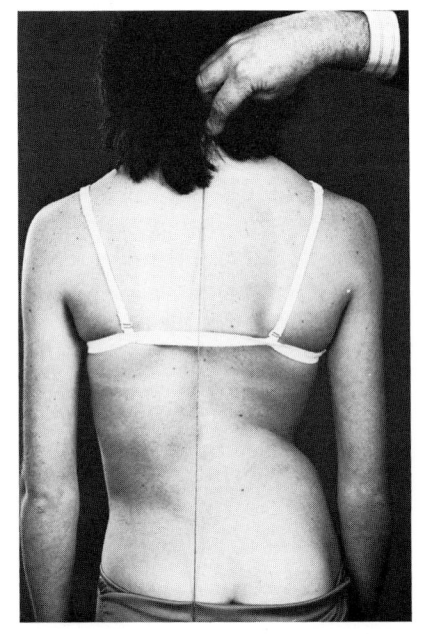

Figs. 4.62 & 4.63 Scoliosis. Clinical evaluation from behind. A left sided thoraco lumbar curve is evident with a prominent right iliac crest. (*Right*) The right arm-to-torso distance is increased; decompensation has caused the plumb line to be displaced to the left.

The Child 205

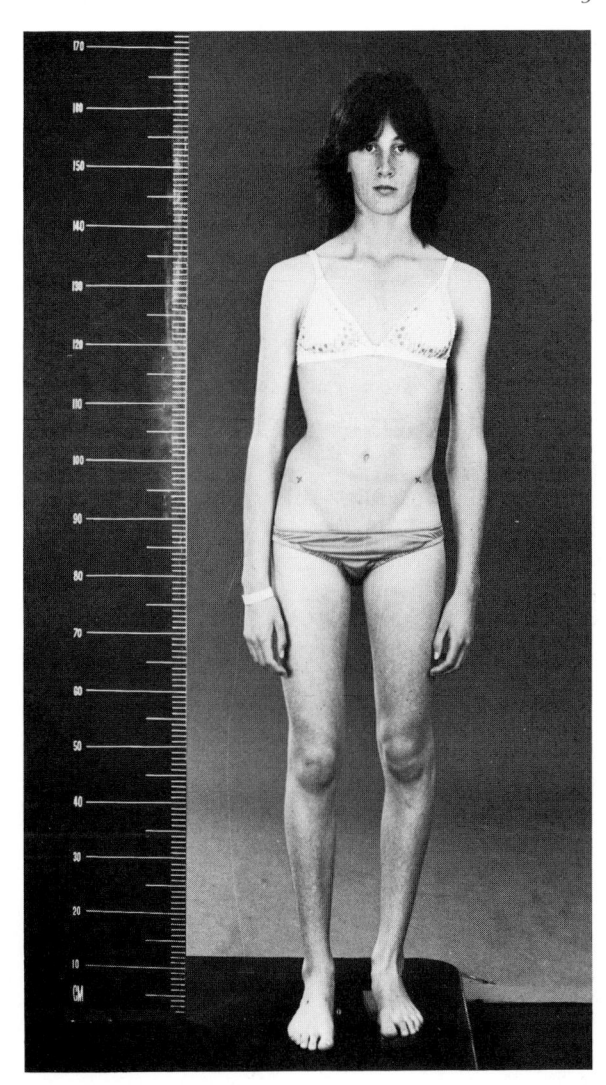

Fig. 4.64 Same patient as Fig. 4.62. Clinical evaluation from the front again demonstrates the deformity and decompensation. Note that a raise has been added under the left leg to compensate for a leg length discrepancy.

thoracic cage is manifest as a prominence of the anterior chest wall to the concave side of the curve. Assessment of the degree of kyphosis or lordosis of the spine must also be made (Fig. 4.67). Tenderness or muscle spasm may suggest a secondary cause in the vertebrae themselves. Such things as cutaneous tumours, hairy patches or the presence of abnormal skin blemishes near the spine should be recorded.

The presence or absence of pelvic obliquity is recorded and the causation of that pelvic obliquity determined by clinical examination of the hip region and the lower limbs.

206   Chapter 4

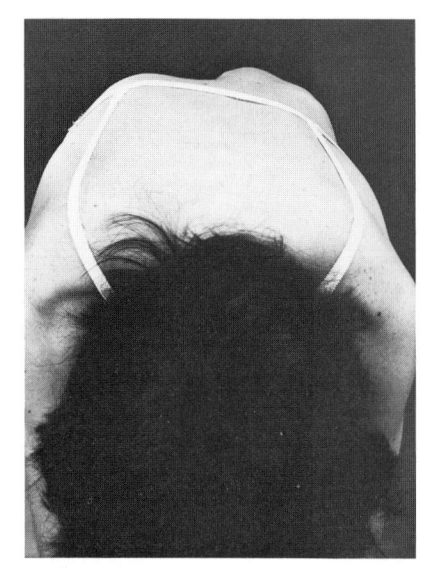

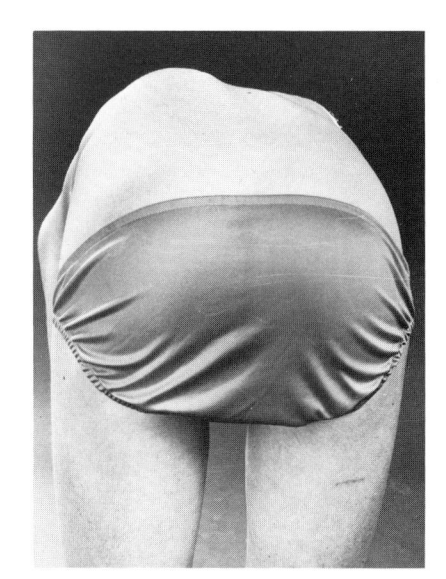

Figs. 4.65 & 4.66 Forward flexion evaluation demonstrates the effect of vertebral rotation resulting in prominence of the lateral structures to the left of the midline at the level of the deformity in the lumbar spine.

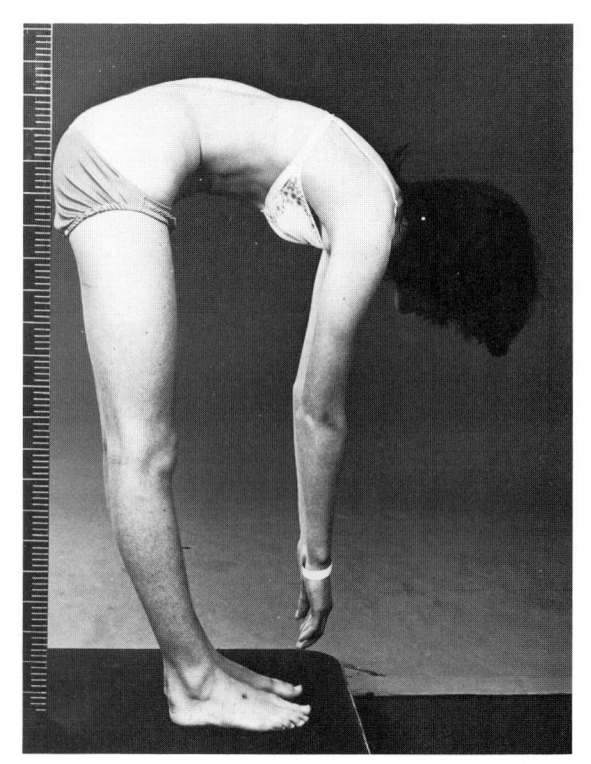

Fig. 4.67 From the side there is no abnormal kyphotic or lordotic element.

RADIOLOGICAL EVALUATION

Radiology provides the most accurate method of measuring the degree of severity of the deformity. The radiographs wherever possible must include the full length of the spine and allow visualisation of both iliac crests (Figs. 4.68 & 4.69). The standard A–P and lateral x-rays of the spine give only a two-dimension impression of the total deformity and it may well be that, in the future, CAT scanning will be employed to give a third dimension to our evaluation.

The films must be done in the erect position wherever possible to provide information about the effects of gravity upon the curve. A lateral erect film is also taken and, in those unable to stand, sitting films are important. Bending films are used where information is required as to the flexibility of minor curves or where information is needed to determine the amount of mobility within the major curve. If there is kyphosis or lordosis, hyperextension and hyperflexion can be used to determine mobility within the curve. In the paralysed patient, traction films may give information regarding mobility.

The recommended method of measuring the curvature is that described by Cobb. The technique entails construction of a perpendicular to the line across the end plate of the uppermost vertebra maximally tilted into the curve and intersection of this line with a perpendicular to a line across the end plate of the lowest end vertebra as determined by the same technique. The angle between

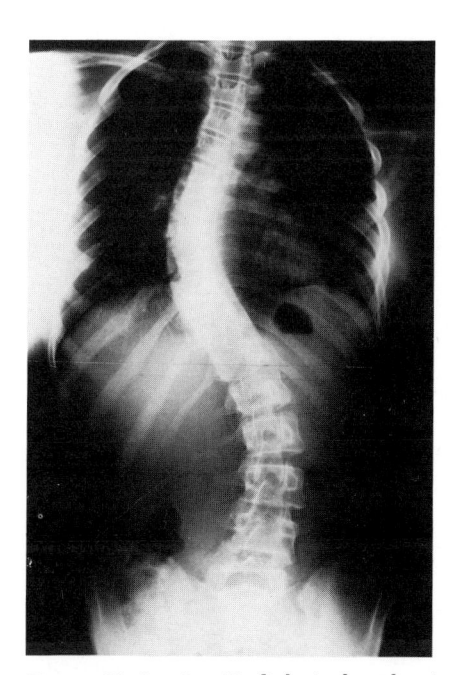

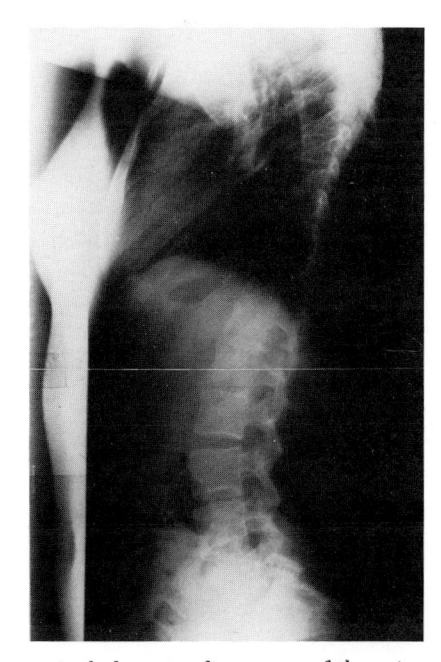

Figs. 4.68 & 4.69 Radiological evaluation must include a standing x-ray of the spine with antero-posterior and lateral views.

208   Chapter 4

these two lines is the Cobb angle. In double curves the transitional vertebra becomes the end vertebra for the upper and lower curves. When comparing Cobb angles it is essential to have comparable films on all subsequent occasions. On a lateral film, using similar techniques to determine end vertebrae, it is possible to measure the angle of lordosis or kyphosis in those cases where kyphoscoliosis or pure kyphosis or lordosis exist.

The x-rays, apart from demonstrating the degree of deformity and the site and type of deformity, in many cases provide a diagnosis as to the cause of the deformity and other information as well. The amount of vertebral rotation can be determined using Moe's classification. The degree of skeletal maturity of the spine can be assessed from the state of ossification of the iliac apophysis (Risser's sign) or from the presence of vertebral ring apophyses and whether these have fused to the body. Another aid to determining skeletal maturity is the use of an x-ray of the wrist and hand and the use of Greulich and Pyle's atlas to assess skeletal age.

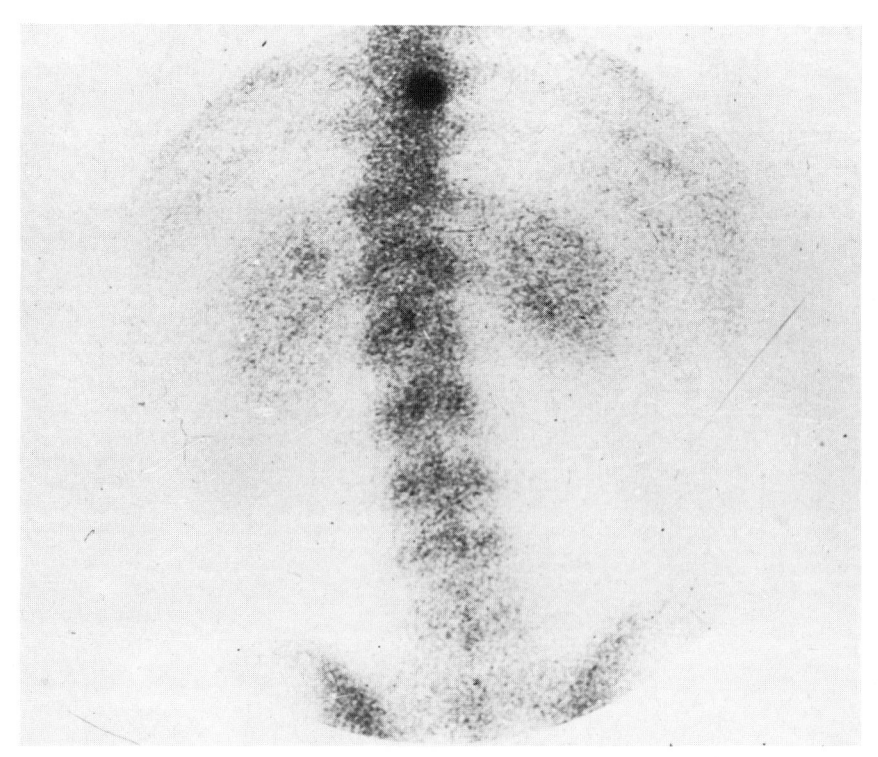

Fig. 4.70 Bone scan of patient with an osteoblastoma in the pedicle of the 7th thoracic vertebra. Note the lesion is at the apex of the curve and in the concavity of the curve.

SPECIAL RADIOGRAPHIC TECHNIQUES

Tomograms can be of use in special situations where more definition is required of the vertebral bodies particularly in congenital scoliosis. Myelography is absolutely indicated whenever congenital abnormalities are present in order to exclude diastematomyelia before undertaking corrective surgery. Bone scanning (Fig. 4.70) has been of assistance in determining the aetiology of certain painful scolioses and on rare occasions a CAT scan (Fig. 4.71) can give more information about the patency of the neural canal and the presence of certain small tumours.

Because of the high incidence of associated anomalies particularly in congenital scoliosis, a chest x-ray and intravenous pyelogram are frequently appropriate.

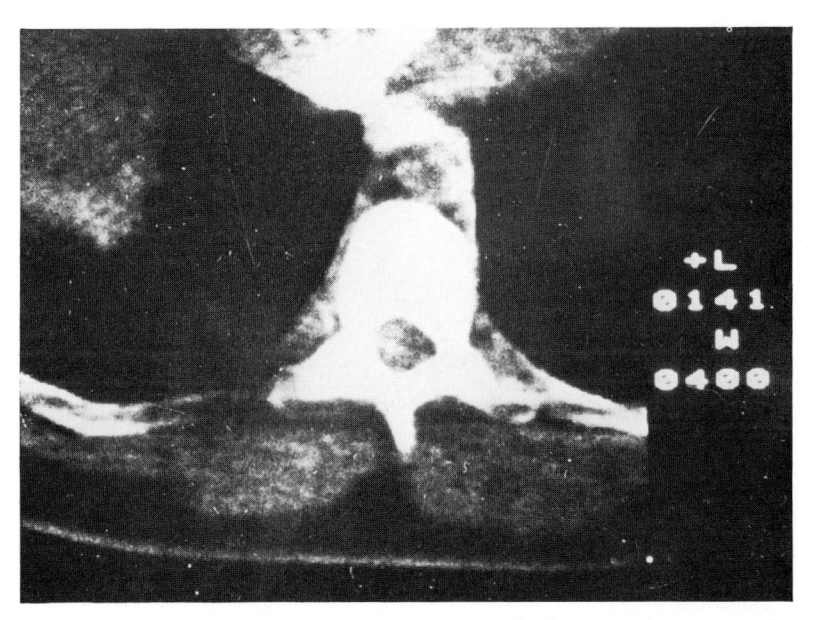

Fig. 4.71 CAT scan of same patient as Fig. 4.70. The lesion is demonstrated at the junction of the pedicle and lamina.

Conservative treatment of scoliosis

The Milwaukee brace with its recent modifications (Figs. 4.72 & 4.73) or the Boston type underarm brace are effective orthoses in the conservative management of scoliosis. In all bracing programmes it is essential that the patient undertakes a programme of exercises as an adjunct to the brace therapy. Recent reports of electrical stimulation, either implanted or applied externally, suggest

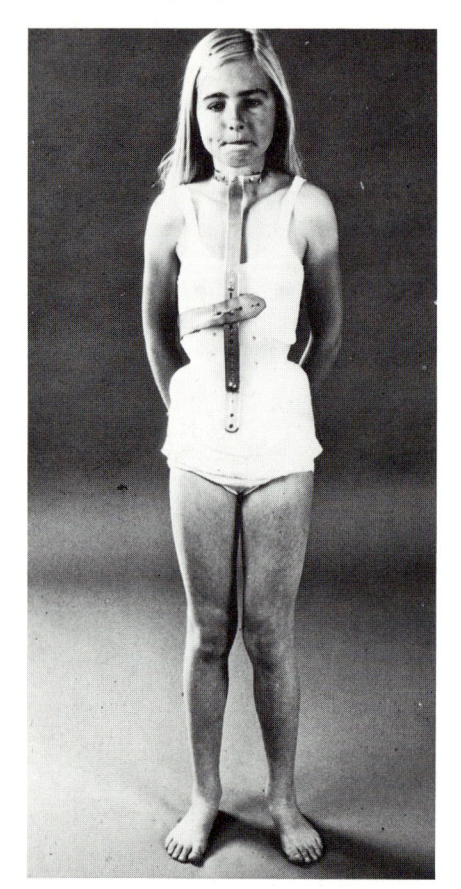

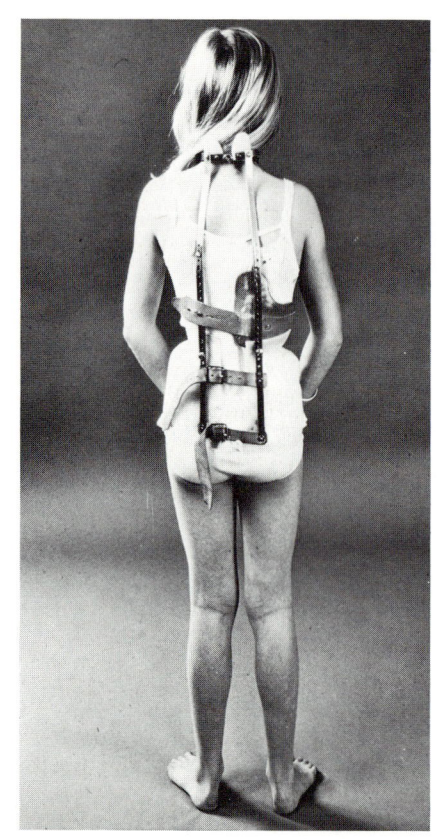

Figs. 4.72 & 4.73 The Milwaukee brace. The brace is constructed on a pelvic girdle which is moulded accurately over the iliac crests, and irons out the lumbar lordosis. The metalic superstructure attaches to the girdle inferiorly and to a neck ring above, incorporating a throat mould and occipital pads. The thoracic pad attaches to the uprights and exerts pressure on those ribs leading up to the apex of the curve.

that these techniques may be as effective as the Milwaukee brace in control of early curves. However they are experimental and should not be considered as part of the routine of conservative management.

The Milwaukee brace originally developed by Blount and Schmidt has been extensively modified over the years. The modern brace is extremely effective in controlling early curve. The fabrication of such braces now includes the use of modern materials which allow a much more satisfactory moulding of the pelvic component over the iliac crest. Also, with pre-fabricated uprights it is possible to produce a Milwaukee brace in a short period of time and allow adjustment to produce an excellent fitting brace.

The indications for the brace should be strictly adhered to and are:
1. Curves greater than 20° demonstrating progression.
2. Curves greater than 30° but less than 40°.

The individual being braced must still be skeletally immature and willing to co-operate in the brace programme. One contraindication to the brace can well be geographical: if the patient cannot easily visit the orthotist, supervision of the brace wearing and adjustment are impossible—this will inevitably lead to failure of the orthosis. It is essential that the orthotist is skilled in the manufacture of these braces. The brace is supplied to the patient with the instruction that it is to be worn 23 hours per day.

The Milwaukee brace is appropriate for curves with an apex above T11 and is also effective in managing double major curves. In the case of thoracolumbar and lumbar curves with an apex at or below T11, the Boston type of orthosis (Figs. 4.74 & 4.75) has proved as effective as the Milwaukee brace and does not require the individual to wear superstructure around the neck.

Braces require constant checking and adjustment and frequent review with x-rays at six-monthly intervals to assess control and to detect deterioration in correction if this should occur (Figs. 4.76–4.78). Long term follow up studies suggest that the ultimate goal of brace therapy is to have a curve which is identical to that at the commencement of therapy. Once skeletal maturity has

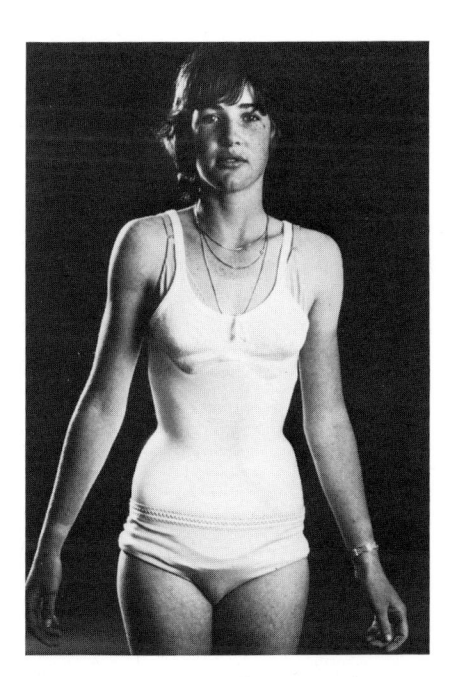

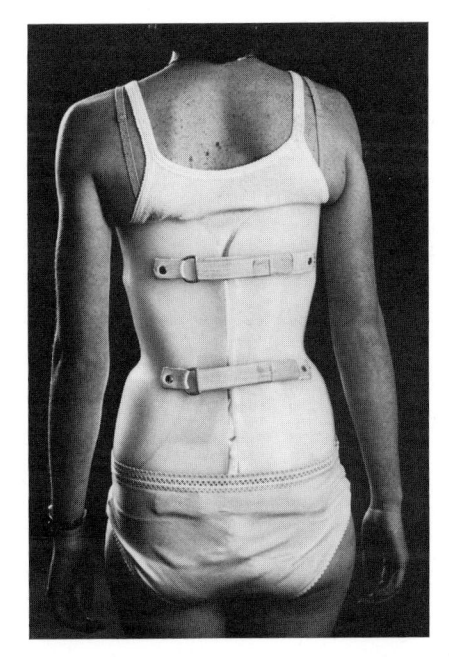

Figs. 4.74 & 4.75 The Boston brace. An underarm orthosis suitable for control and correction of early curves in the thoraco lumbar and lumbar region. It should only be used for curves with an apice at or below T11.

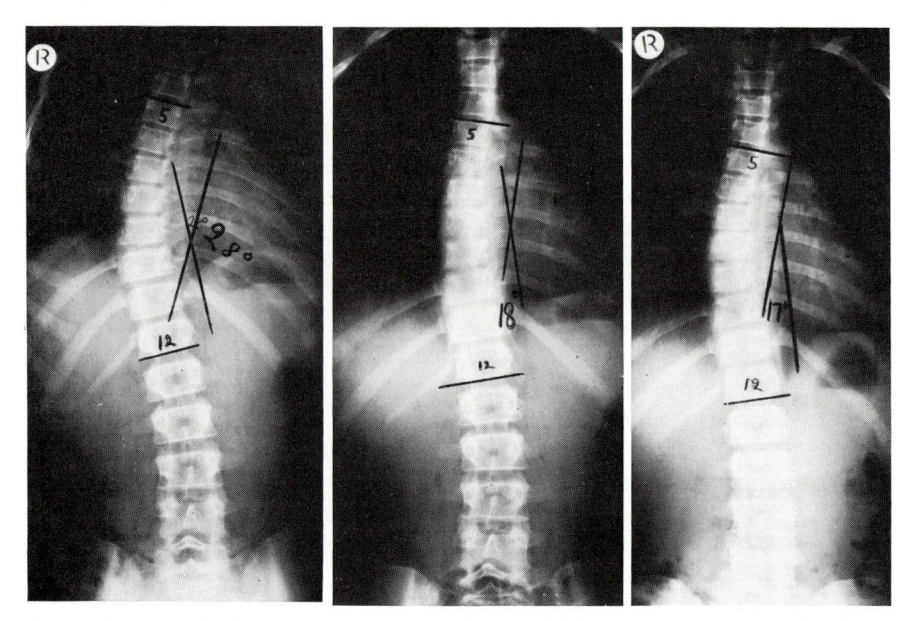

Figs. 4.76–4.78 Antero-posterior radiographs of a child undergoing treatment with the Milwaukee brace. The films are at six monthly intervals and demonstrate the effectiveness of the brace.

been confirmed by cessation of growth and capping of the iliac apophysis, the child is weaned off the brace over a period of 6–12 months.

Infantile idiopathic scoliosis

Infantile idiopathic scoliosis is an uncommon condition in the Australian community and most of the literature on the subject emanates from the United Kingdom. In particular the articles by James and also those of Lloyd-Roberts and Pilscher and James have given us a far broader knowledge of the subject and demonstrated the clinical features.

The condition is most commonly seen in males in a ratio of 3 : 2 and the vast majority of the curves are thoracic curves to the left side. Wynne-Davies showed that the incidence of plagiocephaly was 100% with the flat side of the head to the concave side. She also reported a high incidence of non-spinal congenital anomalies.

The natural history of infantile idiopathic scoliosis is for the curve to resolve in a high proportion of cases (90%). The work of Mehta has suggested a radiographic technique to determine which cases are likely to be progressive by measurement of the rib vertebral angle.

Management of the non-progressive type is by observation. Usually resolution to normal occurs over 2–3 years. The progressive form of infantile scoliosis poses a most difficult problem as the amount of time available for deterioration of the curve is great. Observation alone is unacceptable and vigorous forms of treatment are indicated in an endeavour to prevent progression. The Milwaukee brace can be effective in controlling these curves but there are considerable difficulties in making a satisfactory brace for very young children and the availability of a skilled orthotist is essential. The Milwaukee brace programme must be continuous and aim to prevent curve progression. The use of serial casting on a Cottrell table followed by Milwaukee bracing appears to offer some help in controlling progression.

If a curve progresses to a severe degree or, as sometimes happens, the curve at presentation is already severe then correction and fusion must be attempted irrespective of the age of the child. Following fusion, if done at a young age, it is essential to provide protection to the graft with a Milwaukee brace until skeletal maturity. The place of re-exploration and regrafting is debatable. If there is doubt as to the existence of solid fusion then re-exploration should be undertaken.

If the patient is very young, correction without fusion should be considered, using Harrington instruments with continued correction in a Milwaukee brace (Figs. 4.79–4.81).

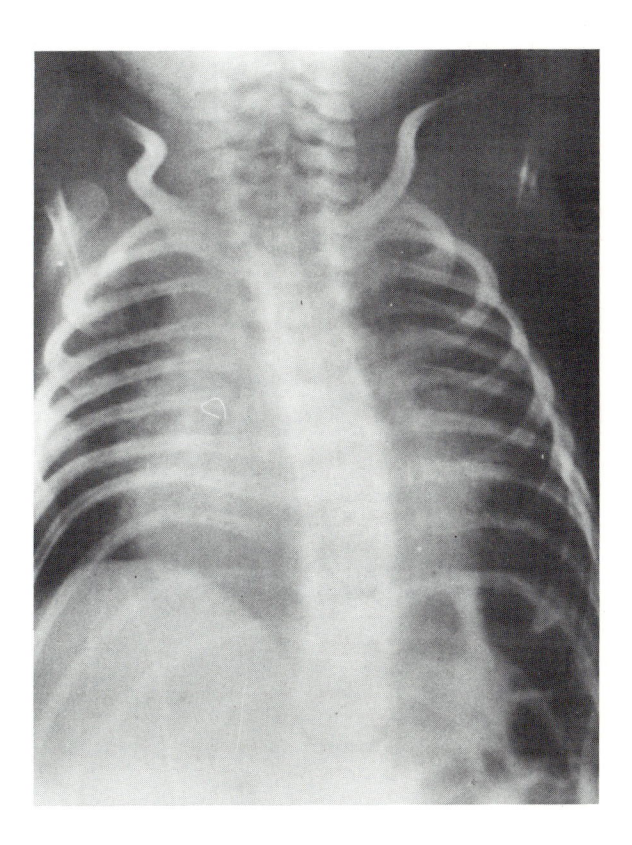

Fig. 4.79 (*See p. 215 for caption.*)

Juvenile idiopathic scoliosis

Structural scoliosis developing in children between the skeletal age of 3 years and the onset of puberty is classified as juvenile idiopathic scoliosis. The pattern of the curves mirrors those of adolescent idiopathic scoliosis but the incidence of the condition is much lower than the adolescent group, comprising approximately 10% of all cases.

The curves in this group of patients can progress with time. Efforts should be made to manage them conservatively with a Milwaukee brace until skeletal maturity.

In those cases where progression occurs beyond 40°, surgery is likely to be required. The Milwaukee brace is retained in an endeavour to hold the curve until the patient is in the second decade so that maximum spinal growth can occur before surgical fusion is performed. If the curve remains uncontrolled and progresses beyond 60°, fusion is indicated by Harrington's technique.

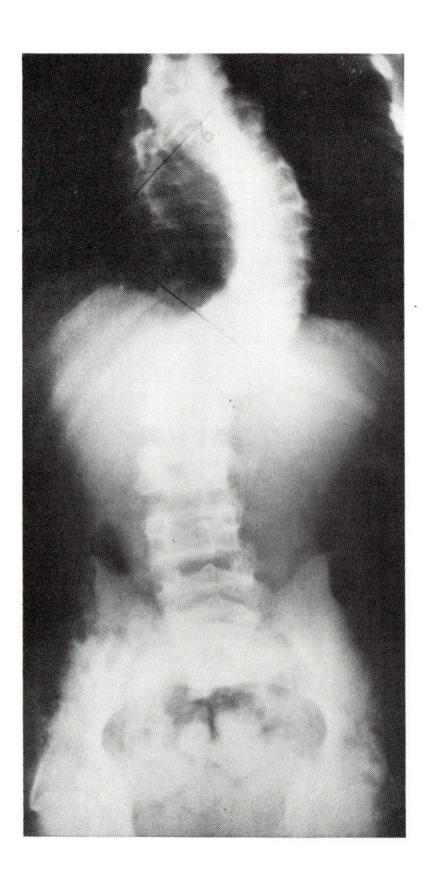

Fig 4.80 Same patient as Fig. 4.79. (*See opposite for caption.*)

Adolescent idiopathic scoliosis

Idiopathic scoliosis makes up 65% of the cases presenting to a scoliosis clinic and the adolescent variety (of whom 90% are females) constitutes the vast majority of these cases.

The curve patterns in idiopathic scoliosis conform to several major subgroups. The classification outlined by Ponseti and Friedman uses five different classes of curve.

1   Major lumbar—the apex is at L1 or 2 and the curve extends from T11/12 down to L4/5 (24%).
2   Thoracolumbar—the apex is at T11 to 12 with end vertebrae at T6 or 7 above and L1 and 2 below (16%).
3   Combined thoracic and lumbar double major curves—an apex at T6 or 7 for the thoracic curve and at L2 for the lumbar curve (37%).
4   Major thoracic curves with an apex at T8 or 9 and end vertebra at T6 above and T11 below (22%).
5   Cervicothoracic curves with apex at T3 and end vertebra at C7 or T1 above and T4 or T5 below (1.3%).

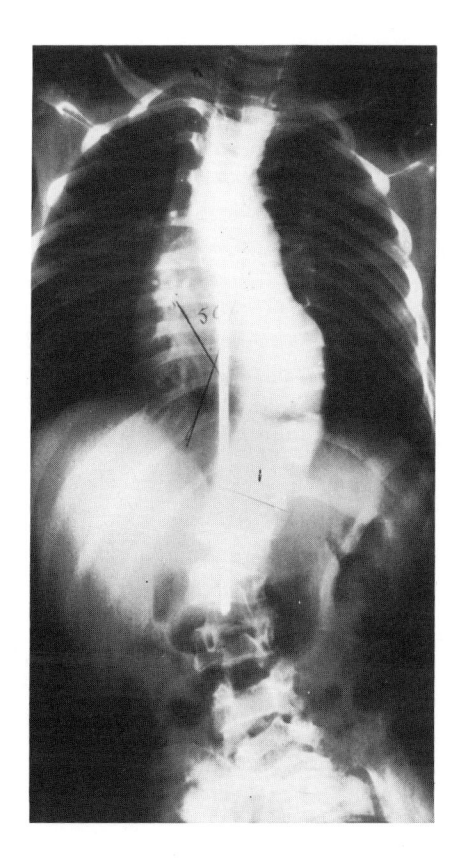

Figs. 4.79–4.81
Infantile idiopathic scoliosis demonstrating progression to an unacceptable level despite conservative treatment. Harrington instrumentation without fusion was performed and when the patient is older Harrington fusion can be contemplated.

More recently Moe and Winter *et al* have classified the curves into a more detailed curve pattern.

These curves are commonly detected during the summer period, when the child is seen in a relatively undressed state. They progress during the rapid growth spurt and an assessment of the state of spinal maturity helps in predicting whether progression is likely. The chronological age, secondary sex development and a history of increasing height all help in an assessment of skeletal maturity. Radiological assessment may also assist in determining whether growth has ceased.

The curves develop minor curves above and below to compensate for the deformity but, despite this, the usual cause of presentation is a cosmetic one. Symptoms from the spine are rare which explains the often late presentation.

Conservative treatment is appropriate for curves greater than 20° showing progression. Operative treatment is only indicated where the curve has progressed beyond 40° with growth still being present or where growth has ceased and the curve has progressed beyond 45°.

Surgery in scoliosis

INDICATIONS FOR TREATMENT

In the adolescent with idiopathic scoliosis, once a curve is greater than 45° the likelihood of progression is so great, particularly in the presence of continued growth, that surgical correction and fusion is indicated. The natural history of this condition suggests that, even after skeletal maturity, if the curve exceeds 50° progression continues and for this reason it is simpler to treat the condition in the adolescent stage rather than to treat a more significant deformity in adult life. Curves greater than 60° can produce sufficient thoracic deformation to cause detectable alterations in respiratory function. For this reason curves should not be allowed to progress to these levels without treatment. Sometimes deformities of less than 45° will be treated surgically because of the degree of rotatory deformity which may produce an unacceptable appearance in an adolescent girl.

PRE-OPERATIVE ASSESSMENT

Routine assessment prior to operation must include a history and examination, radiological investigation of the curve, and adequate investigation of the general health of the patient and of their pulmonary function. Myelography is indicated in congenital scoliosis. Only after the curve has been defined, and the aetiology clarified, should surgical intervention be embarked upon.

PRE-OPERATIVE CORRECTION

The use of traction or plaster cast in the correction of curves pre-operatively has often been employed unnecessarily in the past. As a result of the work of Nachemson and others it is apparent that the correction obtained with or without preliminary traction is identical in curves up to 75° using Harrington's procedure. Preliminary traction is now used only in cases with curves beyond this degree of severity. We have found halo traction with an inclined bed to be quite effective in obtaining correction pre-operatively (Fig. 4.82). Cottrell traction has also proved satisfactory (Fig. 4.83). The halo pelvic apparatus has a very limited place in the pre-operative correction of scoliosis and is used only infrequently for severe late-presenting infantile idiopathic and congenital scoliosis (Figs. 4.84–4.86). The use of corrective jackets can also be effective in appropriate cases.

SURGICAL PROCEDURES

Harrington fusion (Figs. 4.87–4.94). This procedure is employed for the correction of all idiopathic curves with the exception of the thoracolumbar or lumbar curve with hyperlordosis, for which the Dwyer procedure is performed. The area to be fused must include the end vertebra and all vertebrae above and below the end vertebra which are rotated into the curve. This usually means fusing at least one vertebra above and two below the end vertebra. The advantage of the Dwyer procedure is that a smaller number of vertebrae can be fused.

The technique of Harrington fusion can be obtained from more detailed text

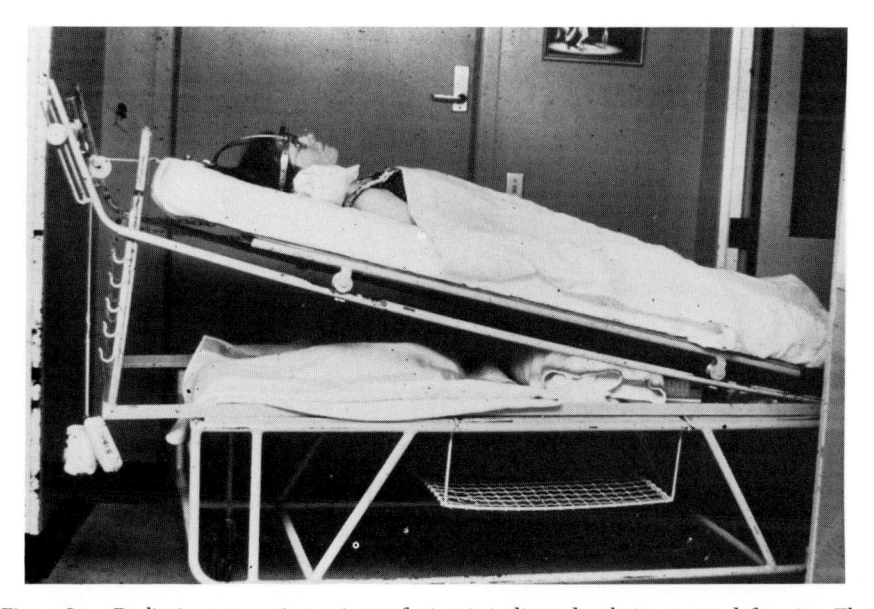

Fig. 4.82 Preliminary traction prior to fusion is indicated only in severe deformity. The halo traction is set up using the body weight as traction on an incline bed and is effective in obtaining correction.

218   Chapter 4

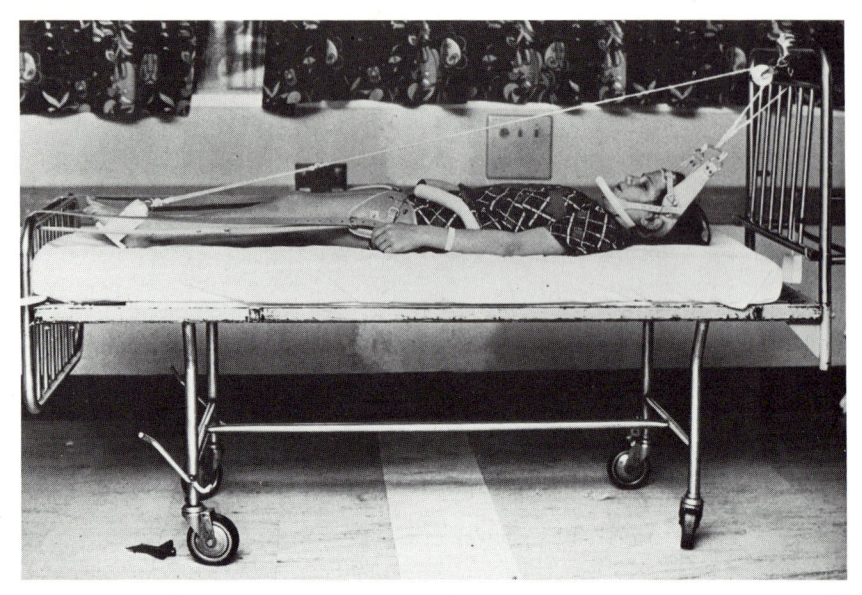

Fig. 4.83   Cottrell traction. This traction technique incorporates a static traction effect with the weight from the head halter over the end of the bed. A dynamic component is also incorporated with the ankle and knee providing the motor power to the spine.

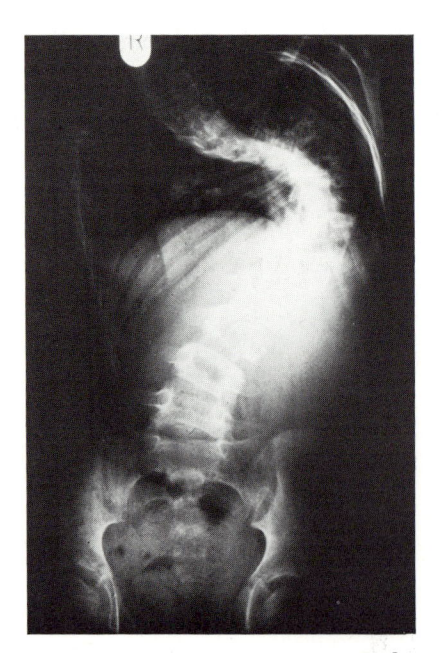

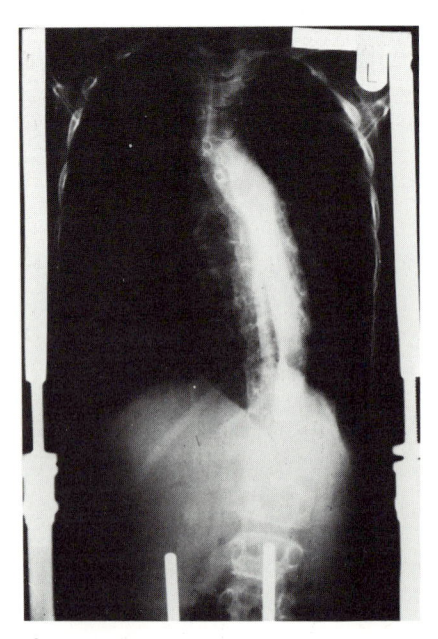

Figs. 4.84 & 4.85   Radiographs of same patient as Fig. 4.86.

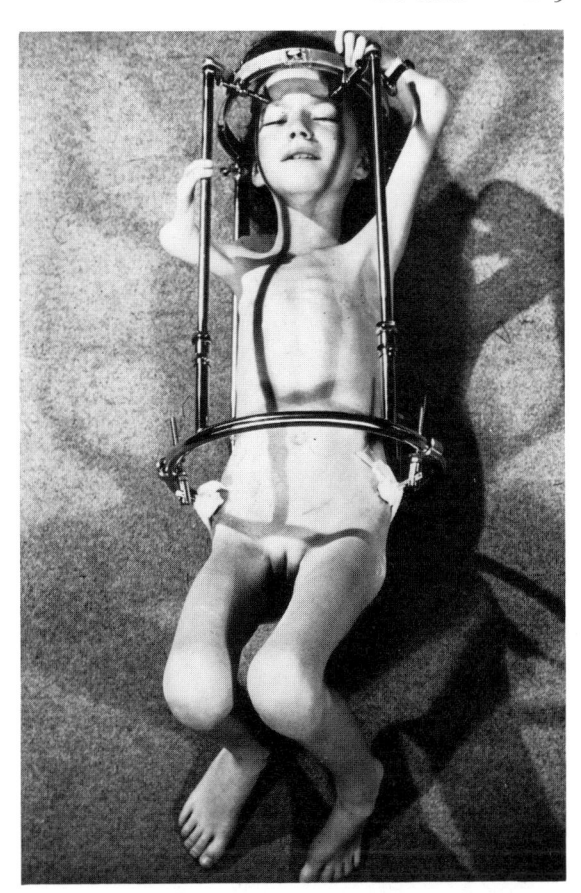

Fig. 4.86 Severe congenital scoliosis in a small child with associated congenital anomalies. Correction was obtained in a halo pelvic apparatus prior to fusion.

books on scoliosis. It is important in the technique of fusion that meticulous care be taken in exposure of the spine. The anaesthetist is a key member of the team and the use of hypotensive anaesthesia can dramatically reduce the amount of bleeding and the time taken to perform the procedure. Adequate exposure is essential as is careful and precise excision of the facet joints and plugging of these joints with cancellous bone. There must be meticulous stripping of the spines, laminae and transverse processes and subsequently complete decortication to obtain fresh bleeding cancellous bone for the graft bed. Autogenous bone taken from the iliac crest or occasionally from the tibial region is preferable to bank bone. If these measures are followed, the incidence of fusion and the complication rates are minimal.

The Harrington distraction and compression system is used wherever possible. The compression device is not used in the presence of thoracic lordosis.

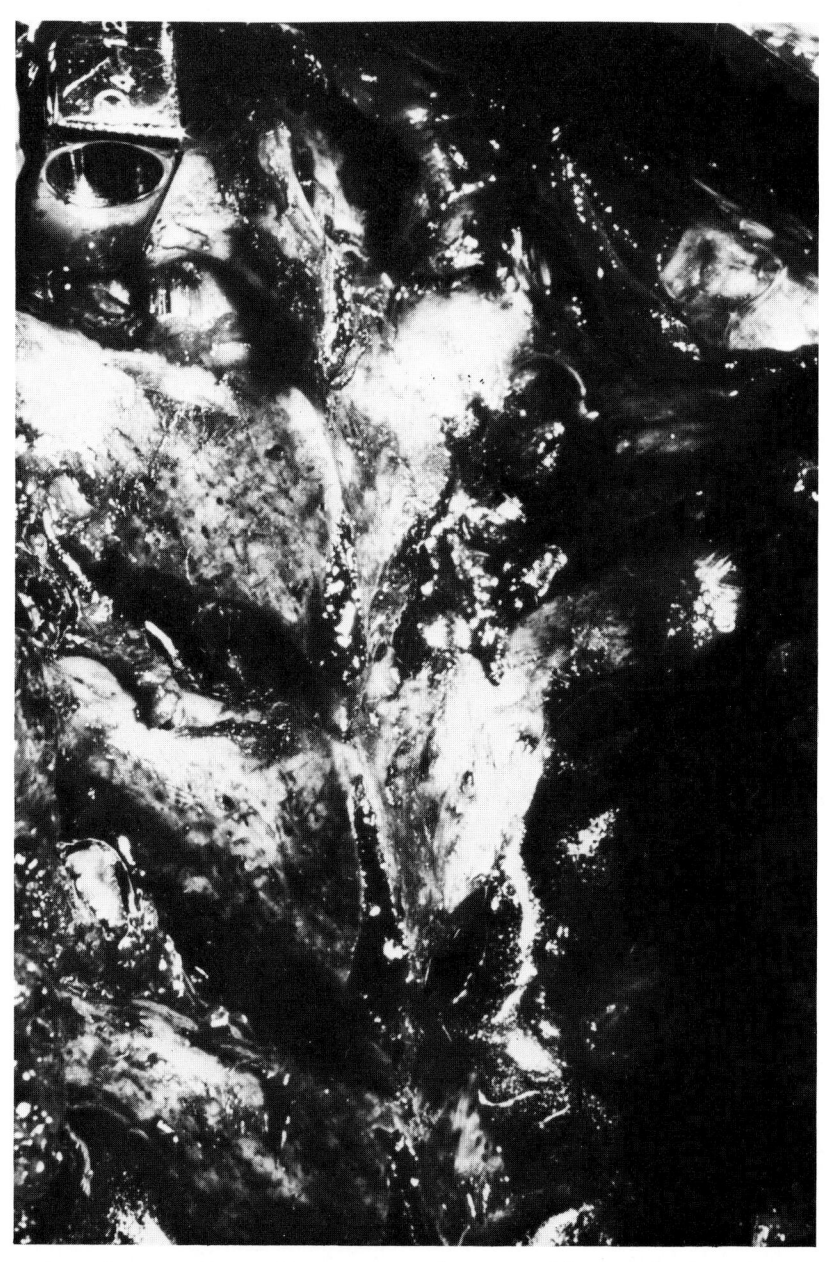

Fig. 4.87 Harrington fusion. Demonstrating placement of the upper hook into a prepared bed under the articular facet in the thoracic region.

The Child 221

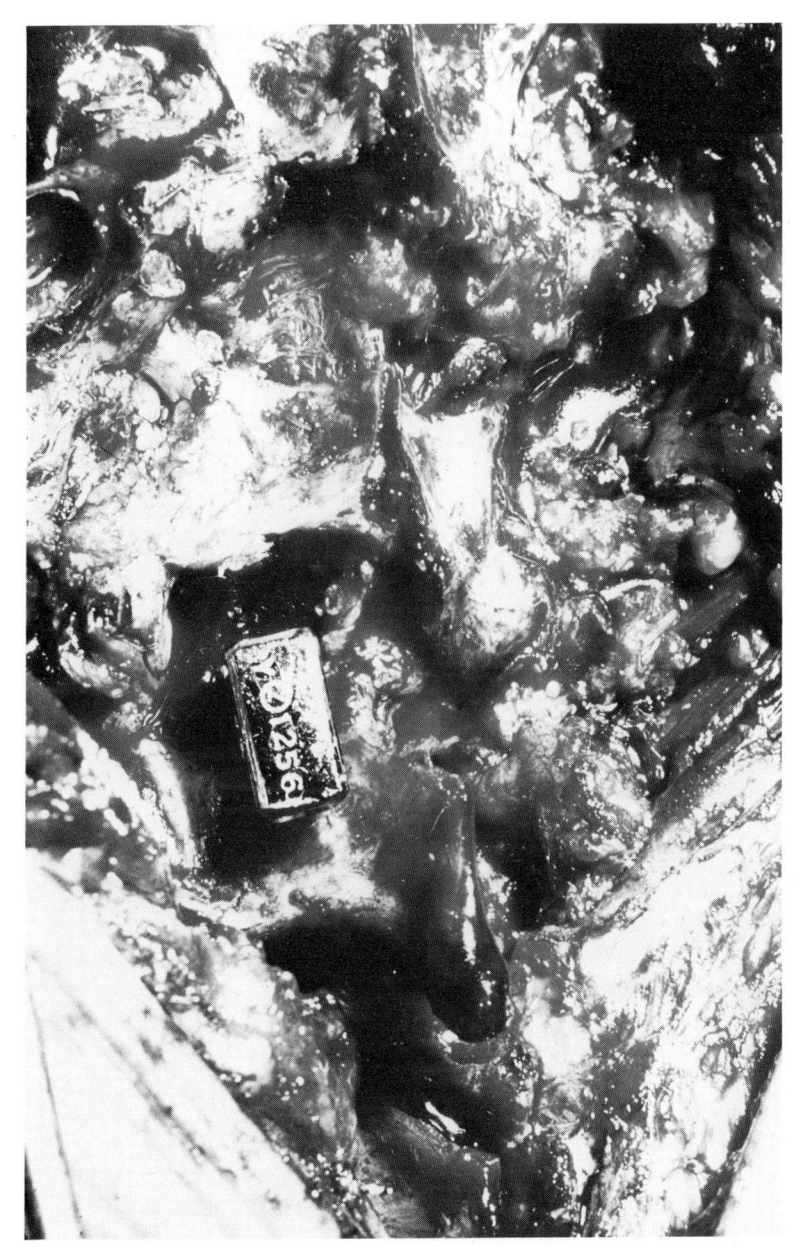

Fig. 4.88 The inferior hook seated over the lamina of the vertebra in the lumbar region after first removing the ligamentum flavum.

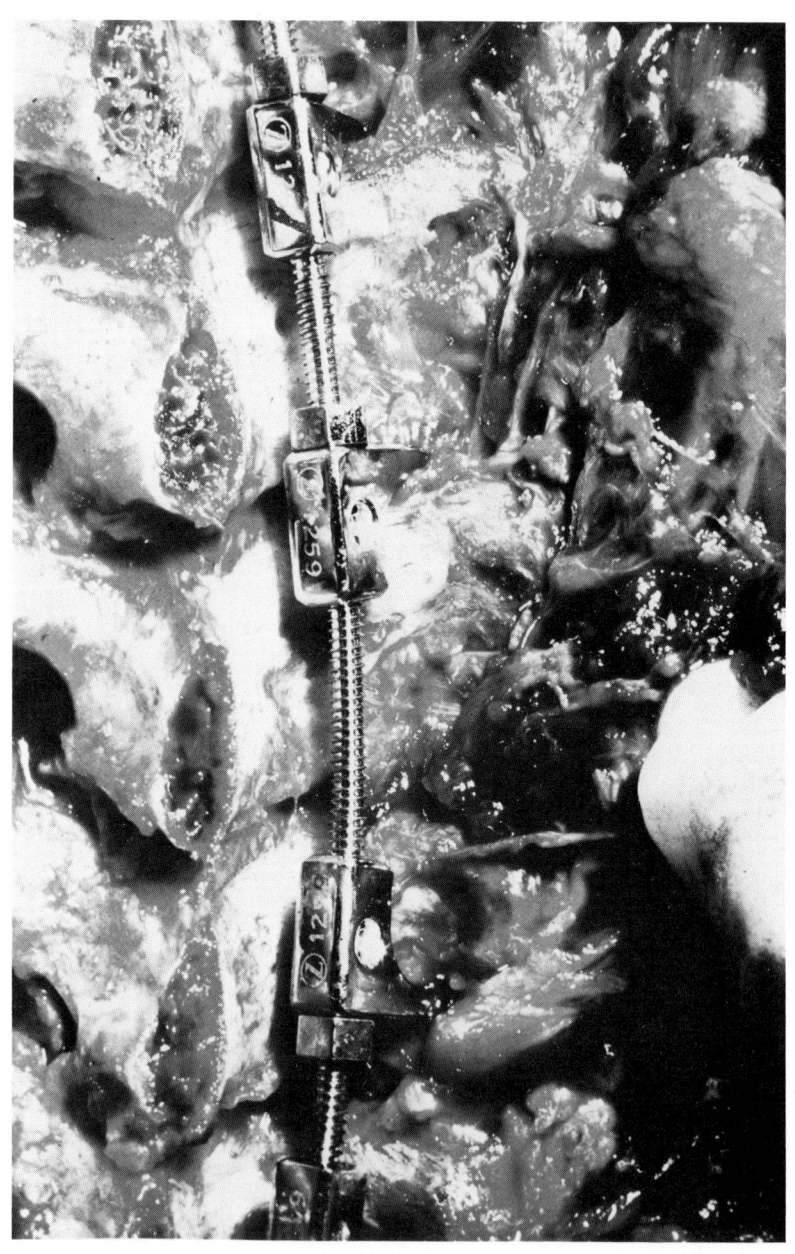

Fig. 4.89 Compression hooks on rod in position. The hook is placed either side of the adjacent transverse processes at the apex of the curve.

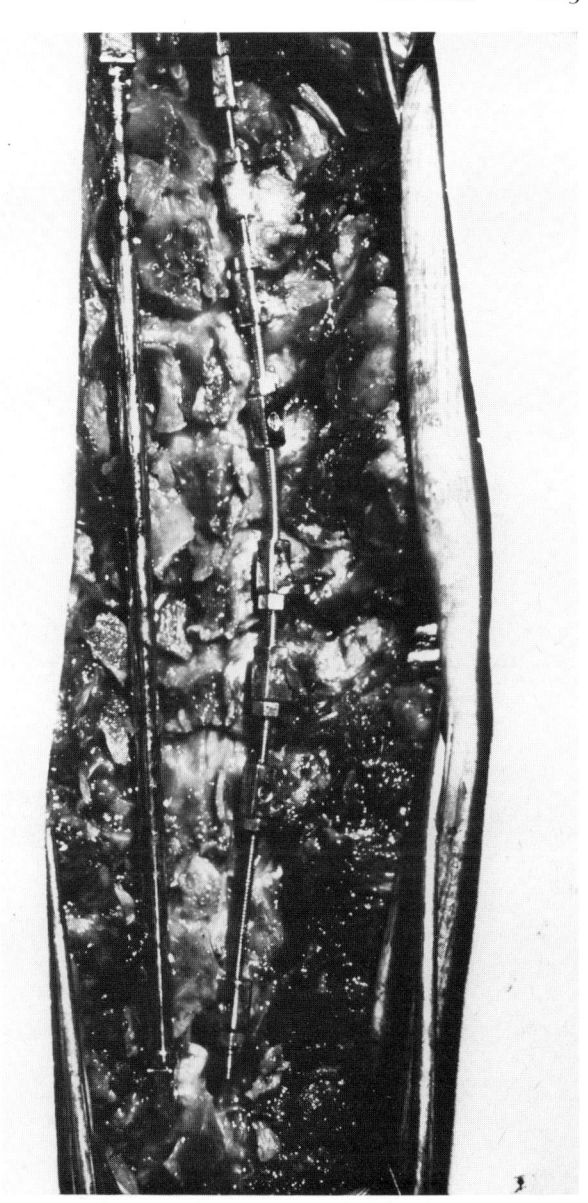

Fig. 4.90 Both distraction and compression apparatus have been placed in position and the correction obtained. Decortication of the posterior elements has been performed. The articular facets within the curve have been excised and some of the autogenous graft is in place.

224   Chapter 4

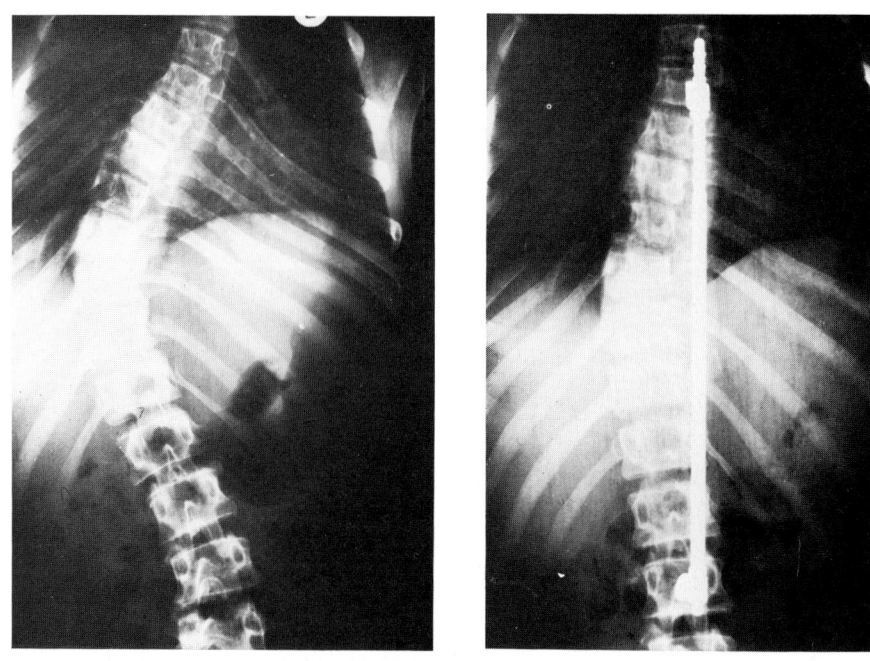

Figs. 4.91 & 4.92   A typical right sided thoracic curve. (*Right*) Treated with distraction rod only.

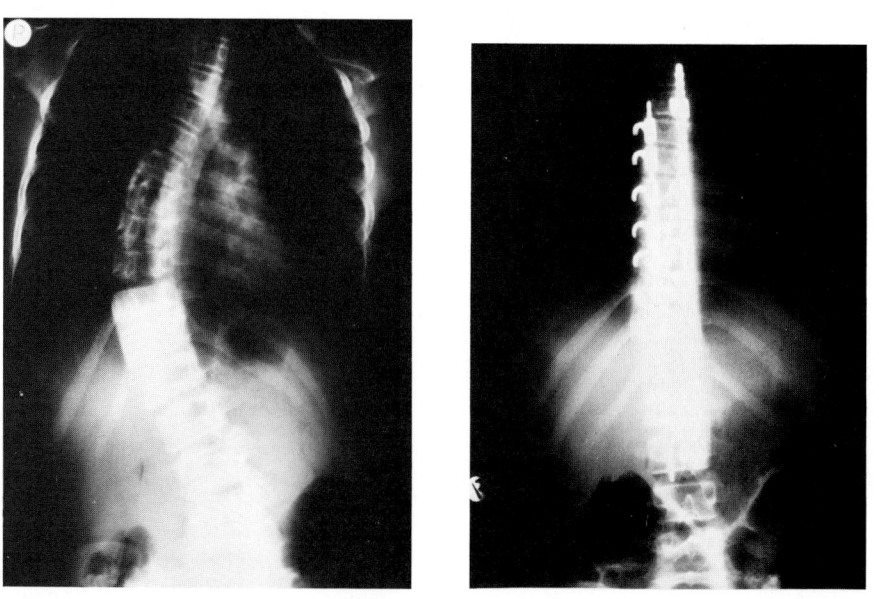

Figs. 4.93 & 4.94   Similar right sided thoracic curve. (*Right*) Treated with distraction and compression. The compression system is always placed inside the area covered by the distraction rod.

Dwyer's procedure (Figs. 4.95 & 4.96). Dwyer's procedure also requires considerable attention to detail in surgical technique and again the full details of the procedure are outlined elsewhere. The essential feature of the Dwyer procedure is the complete removal of all disc space material and vertebral end plates to give a circumferential clearance down to cancellous bone. The potential to produce

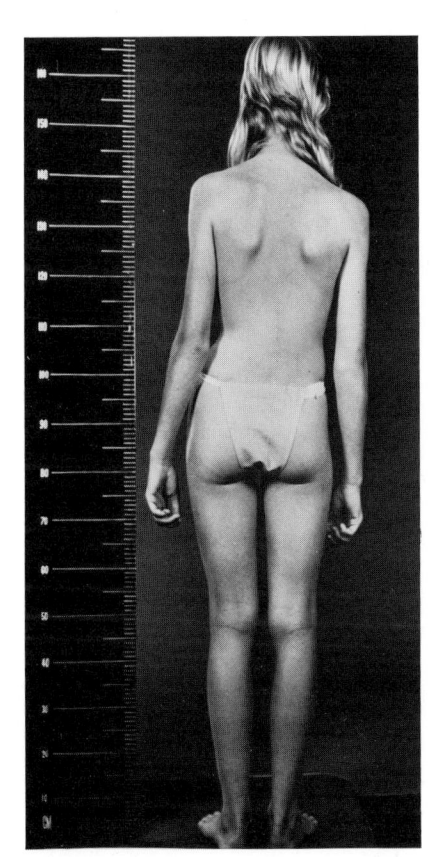

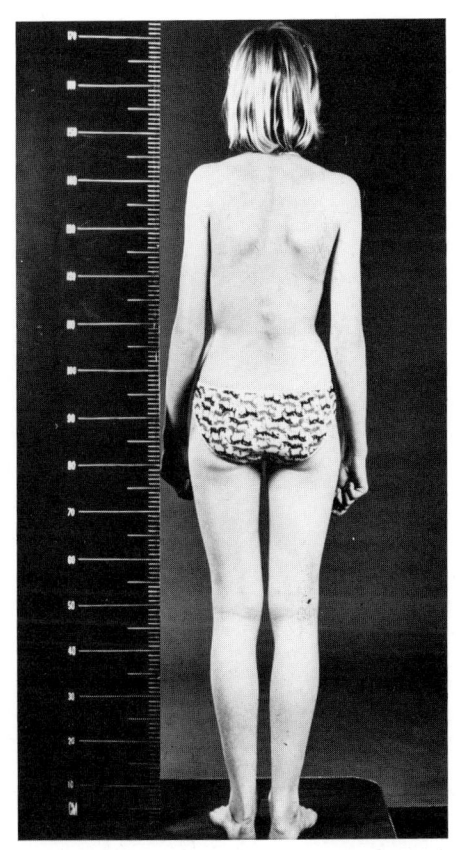

Figs. 4.95 & 4.96 Clinical appearance before and after Dwyer fusion. Note the correction of the list to the left side and the return to a more normal contour to the waist line.

kyphosis when using Dwyer's apparatus is considerable and therefore placement of the screws well back in the vertebral bodies and packing of the anterior disc space with graft material is advised. The new modification of Zilke using a rigid rod may help in this regard.

The best indication for the Dwyer procedure is the adolescent idiopathic lumbar or thoracolumbar curve in the presence of hyperlordosis (Figs. 4.97 & 4.98).

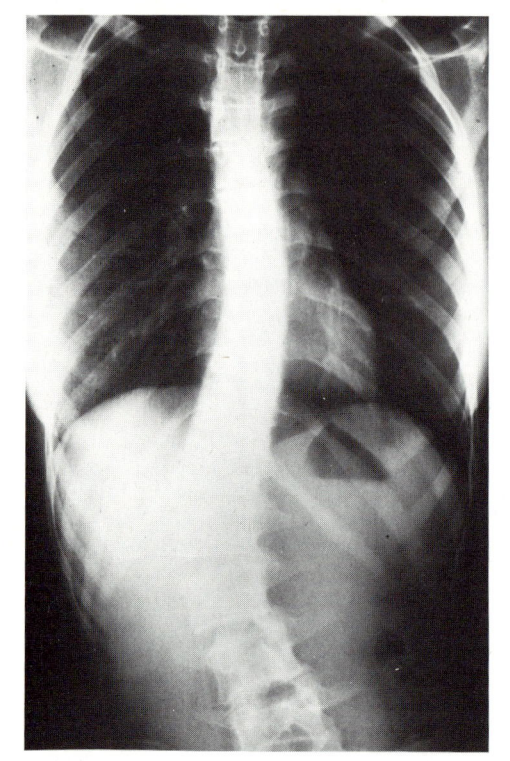

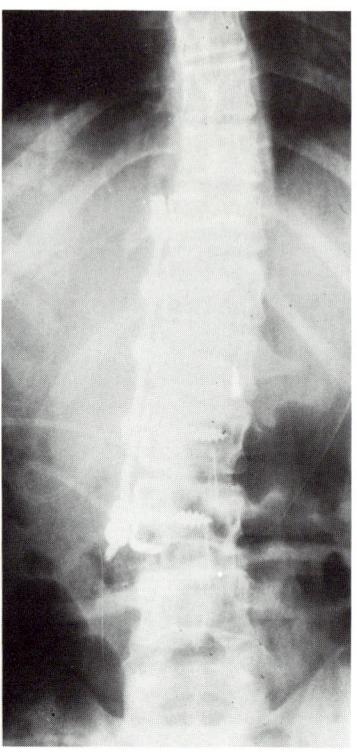

Figs. 4.97 & 4.98 Radiography of the spine prior to and following Dwyer fusion. Access has been obtained through the bed of the 11th rib. The patient had hyperlordosis pre-operatively.

POST-OPERATIVE CARE

In the post-operative phase, routine general care is performed. The patient is nursed on a Stryker frame (Fig. 4.99) following the Harrington procedure and sits free in bed after the Dwyer procedure. The chest drain is removed 2–3 days post-operatively after the Dwyer, the patient is then allowed to sit out of bed and, once able to stand for a sufficient time to allow casting, an underarm cast is applied. It is retained for three months. After the Harrington procedure, the patient remains recumbent on the Stryker bed for ten days and then a Risser cast is applied on the Cottrell table. This cast is retained for six months and the patient is then re-admitted, the jacket removed, and an assessment of the fusion made with x-rays. If soundly united, the patient is managed in a high Taylor brace (Fig. 4.100) which is retained for a minimum of three months (and usually for six) to protect the graft. In very young cases, the use of a Milwaukee brace for a prolonged period may be indicated to protect the sound fusion.

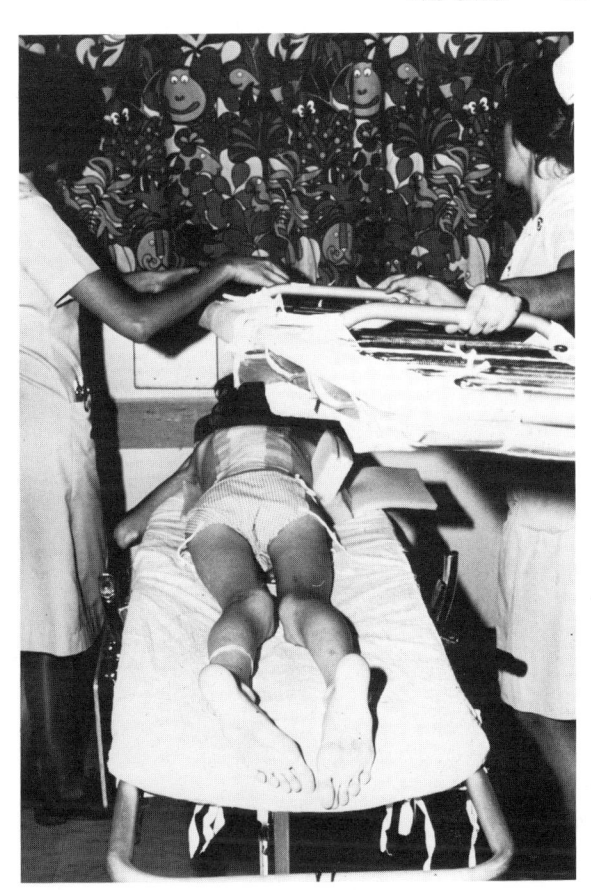

Fig. 4.99 The Stryker frame facilitates nursing care and turning in the post-operative stage.

OTHER SURGICAL TECHNIQUES IN SCOLIOSIS

Excision of the rib hump is a procedure which produces considerable cosmetic improvement. It is essential that very adequate respiratory function be present in those patients on whom this procedure is performed. In cases with neurological disorders where there is a collapsing spine, it is preferable wherever possible to obtain sound fusion both anteriorly and posteriorly. This may entail the use of a Dwyer anterior fusion followed by posterior Harrington fusion. This is particularly applicable in the patient with paralytic scoliosis and associated pelvic obliquity and predominantly when there is a lumbar curve. This is most commonly seen in children with spina bifida.

Neuromuscular scoliosis

The conditions producing paralytic scoliosis present specific problems which make management in many cases more difficult. The presence of muscle

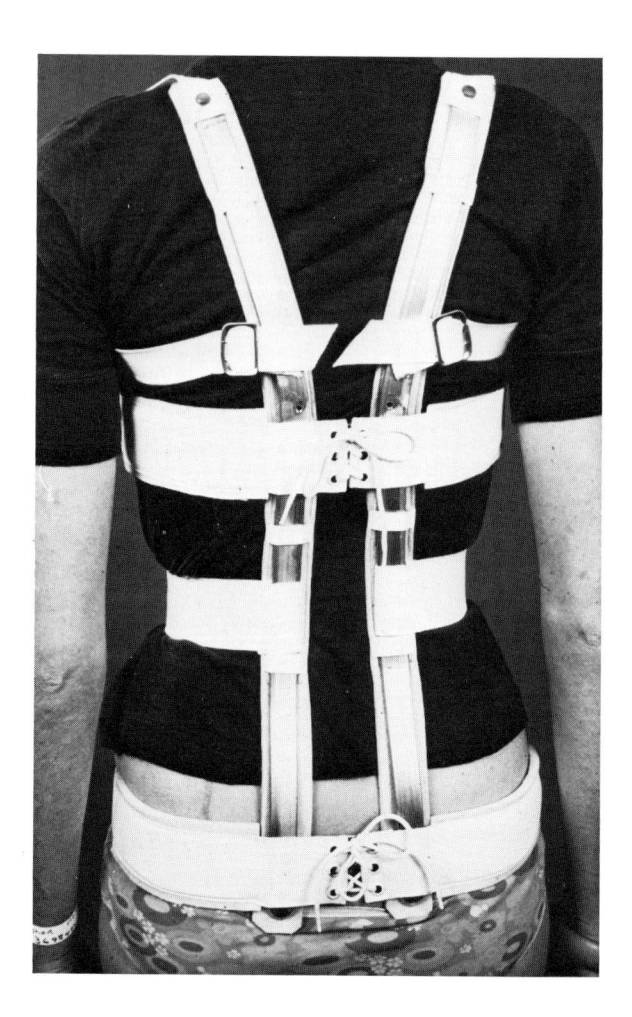

Fig. 4.100 The high Taylor brace is used as an external support after removal of the spinal jacket. The orthosis is worn for 3–6 months to afford protection to the fusion mass during maturation.

imbalance and the tendency for the curves to collapse results in a more rapid progression. If there is also a progressive neurological or muscular disorder, the rate of progression can be extremely rapid (Figs. 4.101 & 4.102). The presence of paralysis affects not only the muscles of the spine, but also the muscles of respiration and therefore one has to be more cautious in the management of this group of patients. Neuromuscular dysfunction also affects the patient's capacity to co-operate in the treatment programme making conservative management difficult and also complicating the operative and post-operative care.

Intra-operative problems are also increased due to osteoporosis and the necessity for long fusions. Pelvic obliquity is a common occurrence in paralytic curves due either to the curvature or contractures around the hip joint. Before embarking on surgical correction of the spinal deformity, it is imperative to correct any hip contractures by surgical means. If pelvic obliquity is present,

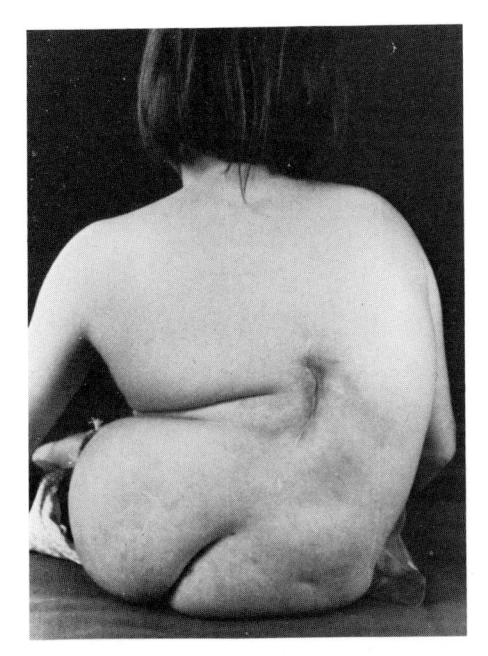

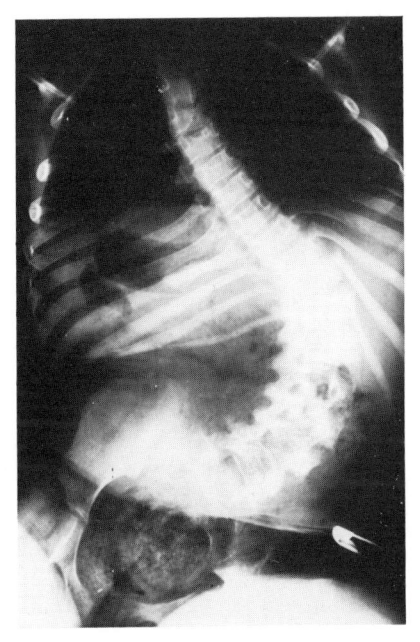

Figs. 4.101 & 4.102 Clinical photograph and x-ray demonstrating a typical paralytic scoliosis in a child with spina bifida. The pelvic obliquity produces sitting balance difficulties and increases the likelihood of pressure sore problems. The pelvic deformity was due to the spinal deformity and not related to hip joint contractures.

fusion to the pelvis is indicated. The poor musculature attaching to the wing of the ilium often produces rather poor bone stock for bone grafting and it is frequently necessary to resort to bone bank supplies to supplement autogenous bone graft in paralytic fusions.

In the post-operative phase, management is modified because of the need to provide longer periods of protection to the fusion area. The post-operative complications of pseudarthrosis and infection are higher in this group of patients. To avoid pseudarthrosis attempts are often made to obtain a 360° fusion, that is anterior and posterior fusion (Figs. 4.103 & 4.104). Infection in the post-operative phase is very common in spina bifida patients but can be reduced if attention is paid pre-operatively to the erradication of foci of infection, notably in the urinary tract.

In assessment of these patients it is often difficult to obtain erect films and, in many cases, sitting films are employed to assess the effect of gravity. Correction films are more appropriately done with the patient recumbent and in traction.

Conservative treatment of scoliosis in patients with neuromuscular disorders is a neglected area but more recently attempts have been made to control curves

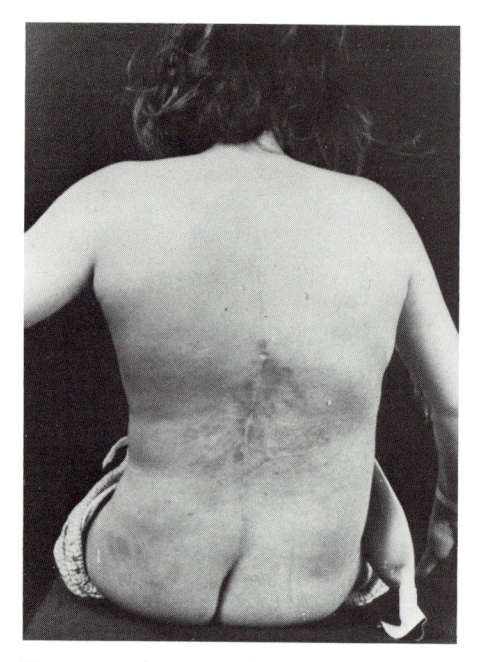

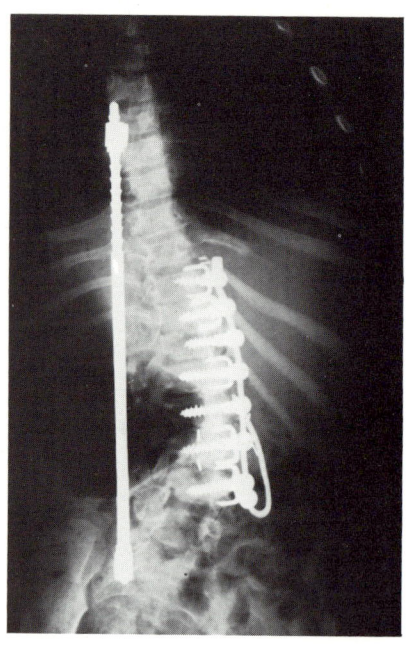

Figs. 4.103 & 4.104 Same patient as Fig. 4.101 following surgery employing both the Harrington and Dwyer procedures for correction, with a fusion both anteriorly and posteriorly. Employing the Moe sacral hook allows fusion to the ala and facilitates correction of pelvic obliquity.

in this group using orthoses and seating devices. It is hoped that this will result in fewer patients with paralytic scoliosis progressing to severe deformity. A limiting factor in conservative management is the presence or absence of skin sensation which can make orthotic care extremely difficult.

Progression of the primary pathology causing the scoliosis has a very marked bearing on the decision about treatment; the indications for surgery in this group are complex and not easily defined.

Problems such as sitting balance, pressure sores and pain may well determine that surgery is needed regardless of the degree of severity of the curve. Respiratory function also has a marked bearing on the decision for or against surgery. Surgery may be indicated to help preserve respiratory function.

The surgical management is complex and large fusions are required in most cases. The post-operative phase is difficult and, in unco-operative patients, immediate post-operative casting may be necessary. With all these precautions, the result of fusion in neuromuscular scoliosis can be most gratifying.

Congenital scoliosis

Congenital scoliosis is that curvature resulting from abnormal development of the bony architecture. The curve may be present at birth or may develop during growth. The abnormality of bone development may be single or multiple and may have associated involvement of the neural structures and other organs, in particular the renal tract and cardiac system. Many single abnormalities do not produce significant problems but there is a group in which severe progression can occur. As a result of the work of Winter, Moe and Eilers the congenital spinal anomalies have been classified into two: failure of segmentation and failure of formation. The failures of segmentation may be total and bilateral producing vertebral fusion or unilateral unsegmented bar (resulting in a considerable deformity). Failure of formation can be a partial failure of formation of half the vertebral body producing a wedge vertebra or total failure resulting in a hemivertebra. There is a group of congenital curvatures in which a mixture of failures of segmentation and formation occurs, so making classification impossible. In many of these groups, and particularly the latter, there may be congenital fusions of the ribs.

In those who have progressive scoliosis with congenital abnormalities, the shortening of the trunk is a frequent feature and the curves may progress to a very severe deformity. The association with diastematomyelia makes it mandatory to perform myelography in any patient with congenital scoliosis if surgical correction is contemplated. The condition of unilateral unsegmented bar is one which is always associated with progression and can produce very severe deformation. In this group surgical fusion at an early stage is indicated to stop growth on the convexity of the curve and so avoid severe deformity. The use of the Milwaukee brace in congenital scoliosis is often associated with failure of control.

Scoliosis associated with other causes

MARFAN'S SYNDROME

Marfan's syndrome is a dominantly inherited condition and has a 45% incidence of scoliosis. The scoliosis usually appears in the 10–12 year group, develops rapidly, and can progress to quite a severe curve. Patients with Marfan's syndrome can expect a life span into the fourth decade, however they should anticipate continued difficulties since it is a feature of the scoliosis in this condition that it can progress even after skeletal maturity.

The indications for surgical correction are as for adolescent idiopathic scoliosis and the Milwaukee brace also is employed, although it is often not effective. One must be aware of the condition of homocystinuria which produces a syndrome similar to Marfan's syndrome, but is an inherited condition which is often associated with mental retardation. In this, surgical intervention can result in coagulation problems and thrombosis.

232   Chapter 4

NEUROFIBROMATOSIS

This is an autosomal dominantly inherited condition with an incidence which has been variously reported to be as high as 75% and as low as 2%. There are several curve patterns recognised in the disorder. The condition may be associated with a typical curve of idiopathic scoliosis. The classical deformity, however, is a severe, sharp, angular deformity usually associated with a kyphotic

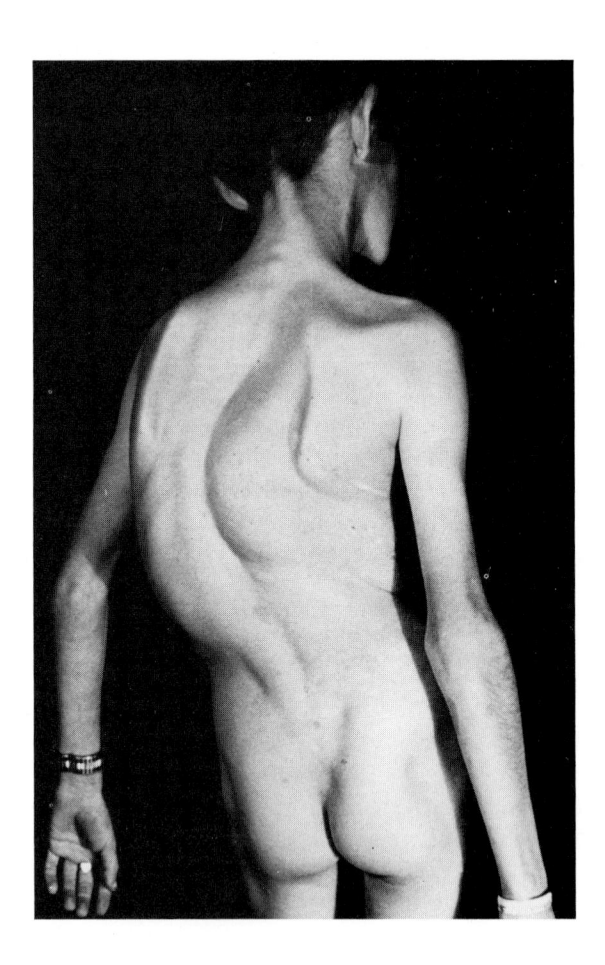

Fig. 4.105   A boy with the characteristic kyphoscoliosis of neurofibromatosis.

element (Figs. 4.105 & 4.106). These curves progress rapidly to a rigid and fixed deformity.

In the idiopathic type, the treatment of this curve is along identical lines to those for the adolescent idiopathic scoliosis. In the very severe classical curve one associates with neurofibromatosis, bracing is usually ineffective and early surgical fusion is recommended.

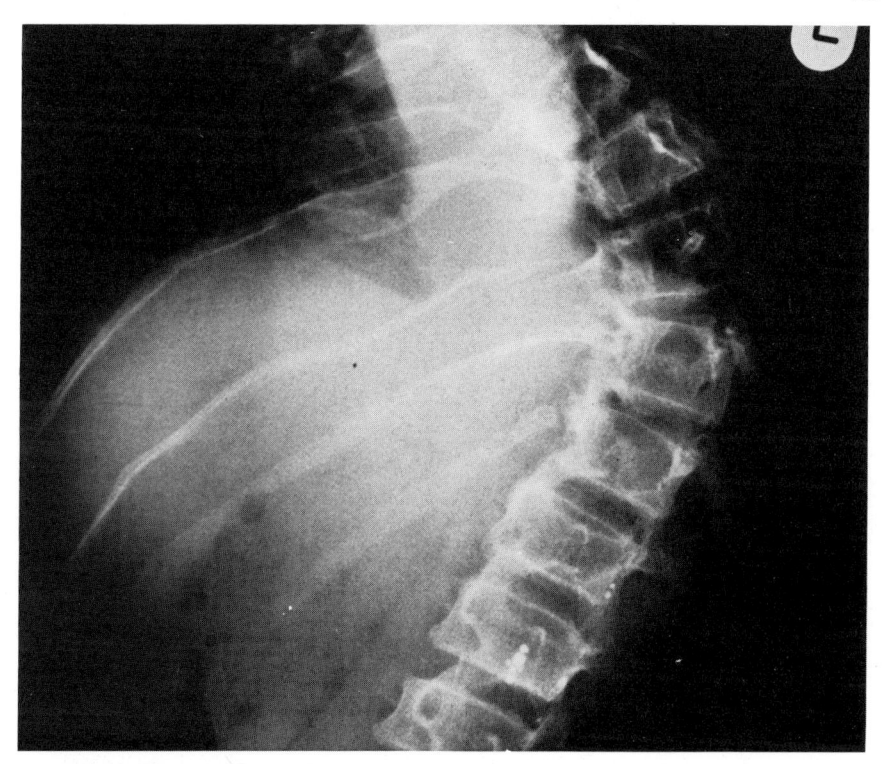

Fig. 4.106 The angular scoliosis of neurofibromatosis. Note also the characteristic ribboning of the ribs.

Scheuermann's disease

The condition of Scheuermann's disease, or juvenile kyphosis, is a condition of obscure aetiology. Abnormalities of the ring apophyseal growth plates, end plate disruption due to disc protrusion, contracture of muscles, and osteoporosis have all been suggested as possible reasons for the tendency for these vertebrae to collapse anteriorly.

CLINICAL PRESENTATION

Children usually present because of deformity; pain is not a feature of the disorder in the early phase. The appearances of the spine are those of an accentuation of the normal thoracic kyphosis and lumbar lordosis (Figs. 4.107 & 4.108). This is much more obvious in the forward flexed position where there is an angular deformity at the apex of the affected segment. Frequently there is a mild associated scoliosis of a structural type with rotation producing a slight prominence of the ribs on forward bending (Fig. 4.109).

234 Chapter 4

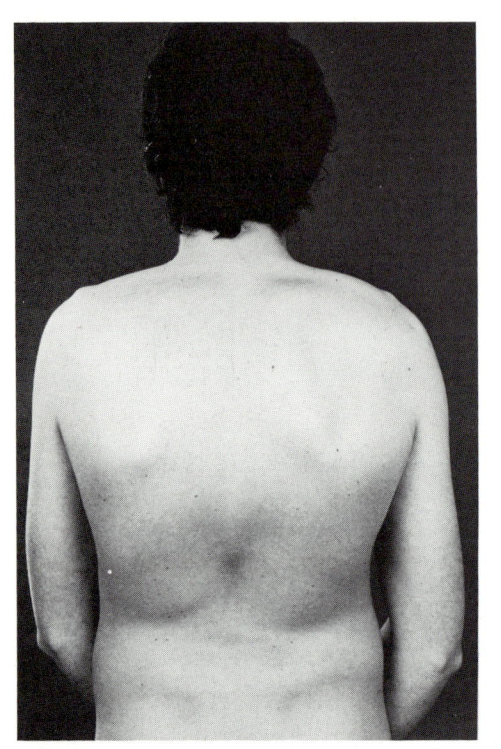

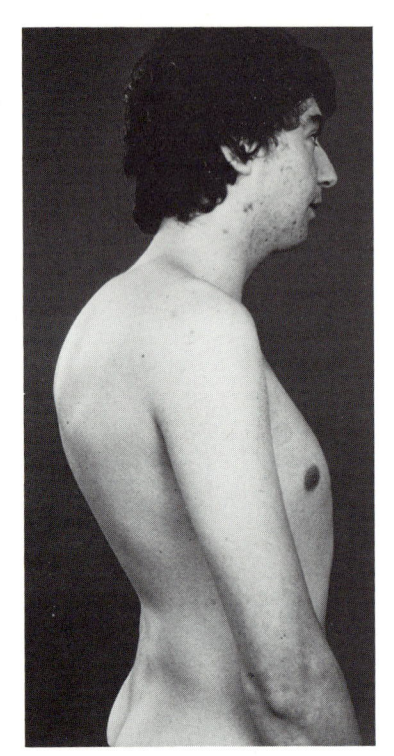

Figs. 4.107 & 4.108 Scheuermann's disease—characteristic appearances.

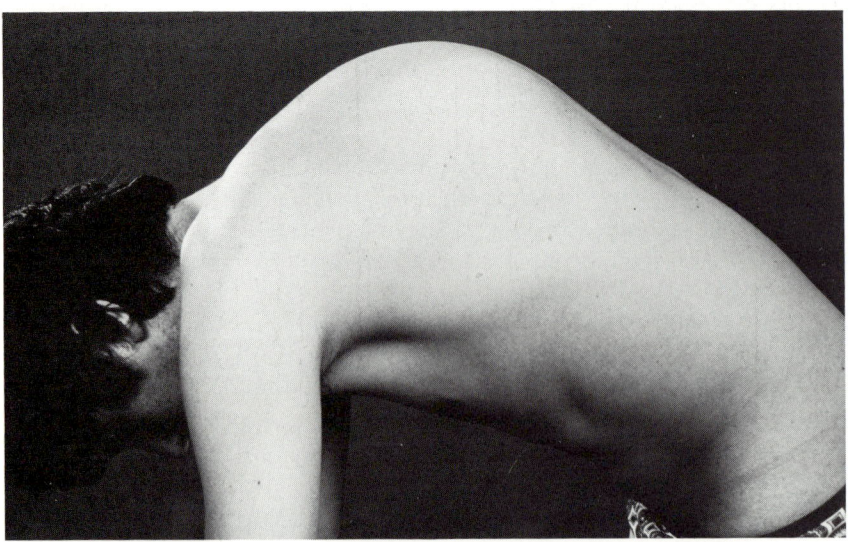

Fig. 4.109 Same patient as Fig. 4.107. The accentuation of the thoracic kyphosis is more marked on forward flexion when viewed from the side. Compensatory lumbar lordosis is also evident but is not fixed and corrects with forward flexion.

The Child 235

RADIOGRAPHIC EVALUATION

Routine full length A–P and lateral films should be taken with the patient standing. They must include the iliac crest to assess skeletal maturity. Measurement of these curves is by the Cobb technique, as described for scoliosis (p. 207). The classical x-ray appearances are wedging of the vertebral body (Fig. 4.110),

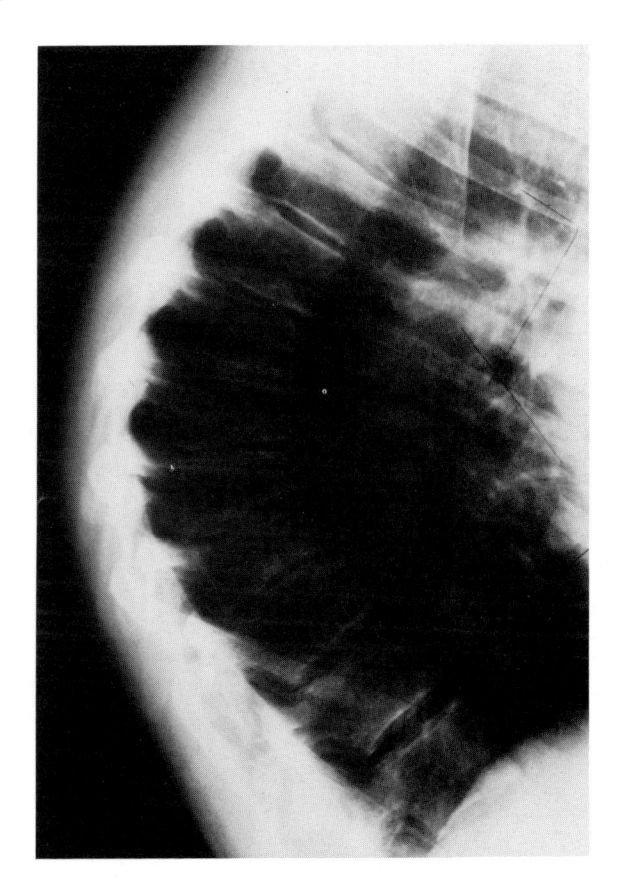

Fig. 4.110
Radiograph of the spine demonstrating wedging of vertebral bodies on the lateral (erect) view.

often associated with disc protrusion into the vertebral body (Schmorl's nodes), and an irregular, moth-eaten appearance in the growth plate.

A Cobb angle of kyphosis greater than 40° is regarded as an abnormal kyphosis.

INDICATIONS FOR TREATMENT

In those patients with a fixed dorsal kyphosis in which skeletal growth still remains, a Milwaukee brace has proved most effective in correcting the curve. The brace usually has its effect over a very short time and once correction has

236 Chapter 4

been obtained the patient can be weaned out of the brace quite early on. The indications for Milwaukee braces are curves between 40 and 60° producing a significant cosmetic deformity in a child who has an immature skeleton.

If the curve is greater than 60° it is unlikely that the Milwaukee brace will be effective and, under these circumstances, surgical correction using Harrington compression systems can be undertaken (Figs. 4.111 & 4.112).

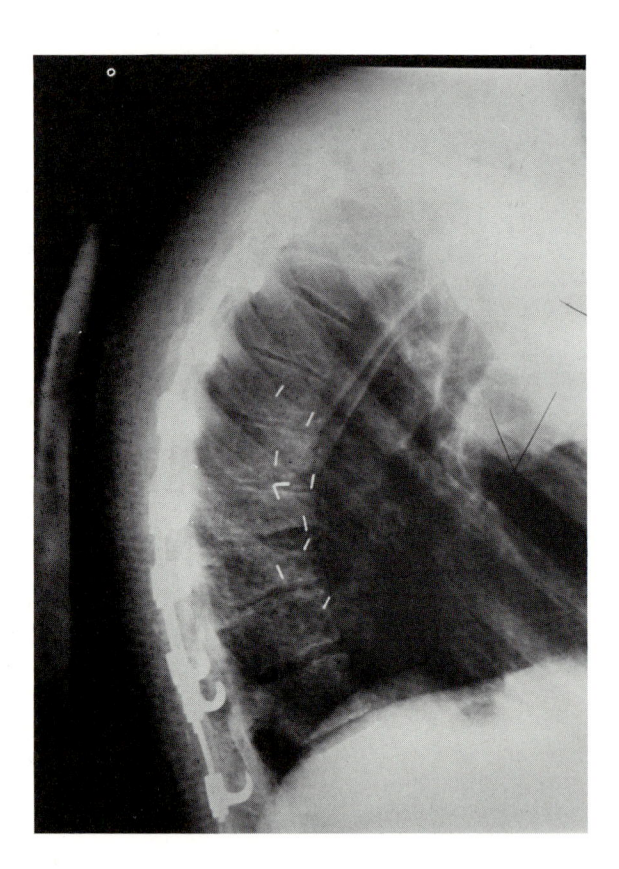

Fig. 4.111 Surgical correction of Scheuermann's disease with marked kyphosis.

SPINAL DYSRAPHISM

The term spinal dysraphism was first employed by Lichtenstein in 1940. He used the term to describe the conditions in which there was incomplete fusion in the midline of various embryonic structures related to the spinal cord and its coverings. The term was extended by Garceau in 1953, to include conditions in which there was tethering of the conus and, in 1960, James and Lassman described the orthopaedic manifestations of the condition in considerable detail. They were able to describe the operative findings in a large series of patients.

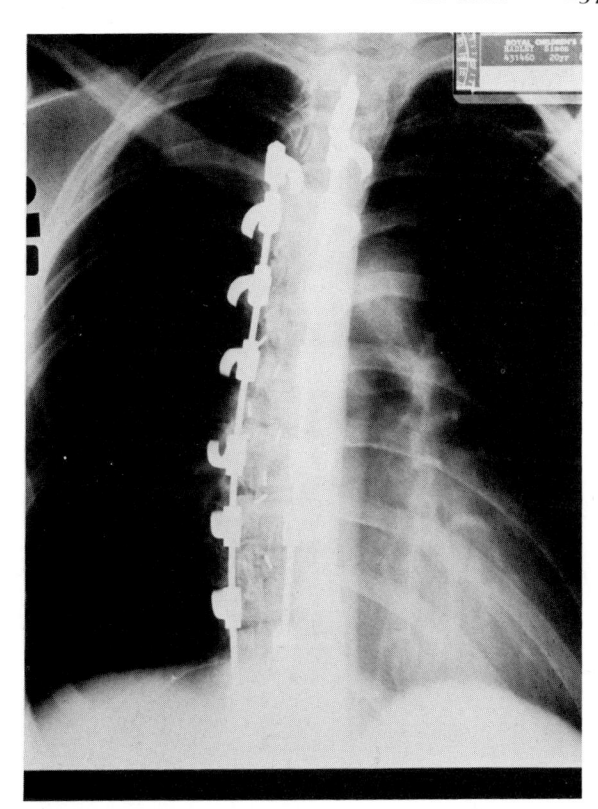

Fig. 4.112 Same patient as Fig. 4.111. Harrington compression rods have been employed posteriorly to obtain correction following a preceding anterior spinal release.

Pathology

Various forms of pathology are associated with spinal dysraphism. Most commonly there is some abnormality which results in a traction lesion on lumbar or sacral nerve roots. Normally the level of the conus is at the tip of the coccyx in the fetus, at the upper level of the third lumbar vertebra at birth, and at the upper level of the second lumbar vertebra at the age of 5 years. Those patients with tethering of nerve roots may have the conus at a lower level than is appropriate for their age as well as a thickened, tight filum terminale. The second most common cause of the condition is an intraspinal lipoma and the third is diastematomyelia—here there is a midline spur (either of bone or fibrous tissue) which splits the spinal cord into two parts which pass on either side of it. Other forms of pathology which may be present are a dermal sinus, abnormalities in the composition or level or mobility of nerve roots, and dermoid cyst formation.

Clinical features

Deformity of one foot is the commonest presenting complaint and examination

238   *Chapter 4*

may then reveal changes in the low back. These may consist of a pit, sinus, pigmented area, lipoma, or patch of hair in the midline of the back (Fig. 4.113).

The orthopaedic manifestations of the condition may be one or several of the following:

A short leg
A small foot
Cavo-varus deformity of the foot
Paralytic valgus deformity

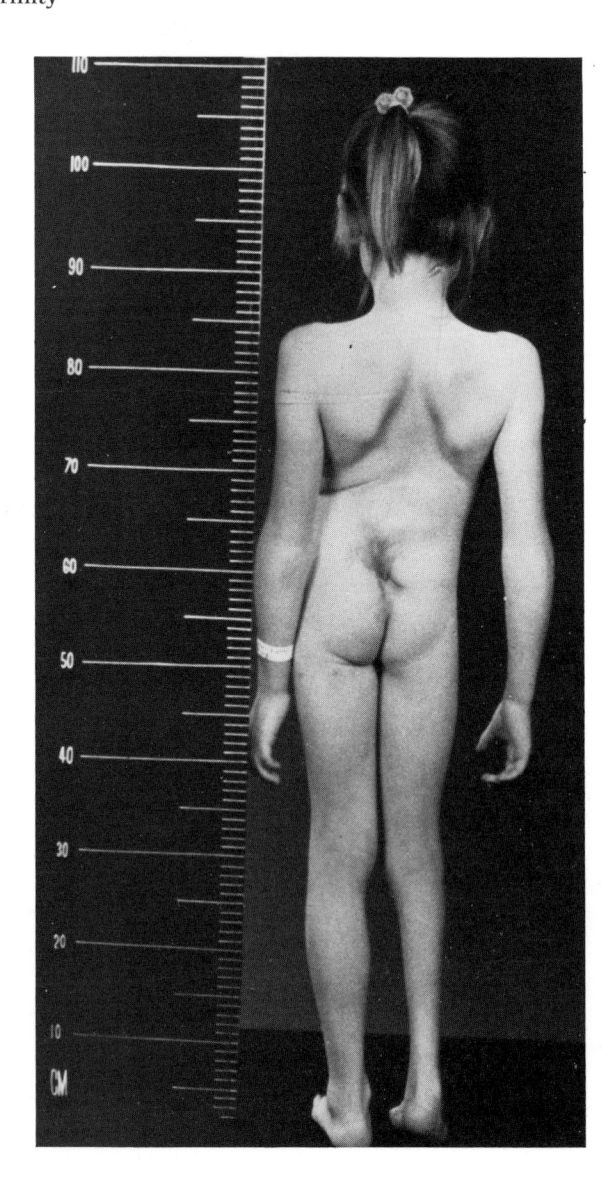

Fig. 4.113 Spinal dysraphism presenting at the age of 5 years. There is a tuft of hairs in the lumbo-sacral region, gross wasting and shortening of the right leg, and increasing cavo-varus deformity of the right foot.

Trophic ulceration
Minor abnormality of gait
Pain in the foot or back

On neurological examination there may be depression of reflexes, analgesia to pin prick, and muscle weakness in areas depending on the nerve roots affected.

INVESTIGATIONS

X-rays

Any child who presents with any of the clinical features listed above should have an x-ray of the entire spine. This may show spina bifida, a widened canal (with an increase in the interpedicular distance), a bony spur, abnormal laminae, or abnormalities of segmentation of the vertebral bodies.

Myelography

Air or metrisamide myelography is preferred. It is indicated in any patient in whom there is a high index of suspicion of spinal dysraphism, especially if there are radiographic abnormalities in the plain x-rays. However, an unexplained foot deformity or neurological abnormality in the lower limb (with or without skin manifestations) may lead the clinician to perform myelography. The myelogram will define the nature and extent of the lesion, locate the conus and demonstrate whether or not the cord and nerve roots are normally mobile.

Urological function should be assessed by an intravenous pyelogram and micturating cystourethrogram in all patients.

INDICATIONS FOR SURGERY

An absolute indication for spinal exploration is the combination of progressive loss of function with a recognised abnormality on myelography which, in whole or part, could be corrected by surgery.

If distal tethering is discovered in a patient with scoliosis this must be corrected prior to surgical intervention, particularly if a spinal lengthening procedure is to be employed. Without prior correction, acute deterioration in function can complicate the scoliosis operation.

The combination of myelographic anomaly and a stable state of lower limb function is a less clear indication for surgical exploration. The bone or fibrous septum in diastematomyelia should always be excised because of the high risk of late deterioration, and a dermal sinus should be similarly dealt with to prevent intraspinal sepsis.

With all other lesions a conservative course involving careful repeated examination is advisable. Spinal surgery is only advisable if definite neurologic deterioration is documented.

SURGICAL MANAGEMENT

The aim of surgery is to relieve traction on the terminal neural tissues and thereby restore their normal mobility. In the case of a dermal sinus, the elimination of a source of infection is an additional important consideration. It is generally possible to achieve mobility of the nervous tissues without risk of further damage but, in the case of an intraspinal lipoma, great care and careful judgement are required.

The outcome of a successful operation would be the absence of any further neurologic deterioration. In a small number of cases, some improvement may occur although this is generally minimal. Any subsequent orthopaedic treatment to correct foot deformity should therefore not face the risk of late deterioration. It should be noted that neurological deterioration is only to be expected during the period of spinal growth. In children presenting close to maturity it is therefore legitimate management to ignore the spinal lesion and to treat the orthopaedic complaint on its merits.

TORTICOLLIS

The term torticollis means a twisted neck. Generally there is lateral flexion of the head towards the shoulder with rotation of the face towards the opposite shoulder. The causes can be conveniently categorised into neonatal, sternomastoid, and secondary.

Neonatal torticollis

This is due to the posture of the baby in utero. It may be associated with a postural scoliosis with the convexity of the curve in the same direction as the convexity of the curve of the torticollis. Such children commonly have limited abduction in flexion of the hip on the concave side of the curve. This syndrome always recovers spontaneously without treatment but may persist for as long as twelve months.

Sternomastoid or infantile torticollis

This condition is associated with abnormalities within the sternomastoid muscle and will be considered in detail below.

Secondary torticollis

TRAUMA

Following falls and motor vehicle accidents, children between the ages of 4 and 10 years are commonly admitted to hospital with a severe stiff neck which may be held a little asymmetrically and in flexion. There is considerable discomfort on movement of the neck. Radiographs may show an acute angulation between two adjacent vertebrae in the upper cervical spine—usually C_2 on C_3. This is a normal appearance in children when they are x-rayed with their neck in full flexion.

These patients are presumed to have a ligamentous injury which settles with a period of rest in bed followed by the use of a soft collar until the symptoms settle, about two weeks later. Rarely children take very much longer to get better following an incident of trauma to the neck. If they hold their head with marked asymmetry, antero-posterior views of the atlanto-axial joint may suggest subluxation of these joints (rotary atlanto-axial dislocation). This is a radiological appearance resulting from the posture of the upper two cervical vertebrae (Fig. 4.114). Such children have presumably suffered a more major ligamentous injury to the cervical spine (the nature of which is yet to be defined) and the recovery may take many months. These patients may obtain greater comfort and quicker recovery if they are placed on neck traction for several days. Once the posture of the cervical spine has been restored to normal the radiological appearance of the atlanto-axial joints returns to normal.

INFECTION

Torticollis may result from external compression of the spinal cord or its nerve roots by chronic pyogenic osteomyelitis or tuberculous osteomyelitis of the spine. Chronic sepsis in lymph glands adjacent to the cervical spine may also result in this deformity. These inflammatory conditions may proceed to osteomyelitis of the spine.

TUMOUR

Extramedullary spinal cord tumours such as fibromata, epidermoid cysts, or dermoids may cause external compression on the spinal cord or on nerve roots which then results in torticollis.

MUSCLE SPASM

Children may present with torticollis of an acute onset without any underlying cause being apparent. The reason may be that one sternomastoid muscle is in a state of acute spasm which passes off over a period of several days. Sometimes this condition is attributed to exposure to cold.

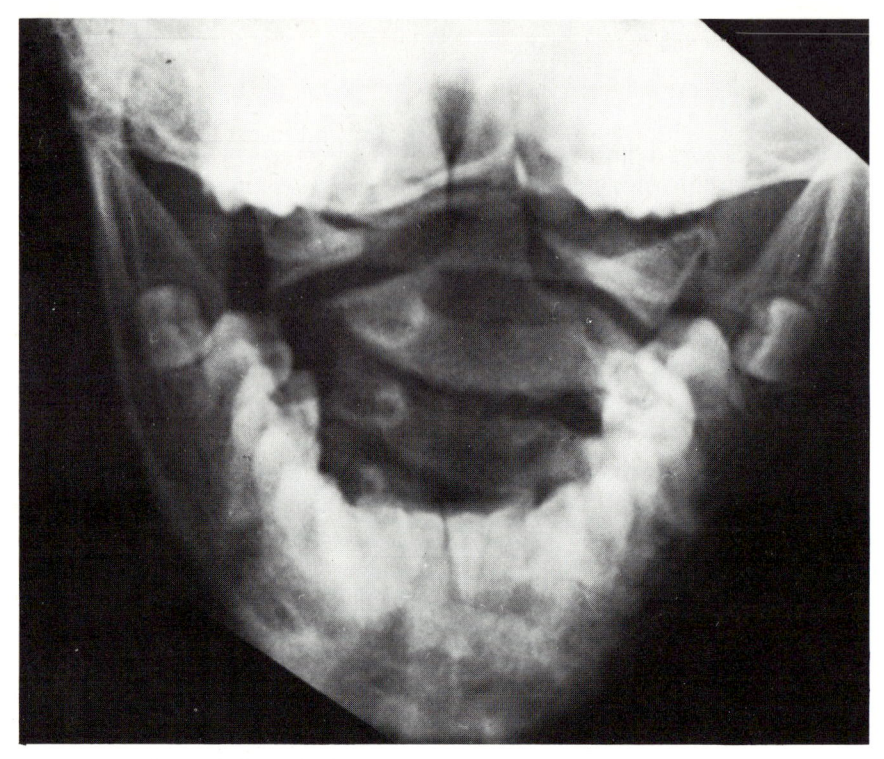

Fig. 4.114 The radiological changes in the condition which has been designated atlanto-axial rotary instability. These changes may simply reflect the altered posture of the upper cervical spine rather than imply any primary pathology in the atlanto-axial joints. There is asymmetry of the atlanto-axial joints with lateral displacement of the lateral mass of the atlas on the side of the widened joint (right side). If the neck can be placed in the anatomical position (and it may require anaesthesia to do this) the radiographs then show a normal appearance of these joints.

VERTEBRAL ANOMALIES

Congenital vertebral body anomalies may produce torticollis.

OCULAR

Muscle imbalance of the external ocular musculature may lead to torticollis. Usually the imbalance affects those muscles responsible for movement in the vertical direction.

HYSTERIA

Hysteria is a cause of torticollis in adults and rarely in childhood.

Sternomastoid or infantile torticollis

This is the most common form of torticollis. At some time between birth and the age of 3 years the characteristic deformity is noted. In one in five cases a sternomastoid tumour is present between the ages of 1 and 4 weeks. The tumour always resolves without treatment and only one-third of these cases subsequently require treatment for torticollis.

AETIOLOGY

The cause of the condition is unknown and no explanation is convincing. Trauma due to birth injury has been suggested and is supported by the high incidence of breech and forceps deliveries in patients with this condition. However a sternomastoid tumour may be present at birth in a child born by Caesarean section. Sternomastoid tumours have been reported in identical twins. Ischaemia has long been considered a cause; both arterial and venous occlusions have been implicated. It may be that both trauma and ischaemia occur during the birth process.

PATHOLOGY

A sternomastoid tumour may occupy either the sternal head or both heads of the sternomastoid muscle. Microscopy displays degenerating muscle and cellular fibrous tissue. In established torticollis, biopsy shows mature fibrous tissue in various portions of the sternomastoid muscle. There may also be thickening and shortening of the surrounding fascia.

CLINICAL FEATURES

The condition may present in a number of different manners. Between the first and the fourth weeks of life the child may present with a swelling in the neck which is large and discrete and can be felt to be within the sternomastoid muscle. In addition, the lump is tender and the child exhibits signs of discomfort if the muscle is stretched. There may be accompanying torticollis deformity. By the seventh month of life the sternomastoid tumour has generally disappeared. At some time after this the child may present with the characteristic deformity of torticollis with lateral flexion of the head towards the side of the tight muscle and rotation of the face towards the opposite shoulder. The affected muscle may be deformed as well as shortened with abnormal bands passing to the clavicle well lateral to the lateral extent of the normal muscle. Whilst the majority of children present within the the first three years of life, a few patients have such a minor degree of deformity that they do not present until adolescence.

With well established deformity there is a full range motion in the direction of the deformity but limitation of motion in the opposite direction. Facial asymmetry

244   Chapter 4

is generally marked in the infant with torticollis, though it may not be present in the child with a sternomastoid tumour. Later, facial asymmetry gradually increases as does the neck deformity. The face on the side of the deformity is smaller in all its features and the eye is smaller and lower than the opposite side (Fig. 4.115). Affected children at birth commonly have marked plagiocephaly which improves spontaneously.

DIFFERENTIAL DIAGNOSIS

If there is a characteristic sternomastoid tumour or if the sternomastoid muscle can be felt to be contracted then the diagnosis is certain. Difficulty arises when a patient presents with the head tilted to one side but the sternomastoid muscle is not definitely abnormal. In these circumstances the various forms of secondary torticollis (outlined above) are excluded by careful physical examination, radiology of the spine, and consultation with an ophthalmologist.

MANAGEMENT

If a child presents in the first year of life with a sternomastoid tumour or torticollis,

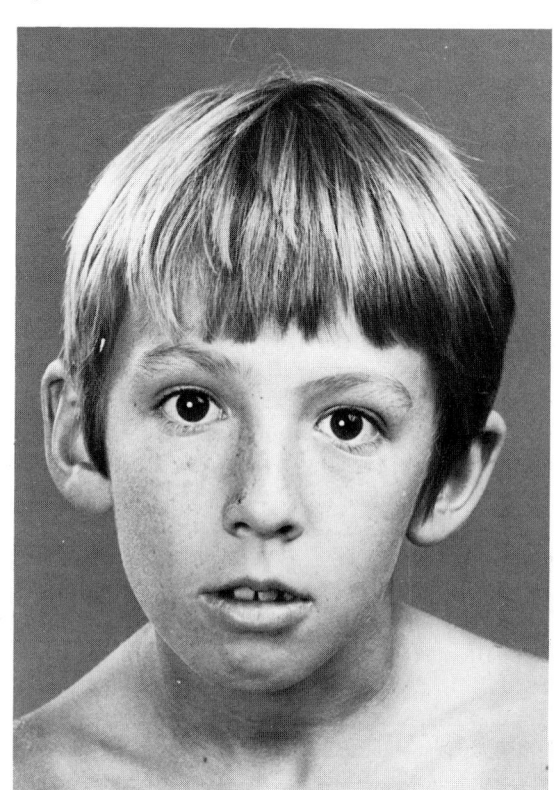

Fig. 4.115   Left sternomastoid torticollis in a boy who presented at the age of 7 years. Note the posture of the head and the facial asymmetry as evidenced by the lower eye, flatter cheek and nasal ala, and narrower mouth on the left.

or both, then the management consists of parental reassurance and observation of the child over a prolonged period. The parents must be told that there is a possibility that surgery will be necessary but that, in any case, there will be no significant persistent deformity. The child is observed at four-monthly and then yearly intervals until it becomes clear that there is either progressive deformity requiring surgery or that there will be no deformity.

There is no evidence that physiotherapy or passive stretching or manipulation alter the course of the condition.

Surgical correction is performed by dividing the muscle at its origin from the mastoid process. The operation is performed through an incision parallel to and just distal to the lower border of the mastoid process. Adrenalin, 1:250 000, is injected along the line of the incision and the use of cutting and coagulating diathermy ensures that the muscle can be divided completely under vision with a minimum of haemorrhage. The muscle retracts distally as it is divided. The wound is sutured in two layers with subcuticular Dexon to the skin. If there is a persistent tight band above the clavicle then this can be safely divided by subcutaneous tenotomy with the tenotomy knife passed deep to the band.

This technique of high–low division of the sternomastoid has been performed over 100 times without complications and is preferred to other methods because the sternomastoid muscle does not retract excessively and a normal neck contour results. The scar is never unsightly.

THE SHOULDER

DISLOCATION OF THE SHOULDER

Dislocations of the shoulder in childhood and adolescence are classified as congenital, paralytic, traumatic, recurrent, voluntary, or contractural.

Congenital dislocation is seen in Larsen's syndrome associated with dislocation of other joints. It also occurs in otherwise normal children and the dislocation may be either anterior or posterior. In childhood, reduction can be achieved manually without force but by adolescence the dislocation is usually irreducible. These children do not have any disability and treatment is unnecessary.

Paralytic dislocation occurs in conjunction with obstetrical paralysis and is either seen at birth or occurs later due to splinting in the 'Statue of Liberty' position. The condition is preventable by less traumatic obstetrics and by abandoning the use of the traditional splinting. If recognised early, the dislocation is easily reduced. Late presentation may necessitate open reduction. Paralytic dislocation, usually inferior, is common in poliomyelitis.

Traumatic dislocation is uncommon before adolescence as, in the younger age group, trauma to the shoulder is more likely to cause fracture of the clavicle or an epiphyseal injury to the upper humerus or outer end of the clavicle. Traumatic dislocations are easily reduced and the joint is immobilised in a sling for three weeks.

Recurrent dislocation is only seen in adolescence, follows a definite traumatic incident of dislocation, and is more often posterior than anterior. In both cases surgical repair is indicated. If anterior, the Putti–Platt type repair is effective and should be done through an axillary approach so as to avoid ugly scarring. If posterior, osteotomy of the neck of the scapula is combined with posterior capsular reefing and this combination has a high rate of success.

Voluntary dislocation is seen in childhood and may be either inferior or posterior. It is regarded as a clever trick and becomes irritating for the parents. Management consists of a period in a collar and cuff sling with the arm under the clothing (more punitive than therapeutic) followed by dire warnings to the child should he continue the habit. Resolution is the rule.

Contractural dislocation may occur in association with burn scars or deltoid fibrosis. In either case, release of the contractures may be indicated but the management of the dislocation will depend on the circumstances.

HEAD INJURIES IN CHILDHOOD

The neurosurgical sequelae of head injuries in childhood and the pattern of recovery are often very different from those seen in adults. There is often a more severe early disturbance followed by a more rapid recovery and even children with decerebrate rigidity have a surprisingly good prognosis. However, permanent intellectual disability is the rule and good progress at school after head injury is exceptional.

There are five distinct problem areas in rehabilitation. 1 Prolonged behavioural disturbance especially irritability, tantrums, and general antisocial behaviour. 2 Speech defects which prevent adequate communication by the child and further aggravates the frustration and depression. 3 Motor defects, especially hemiplegia and ataxia. 4 Visual defects which range from monocular visual loss to actual blindness. 5 Epilepsy which is usually easily controlled.

MANAGEMENT

In general, the management of the child with head injuries is similar to that in the adult but with three important variations.

SPASTICITY

In the early management, if fractures of the limbs are present, these must be immobilised as efficiently as possibly. Fractures of the upper limb can usually be managed in plaster casts, but traction is usually necessary in the lower limbs and skeletal traction is preferable to skin traction. In severe cases with fits or clonic spasms, internal fixation may be required but further protection from braces or casts will be required to protect the implant from breaking or bending. Experience has shown that the external fixateur can be used most effectively in these circumstances. Whatever method is used it must relieve pain as pain initiates spasm and a vicious cycle is established. Later when consciousness and co-operation return, relaxation physiotherapy techniques are used to overcome spasticity. Splints, braces and plaster should not be used to control spastic deformity as these will inevitably produce pain and pressure sores.

EMOTIONAL NEEDS

All concerned with the care of the brain-injured child must understand the reason for his poor behaviour, they must learn to communicate, to reassure, and to see that they do not hurt him physically or emotionally. Many of these children cannot speak but can hear and understand. On every bed card there should be written 'Speak to me not about me'.

ORTHOPAEDIC SURGERY

The question of surgery to relieve spasticity should not be raised for at least two years post-accident as spontaneous improvement can occur up till this time. When surgery *is* indicated, the principles are the same as those applying in cerebral palsy of non-traumatic origin.

CHAPTER 5

The Adolescent

Special characteristics of the adolescent patient, 248
Management

Backache, 249

Slipped upper femoral epiphysis (epiphysiolysis), 256

The knee, 259

Peroneal spasmodic flat foot (congenital tarsal coalition), 274

Hallux valgus, 276

Hallux rigidus, 277

Plantar warts, 278

Ingrowing toe nails, 278

Recurrent instability of the ankle, 278

Adolescence is that phase of growth and development in the age group of approximately 10–19 years, that is between childhood and maturity. It is a period of rapid change producing physical, intellectual, emotional, and social maturation. An understanding of these changes is essential if the surgeon is to gain the trust and co-operation of his patient.

SPECIAL CHARACTERISTICS OF THE ADOLESCENT PATIENT

Physical

During adolescence there is a rapid increase both in height and weight. The fuel for this is provided by a large increase in food consumption. Some children, especially girls, become rather fat in early adolescence and become much thinner later. Because both physical activities and school studies escalate during this period, adequate sleep is necessary to prevent fatigue. Fatigue is often the basis of poor posture presenting at this age.

Psychological

Although the adolescent may appear to be self assured and asserting his independence, this is in fact a very fragile covering for a whole host of anxieties. The adolescent patient is greatly concerned about the possible effects of injury or illness on his or her personal appearance and may have hidden fears regarding death and mutilation. Girls are particularly distressed by the loss of hair which may follow cytotoxic therapy. Most intelligent students are concerned about loss of school time, others with any possible interruption to their athletic activities or interference with social occasions.

MANAGEMENT

The Consultant

In childhood it is usual for the surgeon to communicate briefly with the patient and reserve most of his time for the parents both in history taking and in explanation. In adolescence the process must be reversed—the conversation being largely conducted with the patient while the parents act as observers and occasional prompters. Finally, the parents are brought into the act to discuss diagnosis, details and timing of treatment, the anticipated costs, and so forth. The approach should be sufficiently sensitive that the patient feels he is participating in the decisions rather than having them thrust upon him and that the surgeon is able to appreciate his special problems and attitudes.

Hospitalisation

The following observations might apply to hospitalisation at all ages but they seem more important in adolescence. Most hospitals are architecturally unsuited to the adolescent patient but, so far as is possible within these limitations, attention should be given to the proper provision of facilities for privacy, recreation, food, odd eating habits and eating times. Adequate care for the adolescent will be achieved only if all medical and nursing staff accept that he has the right to know the reason for his admission, for his treatment and for any investigations that are proposed. A scoliotic girl who wakes up in the recovery room surrounded by noisy monitors and with an i.v. drip running will immediately assume that something has gone wrong if she has not received prior warning.

BACKACHE

In marked contrast to the adult, not only is backache a fairly uncommon presenting symptom in adolescence but the range of pathology seen is also somewhat different. In a given case it is almost always possible to make a firm diagnosis whereas, in adult practice, vague guesses such as 'back strain' and 'torn ligaments' are often made when positive signs of injury or disease cannot be demonstrated. The causes of backache in adolescence can be listed as follows:

1 Postural backache
2 Osteochondritis—dorsal spine (Scheuermann's disease), lumbar spine
3 Spondylolysis and spondylolisthesis
4 Lumbar disc herniation
5 Hysteria
6 Rarities—lumbago, osteoblastoma, metastatic tumours

Postural backache

This is a distinct entity usually occurring in girls during their last two years in school. It is usually associated with many hours of studying for examinations, worries about passing, and parental pressures. Management consists of giving advice about taking regular exercise and sufficient sleep—both of which have usually been neglected. Resolution can be anticipated once the examinations and stresses are over.

Osteochondritis (synonym: osteochondrosis, avascular necrosis)

The vertebral bodies grow from the ring epiphyses on their upper and lower surfaces. A growth disturbance of these plates may occur and has been given a variety of names, but since the actual cause is unknown an accurate title is not possible. At first considered to be a primary abnormality of the cartilage, it seems more likely that the cartilage plate is injured and allows the passage of intervertebral disc material into the adjacent vertebral body. Clinically and radiologically two varieties are seen.

DORSAL OSTEOCHONDRITIS (SCHEUERMANN'S DISEASE, ADOLESCENT KYPHOSIS)

A condition more commonly seen in boys who present in early adolescence with a dorsal round back and sometimes with pain. There is a fixed kyphosis present and the back is irritable to stress. The radiological appearances are not always easy to interpret. At an early stage there is slight wedging of the middle vertebrae; later, the upper and lower surfaces of the vertebrae become irregular and then fragmented (Fig. 5.1). In several cases these changes go on to further wedging of the bodies and narrowing of the disc spaces.

Management. More than half of the children who present with an early

The Adolescent 251

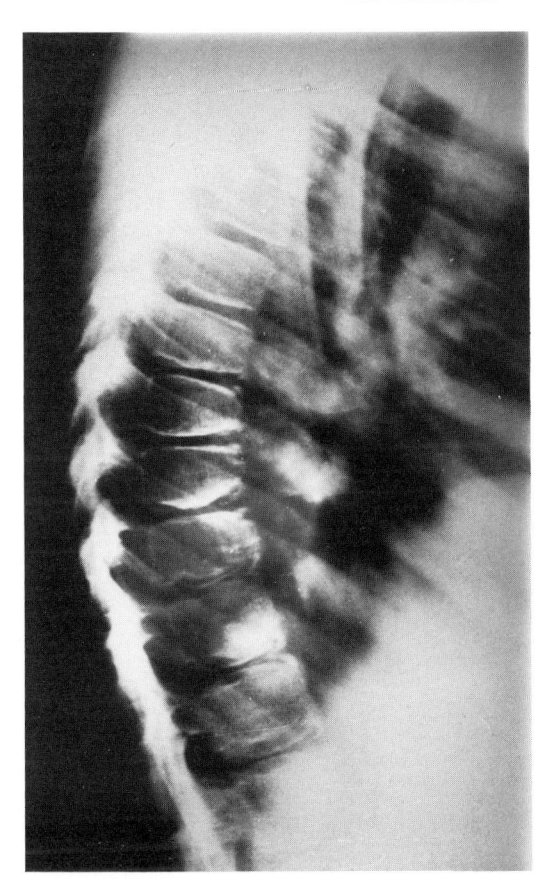

Fig. 5.1 A lateral x-ray showing the typical changes of Scheuermann's disease, i.e. wedging of vertebral bodies, scoliosis, and fragmentation of the ring apophyses.

adolescent kyphosis have a postural problem and this will respond to exercise and future growth. The others who have rigid kyphosis will tend to progress although, even in these, perhaps only one-third will declare themselves as sufficiently severe to warrant bracing. The difficulty is that it is not possible to pick the good from the bad in the early stages. This being so, all early cases should be treated expectantly with a combination of rest and exercise. The child must get sufficient sleep so that he is not always tired and should sleep on a firm mattress. He should be encouraged to play sports and indulge in as much outdoor activity as possible—swimming is especially helpful. If, despite these measures, serial x-rays show that the kyphosis is increasing, a Milwaukee brace should be prescribed and this will have to be used for a prolonged period. The use of this brace is so effective in this condition that care must be taken that the spine is not made too straight. The brace is worn full time until correction is achieved. It may then be discarded for sleeping and later for exercise periods such as swimming. When growth is almost complete, the brace may finally be discontinued.

LUMBAR OSTEOCHONDRITIS

When osteochondritis occurs in the lumbar spine it tends to cause pain without deformity. It is almost invariably seen in boys who complain of backache and stiffness which is bad enough to interfere with sport and other outdoor activities.

The x-ray changes are also quite different to those seen in the dorsal spine. The antero-superior corner of one or more vertebral bodies looks eroded and the disc space is narrowed (Fig. 5.2). There is no wedging. The changes are sometimes confused with inflammatory disease such as tuberculosis.

Management. The natural history of lumbar osteochondritis is for full recovery to occur either at maturity or soon afterwards. Restriction of activity may be all that is required but some will require lumbar bracing for a few months to achieve comfort. Activity can be resumed when the back is comfortable and mobile regardless of the radiological changes.

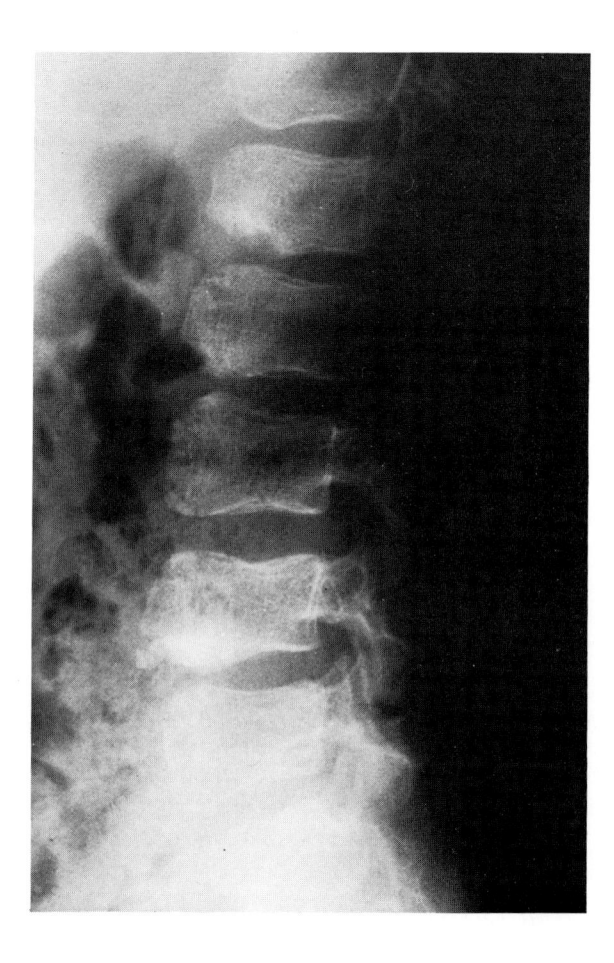

Fig. 5.2 Lumbar osteochondritis juvenilis. Note the anterior erosions of the upper lumbar vertebrae, the irregular narrowing of several disc spaces, and the increased antero-posterior diameter of the fourth lumbar vertebra.

Spondylolysis and spondylolisthesis

Spondylolysis is a term used to describe a defect in the pars interarticularis which may be uni- or bilateral. Perhaps 80% occur in the fifth lumbar vertebra and the remainder in the fourth lumbar vertebra. The defect is only well shown by oblique radiography.

Aetiology. For many years the lesion of spondylolysis was considered congenital but it is now considered more likely to occur in post-natal life as a stress fracture. It is an incidental radiological finding in about 10% of adults.

Clinical features. Adolescents present fairly frequently with backache associated with spondylolysis. This is becoming more common since trail walking and mountaineering carrying heavy packs has become a popular form of exercise in the school curriculum. The condition usually responds to some restriction of physical activities and the use of a lumbar corset. Surgery is rarely required.

SPONDYLOLISTHESIS

This term means a forward displacement of the vertebra on the vertebra below. Again, it is more common at the lumbosacral junction.

Aetiology and pathology. In adolescence the only type seen is that associated with a bilateral defect of the pars (spondylolysis). Slipping may commence in childhood and accelerate during adolescence (Fig. 5.3). In severe cases the fifth lumbar body may fall off the sacrum and lie in the pelvis applied to the front of the sacrum. Even with this degree of displacement, cauda equina involvement is rare although in all degrees of displacement sciatica can occur from root irritation. There is often marked hamstring spasm, the cause of which is not fully understood.

Backache is the usual presenting symptom. All patients with symptoms have some back stiffness and, in severe displacements, there is excessive lordosis with a characteristic shortening of the trunk.

Management. Spondylolisthesis may be discovered as an incidental finding in a patient without symptoms of backache, and treatment is therefore unnecessary. Mild and intermittent back pain will usually respond to restriction of activities and perhaps a corset. Persisting backache, especially with referred pain, should be treated by postero-lateral (intertransverse process) fusion. The operation is best done through a single transverse incision and, if necessary, the loose posterior element removed. The bone grafts are obtained from the posterior ilium on one side.

Decompression of nerve roots is not usually necessary even in the presence of root signs. Plaster immobilisation is unnecessary although activities must be

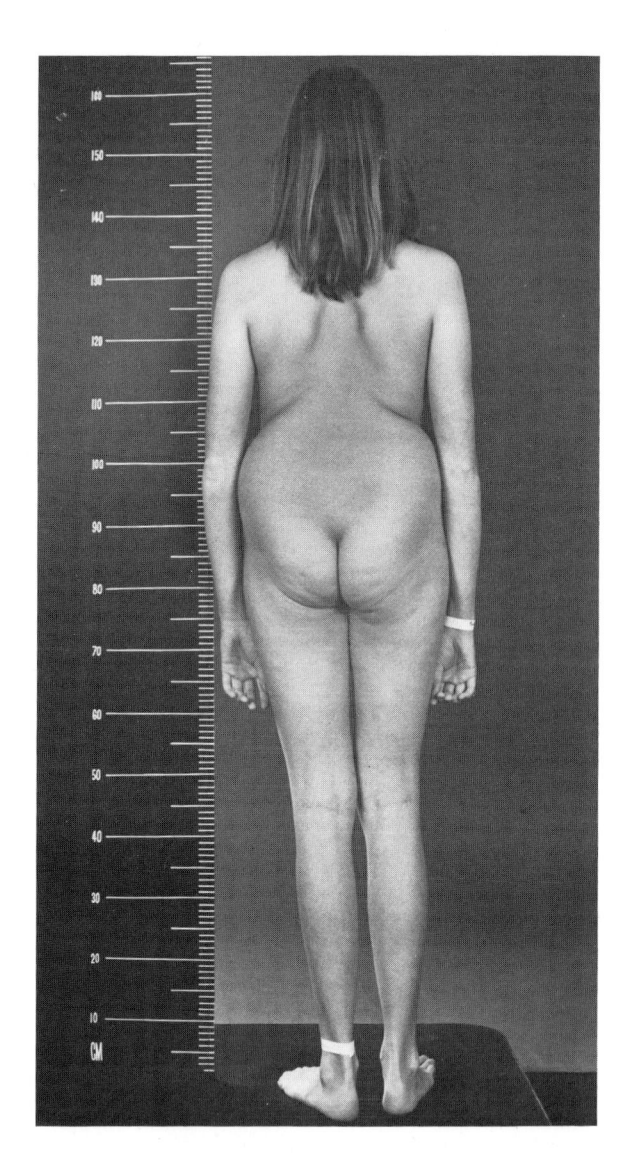

Fig. 5.3 An adolescent girl with a severe grade of spondylolisthesis. The classical shortening of the trunk is well shown as well as the heart shaped buttocks (Tschirkin's sign).

severely restricted for the first three months and until there is radiological confirmation of fusion. The success rate is very high indeed and approaches 100%.

Lumbar disc syndrome

The syndrome of low back pain and sciatic radiation is virtually never seen in childhood and only very rarely in adolescence. The clinical picture is similar to that of the lumbar disc prolapse seen in the adult and the pathology is probably the same. However, since very few are treated surgically this is largely an inference.

Clinical features. There is usually a definite history of injury followed rapidly by pain and stiffness. After the onset, stiffness is often a more striking feature than pain and may persist for many months. Examination reveals a stiff back especially in forward flexion. Straight leg raising may be very restricted on one or both sides. Signs of root compression are rarely present.

Diagnosis. The diagnosis is usually easy but care must be taken to exclude a spinal cord tumour which occurs with equal frequency in this age group. If the onset has been gradual and there are root signs present, a lumbar myelogram should be performed. This will exclude a tumour but will rarely show a disc herniation.

Treatment. Treatment is conservative. After an initial period of bed rest a lumbar brace or corset is fitted and is worn during the day until pain and stiffness have disappeared. This may take up to twelve months. In the over-16 age group, an occasional case will be seen with signs of root compression and this may require surgical relief.

Hysterical back pain

True conversion hysteria is seen surprisingly often in adolescents. The patient is nearly always a girl who complains of pain and this will be associated with stiffness and a curious gait for which there is no adequate explanation. A careful examination and subsequent observation will easily reveal inconsistencies which suggest the diagnosis. Once the diagnosis is suspected further careful enquiry usually reveals a conflict in the home or at school. Separation of the parents is often an initiating factor but difficulties in learning or in sporting activities at school are equally common. Sometimes it is not possible to identify the main causative factor. The condition is best handled by explaining to the parents that the child is not malingering but is subconsciously converting one set of problems into another. If the problem can be identified and attended to, this is obviously the first step in management. Otherwise the parents or the surviving parent can usually cope with the problem by understanding its nature. It is important that psychiatric treatment be avoided and only the simplest orthopaedic measures suggested. A sympathetic physiotherapist can often be of great value in management. Complete resolution is the rule although recovery may take some months.

Rare causes of back pain

LUMBAGO

The clinical syndrome of acute backache of sudden onset lasting about a week is well known in the adult and recurrent attacks may occur over many years. A similar picture is occasionally seen in the child in whom resolution may occur rather more slowly. The pain can be severe at the onset and the back extremely stiff with widespread muscle spasm. Treatment consists of rest and local heat followed by gradual resumption of activities.

OSTEOBLASTOMA

This benign tumour has a predilection for the neural arches of the vertebral column and, as such, is an important cause of backache in adolescence. Unless the possibility is borne in mind the diagnosis is likely to be missed as the lesions are not readily demonstrated in routine radiographs. Once suspected, tomography is very useful to demonstrate the lesion and to accurately localise it so that surgical excision can be planned. A bone scan will also give a very dramatic picture. Relief of pain is complete when the tumour has been removed and recurrence rarely occurs.

SPINAL METASTASIS

In leukaemia and in the terminal stages of neuroblastoma and rhabdomyosarcoma, spinal metastasis may occur and their presence is usually made obvious by back pain. Bracing is poorly tolerated but radiotherapy will often provide useful palliation.

SLIPPED UPPER FEMORAL EPIPHYSIS (EPIPHYSIOLYSIS)

Spontaneous epiphysiolysis occurs at the upper end of the femur as a fairly common event in early adolescence. It is more common in boys and about 20% are bilateral. The age group is approximately 10–15 years in boys and 9–13 years in girls. Many are overweight and the girls are often tall. The aetiology is unknown but the work of Harris suggests that it is due to an imbalance between growth hormone which decreases the shearing strength of the plate, and sex hormone which increases that strength.

Pathology

The epiphysis slowly slips posteriorly and, as it does so, the leg rotates into external rotation. A progressive coxa vara deformity develops with secondary remodelling of the femoral neck. Since the blood supply to the epiphysis is supplied from vessels running along the posterior aspect of the femoral neck these are usually undamaged during the slipping process. However, at any time an acute slip may be superimposed and, in these circumstances, the blood supply may be damaged to produce avascular necrosis of the epiphysis. The degree of slip may be arrested either spontaneously or by surgical pinning when the plate will close prematurely and no further slip may occur. However, all severe grades of slipping alter the mechanics of the hip joint so that degenerative arthritis can be anticipated in later life.

Clinical features

Any adolescent who develops a limp usually without a history of significant injury should be considered to have a slipped epiphysis until proven otherwise. Pain is not a significant feature and may be felt in the knee rather than the hip. There is no such thing as a sprained hip or a torn muscle around the hip—diagnoses which are often used to pass off the condition. Early diagnosis is essential so that surgical treatment can be instituted at an early stage of the slipping process. The cardinal physical sign is loss of internal rotation movement at the hip and pain when the hip is forced into this position. As the slip progresses, a fixed external rotation deformity develops and the hip becomes Trendelenburg positive. If the patient presents with an acute slip, the clinical feature is the same as that of a fracture of the neck of the femur. A history of prior limp and pain can usually be obtained in these cases.

X-ray diagnosis

Three clinical types can be defined and this classification is also useful in planning treatment.

Pre-slip. The epiphysis has only moved a millimetre or so and this may only be visible in the lateral projection. Widening of the epiphyseal line may be present.

Chronic slip. With further slipping, the change will be obvious in both projections. On the antero-posterior projection, if a line is drawn along the upper border of the neck it normally cuts off a small segment of the epiphysis and, when it does not do so, slipping is assumed. In the lateral projection the displacement will be obvious (Fig. 5.4). Changes of avascular necrosis (increased density) may be present.

Acute slip. The epiphysis remains in the acetabulum and the neck is widely displaced from it as the leg rolls out into external rotation.

Management

There is no place for conservative treatment in this condition. Neither bed rest nor traction can be guaranteed to prevent continued slipping and, in any case, such treatment would need to be continued until spontaneous fusion occurred, which may not be until puberty. The details of treatment and after-care will vary according to the clinical type.

Fig. 5.4 Trethowan's sign. (A) In the A–P radiograph of a normal hip a line drawn along the upper border of the neck cuts off a sizeable piece of the head. (B) When the epiphysis has slipped, the line does not cross the head.

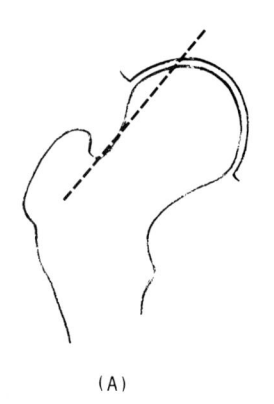

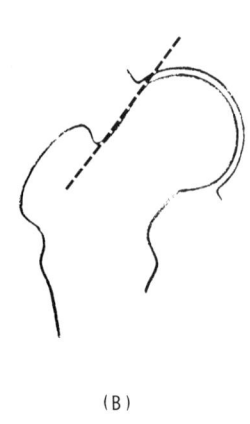

Pre-slip. Immediate fixation using one or two threaded Knowles pins is the treatment of choice. After wound healing, weight-bearing can be resumed at once, although contact sports should be avoided until radiological fusion of the growth plate can be demonstrated.

Chronic slip. In mild to moderate cases the degree of deformity can be accepted and the epiphysis fixed in situ with two pins. As a guide to selection, if the hip will rotate to neutral when the hip is examined under anaesthesia immediately prior to pinning then the deformity can be accepted. In more severe cases with fixed external rotation deformity, three courses of action are possible. 1 *Pinning in situ*—the external rotation deformity produces an ugly gait, difficulty in running, and often secondary foot strain. 2 *Cervical osteotomy*—removal of a wedge of bone from the neck to correct the deformity is theoretically sound but in practice is complicated by avascular necrosis in more than one-third of the cases. 3 *Subtrochanteric osteotomy* is safe and effective but will only be indicated in a very small percentage of cases presenting late with extensive slip. It is best done in two stages. First pinning is carried out to prevent further slip. Once the growth plate is fused, the pins can be removed and the osteotomy done and fixed with a nail and plate. In practice, the second stage is often cancelled as the patient develops much better function than anticipated.

MANAGEMENT OF THE OPPOSITE HIP—PROPHYLACTIC PINNING

The opposite hip is involved in over 20% of cases and the question arises whether prophylactic pinning is justified. Opinion is divided on the issue but our own practice is to pin the opposite hip if one or more of the following apply: if the patient is overweight; if the patient is young; if the problem on the first affected hip was acute slip or late-presenting chronic slip; and if the child lives in an isolated country area where follow up will be difficult. Should it be decided not to pin the opposite hip, the parents must be warned to be on the alert for hip or knee pain or

The Adolescent 259

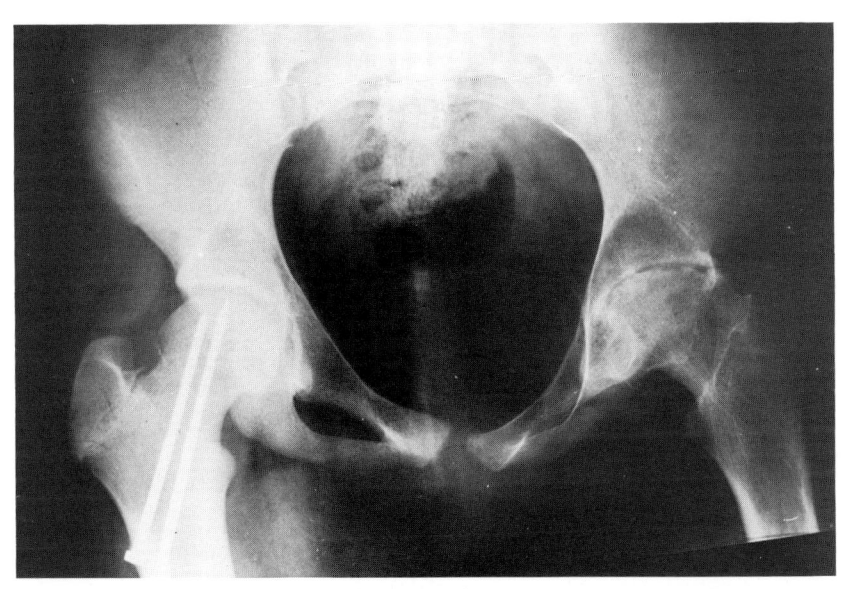

Fig. 5.5 Antero-posterior x-ray of the pelvis of a girl who had undergone pinning of slipped upper femoral epiphyses on both sides three years previously. The pins on the left had been removed. This hip was stiff and painful and x-rays show narrowing of the joint space due to chondrolysis.

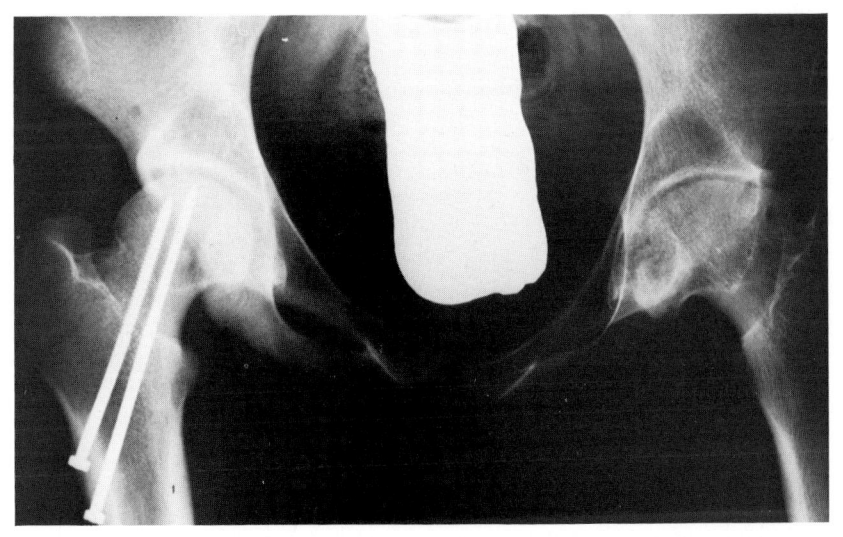

Fig. 5.6 The pelvis of the same girl one year later. She had used crutches for six months of this period and now had a range of flexion of 90° and no hip pain.

the presence of a limp and to report these at once so that an x-ray examination can be arranged.

Chondrolysis

Occasionally chondrolysis may occur as a complication of slipping of the epiphysis and this is much more common in the black races. The hip is irritable and x-rays show progressive loss of joint space (Figs. 5.5 & 5.6). The joint must be protected from weight-bearing for a prolonged period and non-weight-bearing exercises encouraged. Salicylates are prescribed to facilitate repair of articular cartilage.

Although there may be an increase in the joint space with this regime, the repair is largely by fibrocartilage and this has a limited life in this situation so that early degenerative arthritis can be anticipated in all cases. If this occurs early, only arthrodesis is available to restore function.

THE KNEE

Osgood–Schlatter disease (Synonym: osteochondritis of the tibial tubercle)

This name is given to a clinical syndrome in which a painful bony swelling appears over the tibial tubercle usually in boys between the age of 10 and 15 years. There is tenderness over the swelling which is aggravated by kneeling and the child complains of aching pain either during or after exercise. Radiographically, there are irregular areas of ossification in the proximal part of the tubercle giving it the appearance of fragmentation. At various times the condition has been thought to be an apophysitis but the most probable explanation is a partial avulsion of the growing tibial tubercle with subsequent avascular necrosis of the fragments.

MANAGEMENT

The natural history of this condition is for spontaneous recovery to occur at or before maturity. However, if a lump has developed this will remain. Children with this condition may present in a variety of ways: the parents may seek advice because they have noticed the swelling, even though the child has not complained. Often they have been told that the boy has Osgood–Schlatter disease and this adds to their worries. When there are no symptoms, explanation and reassurance only are required.

More frequently the boy is a sport fanatic and finds that the knee condition is restricting his activities. Both he and his parents are concerned that continued activity will be harmful. If the disability is not severe an assurance can be given that, while activity may cause discomfort, it is not harmful. It is unnecessary and indeed wrong to restrict the child's activity and so prevent him from enjoying a period of his life which is unique. If he understands the problem he will probably voluntarily restrict his sport to bring his discomfort to an acceptable level.

Occasionally the pain is such that active treatment is desirable and, in these circumstances, immobilisation in a plaster cylinder for a month will usually alleviate most of the symptoms.

Very rarely, symptoms are severe and persistent and may even continue after maturity when the remainder of the tibial tubercle has fused. An x-ray of the region will show a large loose fragment in the tendon just proximal to the bony attachment. These can be treated by splitting the tendon longitudinally; the bone fragment will be found lying almost free in a small fluid-filled cavity in the tendon and is easily removed. Note that the skin incision should be planned to leave a scar to one or other side of the tubercle and not over it!

Chondromalacia patellae

The term chondromalacia patellae is used to denote a condition in adolescents who complain of pain or aching arising from the articular surface of the patella. It is the commonest cause of pain in the knee in this age group.

PATHOLOGY

Until recently it was considered that the degenerative changes which occur in the articular cartilage of the patella were identical to the early lesions of osteoarthritis. Goodfellow and others have shown, however, that this is not so, for the lesion is really one of basal degeneration of cartilage and, if the surface is involved, this occurs very late. This concept is borne out by the well known fact that most cases of chondromalacia patellae have articular cartilage which is macroscopically normal.

AETIOLOGY

With increasing knowledge of the biomechanics of the knee and of the structure of articular cartilage it is apparent that many factors—either singly or in combination—may contribute to the development of chondromalacia. These can be summarised as follows: 1   *direct trauma* (e.g. a blow, fall, or a dashboard injury),   2   *dislocation* (either acute or recurrent),   3   *malalignment syndrome* (e.g. valgus knee, laterally placed tibial tubercle, patella alta, or lax medial capsule) (Fig. 5.7), and   4   *hazardous occupations* (e.g. athletes, recruits to the armed services, or jobs which entail excessive kneeling).

CLINICAL FEATURES

The patient is young, of either sex, and very keen on athletic pursuits. Most are of athletic build and it is unusual to see the condition in fat, knock kneed girls who might otherwise be expected to develop the condition since they combine being overweight and having the malalignment syndrome.

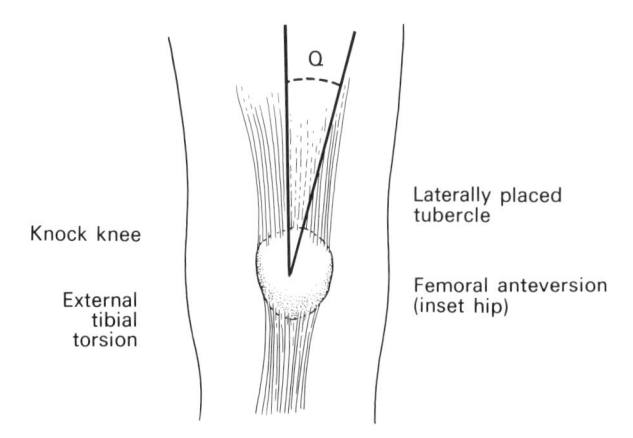

Fig. 5.7 The malalignment syndrome.

The most important complaint is *pain* felt in front of the knee particularly after exercise or when rising from sitting for long periods. It is noticed when walking up and down stairs or when climbing. Associated symptoms such as grating, catching, giving way and locking are also common, but swelling is unusual. Many of the symptoms of chondromalacia patellae suggest an internal derangement and care must be taken that an incorrect diagnosis is not made. Fortunately meniscus injuries are very uncommon in this group and this diagnosis should not be considered in the first instance unless there is a block to movement.

The diagnosis is made in the extended knee pressing down on the patella with the palm of the hand and then skidding the patella forcibly from side to side. This will be accompanied by pain and grating. Sub-patella tenderness is often present. Although a radiograph rarely aids in diagnosis, the investigation should be carried out to eliminate the possibility of osteochondritis dissecans of the patella which may have identical symptoms and signs.

MANAGEMENT

When seen in late childhood and adolescence, the vast majority of cases can be treated conservatively with the expectation of a satisfactory outcome. Conservative treatment consists, firstly, of *reassurance* that the prognosis is good, that exercise is not harmful and that resolution will occur over a prolonged period—maybe several years. Secondly, the condition tends to be episodic and at the onset of a painful period some limitation of pain-producing activities such as kneeling, running, or climbing is advisable. Exercise such as level walking and swimming is encouraged. Thirdly, it is important to realise that resistance quadriceps exercise will only aggravate the pain and that isometric quadriceps exercises are valuable instead. Finally, anti-inflammatory drugs are not very effective in this condition and are not recommended. Aspirin, however, is valuable as it not only relieves pain but appears to have a specific effect in inhibiting cartilage matrix degradation.

Surgical treatment is rarely required in adolescence. The operative procedures available are of three types: 1   *patellar shaving*—the results are variable and on the whole unsatisfactory.   2   *re-alignment techniques*—a whole host of techniques have been described but the most reliable is probably a simple medial transfer of the insertion of the patella tendon. When indicated, good results can be obtained.   3   It is doubtful whether *patellectomy* is ever justified in this age group. Even when pain is relieved, there is usually persisting weakness and quadriceps atrophy.

Dislocation of the patella

Dislocation of the patella in childhood can be considered under the four separate headings of traumatic, recurrent, habitual, and congenital.

TRAUMATIC DISLOCATION

This is usually seen in the overweight, knock kneed girl with a small, high patella. Reduction nearly always occurs spontaneously when the knee is extended and much swelling and bruising is likely to follow. Rarely an osteochondral flake fracture accompanies the dislocation. The pathology consists of a long tear of the medial capsule and expansion, and the logical treatment would seem to be suture of this. However, success can be achieved and an unsightly scar avoided with closed treatment. The important point here is that immobilisation in a plaster cylinder is necessary for a full six weeks to minimise the possibility of recurrence. There is a tendency to treat this injury lightly and merely apply an elastic bandage to control swelling. The convalescence is actually longer and certainly more painful if proper immobilisation is not used.

RECURRENT DISLOCATION

When traumatic dislocation occurs more than three or four times it can be classified as recurrent with the inference that surgical repair is indicated. While many factors which encourage dislocation may be present, we now recognise that the primary defect in the majority of cases is an abnormal directional pull of the quadriceps. This fact has not always been recognised as is witnessed by over 100 different procedures described in the literature. Re-alignment of the quadriceps is the treatment which should be advised in every case of recurrent dislocation to forestall the onset of chondromalacia patellae in later life. The technique will vary with the age of the patient.

Before maturity the patellar tendon must be very carefully removed from the tibial tubercle in such a way as to leave some of the fibres still covering the tubercle. Any dissection or interference with the tubercle will cause premature fusion of the anterior half of the upper tibial growth plate and progressive genu recurvatum. The tendon is sutured under the periosteum 1 cm medially and 1 cm distally.

After maturity a bone block can be moved and the technique described by Hauser (Fig. 5.8a) and modified by McKeever (Fig. 5.8b) is ideal. Although Hauser described moving the tendon far distally as well as medially, this is unnecessary and may well be harmful. The correct alignment is illustrated in Fig. 5.8c. No internal fixation is necessary; plaster can be abandoned after two weeks and the knee mobilised freely.

In each case it is necessary to release the lateral capsule up as far as the top of the patella but medial reefing is unnecessary. Although a medial parapatellar incision is commonly used this produces a very poor scar and a transverse incision below the prominence of the tubercle is preferable in every case.

If the tendon transfer is carried out correctly it rarely fails. Bad results may occur for two reasons: either the tendon is moved too far or the operation has been done too late—the changes of chondromalacia patellae being already established. Transfer in these cases may prevent dislocation but precipitate pain and stiffness.

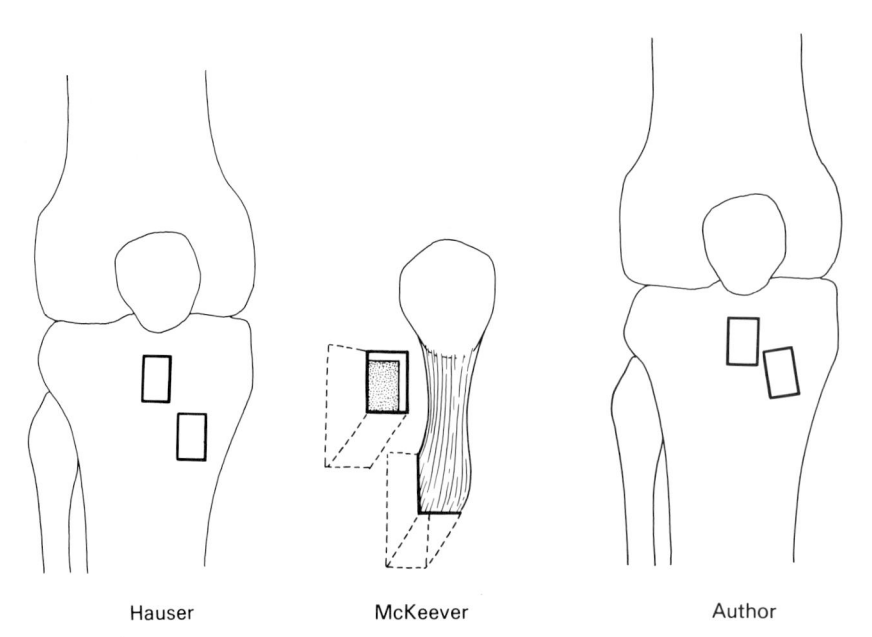

Hauser   McKeever   Author

Fig. 5.8 Diagram showing the distal and medial displacement of the tubercle as described by Hauser; as modified by McKeever to provide self locking of the transplant without internal fixation; and as modified at the R.C.H.

In these circumstances patellectomy is preferable but the repair must be done along the lines suggested by West and Soto Hall for fear of persisting recurrent dislocation of the patella tendon.

HABITUAL DISLOCATION

Here the patella dislocates every time the knee is flexed. The cardinal physical sign here is that if the patella is forcibly held in the midline it is impossible to flex the knee more than about 30° (Fig. 5.9a). Further flexion is then possible if the patella is allowed to dislocate when a full range of motion is readily obtainable (Fig. 5.9b). All these cases have a quadriceps contracture, an abnormal attachment of the iliotibial band, or a combination of the two. Treatment here is the exact opposite to that required in recurrent dislocation, for instead of shortening the quadriceps below the patella it must be lengthened above the patella. The technique of this surgery is as follows:

After the fascial sleeve has been opened, the first abnormality that may be seen is an attachment of the fascia lata to the patella (Fig. 5.10). This is divided. The vastus lateralis is next examined and may be found to have a dense contracted band within the tendon of attachment (Fig. 5.11). This band is divided and the vastus lateralis dissected off the patella and the lateral side of the rectus tendon. Full knee flexion may now be possible without dislocation and in that case the vastus lateralis dissected off the patella and the lateral side of the rectus tendon. possible the tendon of rectus will need elongation.

Whatever the operative details, immobilisation is carried out afterwards for six weeks and a full range of knee motion should be obtainable in every case. If the rectus tendon is lengthened, an extension lag will persist for up to six months after operation.

Habitual dislocation may also occur in extension; the patella dislocates laterally in the last few degrees of extension—when the knee is now flexed it immediately flips back into the midline and remains tracking correctly through the full range of flexion. Patella alta is usually present and it appears that, in full extension, the patella escapes from the femoral groove and falls laterally. If this is associated with symptoms such as recurrent instability the position can be rectified by a Hauser-type tendon transfer. This operation brings the patella down and re-directs the pull of the quadriceps.

CONGENITAL DISLOCATION

Here the patella lies on the lateral aspect of the knee and is irreducible. The condition is often bilateral and familial and there is an extension lag of about 30° which later becomes a fixed flexion deformity. The pathology consists of a very laterally orientated quadriceps, contracture of the vastus lateralis, and a strong fibrous connection between the patella and the fascia lata. The operative treatment consists of an extensive lateral release of the vastus lateralis from the

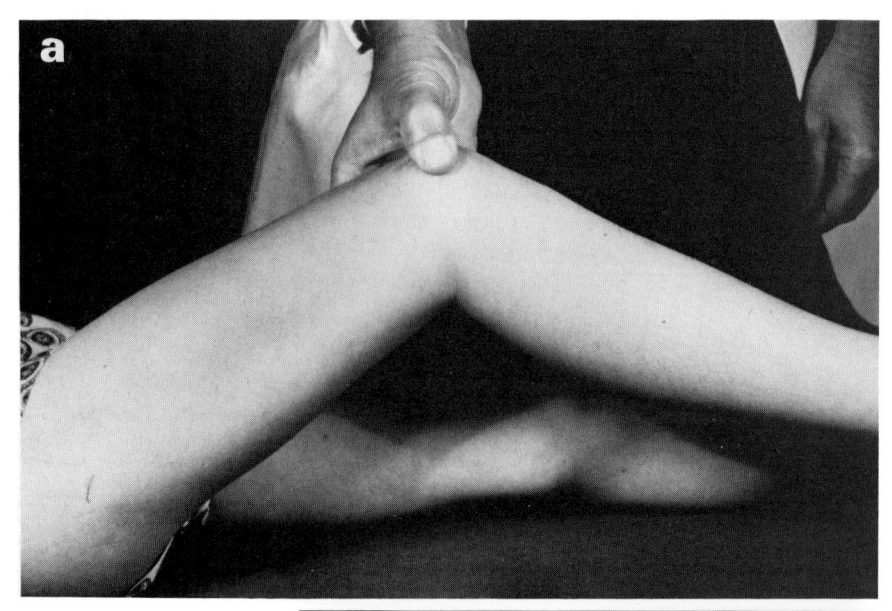

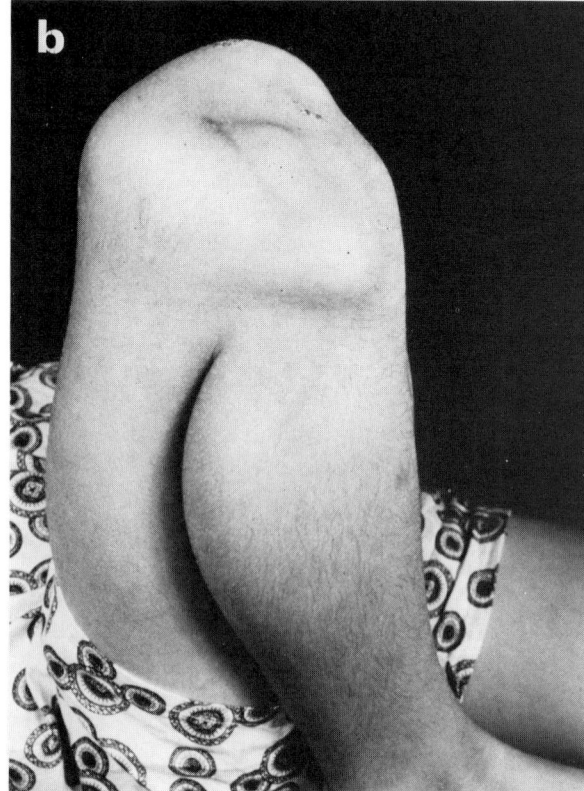

Fig. 5.9a Habitual dislocation of the patella. If the patella is forcibly held in the midline the knee will only flex 30°.
b When the patella is released, full flexion of the knee is possible and the patella dislocates

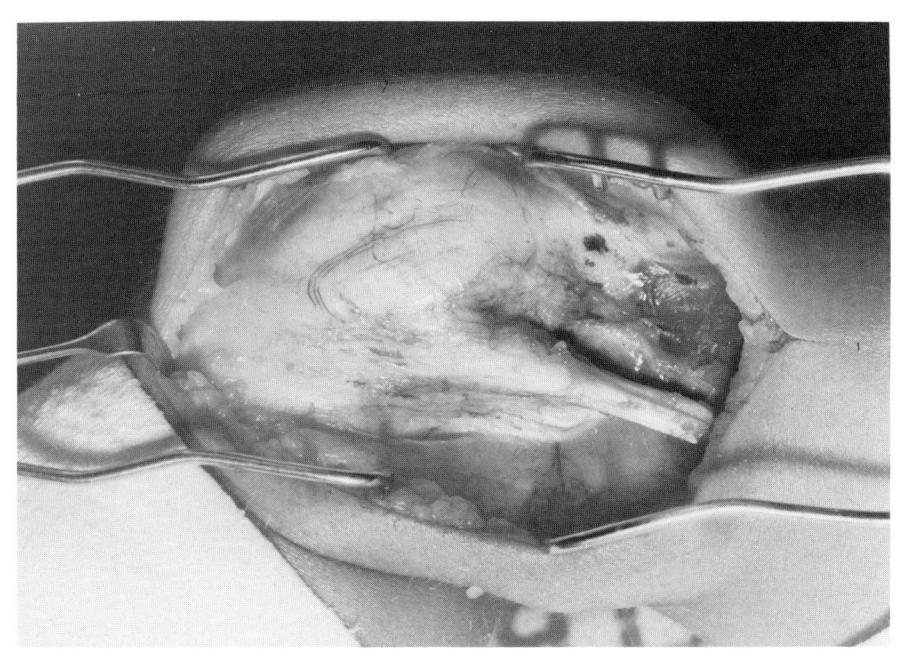

Fig. 5.10 Habitual dislocation of the patella. The left knee is illustrated seen from the lateral side. Note that the fascia lata has a rolled anterior edge like a tendon and this attaches directly to the patella instead of the tibia.

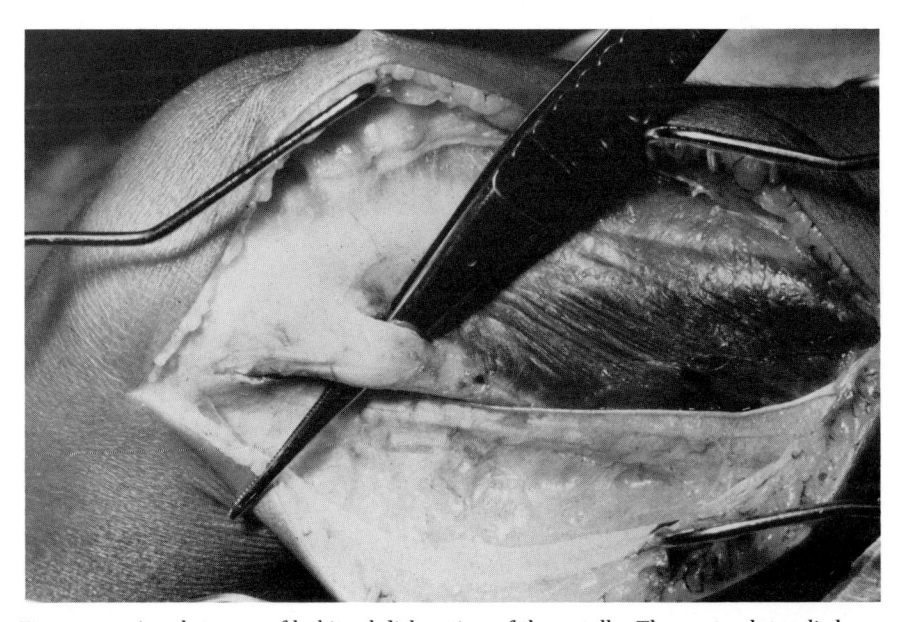

Fig. 5.11 Another case of habitual dislocation of the patella. The vastus lateralis has a dense tendinous band occupying its posterior border and attached to the patellae.

lateral intermuscular septum and the patella to allow the whole bulk of the quadriceps to be re-orientated on to the front of the thigh. It may be necessary to move the patella tendon insertion medially to successfully complete the re-orientation. It is debatable whether cases of congenital dislocation should be treated at all. A good case may be made for surgery as the leg is made stronger and the onset of late osteo-arthritis deferred. However, considerable skill and experience is needed to obtain a satisfactory result and satisfied parents.

Knock knee

As has been indicated in Chapter 4, knock knee frequently occurs between the ages of 2 and 7 years, and in this age group it is to be regarded as a minor variation in posture which corrects spontaneously. In the adolescent, knock knee is less common and spontaneous correction will not occur.

CAUSES OF ADOLESCENT KNOCK KNEE

1. Idiopathic
2. Trauma to the lateral portion of the lower femoral or upper tibial growth plate
3. Malunion of a high tibial fracture
4. Ollier's disease, fibrous dysplasia, dysplasia epiphysealis hemimelica, renal rickets, neurofibromatosis, juvenile chronic arthritis, and some forms of dwarfism

MANAGEMENT

Clinical examination and x-rays are taken to exclude general or local disease as listed above. If none of these conditions is present then the child has idiopathic knock knee of adolescence. This condition is generally accompanied by considerable obesity which should be controlled by diet. This alone may suffice to provide legs which are cosmetically acceptable.

Whatever the cause of the adolescent knock knee, a decision must be made as to whether surgical correction is warranted. This decision will be influenced by the degree of the deformity and by the age and sex of the child. If the deformity is considered to be unacceptable, then it is treated by stapling of the medial aspect of the lower femoral epiphyseal plate (if the child is still growing), or by femoral osteotomy (if maturity has been reached) (Figs. 5.12 & 5.13).

Osteochondritis dissecans

Osteochondritis dissecans is a condition which affects many joints but is most commonly seen in the knees. A localised piece of articular cartilage on the

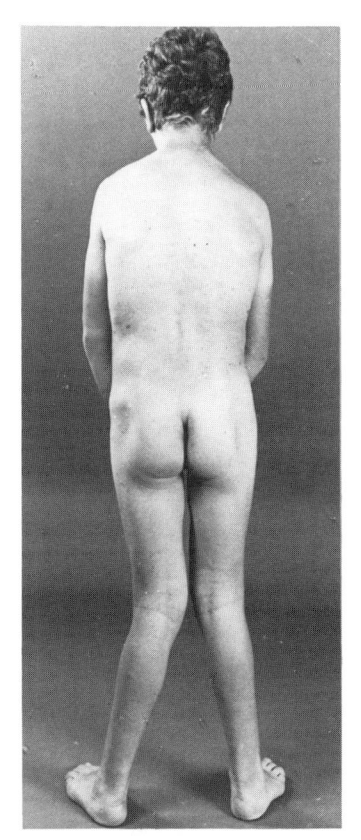

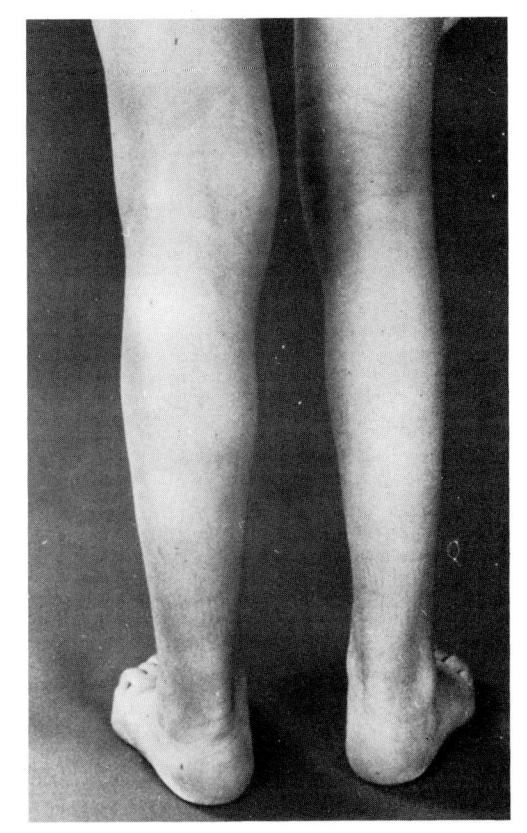

Figs. 5.12 & 5.13 Knock knee deformity at the age of 15 years in a boy with neurofibromatosis. Note the café-au-lait pigmentation of the skin. (*Right*) The appearance one year after stapling of the medial aspect of the lower femoral epiphyseal plate.

infero-lateral aspect of the medial femoral condyle becomes delineated and may separate with a small piece of underlying bone to form a loose body in the joint (Fig. 5.14–5.16). Alternatively, in the younger age group, healing may occur without loose body formation.

AETIOLOGY

The cause is unknown but several factors are thought to play a part. They include 1 *trauma*—rotational strains may cause the tibial spine to impinge against the femoral condyle; 2 *ischaemia*—possibly due to a localised interruption to the blood supply of the subchondral bone; 3 *familial factors*—a familial tendency is uncommon but well known. Multiple joint involvement occurs.

270 Chapter 5

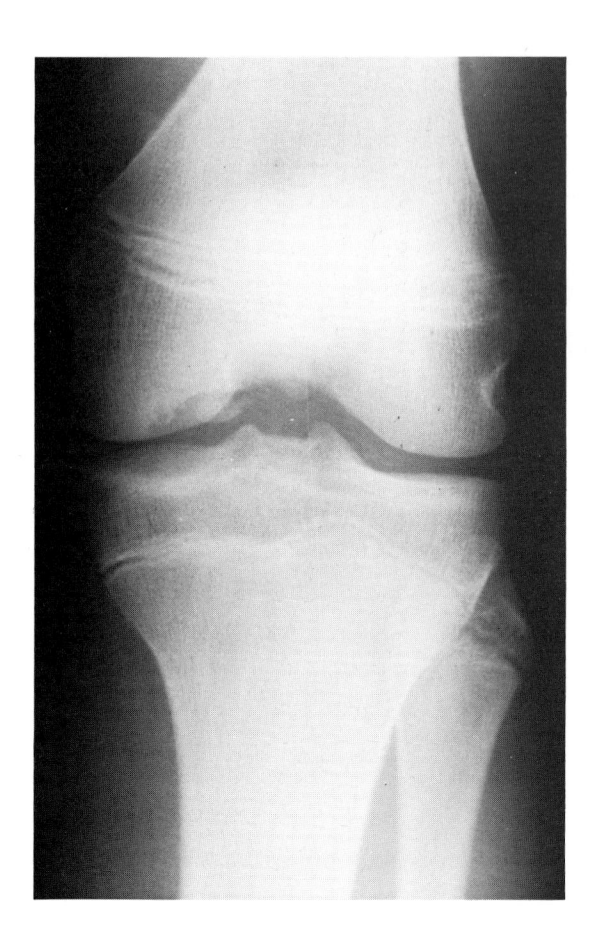

Fig. 5.14
Osteochondritis dissecans of the medial femoral condyle.

CLINICAL FEATURES

Locking from a loose body may be the first symptom especially in late adolescence but more usually the onset is vague with discomfort and intermittent swelling. Athletic children are unable to reach their full potential and the knee often aches after exercise. Physical signs are usually absent although there may be a small effusion of localised tenderness over the affected area when the knee is examined fully flexed.

X-RAY APPEARANCE

Osteochondritis dissecans is a condition which can only be diagnosed by radiological examination and it is therefore important to recognise the normal variant. In the first six years of life irregular ossification near the articular surface is almost universally present and ragged looking areas are seen which must not

The Adolescent 271

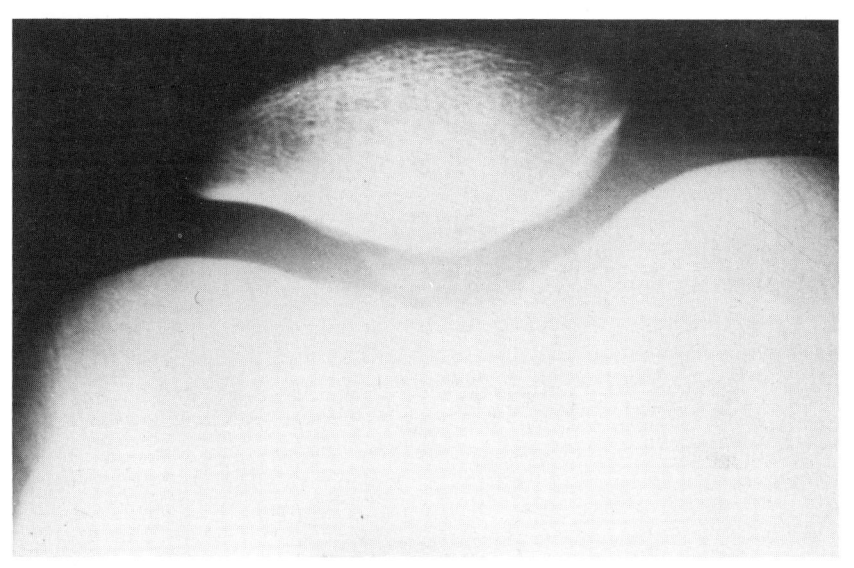

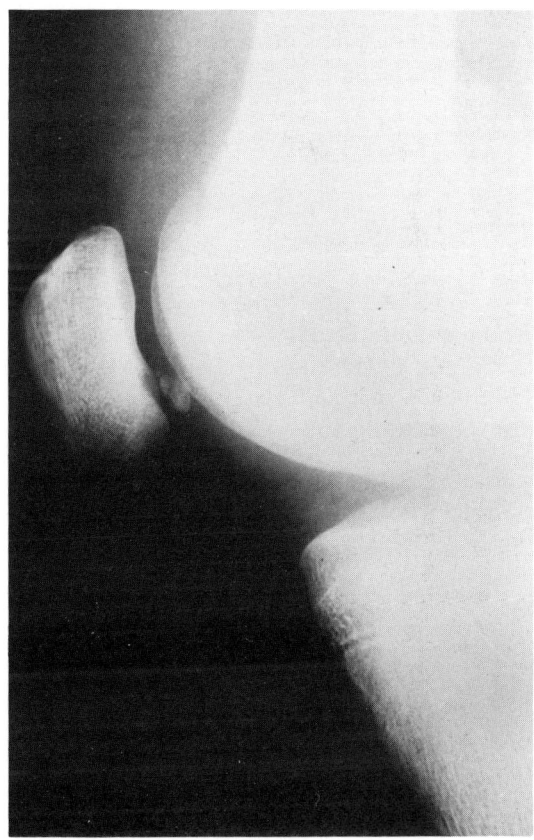

Figs. 5.15 & 5.16 Osteochondritis dissecans of the patella. A similar osteochondral fragment may be produced by the trauma of dislocation of the patella.

be confused with osteochondritis dissecans. In the 6–12 year age group similar irregular ossification is common and separate ossific nuclei may be present suggesting a true osteochondritis dissecans. Since these usually heal without treatment, there is considerable doubt as to whether the true condition exists at all in young children.

MANAGEMENT

Under the age of 12 years the lesion will usually heal without treatment or restriction of activity. In adolescence this is not normally the case and x-ray examination should be carried out every four months to follow the progress of the pathology. In most cases nothing need be done until a loose body forms when arthrotomy is undertaken. The loose body is removed and the edges of the crater bevelled off. After wound healing, normal activity can be resumed and the crater will subsequently fill with fibrocartilage in such a way that it may be difficult to find.

Occasionally the level of disability is such that earlier arthrotomy is demanded but this should be resisted as far as possible because, in the early stages, the area is covered with normal looking cartilage and may be difficult to define.

Multiple drilling to increase the blood supply or replacement of the loose body by pinning are not recommended due to the inconsistent results obtained compared with the consistently good results of simple excision.

Meniscus injuries

Injuries to the menisci are distinctly uncommon in children. Under the age of 15 they are rare and most of these involve an abnormal meniscus usually a discoid lateral meniscus. From 15 to 20 years these injuries are also uncommon, most occurring in males and involving the lateral meniscus. The usual lesion is a bucket handle tear and next in frequency are posterior horn tears. If these tears cause a block to motion of the knee, articular erosions follow and can be quite extensive.

SYMPTOMS

There is usually a history of a rotation weight-bearing strain on the knee and this is accompanied by pain which continues to be the predominant symptom. Swelling is usual but often not severe. While giving way is a common complaint, true locking is rare.

SIGNS

Joint line tenderness is the most reliable and consistent physical sign and many have a positive McMurray's sign. An effusion may be present and a block to complete extension is an important finding.

EFFECTS OF MENISCECTOMY

There is abundant evidence that meniscectomy in early life leads to early degenerative changes and thus it cannot be regarded as a benign procedure. However, it is equally true that a badly torn meniscus causing a block to motion will, if left in situ, also cause premature degeneration of articular cartilage. In view of these facts the following principles of management can be laid down. Firstly, when a meniscal tear is diagnosed, it should be treated conservatively if possible, and meniscectomy only advised if a mechanical block can be demonstrated. Secondly, partial meniscectomy should be practised wherever possible. If the bucket handle only is removed, there is evidence that the remaining meniscus will have some effect in preventing premature degeneration. In doubtful cases, arthroscopy in skilled hands may make it possible to avoid meniscectomy.

MENISCECTOMY IN CHILDHOOD

The same technique is used as in the adult, but somewhat smaller instruments may be required. An adequate exposure is necessary to see as much of the meniscus as possible and, if no tear can be demonstrated, the meniscectomy should be abandoned. If partial meniscectomy is possible, this should always be carried out. After closure, a crepe bandage is used to control effusion and it is wise to immobilise the knee in some form of splint. (These patients do not understand what is meant by rest and are liable to move the knee excessively, producing an effusion or a haematoma under the wound.) The patient should be allowed up on crutches, non-weight-bearing after several days, but exercises are discouraged. At ten days, the dressings can be taken down and, if all is well, weight-bearing allowed. A crepe bandage is worn until such time as there is no further effusion. It is quite illogical to do exercises, and especially resistance exercises, in the early days before the wound and the quadriceps expansion has healed. At the end of the third week an exercise programme can be instituted and recovery of function will occur very rapidly.

DIFFERENTIAL DIAGNOSIS

Chondromalacia patellae—this condition can mimic practically all the symptoms of a meniscal injury and the knee must be very carefully examined to elicit the presence of retropatellar pain and crepitus.

Ligamentous injury—in the older age group ligamentous injury, especially on the medial side, may mimic an injury to the medial meniscus. This injury is common in skiers and, in the first week or so following injury, there is usually a block to full extension. The tenderness however, is more likely to be on the femoral attachment rather than on the joint line.

Osteochondritis dissecans—all injured knees should be submitted to x-ray examination and this should include an intercondylar view.

Chronic synovitis—in chronic synovitis in childhood, pain is not a significant feature but swelling is the rule and this is associated with palpable thickening. A full range of motion may be present although, as the condition advances, some loss of extension commonly occurs.

Penetrating wounds around the knee

The knee joint is very superficial so that penetration of the synovial cavity readily occurs. The most common injuries are caused by kneeling on needles and running into a wooden fence when a large splinter is broken off and penetrates the joint. Sometimes at presentation with a swollen knee no history of a penetrating wound can be obtained. Radio-opaque foreign bodies, such as needles, are readily visualised but the presence of other objects must often be inferred by the presence of an effusion, synovial thickening, and signs of inflammation.

If a child or adolescent presents with a penetrating wound, arthrotomy should always be carried out at once even if there is a history of the foreign body having been pulled out. The needle or splinter may spear into the articular cartilage and break off leaving a piece embedded when the main part is withdrawn. When a wooden splinter is retained it will break up into thousands of small fragments which pepper the synovium and cause a chronic synovitis. Synovectomy will then be necessary as the only way of removing the particles.

PERONEAL SPASMODIC FLAT FOOT (CONGENITAL TARSAL COALITION)

A clinical syndrome exists in which there is a valgus deformity of the foot associated with peroneal spasm and pain. This occurs in inflammatory and post-traumatic conditions affecting the tarsal joints and is especially common in juvenile rheumatoid arthritis. However, the term is now used mainly to describe the condition in which pain and spasm is associated with a congenital tarsal coalition. The most common coalitions are talonavicular and medial talocalcaneal and these may consist of a complete bony bar or the bar may be deficient in the middle, the gap being filled with fibrous tissue or cartilage (Figs. 5.17 & 5.18). Special radiological techniques may be required to demonstrate these bars.

Clinical features

The usual age at presentation is early adolescence but some are seen as early as 8

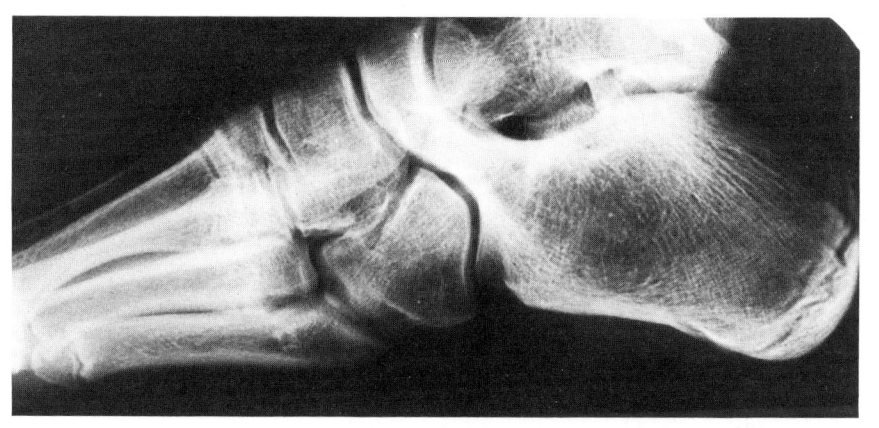

Fig. 5.17 Lateral x-ray of a foot showing a complete talonavicular bar.

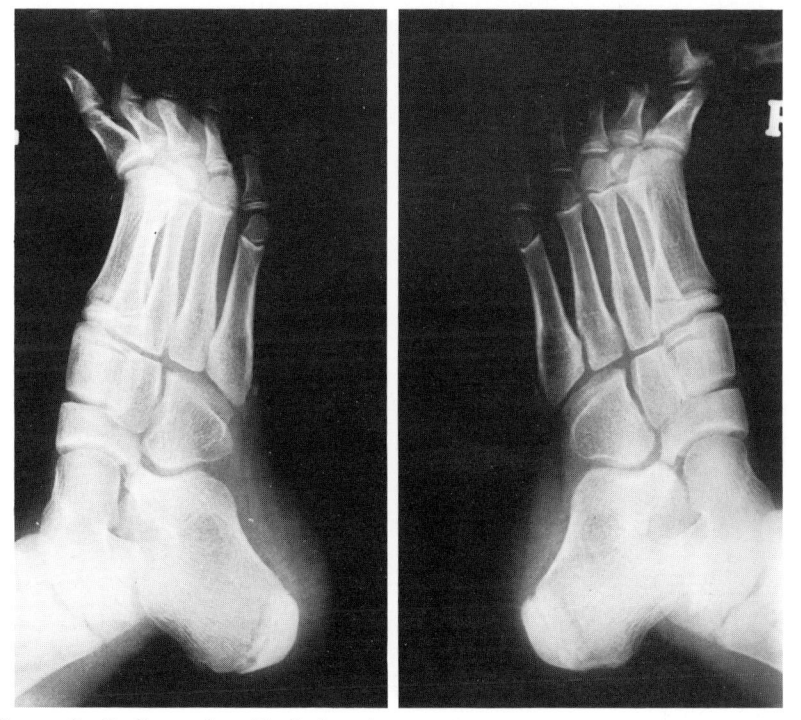

Fig. 5.18 Radiographs of both feet showing incomplete calcaneonavicular bars.

years. Persisting aching, especially after exercise, is the rule; the valgus deformity may also distort the shoe. The foot is fixed in valgus and any attempt to correct this forcibly is not only painful but initiates intense spasm in the peroneal muscles and often in the extensors of the toes as well.

Management

Mild cases can be treated as a foot strain: limitation of activity and the provision of an arch support. All severe cases should be treated surgically. The traditional conservative treatment of prolonged plaster fixation followed by bracing is rarely successful. The type of surgery employed will depend on the age of the child: under the age of 12 years, the bar can be excised, the gap filled with fat or muscle, and the foot mobilised early. There is a very good chance of a good result in this group. Over the age of 12 years, resection is rarely successful and triple arthrodesis using an inlay technique is advisable.

HALLUX VALGUS

Hallux valgus in adolescence is always associated with metatarsus primus varus and both deformities seem to develop together. There is a great preponderance of females and many of these will give a family history of bunions. While poorly fitting footwear and stretch socks and stockings undoubtedly aggravate the deformity, it seems clear that heredity plays the major role in causation. As the deformity increases, the head of the first metatarsal becomes increasingly prominent on the medial border of the foot, a bursa forms and pressure symptoms and signs make their appearance.

Clinical features

Most adolescents with hallux valgus present because their mothers are concerned at the progressive deformity. There may be difficulty in obtaining adequate footwear because of the excessive width of the forefoot and occasionally a complaint of discomfort after much activity. Considerable pressure may be applied to the surgeon either to 'remove the bunions' or at least to prevent the deformity from worsening.

Conservative management

Obviously care must be taken in shoe fitting and a last selected with a straight inner border and a wide toe. Socks that are made out of wool or cotton are superior to those made of synthetic fibres and stretch socks should never be worn. Experience has shown that the use of a night splint to hold the big toe in the straight position does appear to arrest progression if used during adolescence.

Operative treatment

The literature contains over 40 descriptions of different operative procedures for the correction of hallux valgus. It is not surprising therefore that none of these is entirely satisfactory. The authors' experience of these procedures has been unrewarding—even if a good initial result is obtained, relapse occurs very rapidly. If possible, surgery should be avoided as it is very difficult to obtain satisfied patients and parents. In severe cases and especially those in whom drifting of the lesser toes is occurring surgery may be indicated; whatever technique is selected, it should fulfil the following criteria. 1 The metatarsus primus varus must be corrected by proximal or distal osteotomy in such a way that the metatarsal is not shortened. Shortening is likely to produce metatarsalgia under the head of the second metatarsal. 2 The adductor hallucis is removed from the insertion into the base of the proximal phalanx and the lateral sesamoid. This attends to the main deforming force producing the valgus of the toe. 3 The medial ligament and the capsule must be raised on a distal base to allow shaving of the prominent metatarsal head medial to the annular groove and then re-sutured further proximally so as to hold the big toe in the neutral position. 4 Bone resections involving the joint (e.g. Keller arthroplasty) are contraindicated in adolescence as they produce an unacceptable cosmetic appearance and the new joint is often stiff and painful. 5 Plaster fixation is required for at least a month post-operatively to allow adequate soft tissue healing.

The operations described by McBride and by Menelaus and Simmonds fulfil these criteria.

HALLUX RIGIDUS

Hallux rigidus or stiffness of the metatarsophalangeal joint of the great toe occurs equally commonly in boys and girls. The first metatarsal is often overlong and lies more horizontally than normal (metatarsus primus elevatus) so that weight is borne by the big toe rather than the metatarsal head.

Clinical features

Pain is the presenting feature and may, at times, be acute and associated with redness, heat and swelling. There may be visible enlargement of the MP joint whose motion is very restricted especially in dorsiflexion. At first the x-ray appearances are normal, although the epiphysis at the base of the proximal phalanx is often denser. Later degenerative changes appear in the joints.

Management

Acute episodes will subside with rest. In the chronic phase relief can often be obtained by the use of a heavy soled, low heeled shoe. It may be necessary to stiffen the sole with a steel shank or to add a rocker to the sole. As the condition progresses, operative treatment may eventually be required. Two procedures are available: 1 In children under the age of 12 years if a good range of plantar flexion is still possible, wedge osteotomy of the proximal phalanx to produce extension will allow better use of the painless range. 2 In older children, arthrodesis is the procedure of choice. The big toe is fused parallel to the lesser toes and at an angle of about 20–30° with the metatarsal.

PLANTAR WARTS

Plantar warts are common in children and result from a viral infection which is readily transferable. The normal cauliflower-like wart is compressed by weight-bearing but can be recognised as it is clearly demarcated from the surrounding skin and the base has a punctate appearance due to small haemorrhages in the papillae.

Management

Small warts which are not causing much disability can be ignored as they tend to disappear. Larger and more painful lesions are best treated with 2% formalin. The solution is placed in a container such as the cap of a small bottle and inverted over the wart for five minutes twice a day for several weeks.

These warts, especially on the weight-bearing surface of the foot should never be treated by cauterisation, surgical excision, or irradiation as the scar produced may well be more serious than the wart.

INGROWING TOE NAILS

Painful ingrowing nails usually affect the big toe in boys with large feet which sweat excessively. The nail is very curved so that the edges abrade the sodden nail grooves producing a granuloma which may go on to suppuration.

Management

Tight shoes and socks are avoided and sandals worn whenever possible during the summer months. Mild cases will respond to packing pledgets of wool under the nail edge. If recurrent sepsis is established, excision of the nail and the nail bed (Zadek) is preferable to wedge resection.

RECURRENT INSTABILITY OF THE ANKLE

Ankle instability is not uncommon in adolescents of both sexes. The history is usually given of a severe ankle sprain which was accompanied by much pain, swelling, and bruising and which recovered slowly. Since that event, recurrence has been common with episodes provoking rather less reaction than previous ones. Instability may now occur in bare feet or in a variety of footwear.

Examination usually, but not always, reveals a pes cavus with some hind foot varus. There is an excessive range of inversion at the ankle and strain views occasionally reveal tilting of the talus in the mortice.

Management

The best management is prevention and all severe ankle injuries should be treated in a walking plaster for at least three weeks to allow adequate healing of the tear in the lateral ligament. Once the instability is established, the vicious circle must be interrupted by either the use of boots or a float on the heel. In some cases an ankle–foot orthosis will be indicated. If instability continues despite these measures, surgery may be required.

The following operations are available.

Peroneal tenodesis (Evans). The tendon of peroneus brevis is divided above the ankle and the distal part threaded through a drill hole in the lateral malleolus and sutured to the periosteum. This is a most effective reconstruction and will allow a full range of activities once consolidated.

Dwyer osteotomy of the os calcis (Dwyer). If the foot is cavus with a varus heel, this osteotomy is indicated and will usually correct instability and improve shoe wear.

CHAPTER 6

Fractures and Dislocations

Characteristic features of skeletal injuries in childhood, 280

Characteristic features of fractures in childhood, 281
Types of fracture; Fracture healing; Principles of diagnosis; Principles of treatment; Complications

Treatment of specific fractures and dislocations, 294
Clavicle; Humerus; Elbow; Forearm; Wrist; Hand; Pelvis; Hip; Femur; Tibia; Ankle; Foot; Spine; Fractures in special circumstances

Children are susceptible to injury because of their carefree play habits and skeletal injuries are extremely common. The following is a brief account of the characteristic features of skeletal injuries in children, the general principles of treatment, and the treatment of specific fractures and dislocations.

CHARACTERISTIC FEATURES OF SKELETAL INJURIES IN CHILDHOOD

Sprains

For practical purposes sprains do not occur in children so that post-traumatic pain, swelling, and loss of function are nearly always the result of a fracture or growth plate separation.

Dislocations

Dislocations are also rare in childhood. The types of injury which often produce a dislocation in an adult, usually give rise to a fracture or growth plate separation in a child. The few dislocations that do occur in children usually affect the elbow, superior radio-ulnar, and hip joints.

Fractures

Fractures are the commonest type of skeletal injury in children. They commonly result from low velocity trauma such as falls from play equipment, but a small number of children receive high velocity injuries from motor vehicle and bicycle accidents and a small group have pathological fractures.

CHARACTERISTIC FEATURES OF FRACTURES IN CHILDHOOD

Fractures in children differ in many respects from fractures in adults. In addition to the obvious difference—that growth plate injuries are confined to the growing child—important differences also exist in fractures at other sites as well as in fracture healing and the re-modelling capacity of bone.

TYPES OF FRACTURE

Metaphyseal fractures

Metaphyseal fractures are commonly seen in the cancellous bone of the distal radius, ulna and tibia. There are three types of metaphyseal fractures:

Buckle fracture—in young children, the compressed metaphyseal bone elevates the cortical surface giving the bone a buckled appearance (Figs. 6.1 & 6.2).

Greenstick fracture—when an angulatory force is applied to the metaphyseal region, the cortex under tension is disrupted while the opposite side, which is compressed, remains intact and acts as a hinge (Figs. 6.3 & 6.4). The periosteum is thick and remains intact on the hinge side of these fractures.

Complete fracture—with more severe trauma, particularly in the older child, the metaphyseal fracture may completely disrupt the entire cortex and produce displacement (Figs. 6.5 & 6.6).

Diaphyseal fractures

The majority of diaphyseal fractures are complete and comminution is rare (Figs. 6.7 & 6.8). Several other types of diaphyseal injury are also seen. Plastic deformation without fracture commonly occurs in the ulna or fibula when there is a displaced or angulated fracture in the adjoining bone. Greenstick fractures of the diaphysis are seen in neonates and infants but they are rare in older children, unless the bones are abnormally fragile (Figs. 6.9 & 6.10).

Growth plate injuries

At least a third of children's fractures involve the growth plate. These fractures are of particular importance because permanent growth plate damage may result.

The types of growth plate injury, as described by Salter and Harris, are

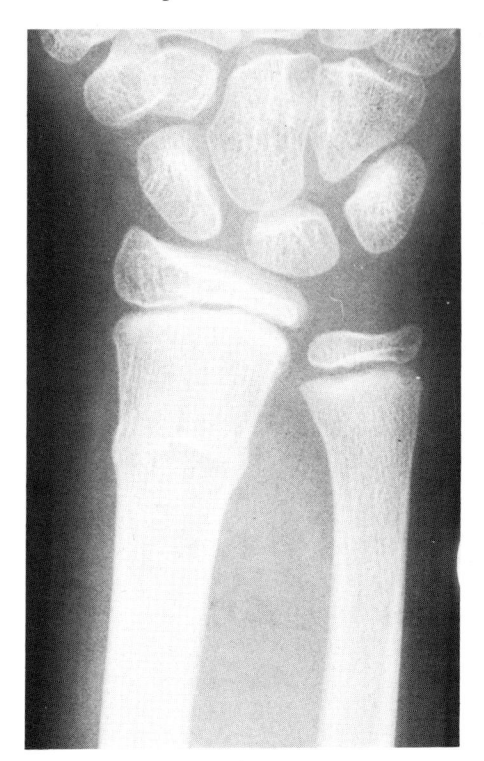

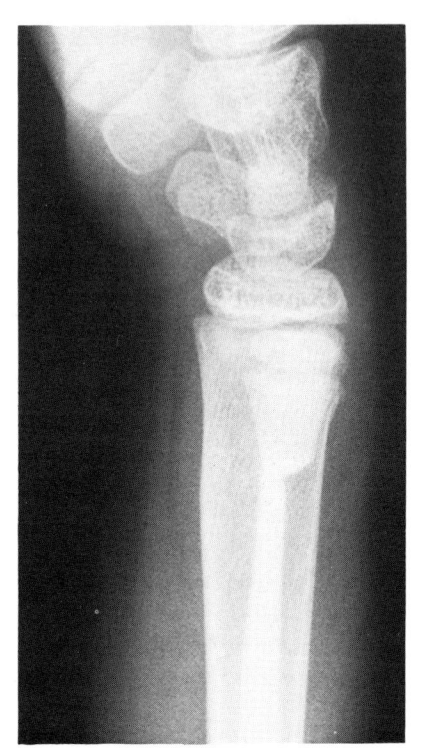

Figs. 6.1 & 6.2 Buckle fracture of the distal radial metaphysis. There is bulging of the medial and lateral cortices of the radius at the site of the buckle fracture. The lateral view shows that the posterior cortex of the radius is buckled.

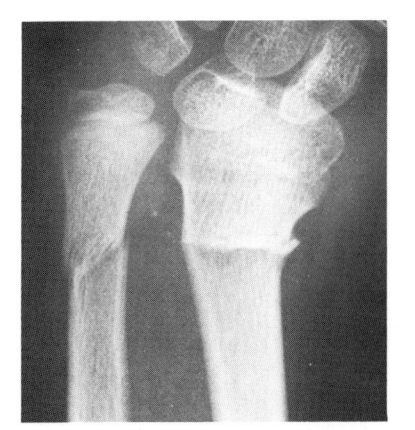

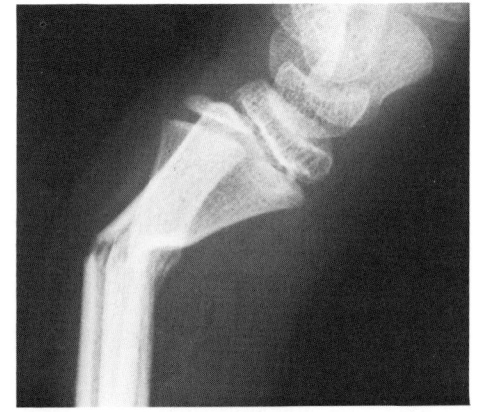

Figs. 6.3 & 6.4 Greenstick fractures through the metaphysis of the distal radius and ulna. There is marked angulation with rupture of the posterior cortices and buckling of the anterior cortices. Recurrence of the deformity is prevented by complete disruption of the intact cortices.

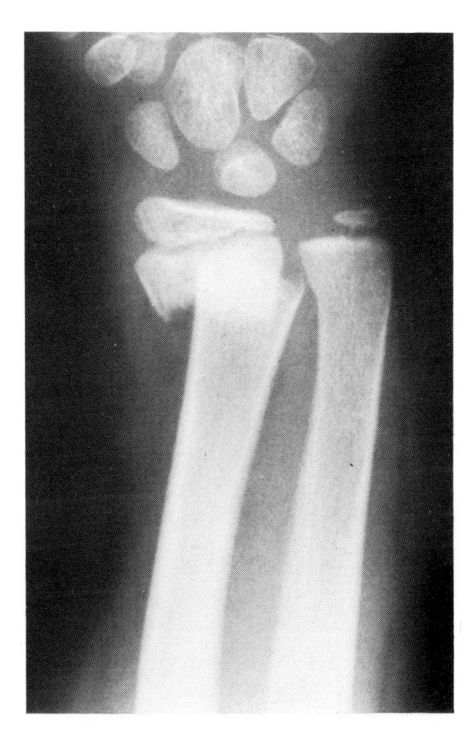

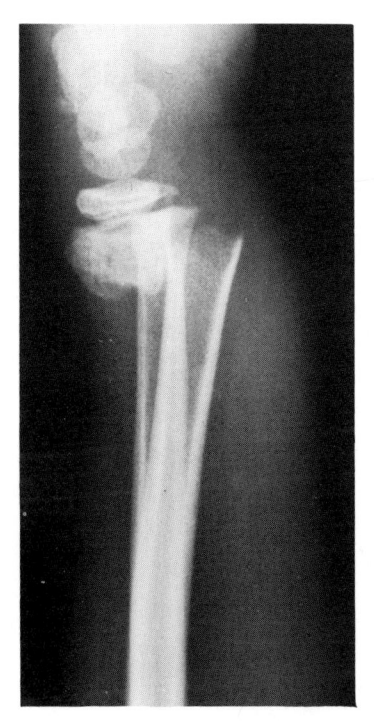

Figs. 6.5 & 6.6 A complete fracture through the radial metaphysis with lateral displacement and angulation of the distal fragment. The lateral view shows that the distal fragment is lying on the posterior surface of the distal radius.

illustrated in Fig. 6.11. This classification aids in the understanding of the nature of the injury and the likelihood of future complications.

TYPE I

In the type I fracture, the growth plate cartilage is cleaved horizontally at the junction between the uncalcified and calcified zone. The paucity of matrix accounts for the weakness of this region of the growth plate. As the germinal layer of the growth plate remains attached to the epiphysis, and is not damaged, future growth is normal. While the epiphysis may be widely displaced, many of these fractures are undisplaced.

This type of growth plate injury is usually seen in infants but also occurs in older children with scurvy, rickets, osteomyelitis, and hormonal imbalance.

TYPE II

This is the commonest type of growth plate injury. The plate is cleaved horizontally, in the same plane as in the type I injury, but the fracture extends across one

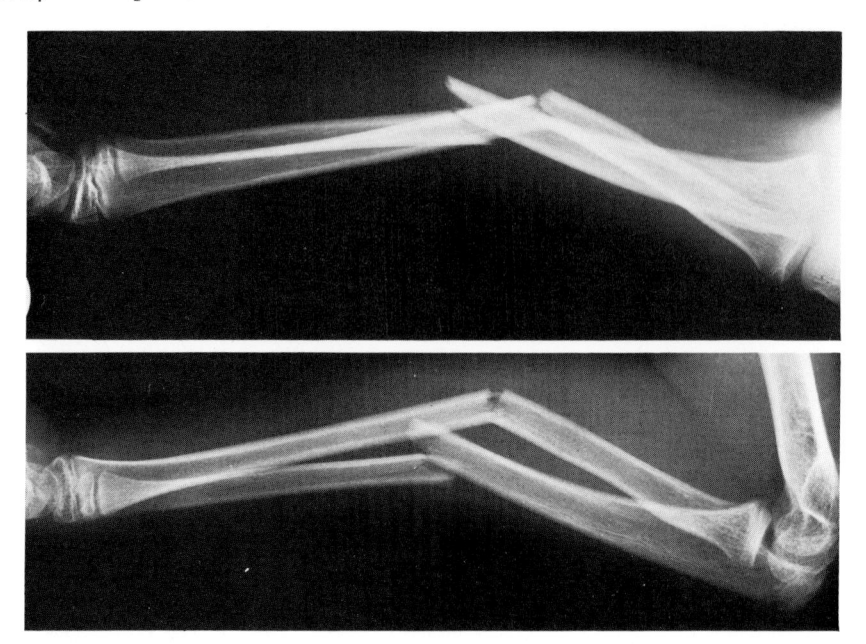

Figs. 6.7 & 6.8 An A–P x-ray of the forearm with complete fractures of the shafts of the radius and ulna with medial angulation. Note the marked degree of anterior angulation of these fractures on the lateral view.

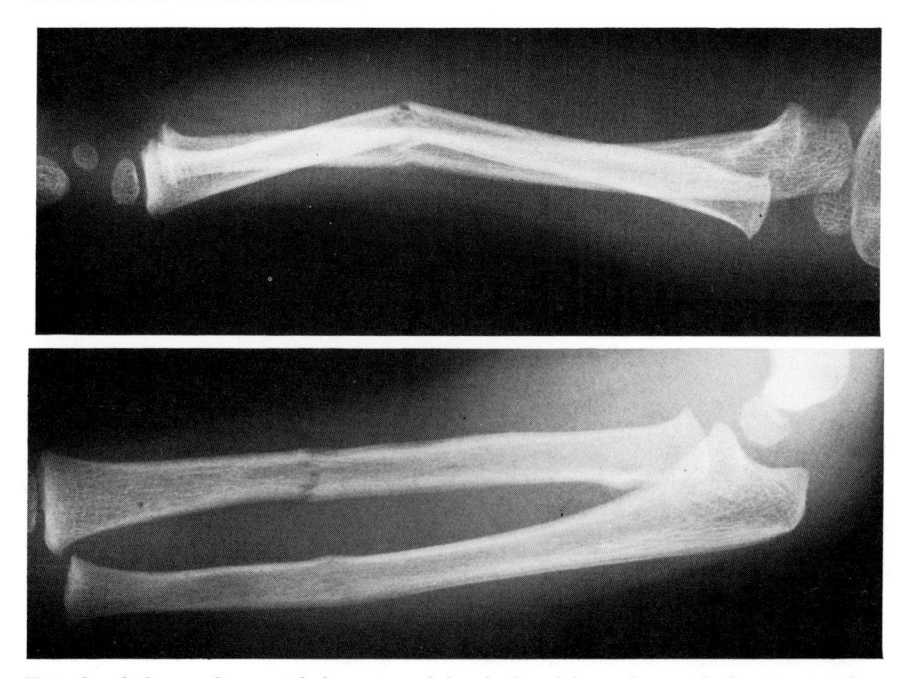

Figs. 6.9 & 6.10 Greenstick fractures of the shafts of the radius and ulna in an infant.

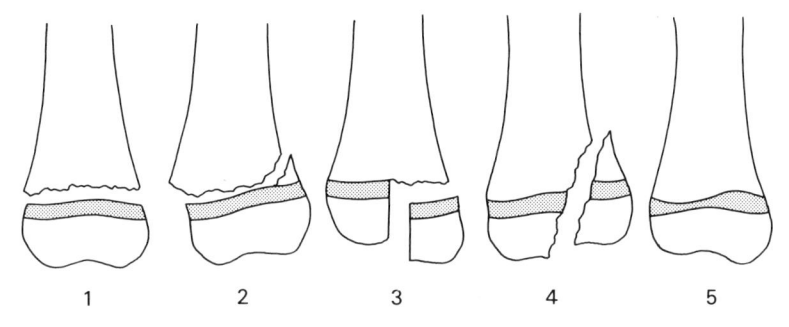

Fig. 6.11 Salter–Harris classification of growth plate injuries.

corner of the metaphysis producing a triangular fragment of variable size. The periosteum is intact over the metaphyseal fragment but is ruptured on the opposite side. As with the type I injury the resting chondrocyte layer is usually undamaged.

TYPE III

This injury is rare but is most commonly seen in the distal tibia. Future growth is usually normal but displaced fractures produce an irregular articular surface.

TYPE IV

The lateral condyle fracture of the humerus is a typical example of a type IV injury. The fracture extends from the epiphysis across the growth plate into the metaphysis. It is one of the few fractures that may lead to non-union and malunion with a progressive disturbance of growth.

TYPE V

Crushing injuries of the growth plate may produce permanent damage to the resting chondrocytes with complete or partial cessation of growth giving rise to limb length discrepancy and deformity. This injury may occur without displacement of the epiphysis and it is also seen as part of the type II injuries of the lower femoral and upper tibial growth plates.

FRACTURE HEALING

It is common for many children's fractures to heal in less than half the time the equivalent injury would take to heal in an adult, and non-union is almost unknown. This difference is most apparent in the infant and young child. Extensive re-modelling follows the healing of fractures in children and involves alterations in both length and shape.

Length

Diaphyseal fractures stimulate longitudinal growth for up to a year following injury so that a small amount of shortening can be expected to correct spontaneously.

Shape

Residual angular deformities usually correct spontaneously but rotary malunion will not correct at any age. Complete correction of residual angulation can be expected when the fracture is located close to the growth plate and when the angulation is in the same plane as the motion of the adjacent joint. Correction will often be complete within 6–12 months in young children (Figs. 6.12–6.14).

PRINCIPLES OF DIAGNOSIS

Clinical features

Displaced fractures are obvious at all ages but undisplaced fractures often produce

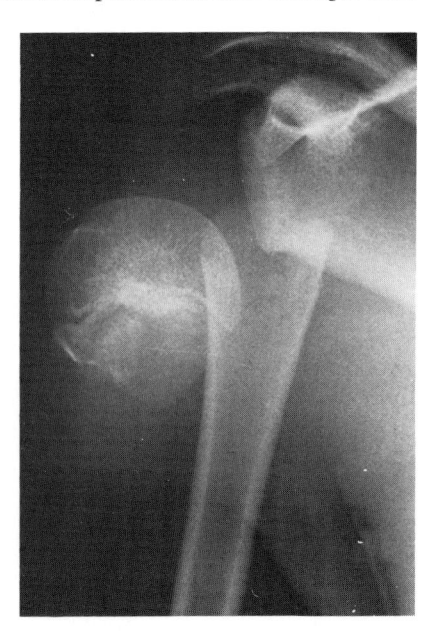

Fig. 6.12 6-year-old child with a completely displaced fracture through the proximal humeral metaphysis. Reduction was not attempted and the arm was supported in a collar and cuff.

Fractures and Dislocations 287

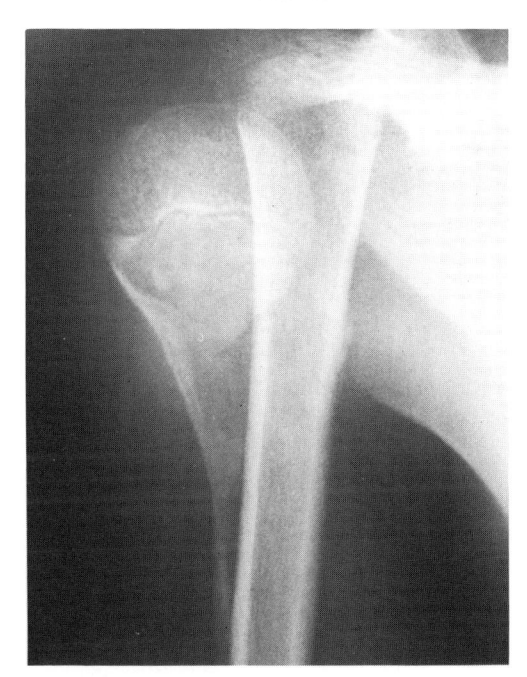

Fig. 6.13 Same patient as Fig. 6.12. Subperiosteal new bone noted six weeks later.

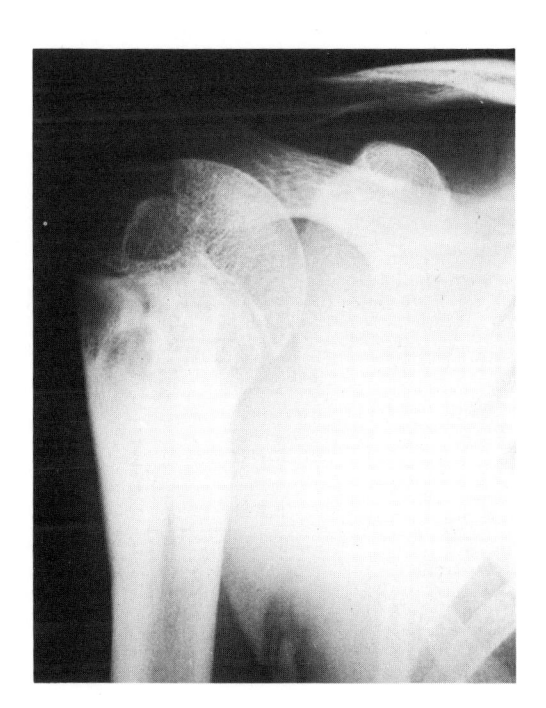

Fig. 6.14 Same patient as Fig. 6.12. Extensive re-modelling of the proximal humerus one year following the fracture.

288   *Chapter 6*

minimal discomfort and disturbance of function. The most important physical sign is local tenderness which localises the site of the fracture and indicates the region to be x-rayed.

Radiological features

Standard antero-posterior and lateral x-rays of the affected bone, extending from the joint above to the joint below, are required. Where difficulty is encountered in interpreting the x-ray it is often useful to x-ray the normal side for comparison. Careful inspection of the films is required in order to detect fine undisplaced fractures and buckle fractures. Problems are often encountered with growth plate injuries as the epiphysis is mainly cartilaginous. Type I injuries may only produce slight asymmetry in the width of the epiphyseal plate and small metaphyseal fragments may be the only sign of type II or IV fractures. A careful search for a fracture is always required when there are radiological signs of soft tissue swelling and haemarthrosis (Fig. 6.15).

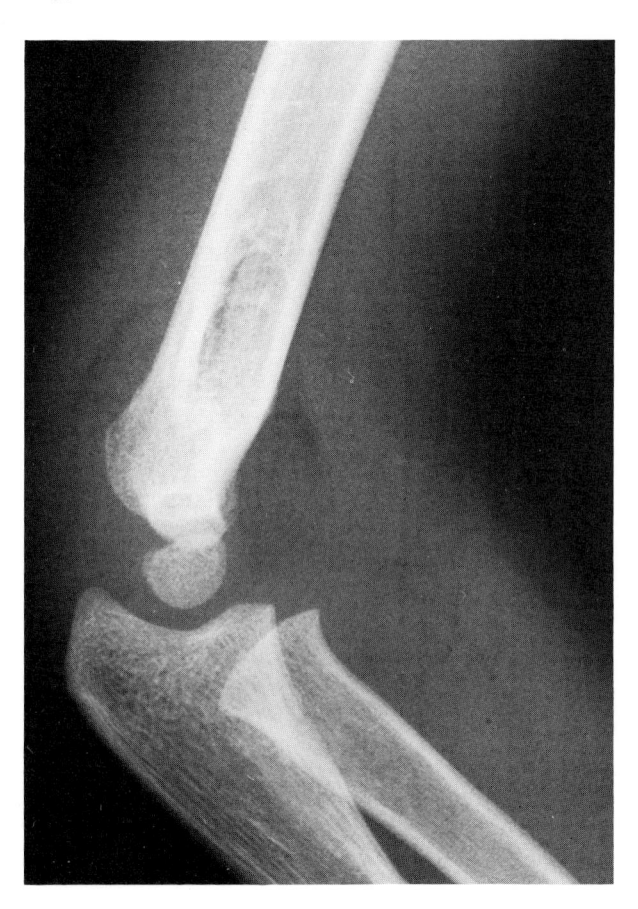

Fig. 6.15 Greenstick supracondylar fracture of the humerus. Note the haemarthrosis with displacement of the fat pads on the front and back of the distal humerus. The condyle of the humerus is deviated posteriorly due to a greenstick fracture through the supracondylar region. The arm was supported for three weeks in a collar and cuff and an elasticised net.

PRINCIPLES OF TREATMENT

The methods of treating fractures include reduction, immobilisation, and rehabilitation.

Reduction

Undisplaced fractures do not require reduction. However, the limb may also have a normal shape when the fracture is mildly angulated. In most instances reduction is not required as it can be anticipated that re-modelling will correct the angulation. When there is clinical deformity or when displacement cannot be expected to correct by re-modelling, the fracture is reduced.

Reduction is usually achieved by manipulation of the fracture under general anaesthesia. As the periosteum is usually intact on the side to which the fragment has been displaced, reduction is best achieved by increasing the deformity so as to relax the periosteal hinge which then enables the fragments to be engaged. The fracture is then closed and, as the periosteal hinge becomes taut, the fragments are kept in position. A sense of reduction is readily felt in diaphyseal and metaphyseal fractures but is less obvious when the fracture involves the cartilaginous growth plate. In correcting angulated greenstick fractures it is necessary to completely fracture the intact cortex which would otherwise act as a hinge leading to recurrence of the deformity.

Displaced fractures may also be reduced by traction. This applies particularly to fractures of the shaft of the femur and to supracondylar fractures of the humerus. Skin traction is usually adequate although skeletal traction may be required in older adolescents with fractures of the femur. Pins inserted across the bone for skeletal traction must not be placed across the epiphyseal plate as permanent growth plate damage and progressive deformity will result. Particular care is necessary in placing pins in the upper end of the tibia as the growth plate descends to the middle of the tubercle in front.

Children's fractures rarely require open reduction. However open reduction and accurate re-positioning of the fragments are required for displaced type III and IV growth plate injuries in order to re-align the articular surface and the growth plate. Care must be taken to avoid damage to the growth plate and to the blood supply of the epiphyseal fragment. Open reduction with internal fixation is also occasionally required in children with head injuries and pathological fractures.

Immobilisation

PLASTER CAST

The majority of children with undisplaced or minimally displaced fractures of the long bones will be most comfortable in a padded plaster cast which should immobilise the joint above and below the level of the fracture. Where a fracture has been treated by manipulative reduction, a carefully moulded padded plaster cast is applied. Correct three point moulding of the plaster will keep the periosteal hinge taut and reduce the likelihood of subsequent displacement. Plaster back-slabs should not be used for fractures but are useful in soft tissue injuries to immobilise adjacent joints.

SLING

Immobilisation of the arm in a sling is used for treating fractures of the clavicle and to support plaster casts.

COLLAR AND CUFF

This form of immobilisation, which is commonly used in treating fractures of the

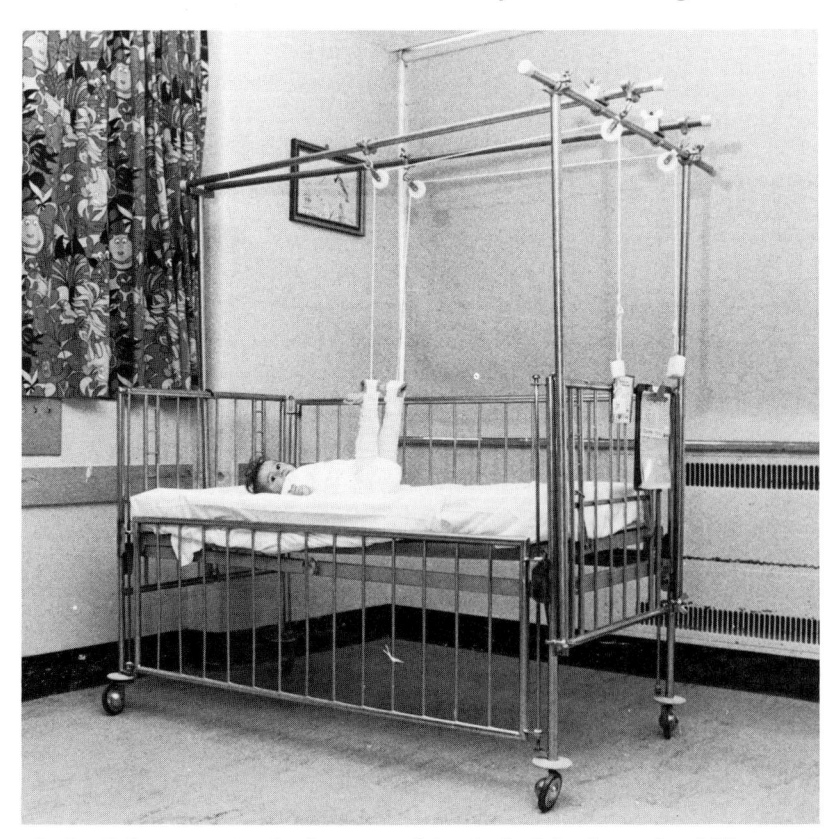

Fig. 6.16 Gallows traction for fractures of the shaft of the femur for children under 2 years of age.

Fractures and Dislocations 291

humerus, allows gravity to maintain the position of the fragments. The collar should be well padded at the wrist and behind the neck; an elasticised net provides further support by holding the arm against the chest.

TRACTION

In children, traction can be used to reduce and immobilise fractures. For fractures of the femur, gallows traction is used for children under 2 years of age, while Hamilton Russell traction is used in older children (Figs. 6.16 & 6.17). Care is required in using gallows traction as Volkmann's ischaemic contracture may occur if the leg bandages obstruct the arterial supply (Fig. 6.18).

Skeletal traction is reserved for older children with fractures of the femur in whom a satisfactory position cannot be obtained by skin traction.

Follow up

When a child is sent home with a fresh fracture, in particular when a plaster cast

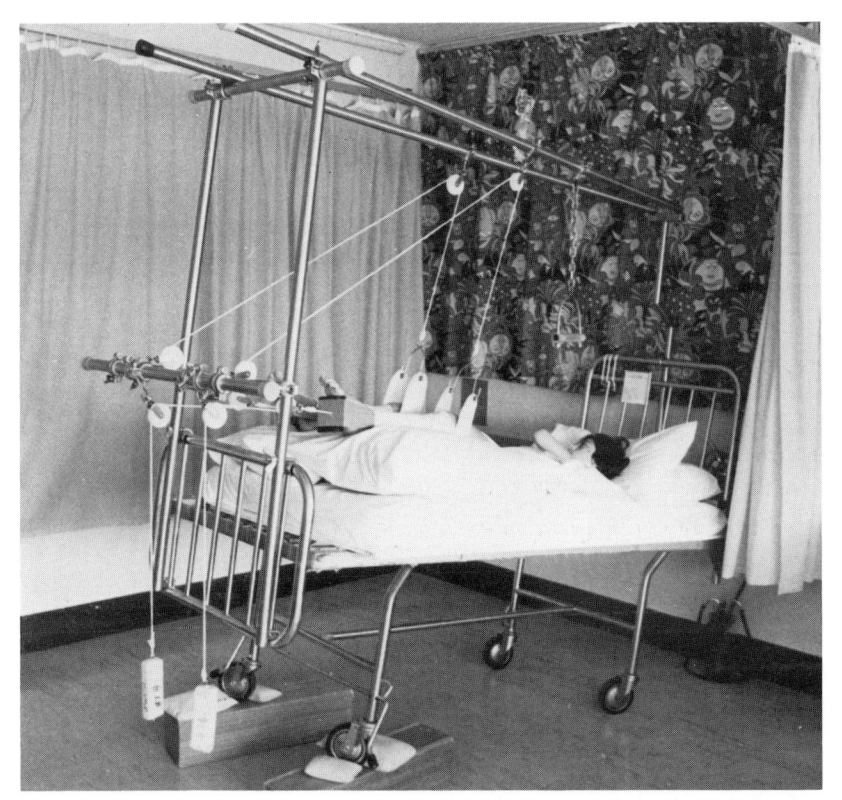

Fig. 6.17 Hamilton Russell traction for fractures of the femur. This form of traction was used to treat bilateral fractures of the femur in this 7-year-old boy with multiple injuries.

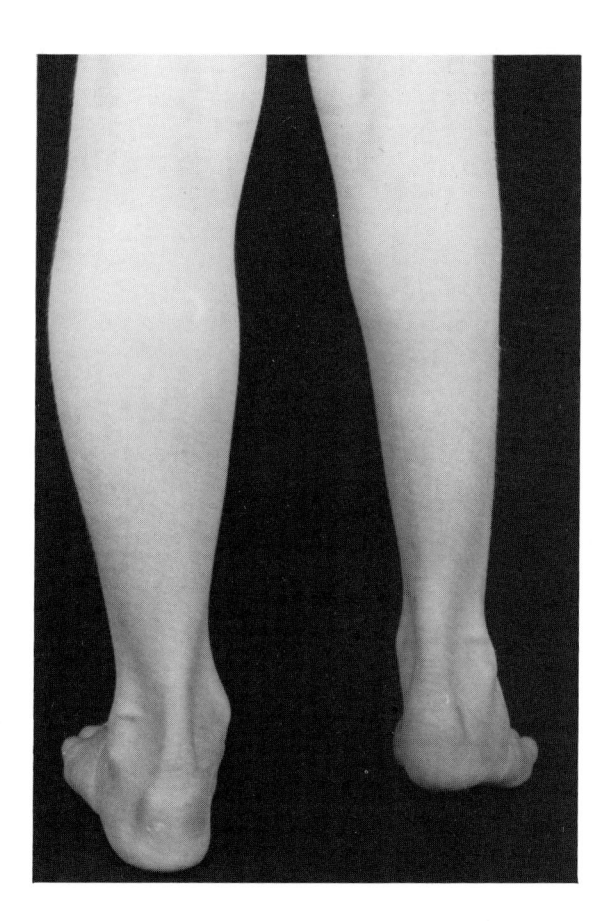

Fig. 6.18 Volkmann's ischaemic contracture from gallows traction. Note the wasted calf and equinus deformity.

has been applied, his parents are provided with a printed set of instructions (*see* page 352) detailing the symptoms and signs which require them to take their child immediately to the doctor. Many children experience some discomfort within the first day but, if pain is unrelieved by elevation of the limb, the plaster is too tight, or producing localised pressure, or there is arterial ischaemia. Other important signs include coldness, swelling and discoloration of the fingers. In each instance, the child should return immediately and the full length of the plaster including the underlying padding should be split. This usually relieves the symptoms but, if not, the entire plaster should be removed. Persistent ischaemia or venous obstruction are usually the result of a tight fascial compartment or a major vascular injury. In these circumstances fasciotomies and arterial exploration are required.

It is more common for the features of a tight plaster cast to become apparent the day following the injury. All children whose fractures are being treated with a plaster cast are therefore reviewed the day following injury.

As the swelling at the fracture site subsides over the following few days, some of the fractures will displace or angulate within the plaster. As children's fractures unite rapidly, it is necessary to correct any unacceptable deformity within the first ten days following the injury. It is our routine to take standard antero-posterior and lateral x-rays of all fractures 7–10 days following the injury and to correct any unacceptable displacement.

The plaster or other means of immobilising the fracture is removed when the fracture is healed. Mobilisation can often be commenced in young children with buckle fractures after 2–3 weeks. On the other hand, displaced fractures in older children frequently require six weeks of immobilisation. Children are usually able to act as their own physiotherapist and, as their limb becomes more comfortable, they will use it during their normal play activities. Physiotherapy is of great assistance for older children with fractures of the femur and for children with multiple injuries, where progress is often slow due to fear of falling and sustaining further injuries.

Review is required whenever permanent growth plate damage is suspected so that treatment can be given before severe deformities have occurred.

COMPLICATIONS

Nerve injury

Before beginning treatment, all children with fractures and dislocations are carefully examined for a nerve injury. In most instances the nerve is damaged by traction at the time of the injury. Nerve palsies are commonly associated with fractures in the upper limb, in particular of the humerus. The majority of nerve palsies recover spontaneously and splintage is usually not required but care is needed to avoid burns and cuts to anaesthetised areas. This applies particularly to the ulnar border of the hand and to the little finger in children with ulnar nerve palsies.

Arterial injury

This is the most important complication of fracture. Unrelieved ischaemia will lead to necrosis of muscles and nerves so giving rise to Volkmann's contracture. Signs of ischaemia include severe and unremitting pain, pallor of the fingers with absence of capillary return, paralysis of the affected muscles, and severe pain on passively extending the fingers or toes. Immediate measures are required to restore the circulation. The steps include bivalving of plaster casts and the underlying padding, removal of any encircling bandages and, if the circulation is not immediately restored, complete removal of these items. If ischaemia still persists, operative intervention is indicated and this may involve fasciotomy and exposure of the main vessels.

With compartment syndromes, the pulse and skin flow through the toes are often normal. Compartment pressures can be measured but, when the techniques are not available, it is best to proceed directly to fasciotomy. An open fasciotomy is required with incision of the full length of the fascia; the overlying skin is left open and is only closed when the swelling has subsided. It is important to decompress the deep as well as the superficial compartments and, in the leg, the four compartments can be easily decompressed through the fibular periosteum. This can be carried out without excising the fibula as resection of the fibula in the growing child frequently leads to a valgus deformity of the ankle. Whenever an injury of a major artery is suspected it is explored first. If arteriograms are required it is preferable to carry these out during the operation in order to save time. It is common for the injured segment of an artery to be collapsed with an appearance suggestive of arterial spasm. However, this appearance is usually produced by intimal rupture with thrombosis. Treatment consists of removal of the thrombosis, resection of the damaged area and insertion of a reversed vein graft. These procedures are most commonly required in the femoral and popliteal arteries. Divided femoral and popliteal arteries also require repair and, in most instances, fasciotomies are also required as compartment syndromes may follow restoration of the circulation.

Complete division of the brachial artery or one of the arteries below the elbow or knee can usually be treated by tying off the artery provided the collateral circulation is adequate.

TREATMENT OF SPECIFIC FRACTURES AND DISLOCATIONS

CLAVICLE

Fractures of the shaft

This is a very common injury which is treated by supporting the arm in a sling. The traditional figure-of-eight bandage is uncomfortable and is not required. After 1–2 weeks the shoulder is usually comfortable and mobilisation is commenced. Parents need to be warned that a lump will appear at the fracture site and that it will gradually disappear over the next year.

Fractures of the medial end

Separations through the epiphyseal plate at the medial end of the clavicle are uncommon. The clavicle may displace either forwards or backwards and occasionally backward displacement will compress the trachea. If this rare complication occurs, the compression can be relieved by closed manipulation.

This fracture also is treated by supporting the arm in a sling and re-modelling can be expected to correct any residual displacement. As a consequence, open reduction is rarely required. Open reduction should also be avoided because scars

Fractures of the outer end

It is common for a fracture at the outer end of the clavicle to be misdiagnosed as an acromio-clavicular dislocation—a rare injury in childhood. The arm is supported with a sling and extensive re-modelling will occur as the inferior part of the periosteum is intact (Fig. 6.19).

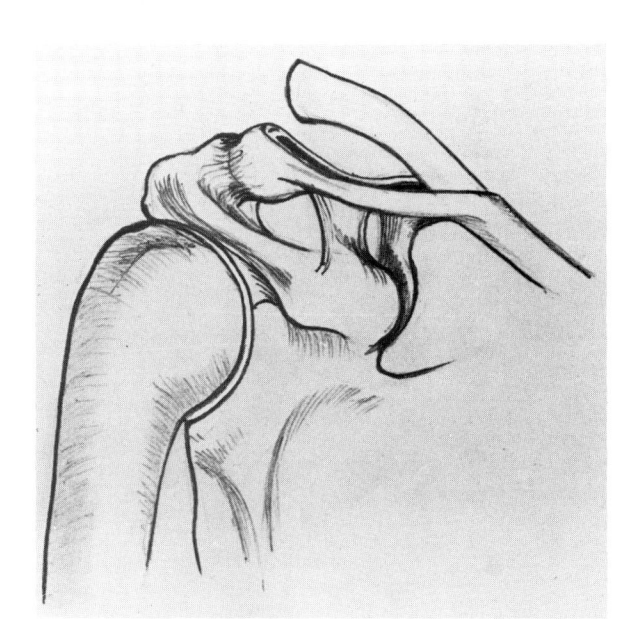

Fig. 6.19 Fracture of the outer end of the clavicle illustrating that the periosteum remains attached to the coraco-clavicular ligaments when the clavicle is displaced. This enables the clavicle to re-model without the need for open reduction.

HUMERUS

Fractures of the proximal humerus

Type I growth plate fractures occur during delivery and in toddlers. Manipulative reduction is rarely required and the arm is supported in a collar and cuff for three weeks. Type II growth plate fractures are common in adolescents and frequently result from a fall from a horse (Fig. 6.20). These fractures may be severely displaced in which case an attempt should be made to improve the position by manipulation. This is not always possible to obtain or to maintain and the use of an abduction shoulder spica to maintain any improvement is unwarranted because of the uncomfortable position of the arm and the possibility of producing a brachial plexus palsy. Open reduction is never required except in those close to maturity where there is considerable displacement which cannot otherwise be

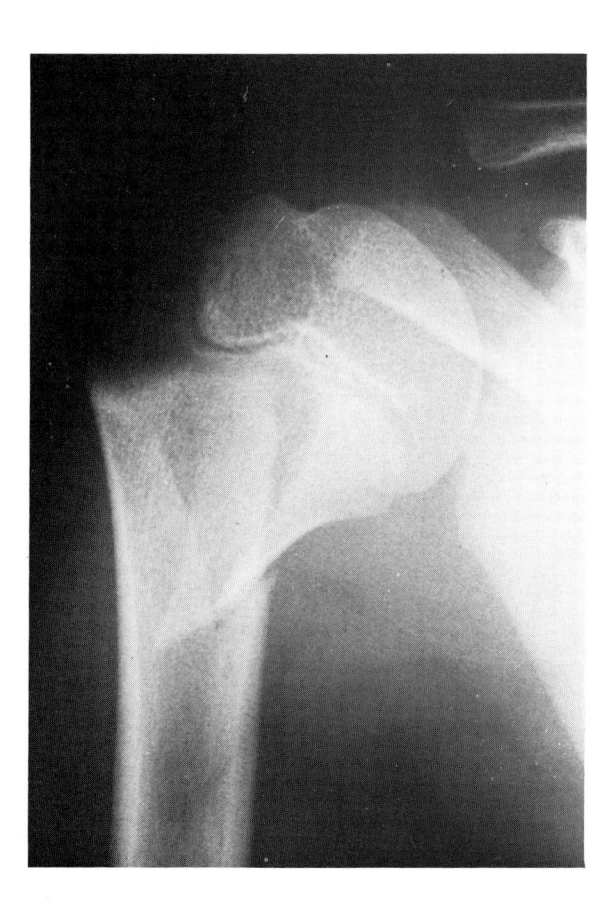

Fig. 6.20 Salter type II fracture of the upper humeral growth plate. The lateral part of the growth plate has been cleaved horizontally but there is a large medial metaphyseal fragment. The arm was supported in a collar and cuff and anatomy was restored by re-modelling over the following year.

improved. The proximal humerus rapidly re-models and full shoulder movement can be expected (see Figs. 6.12–6.14).

Fractures of the upper humeral metaphysis

These fractures are common and are treated with a collar and cuff support. On occasions the shaft will penetrate the deltoid and threaten to penetrate the skin. The position of the fragment can usually be improved by closed reduction but open reduction is never required.

Fractures of the humeral shaft

This fracture is treated with a collar and cuff, and the arm is positioned against the trunk with an elasticised net or a cotton singlet. As the elbow is not supported, gravity will maintain the position of the fracture. A U-shaped plaster slab is rarely required.

ELBOW

Supracondylar fractures of the humerus

Careful assessment of the forearm and hand for signs of ischaemia and nerve palsies is always made. The hand is often ischaemic if the elbow has been splinted in flexion but the circulation rapidly returns when the elbow is extended. Median nerve palsies are common and are readily diagnosed by the typical posture of the hand with the extended index finger.

In the common extension type of supracondylar fracture, the fracture line extends transversely across the metaphysis close to the epiphyseal line. The shaft of the humerus is driven forwards where it may injure the brachial artery or the median nerve and may puncture the skin. The distal fragment is displaced posteriorly and frequently to one or other side. The periosteum is intact posteriorly and on the side to which the distal fragment is displaced.

Undisplaced supracondylar fractures are treated with a collar and cuff and an elastic netting support. This type of immobilisation is continued until the elbow is mobilised three weeks later.

Displaced supracondylar fractures require reduction (Figs. 6.21 & 6.22). This is usually achieved by manipulation under general anaesthesia. The forearm is grasped with the elbow flexed to approximately 20° and traction is applied with an assistant providing counter traction in the axilla. The fragments are disengaged and the sideways displacement of the distal fragment is corrected by direct pressure. Rotary malalignment is corrected by the assistant holding the upper arm firmly while the forearm is internally rotated with the elbow flexed to approximately 45°. Finally the posterior displacement is corrected by flexing the elbow and applying thumb pressure to the olecranon which engages the fragment onto the end of the humerus. As the elbow is flexed the periosteal hinge tightens and the fragments are locked into position (Figs. 6.23 & 6.24).

A strip of two-inch tape is passed around the arm and forearm to maintain the elbow position. An antero-posterior x-ray of the elbow is taken with the humerus on the x-ray plate and the forearm is aligned over it so that the radius and ulna are superimposed onto the humerus. In this way the epicondyles should be clearly visible. A true lateral x-ray of the elbow is also taken. The arm is brought to the side, a collar and cuff support and an elasticised net are applied over the arm to maintain the position against the chest (Fig. 6.25). The capillary circulation of the hand is checked and, if there is any disturbance, the elbow is progressively extended until the circulation returns. Absence of the radial pulse is not important provided the capillary circulation is normal.

The child remains in hospital for several days so that the circulation and the extent of any elbow swelling can be observed. The adequacy of the reduction is checked by repeating the x-ray one week later and, if the position is satisfactory, the elbow is mobilised three weeks following the injury. The full range of elbow

298   Chapter 6

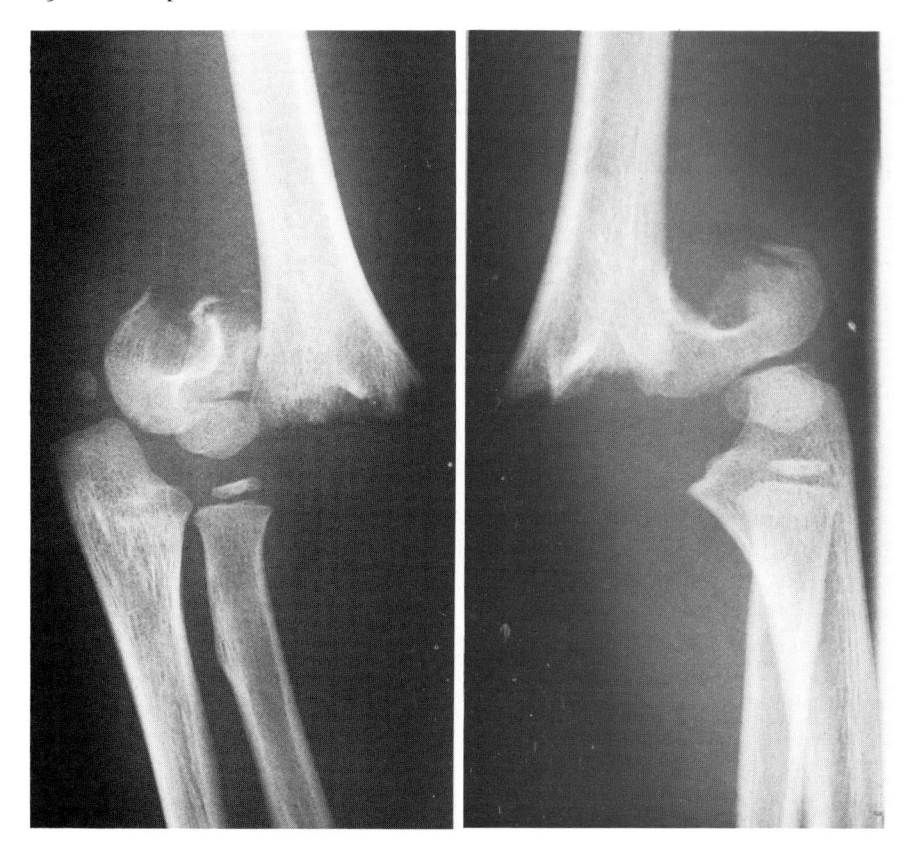

Figs. 6.21 & 6.22 Supracondylar fracture of the humerus with medial and proximal migration of the distal fragment. The lateral view shows the posteriorly displaced fragment. The anterior spike of the humeral shaft was impaled in the brachialis. The fracture was reduced by closed manipulation.

motion is frequently slow to return and full extension may not be achieved for 6–12 months. The parents need to be warned about this and it should be noted that physiotherapy does not increase the speed of recovery.

Problems

FAILURE TO REDUCE THE FRACTURE

This is commonly the result of failure to carry out the reduction in the correct sequence. Unless the sideways and rotary displacements are corrected before the fragment is engaged onto the end of the humerus, the reduction will be unsatisfactory. Furthermore, if an attempt is made to flex the elbow before the fragments

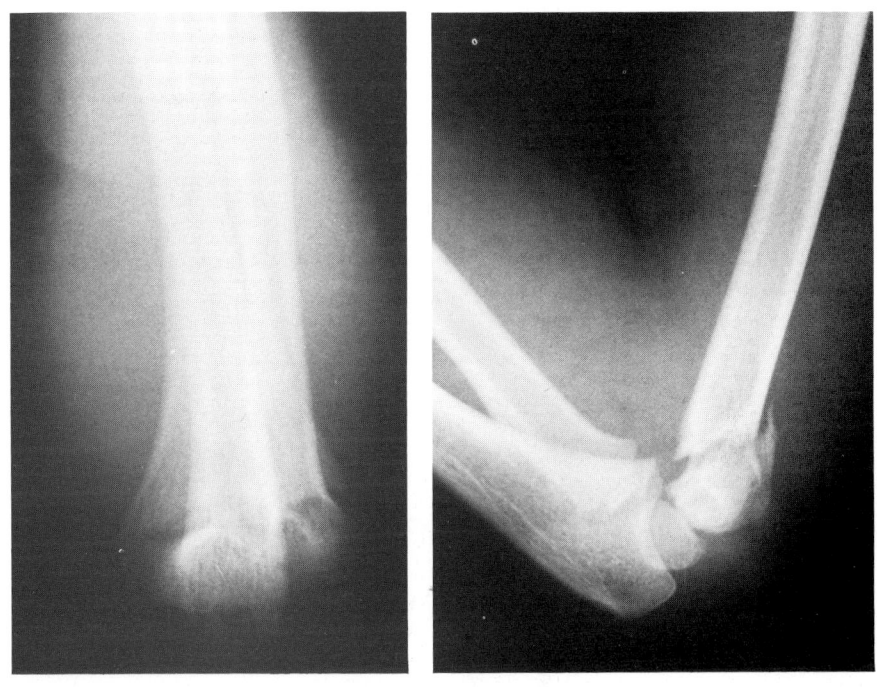

Figs. 6.23 & 6.24 Same patient as Fig. 6.21. An A–P x-ray of the elbow taken following the reduction. The forearm is positioned over the shaft of the humerus so that the medial and lateral margins of the humeral condyle can be examined in order to determine the adequacy of the reduction. This x-ray shows that the condyle is well aligned. The lateral view shows that the reduction is acceptable.

are disengaged, the brachial artery may be trapped between the bone ends. If the fracture cannot be reduced, skin traction is applied to the arm and the child is returned to the ward. Open reduction is not required.

Dunlop skin traction may also be used as the primary method of treatment in children who present with severe swelling of the elbow or in whom a general anaesthetic is contraindicated (Fig. 6.26). The forearm is painted with tincture of benzoin and a strip of Elastoplast is applied to the anterior and posterior surfaces of the forearm. A square spreader situated beyond the fingers keeps the Elastoplast away from the hand and a new crepe bandage is applied to the forearm. An alternative is to use pieces of foam which are also held onto the forearm by a crepe bandage. A rope with a weight attached is passed over a pulley and tied to the spreader. Traction is applied with the arm elevated 45° from the side of the bed and a small canvas sling with an attached weight is suspended from the upper arm over the proximal fragment. Considerable improvement in the position of the fracture and in the carrying angle is usually achieved. This method of traction is simpler and more comfortable than skeletal traction using an olecranon pin. After a week's traction it is frequently possible to improve the position by manipulation

300   Chapter 6

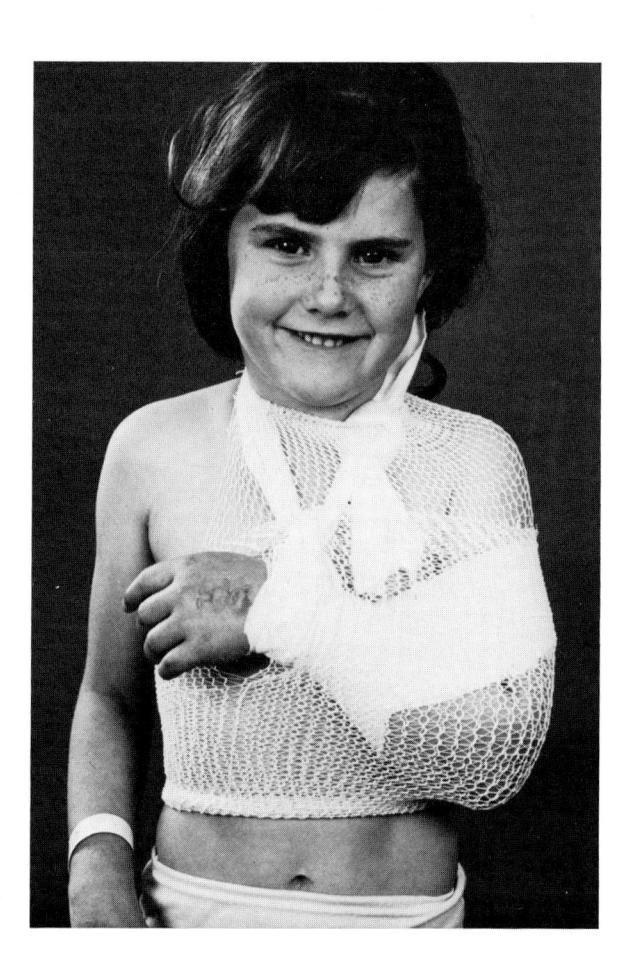

Fig. 6.25 Method of immobilisation of supracondylar fractures of the humerus. The elastic netting has to be removed to enable x-rays to be taken.

under general anaesthesia and then the flexed elbow is immobilised in a collar and cuff with netting support.

FAILURE TO MAINTAIN THE REDUCTION

It may be impossible to obtain a stable reduction because of severe swelling of the elbow. Under these circumstances a short period in Dunlop traction will allow the swelling to decrease so that a further reduction can then be carried out and is more likely to be successful. On occasions, the fracture is unstable because of the direction of the fracture line or because of the severity of the periosteal damage; in these circumstances Dunlop traction can be used as the method of immobilisation. An alternative is to immobilise the arm in extension with a plaster cast. This method has the definite advantage that it is much easier to control alignment. Percutaneous Kirschner wires introduced from each side can be used to transfix the fracture and this is also a useful method of immobilisation in difficult cases.

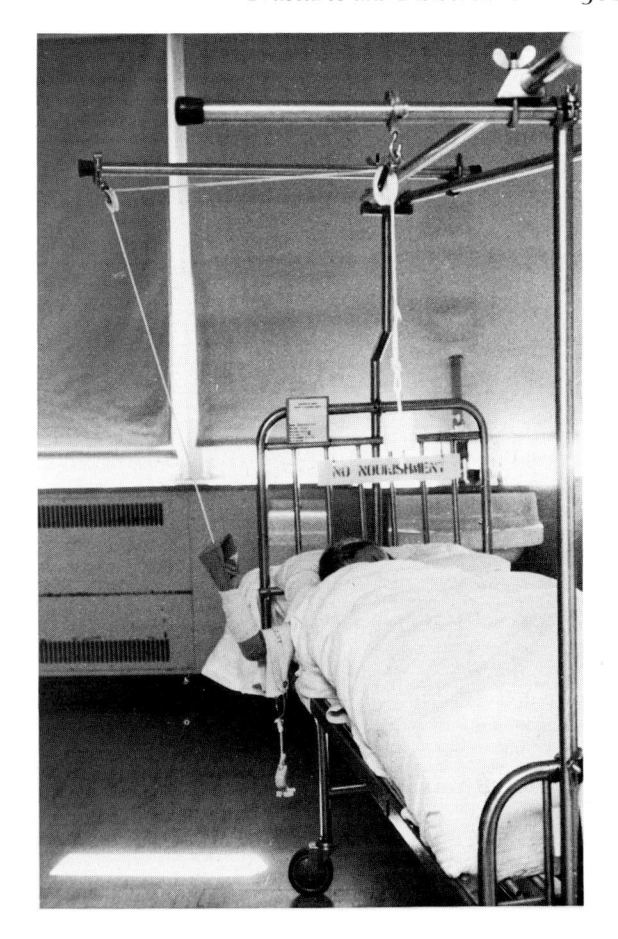

Fig. 6.26 Dunlop skin traction for supracondylar fracture of the humerus. Skin traction was applied with the elbow in 45° of flexion and a counterweight was suspended from a sling located over the proximal fragment. Closed reduction of the fracture was achieved five days later when the swelling had subsided.

OTHER TYPES OF SUPRACONDYLAR FRACTURES

With flexion supracondylar fractures there is anterior displacement of the distal fragment with an anterior periosteal hinge. The fracture is reduced in the reverse manner and the elbow is placed in extension and immobilised in a long arm plaster cast. This is an uncomfortable position for the child and, after a week, the plaster is removed and a further plaster applied with the elbow flexed as much as possible.

MALUNION

In addition to the acute problems of ischaemia and nerve injuries, the other major complication is malunion. The commonest form of malunion produces cubitus varus together with medial rotation and hyperextension of the elbow (Fig. 6.27).

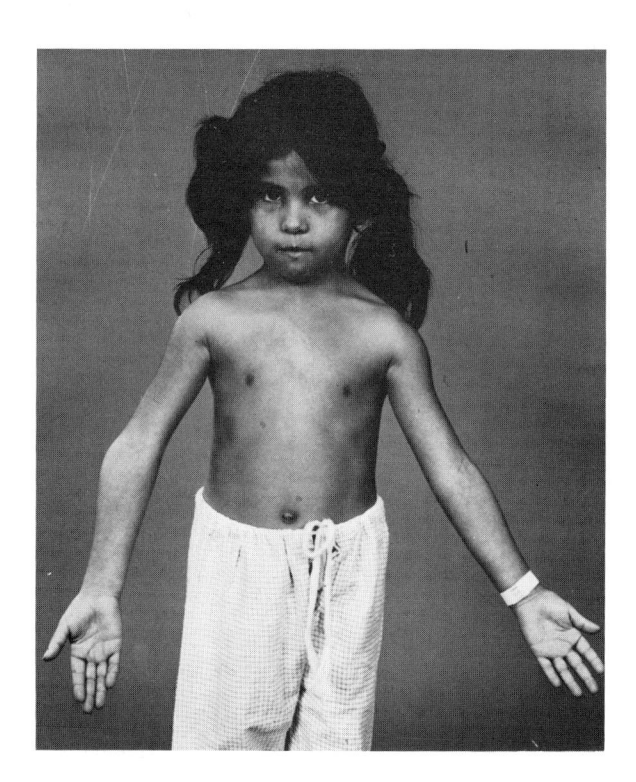

Fig. 6.27 Cubitus varus (gunstock) deformity from a malunited supracondylar fracture of the humerus.

This can largely be avoided by using the techniques and management already described. If manipulative reduction with immobilisation of the elbow in flexion is to be used, satisfactory antero-posterior and lateral x-rays must be obtained to confirm the adequacy of reduction. If problems are encountered, it is preferable to treat the child with skin traction or with the elbow in extension so that the normal carrying angle can be obtained. Ugly cubitus varus deformities (gunstock deformities) frequently require correction by osteotomy.

Fractures of the lateral condyle of the humerus

These are type IV epiphyseal fractures in which the epiphyseal fragment is much larger than would be suspected from the x-ray appearance. On the x-rays the fragment appears only to contain the ossific nucleus of the capitellum and the metaphyseal fragment from the distal humerus (Figs. 6.28 & 6.29). In fact the fragment is largely cartilaginous and contains the capitellum and half of the trochlea (Fig. 6.30). The aim of treatment is to accurately reduce the fracture in order to avoid malunion with a progressive disturbance of growth (Figs. 6.31 & 6.32).

Undisplaced fractures are treated with an above-elbow plaster cast but x-rays must be repeated one week later to confirm that the position has been maintained.

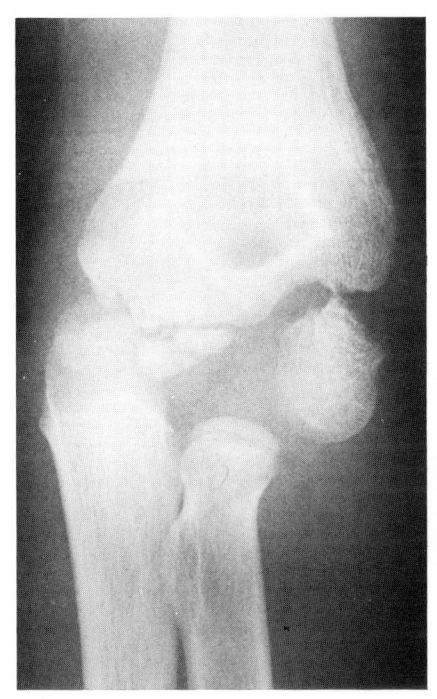

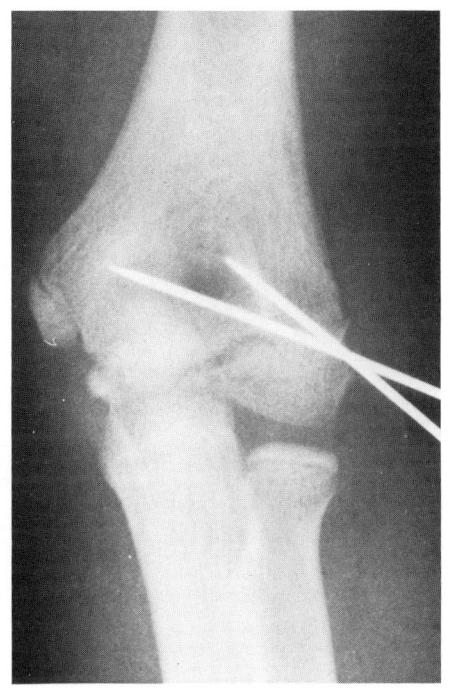

Figs. 6.28 & 6.29 Displaced fracture of the lateral condyle of the humerus which is displaced and rotated from its normal position. (*Right*) An open reduction was carried out. The oblique fracture line indicates that the fragment consisted of the capitellum and the lateral half of the trochlea. The two Kirschner wires were introduced through the metaphyseal fragment and were advanced to engage the opposite cortex.

All other fractures of the lateral condyle require open reduction and internal fixation.

Several points need to be made about the open reduction. The forearm extensors are not dissected from the fragment as the blood supply enters through this attachment. In addition, the fragment should be accurately reduced in order to restore the articular surface to normal as well as align the growth plate and avoid cross-union between the epiphysis and the metaphysis. The reduced fragment is maintained in position with two obliquely placed Kirschner wires which are removed three weeks after the operation (see Figs. 6.28 & 6.29). The elbow is mobilised a week later.

Dislocation of the elbow

Dislocation of the elbow is usually associated with fractures of the medial epicondyle and occasionally with fractures of the lateral condyle, olecranon, or radial neck (Figs. 6.33 & 6.34). Dislocations are reduced by manipulative

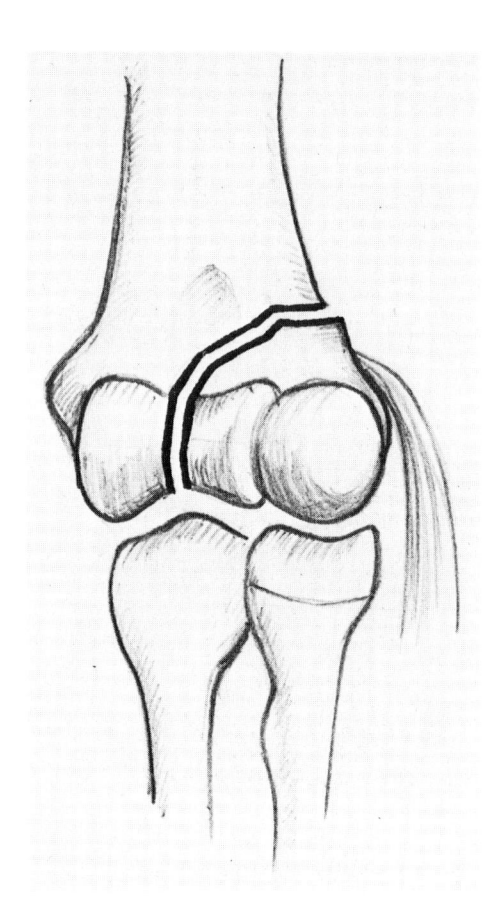

Fig. 6.30 Fracture of the lateral condyle of the distal humerus. The fragment consists of the lateral half of the condyle including the capitellum and the lateral half of the trochlea.

reduction under general anaesthesia and care should be taken to prevent bony fragments, such as the medial epicondyle, from remaining within the joint (Figs. 6.35 & 6.36). If fragments are trapped these are removed at operation.

Fractures of the medial epicondyle of the humerus

These fractures result from a valgus strain to the elbow and are often associated with a dislocation of the elbow and fracture of the neck of the radius. In the young child it is possible to confuse this injury with a fracture of the medial condyle which, like the lateral condyle fracture of the humerus, involves a large portion of the epiphysis.

Undisplaced or minimally displaced fractures of the medial epicondyle are treated by immobilising the arm in an above-elbow cast for 2–3 weeks. Severely displaced fractures of the medial epicondyle can usually be treated in this way although occasionally open reduction and pin fixation is required. If the fractured medial epicondyle is trapped within a joint, it will usually require open reduction

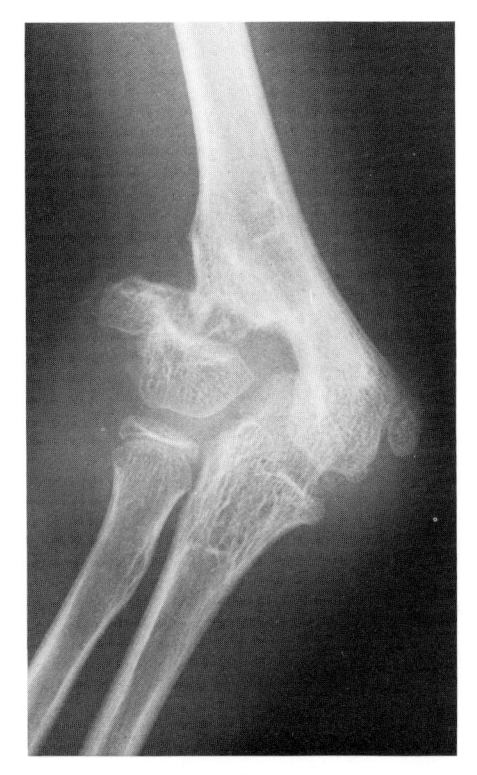

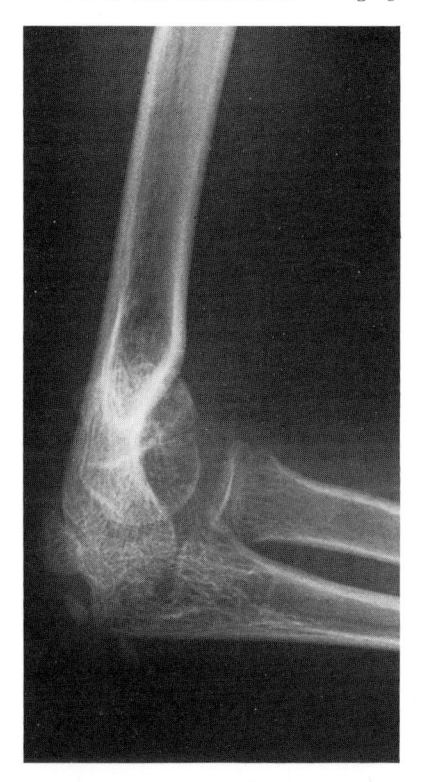

Figs. 6.31 & 6.32 Malunited fracture of the lateral condyle of the humerus. The A–P view shows the malunited untreated fracture with growth arrest and progressive valgus. The lateral view shows the more proximal location of the capitellum. The deformity was treated with a varus closing wedge osteotomy of the distal humerus.

as attempts at manipulative reduction by applying a valgus strain to the elbow with the forearm in supination are usually ineffective. Whatever method of treatment is used, the parents are warned that full extension of the elbow will not be regained for several months.

If there is an ulnar palsy then the ulnar nerve should be moved forwards and the epicondyle reduced and held with a Kirschner wire.

Fractures of the lateral epicondyle of the humerus

This is a very rare fracture and it is common for it to be confused with the more important fracture of the lateral condyle already described.

Fractures of the proximal radius

Valgus injuries of the elbow which fracture the head of the radius in adults

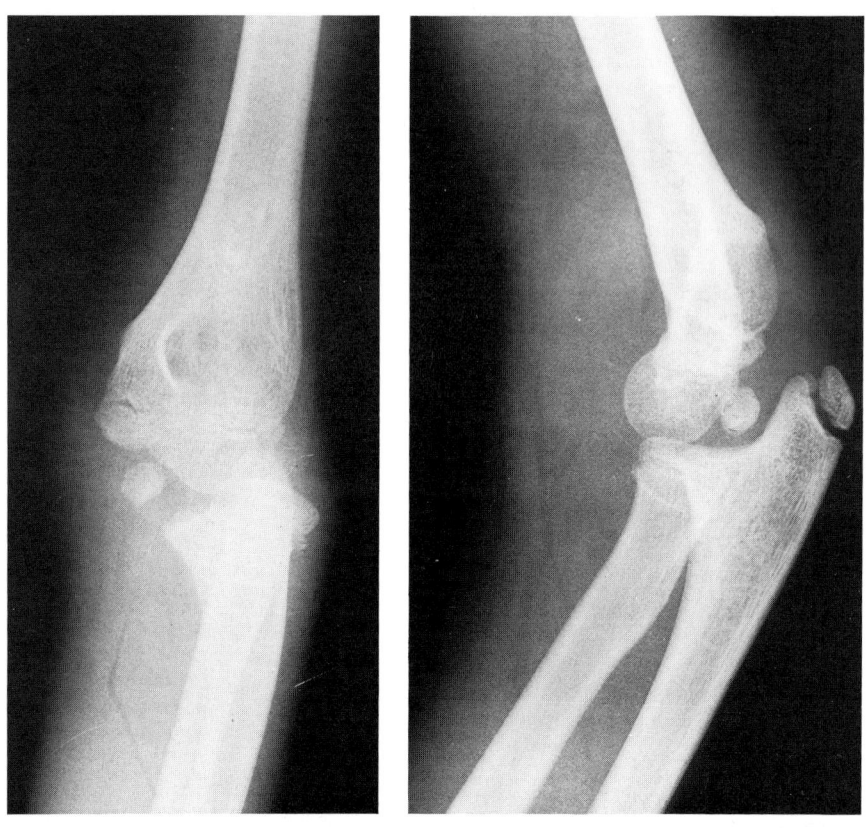

Figs. 6.33 & 6.34 Postero-lateral dislocation of the elbow with an avulsion displaced fracture of the medial epicondyle and a fracture of the neck of the radius. The lateral view shows that the displaced medial epicondyle remains attached to the ulna by the medial collateral ligament.

produce fractures of the neck of the radius and fracture separations of the proximal radial growth plate in children.

In most instances the head of the radius is angulated less than 20°. As re-modelling will correct this degree of angulation, reduction is unnecessary and an above-elbow plaster cast is applied for three weeks.

When the radial head is angulated more than 20°, an attempt is made to improve the position by manipulative reduction under general anaesthesia (Fig. 6.37). A varus force is applied to the elbow while the forearm is pronated and supinated but direct pressure is not applied over the radial head. The position is accepted if less than 20° of angulation remains but greater degrees of angulation require open reduction. There are several points about this procedure. In order to avoid dividing the posterior interosseus nerve, the lateral incision is not extended distal to the neck of the radius. In addition, the intact flap of periosteum and

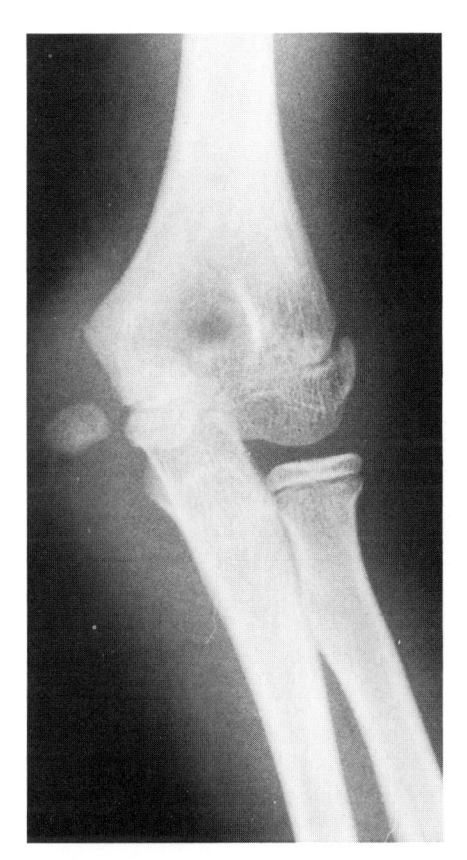

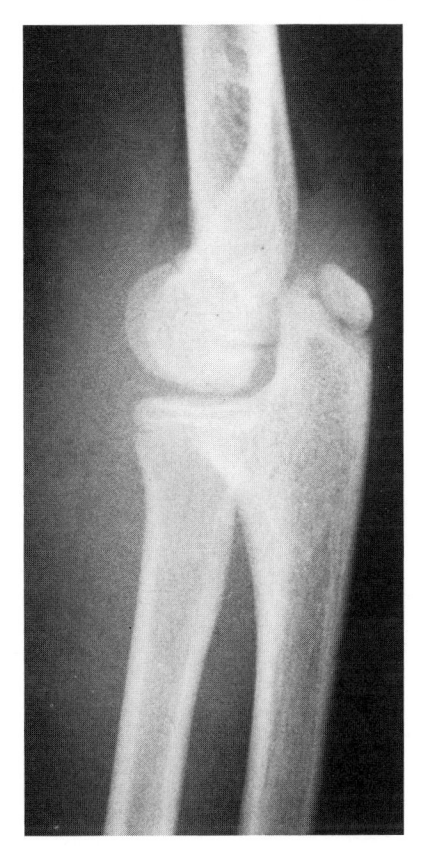

Figs. 6.35 & 6.36 Same patient as Fig. 6.33. A stable reduction was achieved by close manipulation under general anaesthesia. The position of the rotated medial epicondyle was accepted. The lateral view confirms the adequacy of reduction and the absence of any intra-articular fragments. The elbow was immobilised at a right-angle in a plaster cast for four weeks.

synovium, which contains the blood vessels to the head of the radius should be protected. The fracture is reduced by drawing the medially displaced radial shaft outwards rather than by pushing the angulated radial head inwards onto the shaft. The displaced shaft of the radius is drawn laterally with the aid of two small bone levers or a towel clip. The reduction may be stable but internal fixation is frequently required. Fixation may be simply achieved by passing a fine Kirschner wire through the margin of the proximal fragment into the shaft of the radius. The wire is removed after three weeks and the elbow mobilised.

It is preferable not to pass the wire through the capitellum and across the elbow joint into the radius as the wire may fracture at the joint line. The head of the radius is never excised in the growing child as severe progressive valgus deformity will result. If the head of the radius is inadvertently detached during the

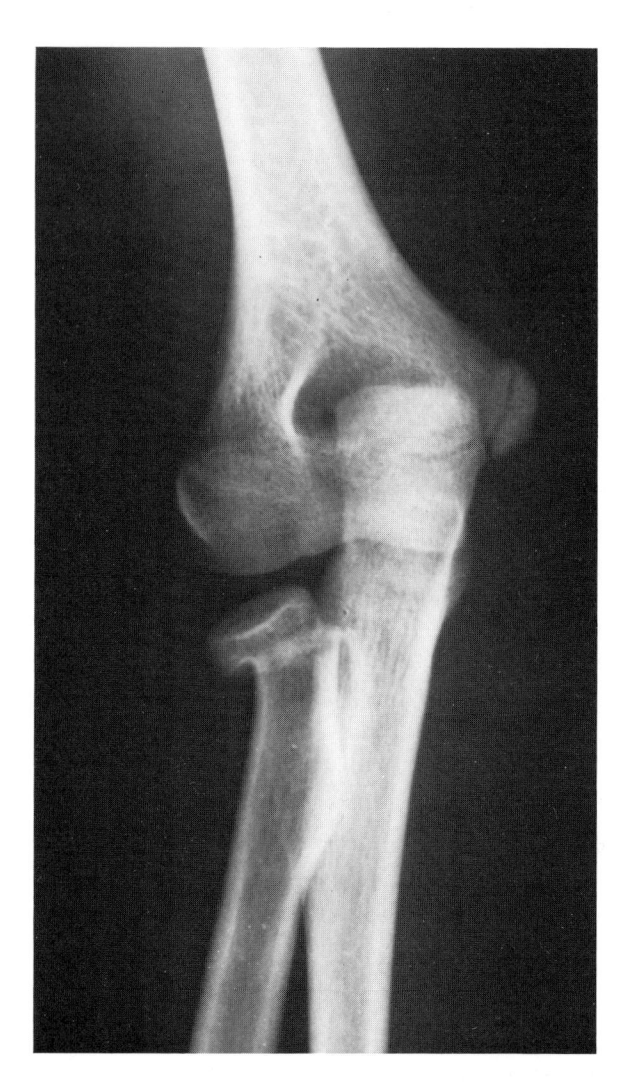

Fig. 6.37 40° angulated fracture of the neck of the radius. The head of the radius is in contact with the capitellum but the shaft is displaced medially. Closed reduction is achieved by pronating and supinating the forearm.

operation, it should be replaced into position and held with an obliquely placed Kirschner wire.

Fractures of the olecranon

Olecranon fractures may occur alone or in combination with either fractures of the neck of the radius or dislocations of the elbow. Adequate reduction is usually achieved by extension of the elbow. A plaster cast is used to maintain this position but, as it is uncomfortable, the elbow is placed in moderate flexion after two weeks. If an adequate reduction cannot be achieved by this method, intramedullary fixation is required.

Dislocation of the radial head

This is rarely an isolated injury in childhood. It is usually seen in association with fractures of the ulna constituting the Monteggia fracture dislocation which will be discussed in more detail below.

FOREARM

Fractures of the shafts of the radius and ulna

In young children greenstick fractures of the shafts of the radius and ulna are common. An above-elbow plaster cast is applied for undisplaced fractures, a check x-ray is taken one week later, and the plaster is removed 3–4 weeks after the injury. When a fracture is angulated to an unacceptable degree, manipulative reduction is required. It is important that the hinge of bone is fractured in order to prevent recurrence of the deformity.

Fractures of the radius and ulna are frequently complete and displaced. Manipulative reduction can usually be readily achieved. On occasions it is difficult to obtain an end-to-end reduction and, in these circumstances, an appositional form of reduction can be accepted, as long as the alignment is otherwise correct. Open reduction is rarely, if ever, required

Monteggia fracture dislocation

Whenever an apparently isolated fracture of the shaft of the ulna is present, one should search for an associated fracture or dislocation of the radius. It is frequent for dislocations of the head of the radius to be overlooked—an error which can be avoided if antero-posterior and lateral x-rays always include the elbow joint. The long axis of the shaft of the radius normally passes through the centre of the capitellum in all views (Figs. 6.38 & 6.39). The ulna may be angulated anteriorly, posteriorly or laterally and the direction of displacement of the head of the radius corresponds with the direction of ulnar angulation.

Reduction of an anterior Monteggia fracture dislocation is achieved by applying traction with the elbow extended and forearm supinated. As reduction of the ulna is achieved, the head of the radius can be pushed back into position and the reduction is maintained by flexion of the elbow. The elbow is immobilised in a plaster cast with the elbow flexed and the forearm supinated. For a posterior Monteggia fracture dislocation, the fracture is reduced with the elbow in extension, the head of the radius is pushed forwards and the elbow is immobilised in extension.

Children with unreduced anterior Monteggia fracture dislocations frequently have good function, although flexion is usually restricted by impingement of the dislocated head of radius onto the humeral shaft. If it is a longstanding dislocation

310   Chapter 6

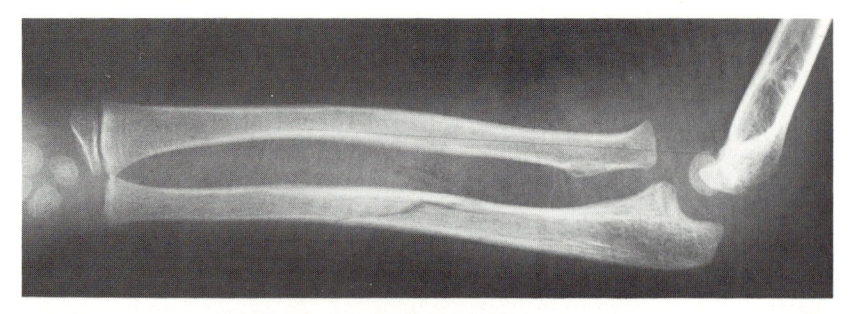

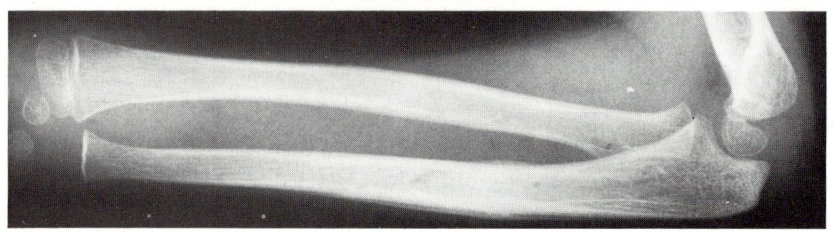

Figs. 6.38 & 6.39   Anterior Monteggia fracture dislocation. (*Top*) A lateral view of the forearm and elbow showing an anterior dislocation of the head of the radius and a fracture of the shaft of the ulna. Closed reduction was achieved by traction with the forearm in supination and the reduction of the head of the radius was maintained with a plaster cylinder with the elbow flexed to a right-angle. (*Bottom*) Six weeks later the fracture of the ulna is seen to be healed and the head of the radius is reduced.

and the elbow is stable it is often preferable to leave the head of the radius in a dislocated position. However, with elbow instability and progressive valgus deformity an open reduction is required (Figs. 6.40 & 6.41). To obtain a stable reduction it is usually necessary to divide the ulna, totally excise the old annular ligament located within the joint and to create a new annular ligament using the triceps.

Galeazzi fracture dislocation

This injury consists of a fracture of the shaft of the radius and dislocation of the inferior radio-ulnar joint. It is less common than the Monteggia fracture dislocation. Although this injury in the adult is best treated by open reduction, closed reduction is always indicated in childhood.

Metaphyseal fractures of the distal radius and ulna

Buckle fractures are common at this level and are frequently misdiagnosed as sprains. An above-elbow plaster is only required for 2–3 weeks.

   Displaced fractures of the distal radius and ulna are also common. Reduction is achieved by increasing the deformity which, by relaxing the intact periosteum,

Fractures and Dislocations 311

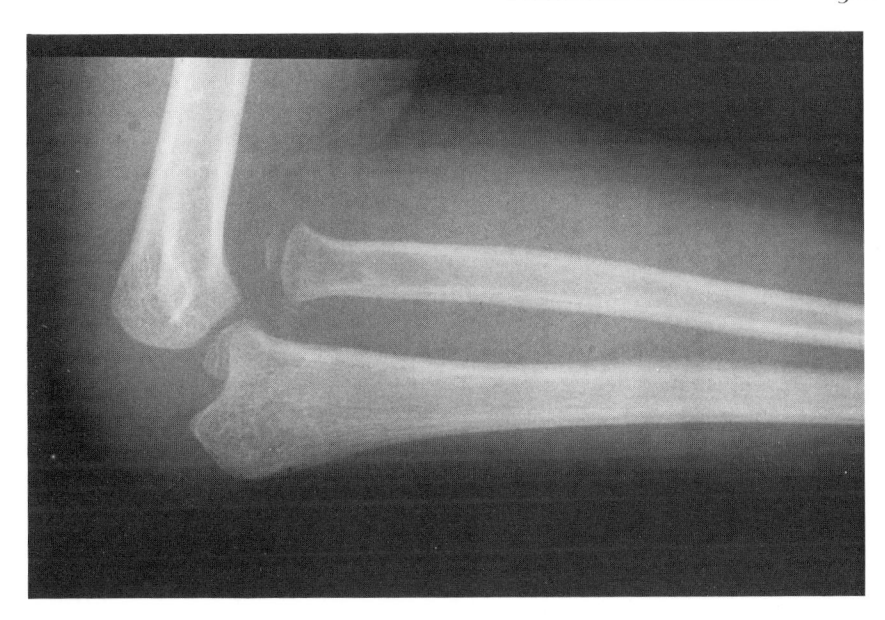

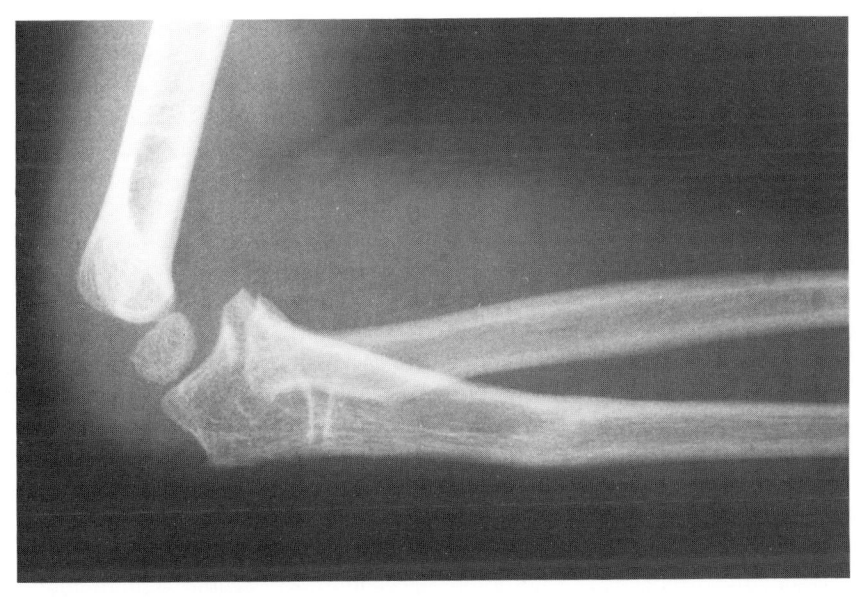

Figs. 6.40 & 6.41 Untreated anterior Monteggia fracture dislocation. (*Top*) The head of the radius is dislocated anteriorly and there is an anterior bow of the shaft of the ulna. (*Bottom*) This two-year-old untreated fracture dislocation was treated by open reduction of the head of the radius and osteotomy of the ulna. An annular ligament was constructed from the triceps tendon.

allows the fragment to be reduced. On occasions, because of severe swelling, an end-to-end reduction cannot be achieved, in which case bayonet apposition is acceptable as long as the alignment in the other planes is satisfactory. This can be easily achieved with the forearm and hand in a neutral position and extreme positions are never required. In the young child the shape of the distal radius and ulna will remodel rapidly producing a forearm of normal appearance and normal function.

Growth plate injuries of the distal radius and ulna

Type II fractures of the distal growth plate of the radius are common and there is often a chip of bone fractured from the ulnar styloid process. Displaced fractures require reduction and this is readily achieved under general anaesthesia. A well moulded above-elbow plaster cast with the wrist held in the neutral position is applied. If the child presents late with an irreducible injury this should be accepted as growth will almost certainly produce a normal appearance.

Type IV fractures of the distal radius are rare. Accurate reduction is required (Figs. 6.42–6.44).

WRIST

Fractures involving the carpal bones are uncommon. Undisplaced fractures of the waist or tubercle of the scaphoid are occasionally seen and are treated in a forearm plaster cast which includes the proximal phalanx of the thumb. Rapid union can be expected.

HAND

Fractures of the metacarpals

The commonest metacarpal fractures are those of the base of the first metacarpal and the neck of the fifth metacarpal. Both injuries are usually the result of fighting.

Fractures of the base of the first metacarpal extend either through the metaphysis or through the epiphyseal plate. Many of the metaphyseal fractures are of the buckle type. The fracture is often angulated but up to 30° of flexion is acceptable as re-modelling can be expected to correct it. The thumb is immobilised in a scaphoid-type cast. Angulation exceeding 30° requires manipulative correction under anaesthesia followed by the application of a similar cast.

Type II growth plate injuries are common and, when undisplaced, are treated in a scaphoid cast. Displaced fractures are treated by manipulative reduction but occasionally the reduction is unstable and percutaneous Kirschner wires are

Fractures and Dislocations 313

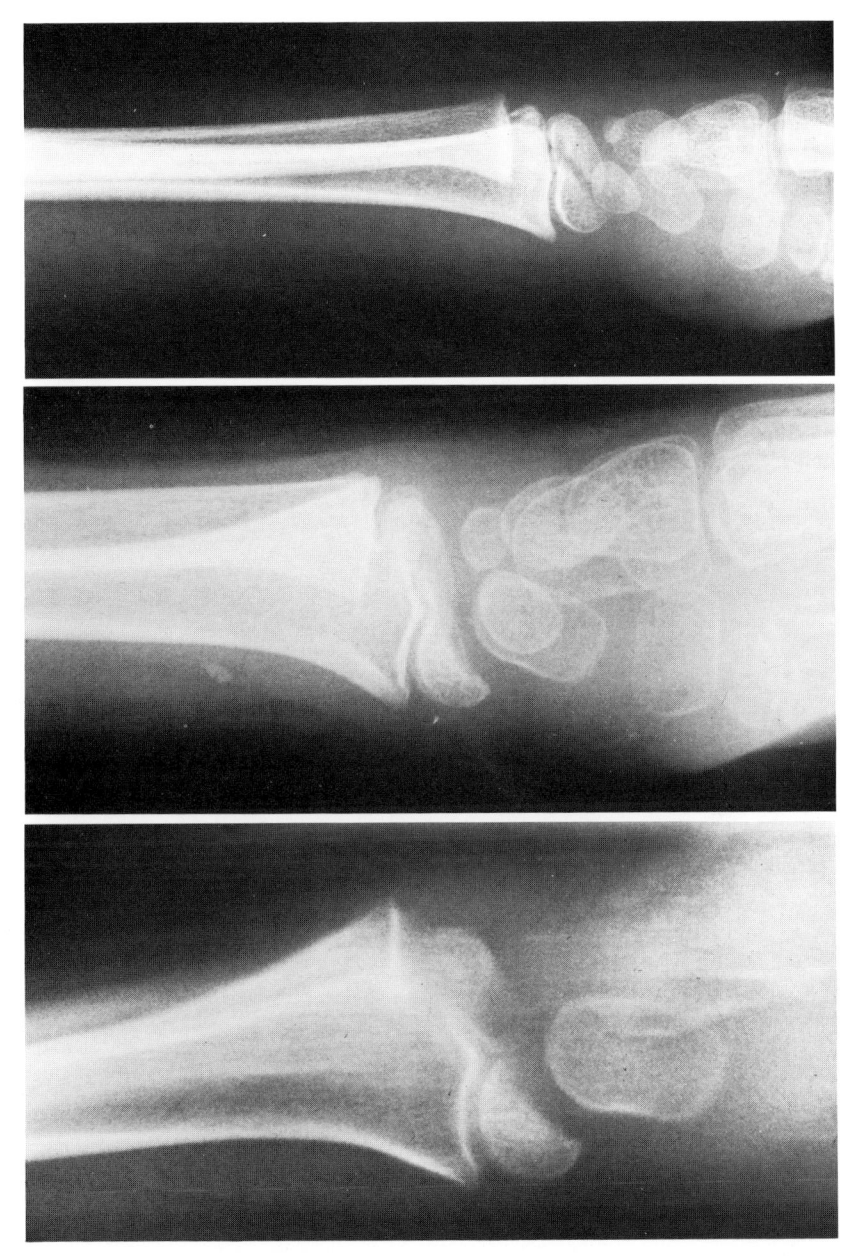

Figs. 6.42–6.44 Type IV fracture of the distal radial epiphysis. (*Top*) An oblique fracture of the epiphysis of the radius, extending across the growth plate into the metaphysis producing a small metaphyseal fragment. The fracture was treated by closed reduction and plaster immobilisation. (*Middle*) An x-ray of the same area three months later. There is premature fusion of the posterior growth plate of the radius. (*Bottom*) The growth plate fusion is shown in more detail in this tomogram.

required to hold it. In adolescence, type III growth plate injuries, equivalent to the adult Bennett's fracture dislocation, are also seen. This involves the medial part of the growth plate which is the last area of this plate to close.

Impacted fractures of the neck of the fifth metacarpal are also common. Mild or moderately displaced fractures are supported in a volar plaster slab. The hand is mobilised three weeks later and re-modelling of the bone will correct the depressed metacarpal head. Manipulative reduction may be required for severely angulated or displaced fractures but the little finger should not be placed in a position of forced flexion in order to maintain the reduction.

Dislocation of the metacarpophalangeal joint of the thumb

This is a common dislocation which can usually be reduced by manipulation under anaesthesia (Fig. 6.45). A scaphoid type of plaster cast with the thumb

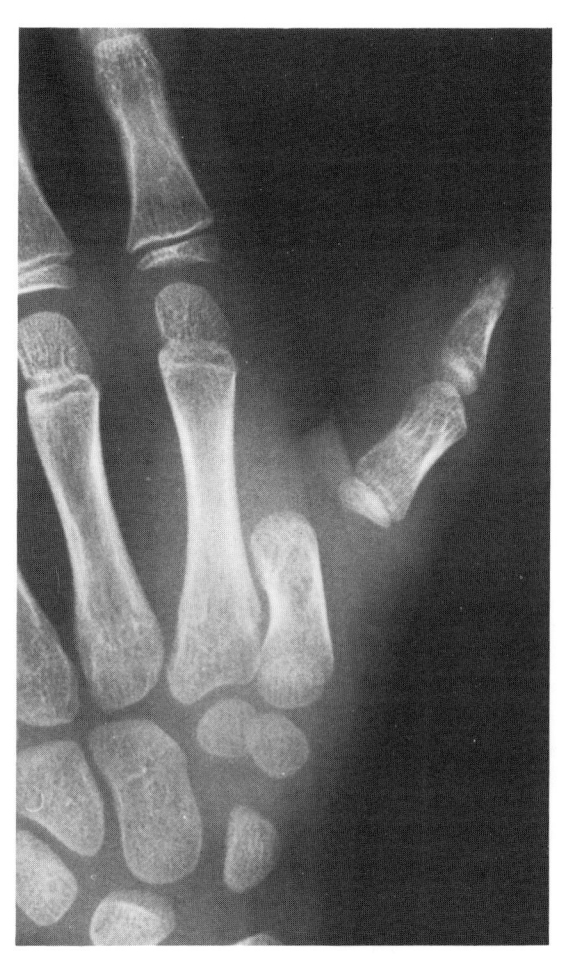

Fig. 6.45 Dislocated metacarpophalangeal joint of the thumb.

flexed is applied for three weeks. Occasionally closed reduction cannot be achieved and, at operation, the metacarpal head may be found to be trapped by the flexor tendons or palmar fascia or the volar plate may be lodged between the metacarpal head and the proximal phalanx.

Phalangeal fractures

Type II growth plate injuries of the base of the proximal phalanx are common. When there is minimal displacement the finger is strapped to the adjacent normal finger; closed reduction is used when the displacement is more severe. These fractures are carefully aligned and angulatory or rotary malunion are avoided if the hand is immobilised in a functional position so that the position of the fingernail can be seen to be in the correct plane. Fractures of the shaft of the phalanx are treated in the same way and similar attention to alignment and rotation is required. Percutaneous Kirschner wire fixation is useful for unstable fractures in which there is risk of malunion.

A mallet finger deformity usually results from a type I fracture separation of the distal phalanx. The angulation is corrected and the distal interphalangeal joint is held in extension with a volar splint for three weeks. This is usually sufficient to prevent recurrence of the mallet deformity. In the adolescent, a type III fracture separation is more common and open reduction of the fragment is usually required.

Condylar fractures are less common but are frequently overlooked and may lead to malunion with angulation and stiffness. Displaced fractures require open reduction to restore the joint surface.

PELVIS

Fractures of the pelvis are usually the result of motor vehicle accidents. The immediate concern is whether there are visceral, vascular, or neurological injuries. Bladder and urethral injuries are more commonly associated with fractures about the pubic symphysis. Urethrograms, cystograms and intravenous pyelograms are required whenever a urological injury is suspected. Haemorrhage from the pelvis may be severe but it usually stops spontaneously.

Careful neurological examination is required as the lumbosacral plexus may be damaged whenever there is disruption of the posterior part of the pelvic ring. Traction on the lumbosacral plexus may also lead to rupture of the cauda equina. Exploration of the sacral plexus does not improve the likelihood of recovery.

There are several patterns of pelvic fractures in children and these are detailed below.

Single fractures of the ring

These fractures usually involve the pubic rami. They are usually undisplaced or

316   Chapter 6

minimally displaced and do not require reduction. The child is rested in bed until comfortable.

Double fractures of the ring

These fractures may involve the pubic rami on both sides of the pubic symphysis but disruption of the pubic symphysis is rare. Careful assessment for urological damage is always required. Reduction of these fractures is rarely required and the child is rested in bed until comfortable.

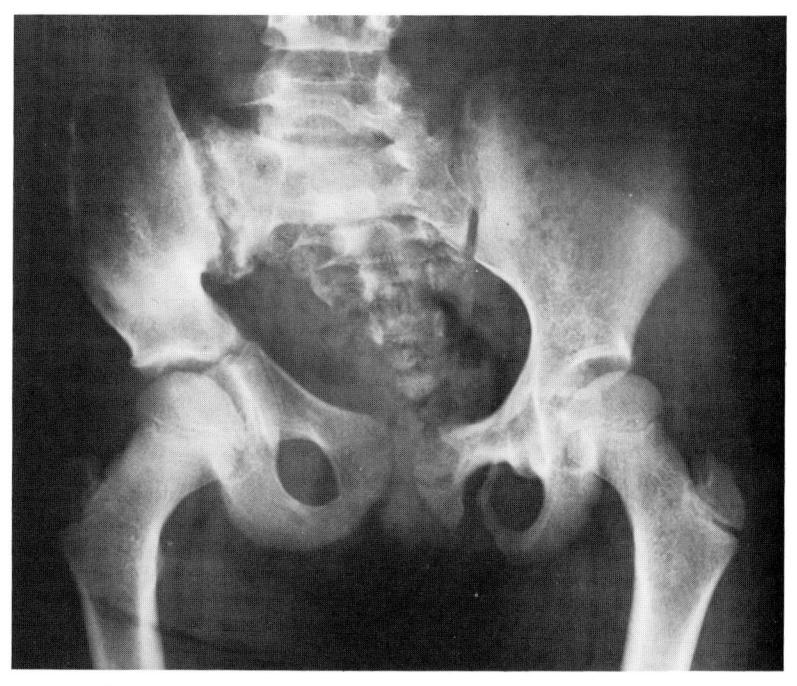

Fig. 6.46 Malunion of pelvic fracture. This distorted pelvis with a scoliosis has resulted from a crushing injury of the pelvis with fractures of the right ilium adjacent to the sacro-iliac joint, the left pubis and ischio-pubic ramus.

Severe displacement of the hemipelvis may occur when fractures of the pubic rami are associated with fractures of the posterior ilium or, less frequently, with disruptions of the sacro-iliac joint (Fig. 6.46). Marked upward displacement of the hemipelvis results in pelvic obliquity and marked inward or outward rotation of the hemipelvis produces a clinical abnormality in the shape of the pelvis and alters the position of the hip joint. In these circumstances, an attempt is made to improve the position of the hemipelvis by manipulative reduction and traction.

Fractures of the acetabulum

These fractures are uncommon and rarely displaced to a degree requiring reduction. Hamilton Russell skin traction is used while the hip is painful and the child is then mobilised on crutches. Avascular necrosis of the femoral head or chondrolysis may occasionally occur.

Fractures outside the pelvic ring

Direct trauma to the pelvis may fracture the wing of the ilium but the child need only be rested in bed until comfortable.

Adolescents taking part in vigorous sporting activity may avulse the apophyses associated with the pelvis. Such injuries include avulsion of the ischial tuberosity by the hamstrings, the anterior inferior iliac spine by the rectus femoris, and the anterior superior iliac spine by sartorius. Reduction is rarely required and crutches are used until the pain has subsided. Persistent discomfort may require open reduction of the fragment.

HIP

Dislocation of the hip

The hip joint of children under the age of 5 years may dislocate with relatively minor trauma. However, in the older child and adolescent, more severe trauma is required and this frequently consists of a severe blow to the front of the knee with the hip flexed.

The head of the femur usually dislocates posteriorly and the leg is flexed, adducted and internally rotated (Figs. 6.47 & 6.48). Fractures of the acetabulum or the femoral neck and sciatic nerve injury may be associated with dislocations in the older child. Closed reduction is readily achieved under general anaesthesia with muscle relaxation. For a posterior dislocation the hip and knee are flexed to 90° and traction is applied with the leg in external rotation. An anterior dislocation is reduced by applying traction with the leg in extension, abduction and internal rotation. Following reduction the hip should move freely and be shown by x-rays to be concentrically reduced.

An open reduction is required whenever a concentric closed reduction is not achieved. On occasions, the head of the femur will be found to be protruding into the buttock through a hole in the posterior capsule of the hip joint. This buttonhole lesion prevents the head from re-entering the joint. A concentric reduction may also be prevented by fragments of cartilage or bone within the joint cavity. These fragments are removed immediately. After achieving a concentric reduction the hip is immobilised in a spica for four weeks. Hip motion usually returns rapidly and full weight-bearing is allowed.

318   Chapter 6

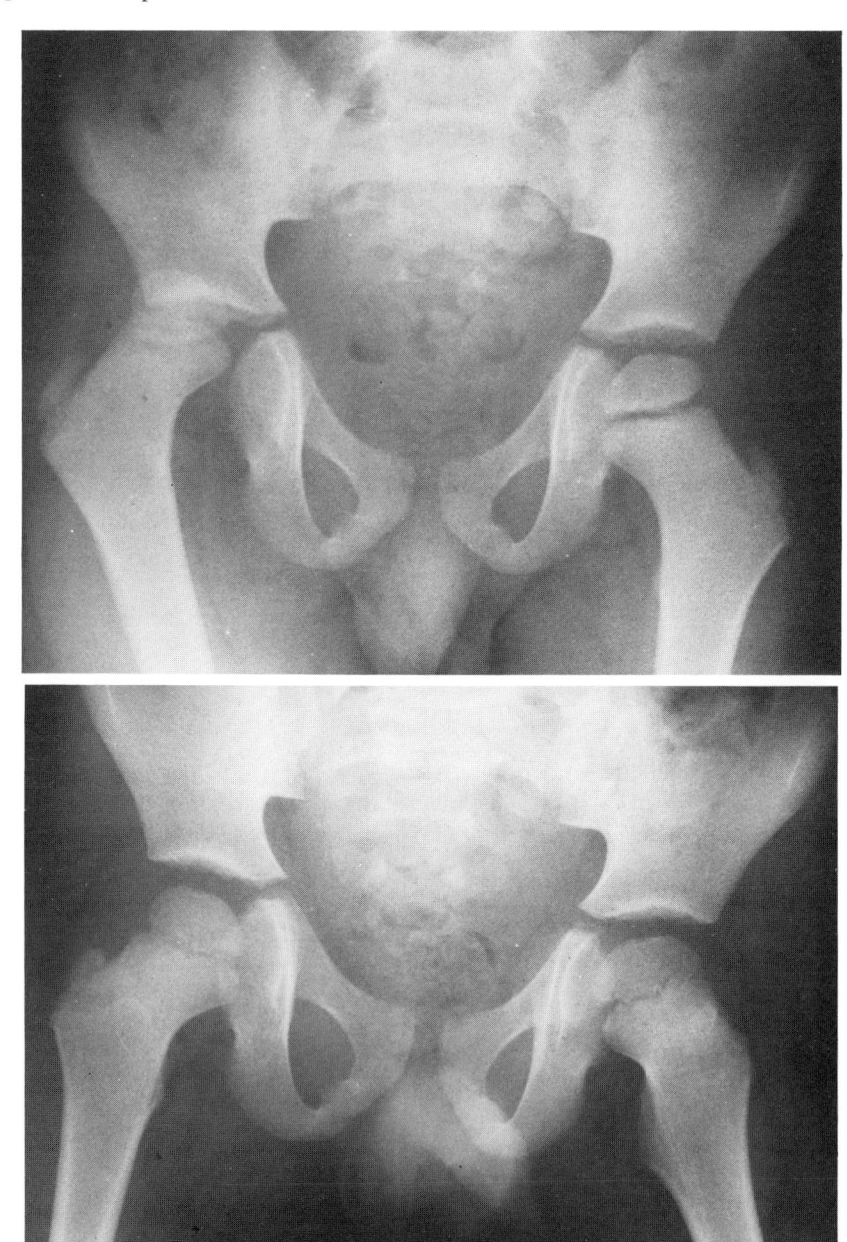

Figs. 6.47 & 6.48   Posterior dislocation of the hip in a 5-year-old child following a fall. This was treated by closed reduction. The lower illustration shows the situation following closed reduction. The apparent increase in distance between the femoral head and the tear drop was due to the poorly centred x-ray and not to fragments within the joint.

Avascular necrosis is a major complication and occurs in approximately 10% of children. Reduction of the dislocation within twelve hours reduces the incidence of avascular necrosis. Radiological evidence of avascular necrosis may be delayed for up to a year but radio-isotope scanning may show at an earlier stage that the head is avascular.

FEMUR

Fractures of the neck of the femur

These fractures are rare in children and usually only occur with severe trauma. The fractures are classified into four groups depending on their location (Fig. 6.49). This classification is useful when planning treatment and is also helpful in predicting the likelihood of complications. These occur in the majority of children with proximal fractures and in fewer children with distal fractures.

TYPE I (TRANS-EPIPHYSEAL FRACTURES)

The fracture cleaves the growth plate transversely in the same manner as type I

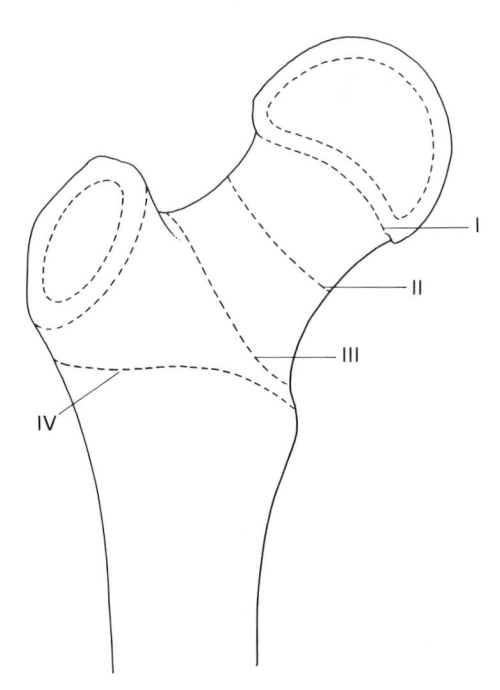

Fig. 6.49 Fractures of the neck of the femur. Undisplaced fractures at all levels have a good prognosis. Displaced type I fractures have a poor prognosis but the prognosis improves as the site of the fracture moves down the neck to the type IV location.

320 Chapter 6

growth plate injuries (Figs. 6.50–6.52). In young children, severe injury is required to produce this fracture while relatively minor injuries may produce an acute slip of this growth plate in adolescents.

For undisplaced fractures a hip spica or traction is used to maintain the position. Frequent x-rays are required to ensure that the position is maintained. For displaced fractures, closed reduction is usually readily achieved and the position is maintained in a hip spica with the leg in abduction and internal rotation. Serial x-rays are also required to ensure that the position is maintained. Fixation of the fracture with Knowles' pins is not required and pinning may increase the likelihood of premature fusion of the growth plate. Occasionally in

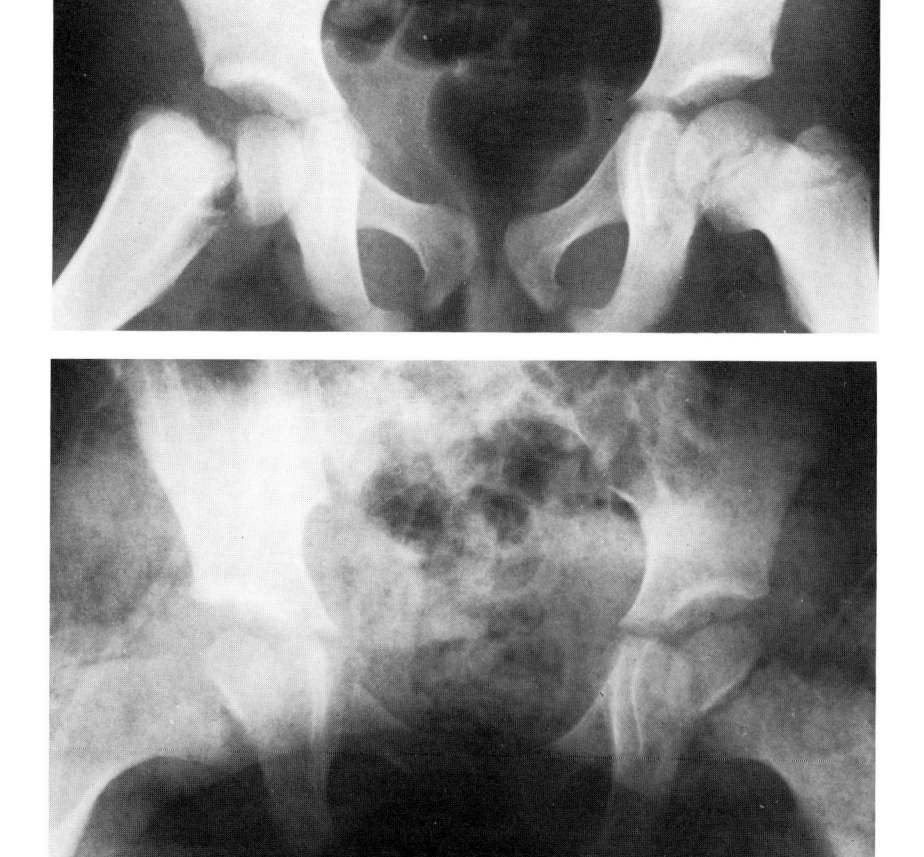

Figs. 6.50–6.51 Type I fracture of the neck of the femur. (*Bottom*) Reduction folllowing gentle closed manipulation. Position maintained with hip spica.

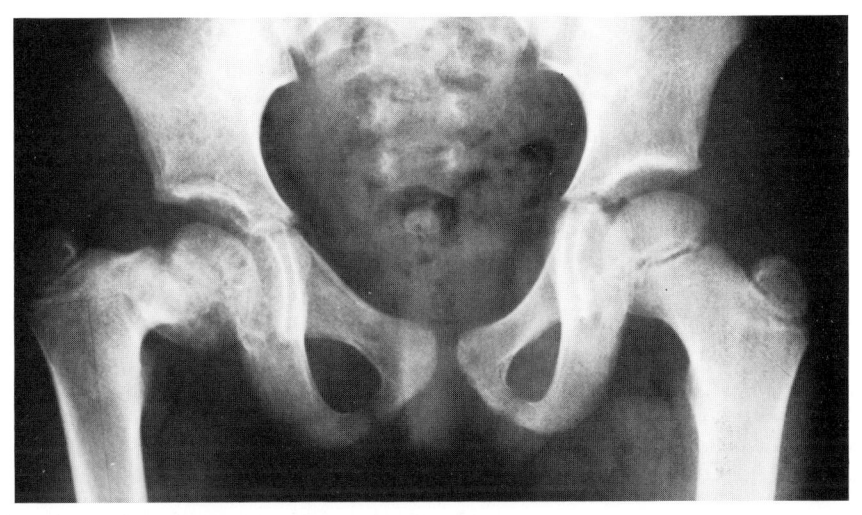

Figs. 6.52 Same patient as Fig. 6.50. X-ray taken two years later. Note the premature arrest of the proximal growth plate with a narrow neck and coxa vara as well as avascular necrosis of the epiphysis.

young children the head of the femur will also be dislocated in which case an open reduction is required.

The majority of the younger children will develop avascular necrosis of the femoral head, premature arrest of the growth plate and occasionally, non-union. These complications account for the poor long term results.

TYPE II (TRANS-CERVICAL FRACTURES)

Undisplaced fractures in young children can be treated in a hip spica, but in older children it is preferable to stabilise the reduction with Knowles' pins in order to reduce the chances of later displacement. Displaced type II fractures can usually be reduced by closed reduction but, if this is unsuccessful, an open reduction can be performed through an antero-lateral approach (Figs. 6.53–6.57). Several Knowles' pins are inserted parallel to each other so that the fracture is not distracted and the pins are not placed across the growth plate. However, in a high trans-cervical fracture it may be necessary to insert the screws across the plate. They are removed as soon as the fracture is united in order to reduce the likelihood of premature arrest. It should be noted that trifin nails, which are commonly used in the management of fractured necks of the femur in adults, are inappropriate in children. It is difficult to drive large nails into the hard bone of the neck of the femur and the fracture is usually distracted and displaced in the process.

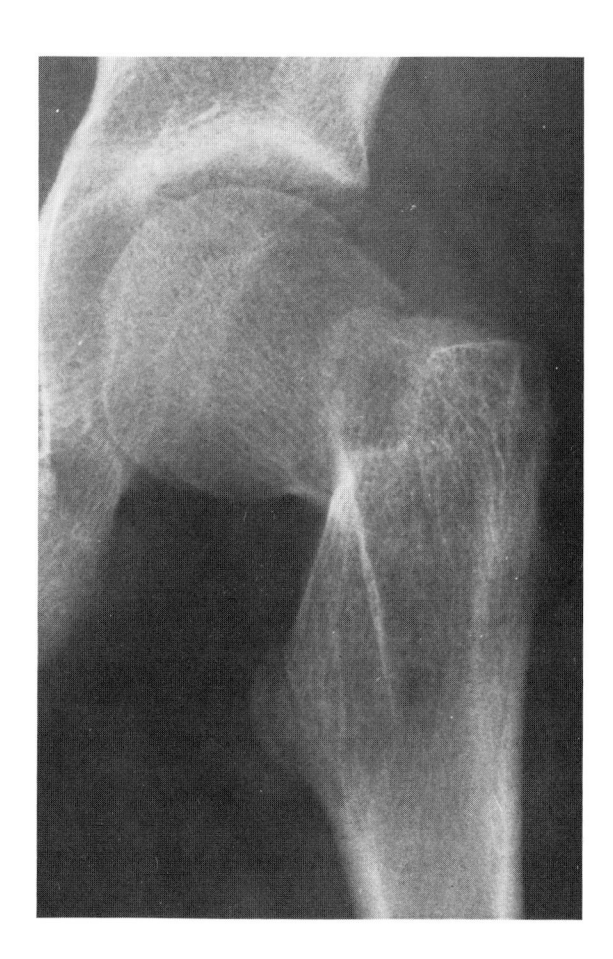

Fig. 6.53 A–P x-ray of the displaced trans-cervical (type II) fracture of the neck of the femur in a 12-year-old girl following a bicycle accident.

Undisplaced type II fractures have a low complication rate but approximately two-thirds of displaced fractures will develop avascular necrosis, coxa vara, premature closure of the growth plate and, occasionally, non-union. The avascular necrosis may occur in the neck as well as in the head of the femur.

TYPE III (CERVICO-TROCHANTERIC FRACTURES)

Undisplaced type III fractures are treated in a spica and serial x-rays are taken to check the position. Displaced type III fractures are treated by closed reduction and Knowles pinning; occasionally an open reduction will also be required (Figs. 6.58–6.60).

Undisplaced type III fractures have a good prognosis. However with displaced fractures 60% develop premature growth arrest, 30% develop avascular necrosis but coxa vara and non-union are less common.

Fractures and Dislocations 323

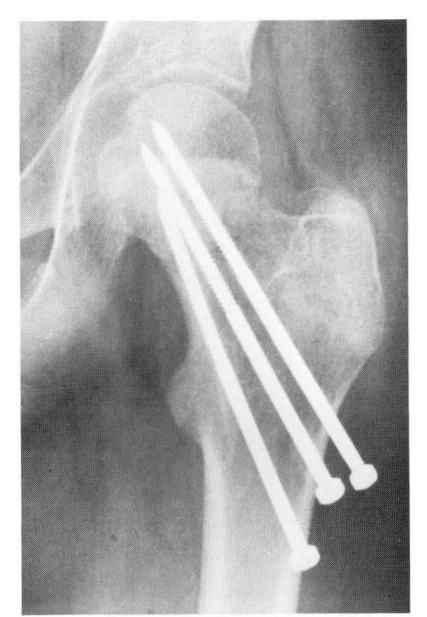

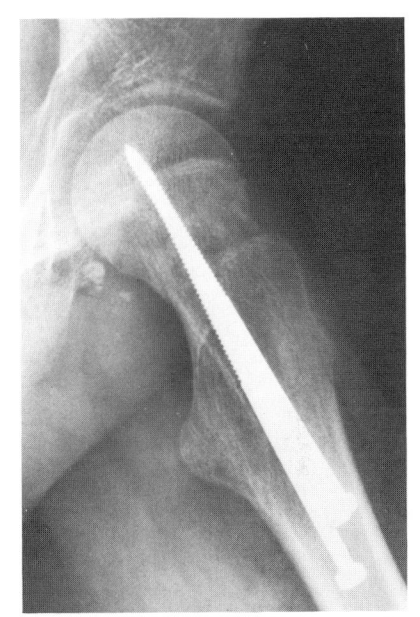

Figs. 6.54 & 6.55 Same patient as Fig. 6.53. A gentle closed reduction was carried out under general anaesthesia and three Knowles' pins were used to hold the reduction. The pins were removed five months later. Lateral view following the introduction of the Knowles' pins.

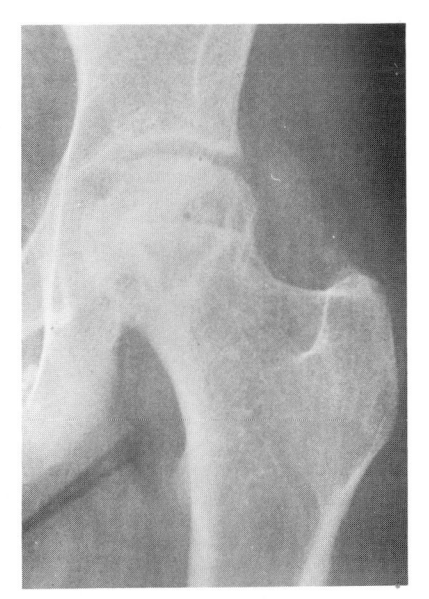

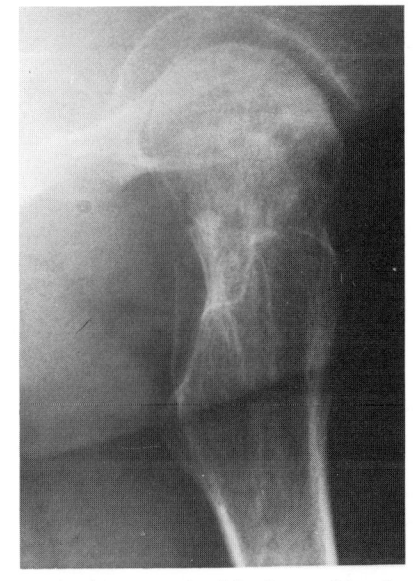

Figs. 6.56 & 6.57 Same patient as Fig. 6.53. Avascular necrosis of the femoral head and neck eleven months following the injury. Lateral view showing the features of avascular necrosis.

324   Chapter 6

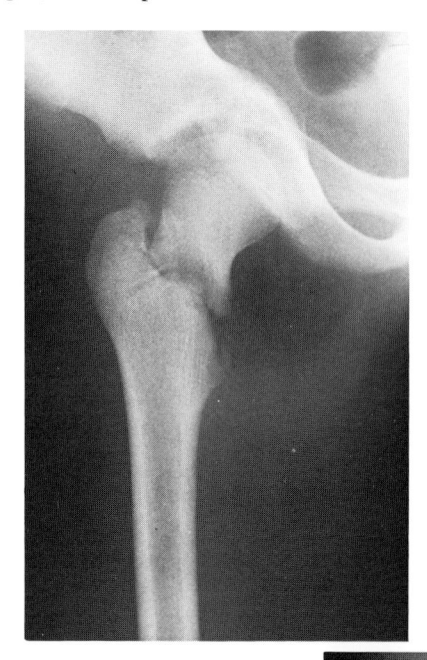

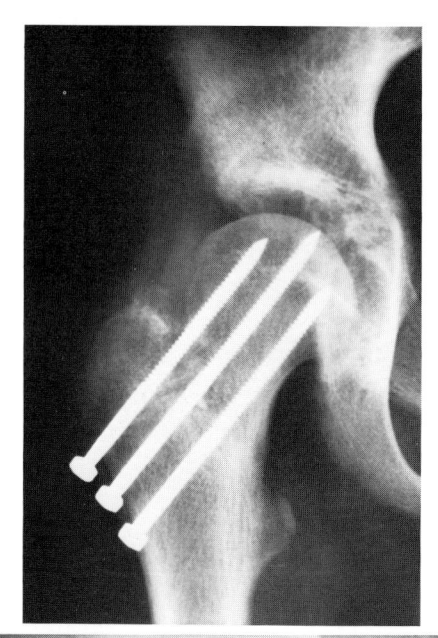

Figs. 6.58–6.60
Displaced type III fracture of the neck of the femur in a 10-year-old child following a car accident. (*Top right*) Closed reduction was incomplete. An open reduction with Knowles' pins fixation was achieved through a lateral approach. The pins were removed five months later. (*Right*) X-rays taken two years later show that hip anatomy and growth were normal.

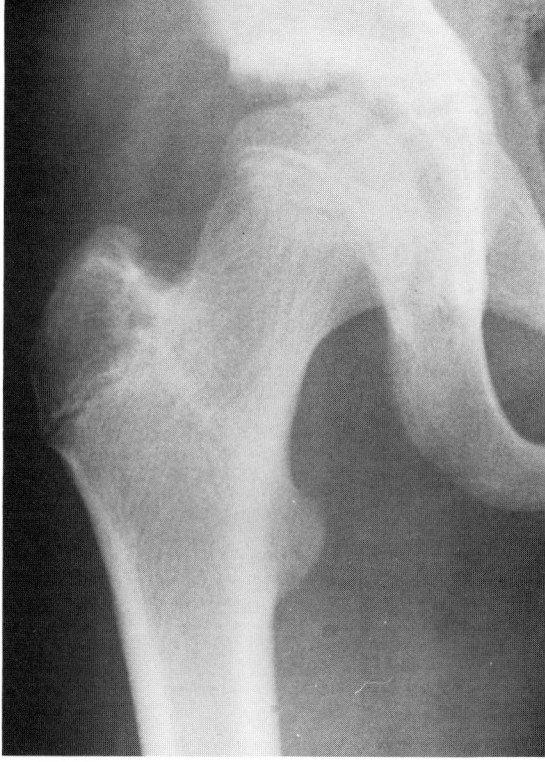

TYPE IV (INTERTROCHANTERIC FRACTURES)

Undisplaced intertrochanteric fractures are treated by skin traction or a hip spica. Most displaced intertrochanteric fractures can be readily reduced by skin traction which is maintained for 3–4 weeks before applying a hip spica. Coxa vara is the main complication of this fracture but it can usually be avoided by allowing the fracture to stabilise in traction before applying the spica. The long term results are good since avascular necrosis, premature growth arrest, and non-union are rare.

Subtrochanteric and upper-third fractures of the femur

Fractures of the femoral shaft are common in childhood and often result from low velocity injuries. In many instances side-to-side apposition of the fragments is obtained but solid union will occur. Re-modelling will correct minor degrees of angulation and in young children shortening of up to 2 cm will correct spontaneously.

Gallows traction (see p. 291) is used initially in treating children less than 2 years of age. Care is required in applying the crepe bandages in order to avoid skin damage and ischaemia. Traction is continued for 2–3 weeks to enable the fracture to stabilise before applying a hip spica since there is a risk of varus angulation if the spica is applied before this time.

For children over the age of 2 years, Hamilton Russell traction (see p. 291) has proved to be a satisfactory method of treatment. Traction is continued for 3–4 weeks before applying a hip spica so as to avoid varus deformities. If the proximal fragment in a subtrochanteric fracture is excessively flexed, it is better to use traction with the knee and hip flexed to 90°. For this form of traction a Steinmann pin is drilled from the medial side across the distal third of the femur, with care being taken to avoid the femoral artery and the distal femoral growth plate. The pin is attached to a stirrup and traction is applied with the hip in 90° of flexion. The knee is allowed to flex to 90° and a sling is used to support the calf in this position. After 3–4 weeks, when the fracture is reasonably stable, the pin is removed and a hip spica applied. The cast is removed and mobilisation commenced six weeks following the injury.

Midshaft fractures of the femur

Varus angulation is not a complication of midshaft fractures of the femur so that prolonged periods of traction are not required before the child is placed in a hip spica. The immediate application of the hip spica has proven to be a better alternative in children up to the age of 10 years (Fig. 6.61). It is suitable for fractures in the middle- and lower-thirds of the femur whether they be transverse, oblique or spiral. The fracture can be reduced and the hip spica applied without anaesthesia or with a femoral nerve block; however, it is usually easier and more comfortable for the child if it is carried out under general anaesthesia. The hip

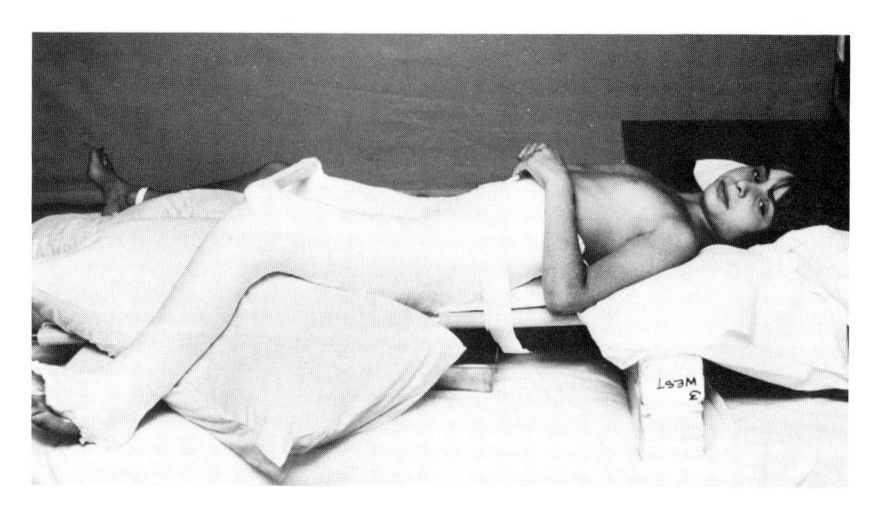

Fig. 6.61 Immediate hip spica for fractures of the shaft of the femur. This 8-year-old girl with a fracture of the midshaft of the left femur was treated by closed reduction and the application of an immediate hip spica. The hip is help in 30° of flexion and the knee in 60° of flexion and the sole of the plaster has been removed. She is nursed on a frame and is also able to move about the house on a trolley.

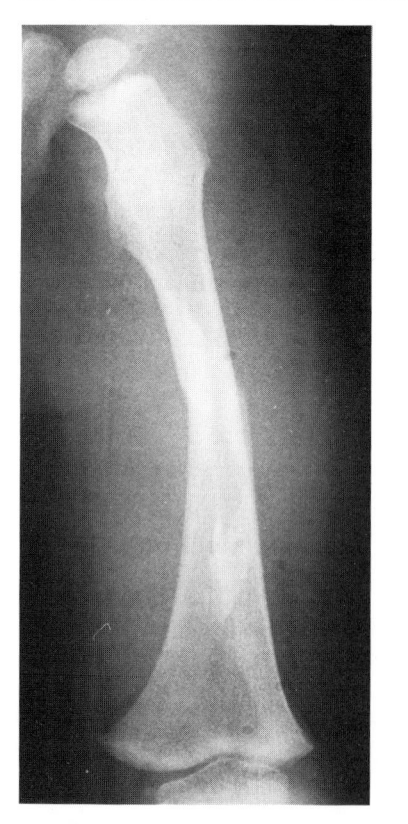

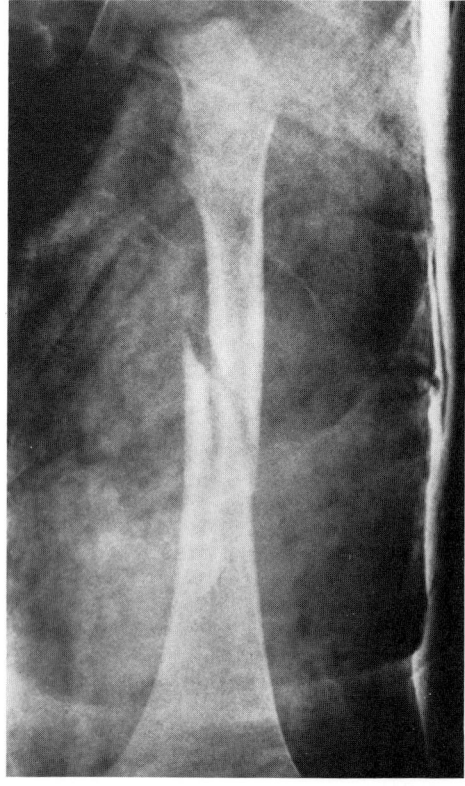

Figs. 6.62 & 6.63 Spiral fracture of the mid-shaft of the femur in a 2-year-old child. A hip spica was applied under general anaesthesia on the day of admission. The length of the femur has been restored to normal and the fragments have been moulded into slight valgus.

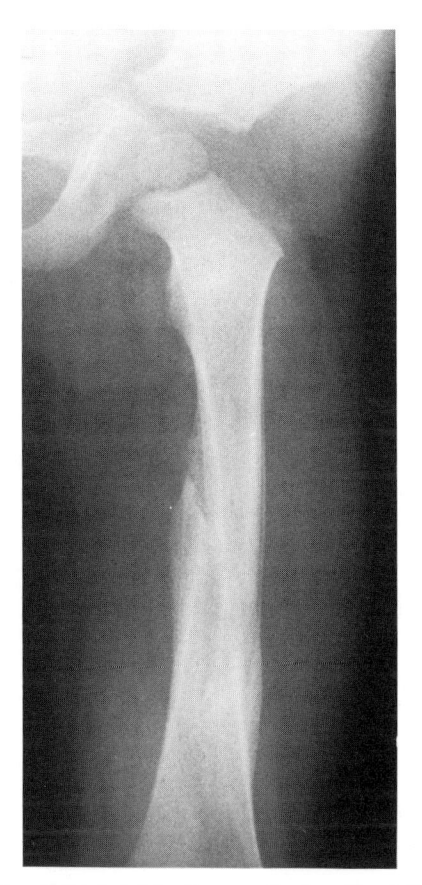

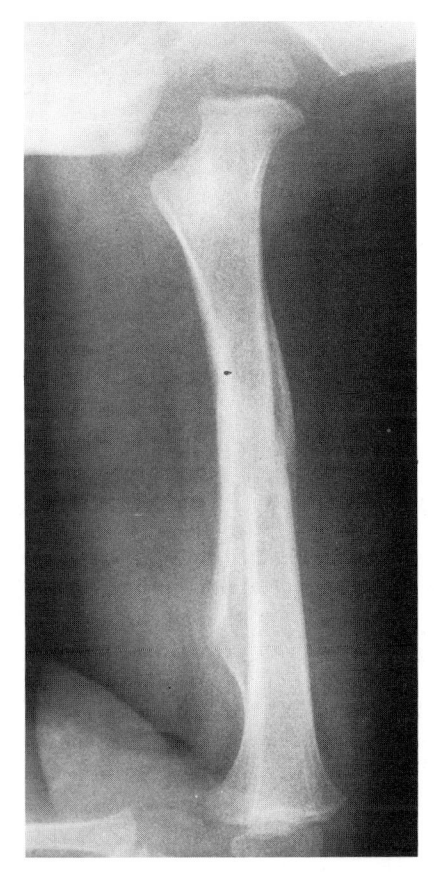

Figs. 6.64 & 6.65 Same patient as Fig. 6.62. Six weeks later the fracture has united and the femur is well aligned. The fracture is also well aligned in the lateral plane and the extent of the new bone formed beneath the periosteum is typical of spiral fractures in childhood. During the period in plaster the amount of shortening increased to 1 cm and this was corrected by growth stimulation over the following six months.

spica is applied in two stages. The child is first transferred onto the spica table where the heel of the fractured leg is grasped in one hand while the calf is held in the other with the knee in at least 60° of flexion. Traction applied to the calf aligns the fracture and reduces the amount of overlap and an assistant then applies a padded long leg cast with the knee flexed to 60°. When the cast is dry, a well moulded 1½ hip spica is completed with the hip on the fractured side in about 30° of flexion with neutral abduction, adduction and rotation. It is easier to nurse a child less than 5 years of age if a double hip spica is applied. At all ages a bar across the legs of the spica improves the strength of the cast as well as making it easier to lift and turn the child. Angulation and increased over-riding of the fragments due to the child pushing his foot against the sole of the plaster are avoided by removing the cast beneath the foot.

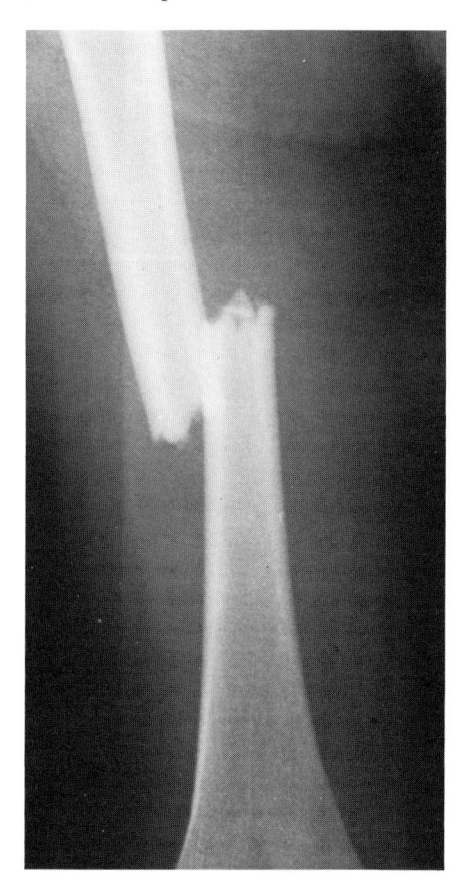

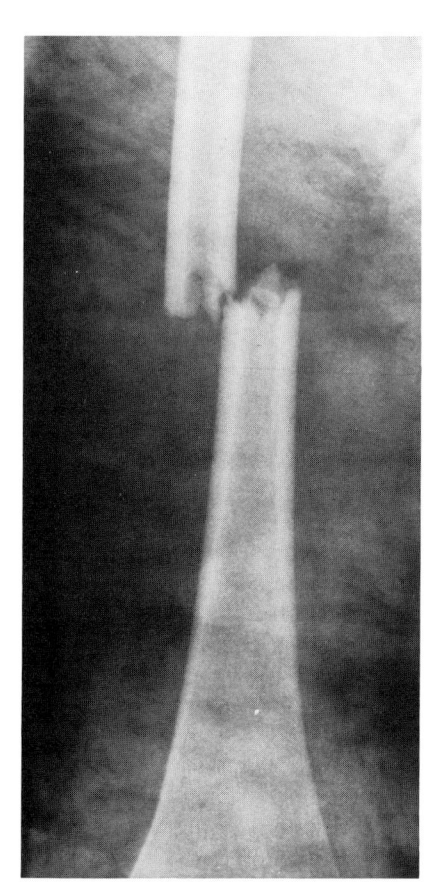

Figs. 6.66 & 6.67 This 5-year-old boy sustained a transverse fracture of the femur in a motor car accident. (*Right*) On the same day an immediate hip spica was applied under general anaesthesia. The alignment is correct with a small amount of overlap.

The reduction is checked by x-rays and anterior angulation of more than 20° or medial angulation of greater than 15° is corrected one week later by wedging of the cast.

Parents are instructed in the methods of nursing the child in the spica and the child is discharged when the plaster is dry—which means that the majority of children return home within 2–3 days of their fracture (Figs. 6.62 & 6.63). The child is reviewed a week later and any unacceptable angulation is corrected by wedging. During the first two weeks it is common for the amount of overlapping to increase but it rarely exceeds 1–1½ cm. The child is re-admitted 6–8 weeks following the injury for removal of the plaster and x-ray assessment (Figs. 6.64 & 6.65). Review of this method of treatment has shown that normal limb function is achieved without angular or rotary abnormalities. The initial leg length discrepancy usually corrects as a result of stimulation of femoral growth but persistent shortening may occur in older children whose initial over-riding was 2 cm or more (Figs. 6.66–6.70).

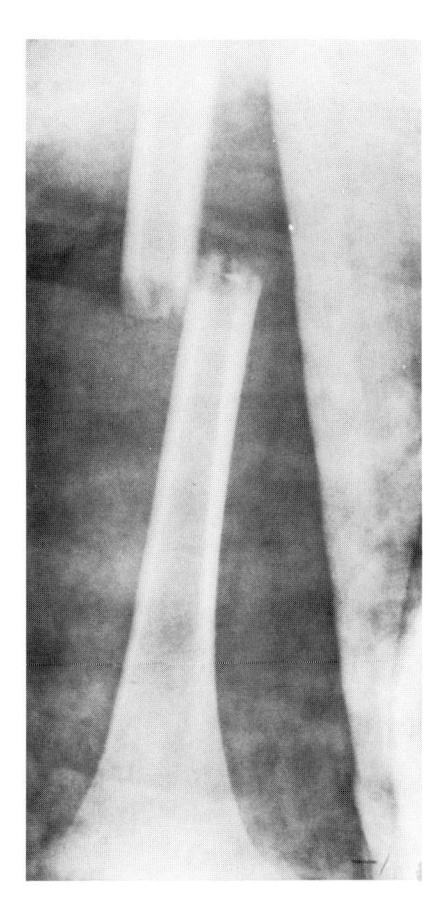

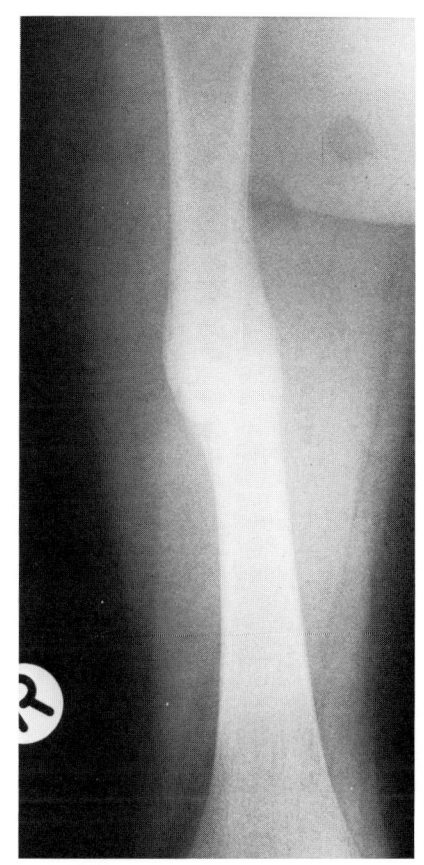

Figs. 6.68 & 6.69 Same patient as Fig. 6.60. The alignment is correct in the lateral plane and there is a small amount of overlap. (*Right*) Seven weeks later the fracture has united in good position (A–P view).

Children less than 10 years of age who have associated injuries (in particular abdominal injuries, compound injuries, or head injuries) are treated initially by Hamilton Russell traction. A hip spica of the same type is applied when the other injuries are no longer of concern.

Hamilton Russell traction is used for children over the age of 10 years for a period of 2–3 weeks to allow the pain to subside and the fracture to stabilise. A femoral cast brace is then applied. The quadrilateral thigh component is best made from plaster with hand moulding and polypropylene knee hinges are used to connect the thigh piece to a below-knee cast. The child is mobilised with crutches and a plaster sandal. Once the child has become confident in the use of the crutches, he may leave hospital. Excessive shortening is avoided by delaying the application of the cast brace for 2–3 weeks. This method has the advantage of allowing the child to return home at an early stage and avoids the problems of nursing the older child and adolescent in a hip spica. The method is also

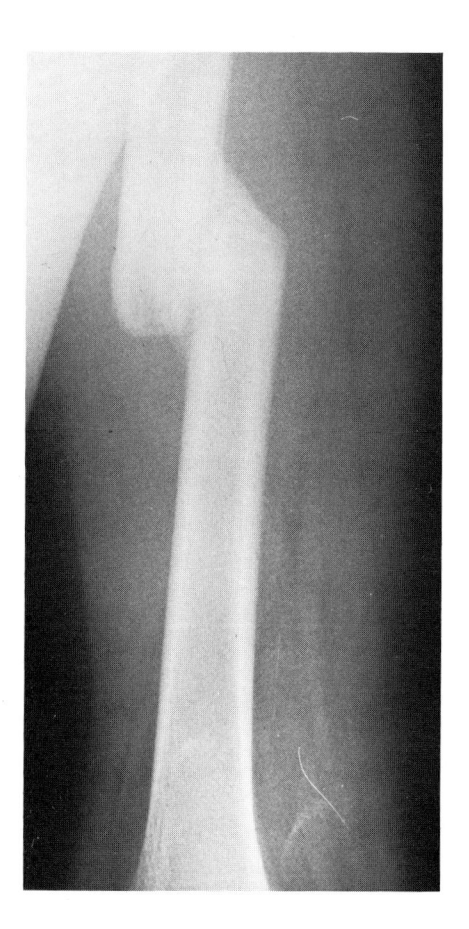

Fig. 6.70 Same patient as Fig. 6.66. Lateral view of the united fracture seven weeks after injury. An increase in the amount of overlap occurred during the period in plaster. Stimulation of growth led to complete correction of this 1.5 cm shortening over the following year.

applicable to children with bilateral fractures of the femur (Fig. 6.71). Skeletal traction may be required in adolescents if the degree of shortening is excessive. However, after 2–3 weeks a cast brace can usually be applied.

Other methods need to be considered in special circumstances. Fractures of the femur are difficult to treat in children with head injuries complicated by spasticity and in children with cerebral palsy. An intramedullary rod can be used to fix many of these fractures but a major operation can be avoided by the use of the external fixateurs. Screws are inserted from the lateral side into the proximal fragment and either screws or Steinmann pins are inserted into the distal fragment. The screws are inserted from the lateral side whilst the Steinmann pins are introduced from the medial side in order to avoid damage to the femoral artery. The protruding ends of the screws and Steinmann pins are attached to the fixateur or are cemented to a rod with methyl methacrylate. An external fixateur is often useful in stabilising difficult compound fractures and, as an alternative to internal fixation, may also be needed to stabilise the fracture when there is an adjoining major arterial injury.

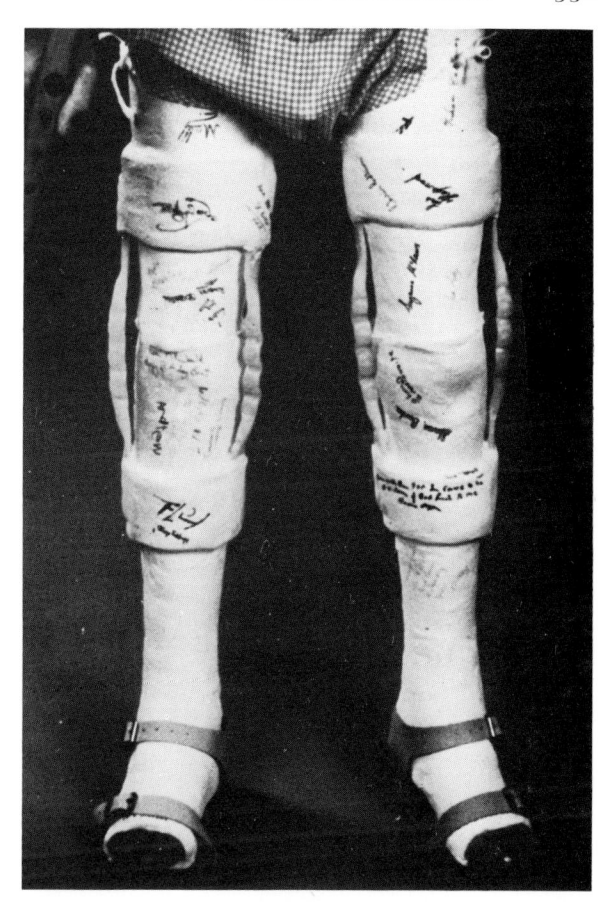

Fig. 6.71 Cast bracing of fractured femur. This 12-year-old child with mid-shaft fractures of the femora began standing and walking in these plaster cast braces two weeks following the injury.

Supracondylar fractures of the femur

Buckle fractures are common in toddlers and are readily treated in a long leg cast with the knee in extension—a technique which is also used for undisplaced fractures in older children (Figs. 6.72 & 6.73). However displaced fractures are often difficult to align and may lead to significant valgus or varus deformities of the leg. As these deformities cannot be expected to correct spontaneously, they should be avoided by supporting the leg on a straight Thomas splint with skin traction. In contrast, moderate flexion and extension deformities can be expected to correct by re-modelling; a long leg cast is applied when callus appears on the x-ray.

Distal femoral growth plate injuries

Severe hyperextension of the knee may produce a type II fracture of this growth plate with displacement of the distal femoral epiphysis. The shaft of the femur is

332   Chapter 6

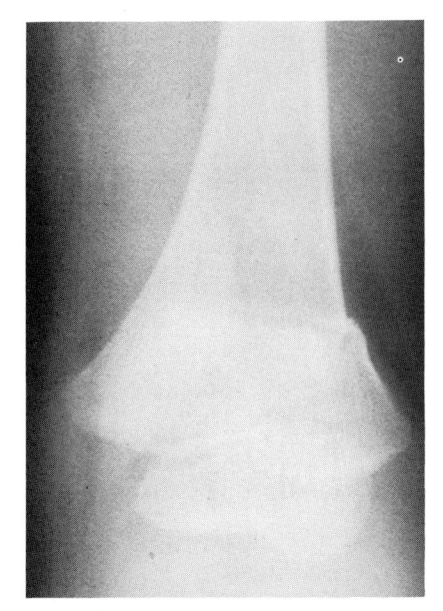

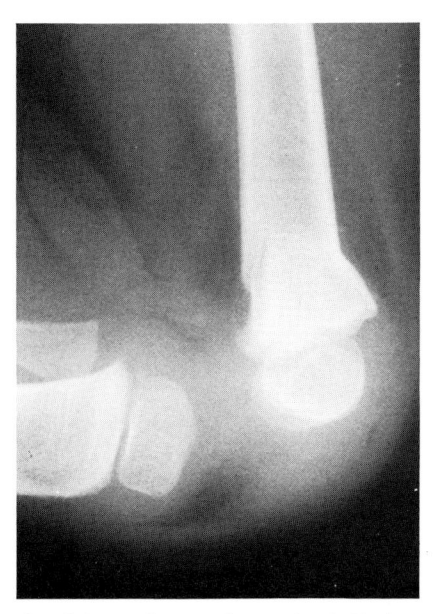

Figs. 6.72 & 6.73 Greenstick fracture of the distal femoral metaphysis. An A–P view shows that the fracture is well aligned. A lateral view indicates that there is a minor degree of anterior angulation which will re-model spontaneously.

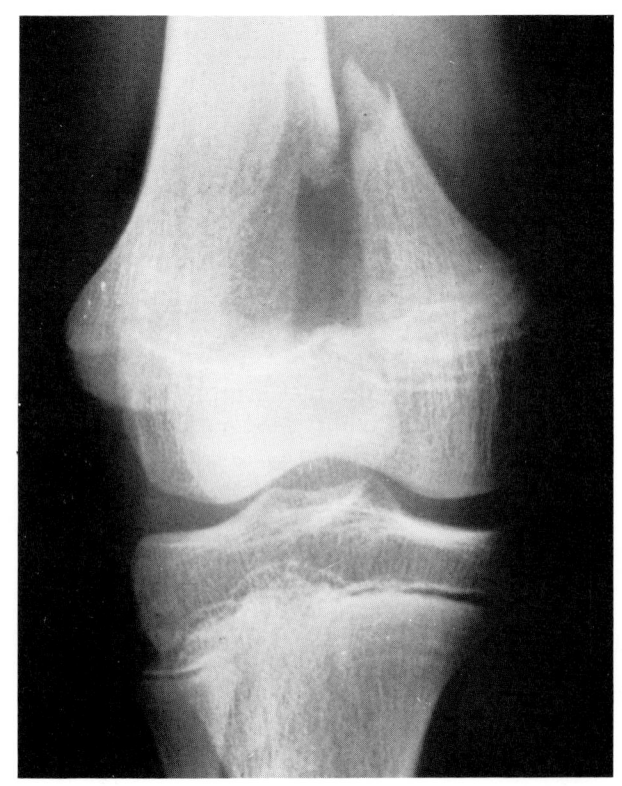

Fig. 6.74 Type II fracture of the distal femoral growth plate. The lateral half of the growth plate closed prematurely but as the patient was close to skeletal maturity there was no significant deformity or leg length discrepancy.

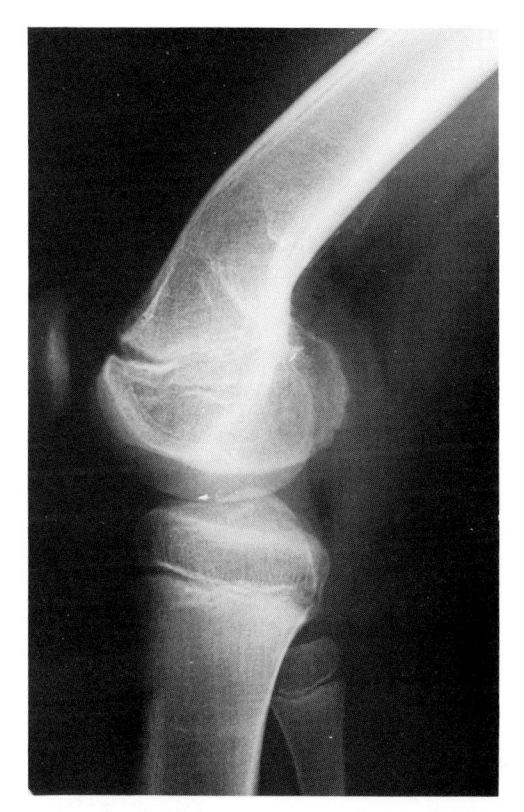

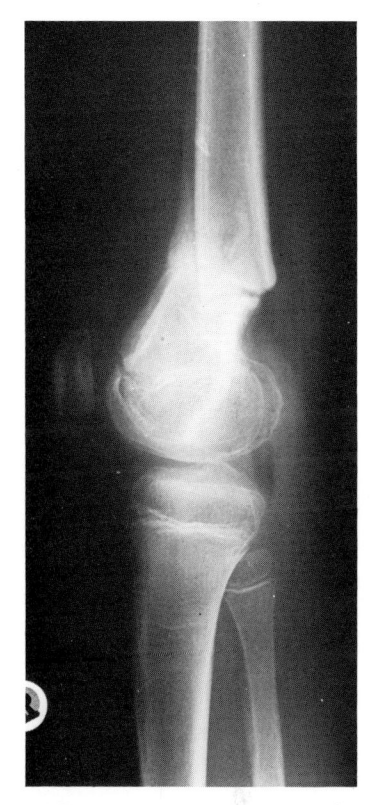

Figs. 6.75 & 6.76 Asymmetrical growth plate arrest following type II fracture of the distal femoral growth plate. (*Left*) A bony bridge has formed across the back of the distal femoral growth plate leading to progressive flexion deformity of the knee. (*Right*) The deformity has been corrected by a supracondylar osteotomy and further deformity has been prevented by an epiphysiodesis of the distal femoral growth plate.

displaced posteriorly and may penetrate the skin of the popliteal fossa and damage the popliteal vessels. The fracture is reduced under general anaesthesia with the child in the prone position. Traction is applied to the leg to disengage the fragments and the knee is flexed while maintaining traction on the foot. The fragments will usually lock into place when the knee is flexed to approximately 100°. A well padded above-knee cast is applied and, after 2–3 weeks, the amount of flexion is reduced to 60°; the plaster is removed four weeks after the injury. The first week after reduction is critical as re-displacement may occur and the fracture must therefore be carefully watched.

If the reduction is initially unstable, percutaneous smooth Kirschner wires can be introduced through each condyle into the shaft of the femur. A plaster cast is then applied with the knee in less flexion. Skeletal traction can also be used to maintain the reduction.

Type II fractures of the distal femoral growth plate may also be produced by varus or valgus injuries to the knee and are also treated by closed reduction and plaster cast immobilisation (Fig. 6.74).

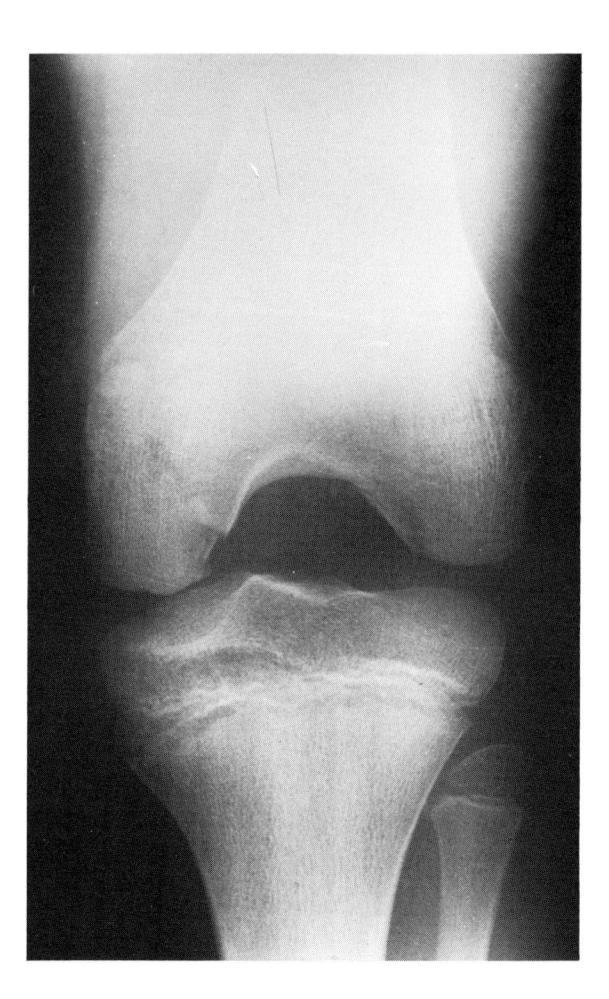

Fig. 6.77 Fracture of the medial condyle of the femur. Note the oblique fracture line extending across the medial femoral condyle. As this fracture was undisplaced it was treated with a plaster cast for four weeks, but displaced fractures require open reduction and internal fixation.

Although the majority of these injuries have the radiological features of a type II fracture of the growth plate, partial or complete arrest of growth in the fractured area is common so that later review is always required (Figs. 6.75 & 6.76). Occasionally these injuries present late and are found to be irreducible by manipulation. The position is best accepted and, if necessary, residual deformity should then be corrected by osteotomy at a later date. If open reduction of the fracture is attempted, premature fusion of the growth plate always occurs.

Intra-articular fractures of the distal femur

There are several types of intra-articular fractures. Fracture of the posterior part of the femoral condyle requires accurate reduction with care being taken to avoid damage to the vascular supply to the fragment (Fig. 6.77). The fragment is held by a compression screw inserted into the adjoining part of the epiphysis. Type III and IV injuries also require accurate reduction and can also be held by a

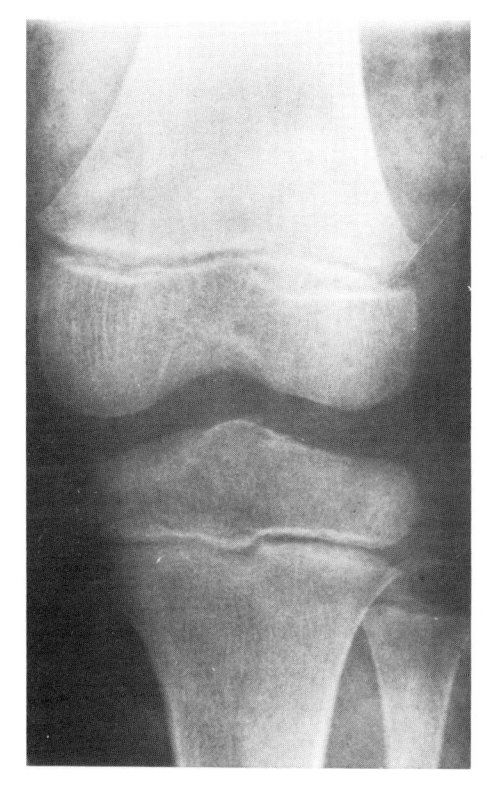

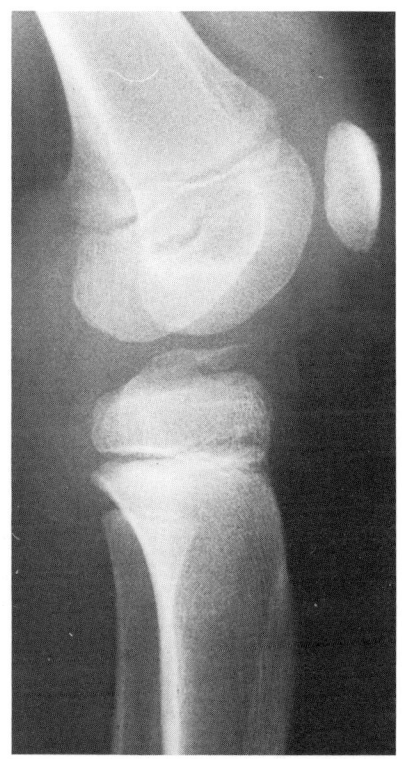

Figs. 6.78 & 6.79 Fracture of the anterior tibial spine of the tibia. On A–P view, the minor elevation of the anterior tibial spine can easily be overlooked. (*Right*) The fragment is displaced on this lateral view.

compression screw introduced from the fragment into the adjoining epiphysis. If fixation is required across the epiphyseal plate, it is preferable to use a smooth Kirschner wire rather than a screw.

TIBIA

Fractures of the tibial spine

This is a frequently overlooked cause of knee swelling following an injury (Figs. 6.78 & 6.79). The anterior tibial spine is avulsed by the anterior cruciate ligament. Extension of the knee under general anaesthesia is usually sufficient to reduce partially displaced fragments which are only detached anteriorly. Aspiration of the haemarthrosis usually makes it easier to extend the knee and has the added advantage of relieving the child's pain (Fig. 6.80). A long leg cast is applied for four weeks.

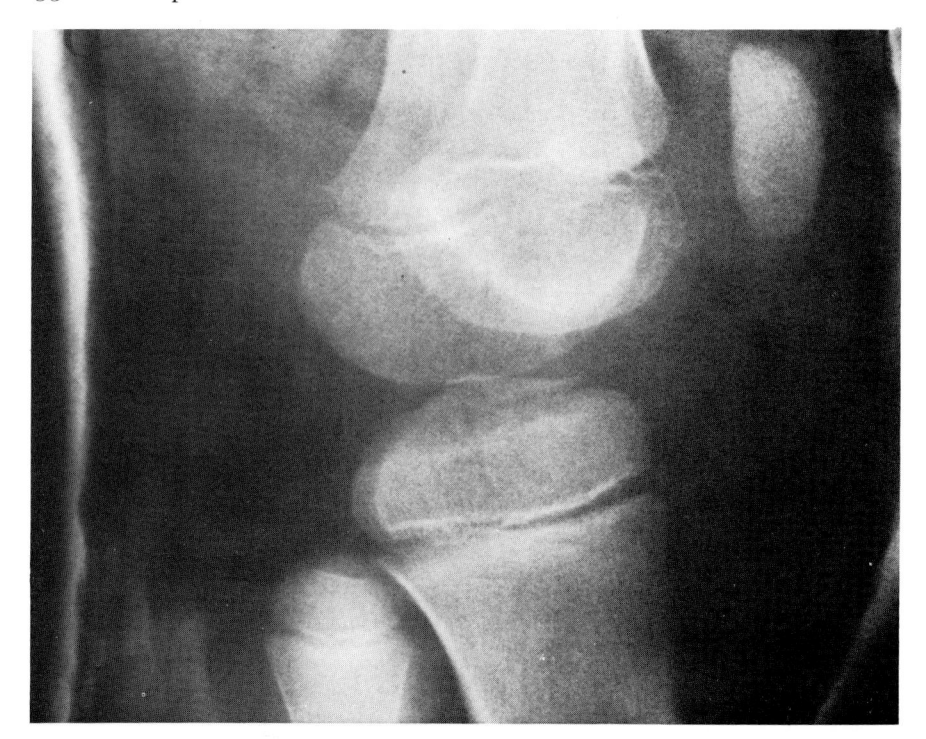

Fig. 6.80 Same patient as Fig. 6.78. Reduction has been achieved following aspiration of the haemarthrosis and extension of the knee.

More marked displacement of the anterior tibial spine may not be corrected by extension of the knee, especially if it presents late, and open reduction may then be required. The fragment is usually found to be much larger than expected and the menisci are often displaced into the defect. The reduced fragment is held in position by a chromic catgut suture passed through drill holes in the epiphysis. Care is taken to place these holes above the tibial growth plate. The leg is immobilised in a long leg cast for four weeks and a good outcome can be expected.

Proximal tibial growth plate injuries

Fractures of the upper tibial growth plate are less common than fractures of the distal femoral plate although the treatment of both is very similar. Furthermore, partial or complete arrest of growth is also a common sequel.

Proximal metaphyseal fractures of the tibia

These fractures usually occur in young children and are often minimally displaced. However, a small amount of valgus angulation may produce an obvious knock knee deformity which usually does not correct spontaneously. As a result, any valgus angulation should be corrected by manipulative reduction with varus moulding of the plaster cast.

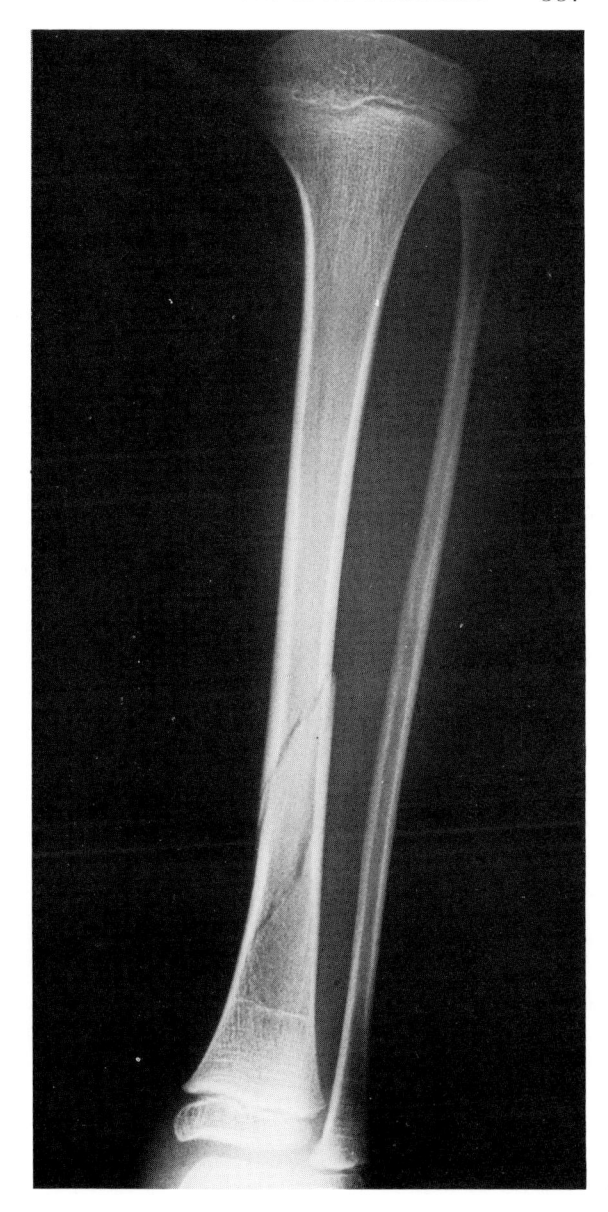

Fig. 6.81 Spiral fracture of the tibia with intact fibula. This is a stable fracture which is readily treated with a plaster cylinder but careful moulding is required to prevent varus angulation.

Diaphyseal fractures of the tibia

A fine undisplaced spiral fracture of the shaft of the tibia is common in toddlers and is referred to as the toddler's fracture. For these, as for undisplaced fractures in older children, the leg is immobilised in an above-knee cast with the knee in extension.

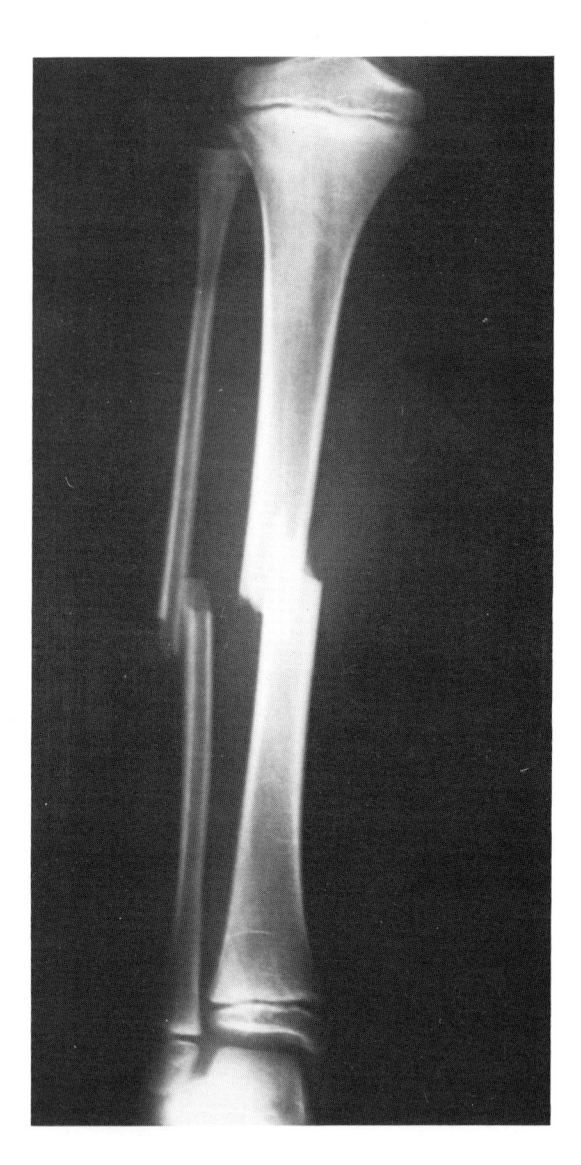

Fig. 6.82 Oblique complete fractures of the midshafts of the tibia and fibula. These fractures are readily treated by closed reduction and plaster immobilisation.

The majority of displaced fractures of the shaft of the tibia can be readily reduced by manipulation under general anaesthesia. The fibula is often intact, although bowed, and it tends to angulate the tibial fracture to produce a bow leg (Fig. 6.81). Careful moulding of the plaster is required to overcome this tendency. When the fibula is fractured the tibia becomes unstable but a satisfactory position can usually be obtained by manipulation, and immobilisation in a long leg plaster cast is usually adequate (Figs. 6.82–6.86). If difficulty is encountered in controlling the position of the fracture, either Knowles' pins placed above and below the fracture and incorporated into the cast or the use of an external fixateur will provide satisfactory immobilisation. Open reduction and internal fixation of a

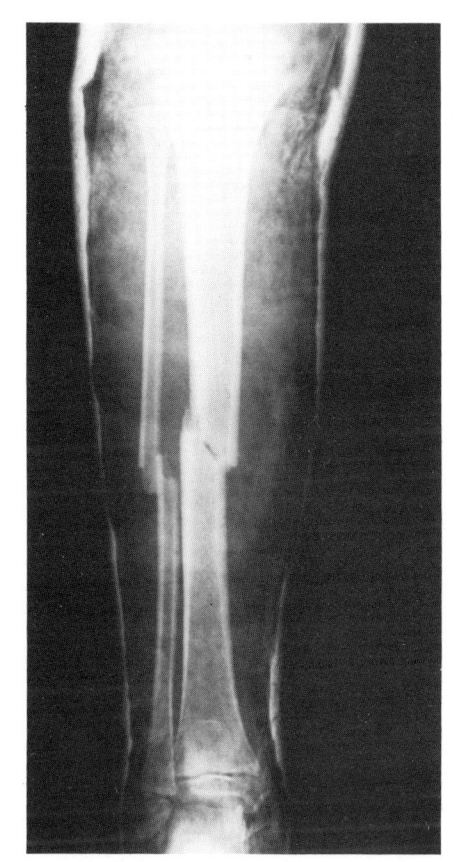

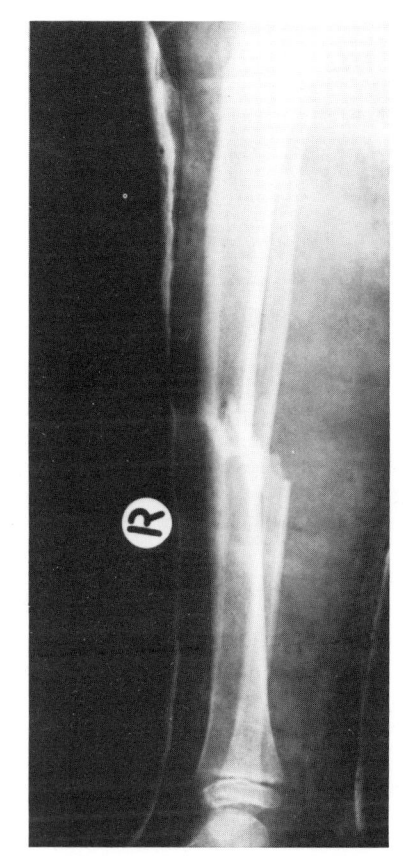

Figs. 6.83 & 6.84 Same patient as Fig. 6.82. The bones are well aligned in the antero-posterior and lateral projections following closed reduction and plaster immobilisation.

fractured shaft of tibia is never required. Whatever method is used it is very important to align the fractured leg so that it looks like the other leg whether this be varus, valgus or straight. Special attention is necessary to ensure that rotation is the same on both sides.

ANKLE

Ankle injuries are common in childhood and usually consist of growth plate injuries of the distal tibia and fibula and their adjoining metaphyses. Ligamentous damage is rarely the cause of ankle injuries in children.

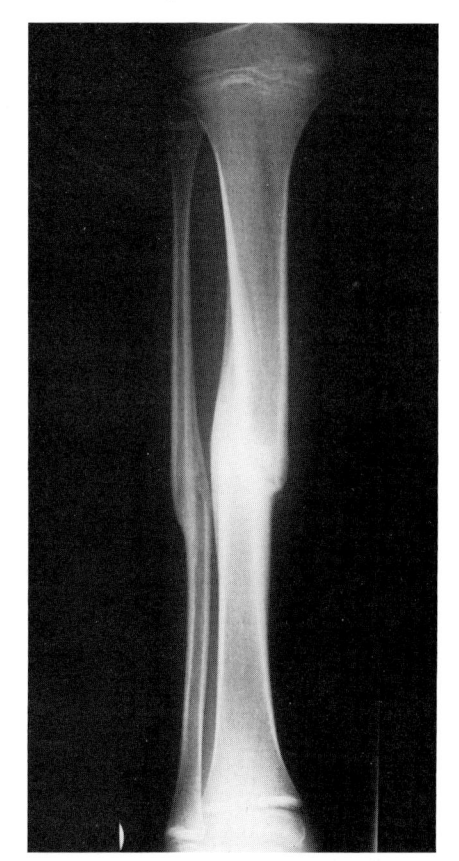

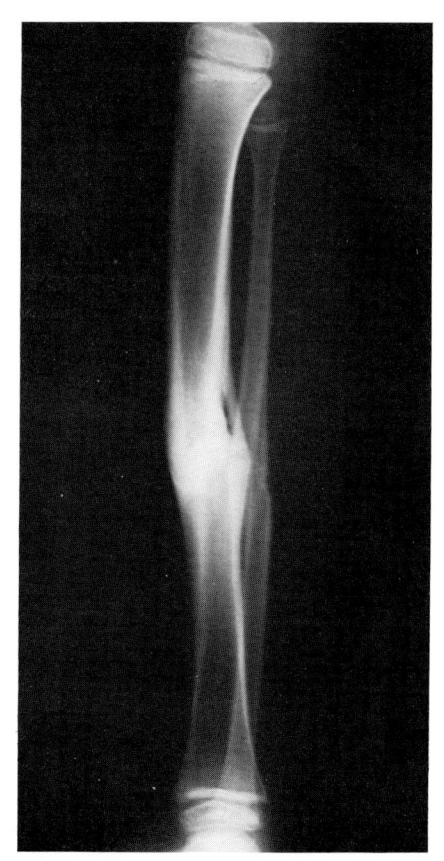

Figs. 6.85 & 6.86 Same patient as Fig. 6.82. X-rays taken nine weeks after the fracture and three weeks after the plaster was removed. The fractures have united and the bones are well aligned.

Metaphyseal fractures of the distal tibia

Buckle fractures and displaced fractures may occur in this area. Undisplaced fractures are treated in a plaster cast for four weeks. Whenever reduction is required, the foot is immobilised in the position giving the most stable reduction. An equinus position will not lead to permanent stiffness of the ankle.

Fractures of the distal growth plate of the fibula

Type I or II fractures of the distal fibular growth plate are the commonest type of ankle injury. Type I injuries are usually undisplaced and slight widening of the growth plate with overlying soft tissue swelling confirm the diagnosis. A walking cast for three weeks is sufficient.

Fractures of the distal tibial growth plate

Type II injuries of the distal tibial plate are common and are usually associated with fractures of the distal fibula. These fractures are readily reduced by

Fractures and Dislocations 341

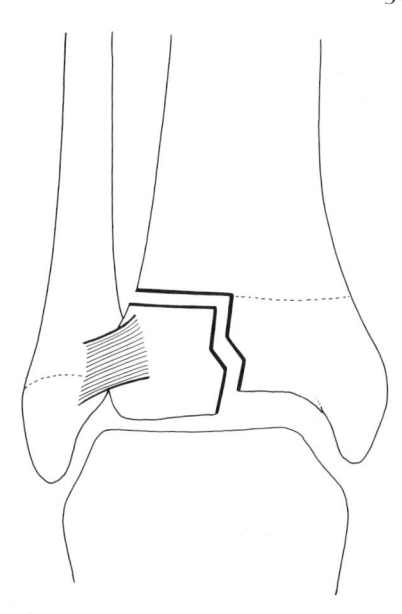

Fig. 6.87 Tillaux fracture of the tibia. The fragment is avulsed by the anterior tibio-fibular ligament.

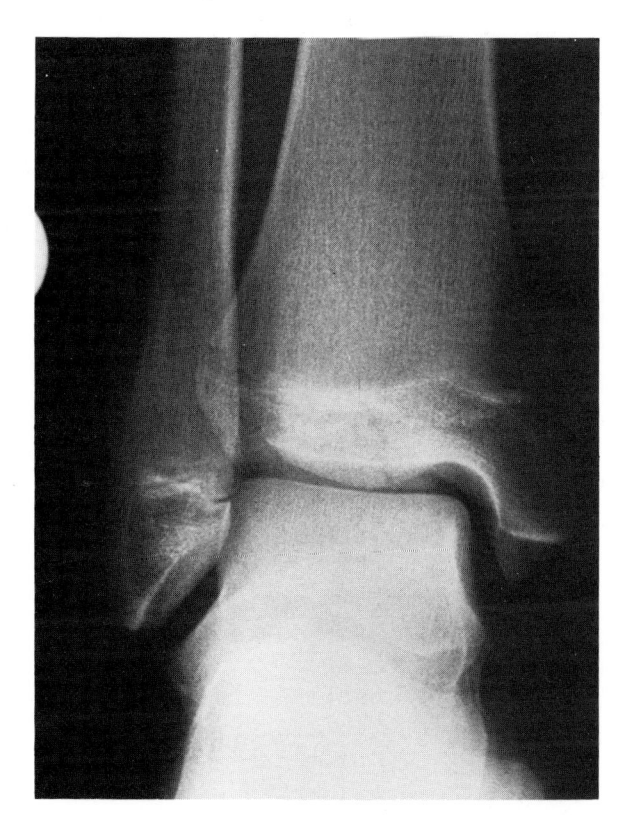

Fig. 6.88 Undisplaced type III fracture of the distal tibial growth plate (Tillaux fracture).

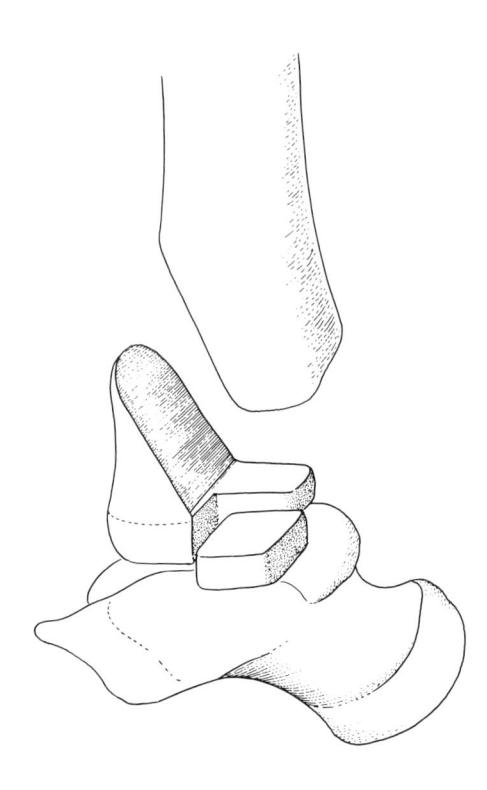

Fig. 6.89 Tri-plane fracture of the distal tibial epiphysis.

manipulation and a long leg cast is applied for 4–6 weeks. Normal growth of this epiphysis can be expected.

Type III injuries of the lateral part of the distal growth plate are seen in early adolescence. The central portion of the tibial plate closes first while the lateral component closes last; as a consequence, external rotation injuries may avulse the anterior portion of the lateral quadrant of the tibial epiphysis and so produce a Tillaux fracture (Fig. 6.87). When the displacement is minimal, a below-knee plaster cast is applied for four weeks (Fig. 6.88). When the fragment is displaced, an attempt is made to reduce the fracture under general anaesthesia. External rotation of the foot is found to increase the displacement due to the attachment of the anterior inferior tibiofibular ligament to the fragment, while internal rotation will often reduce the fracture. If not, an open reduction and fixation with a Kirschner wire is required.

The tri-plane fracture of the distal tibial growth plate combines the Tillaux fragment with a type II injury (Fig. 6.89). Displaced fractures are treated by closed reduction and open reduction is used only if the position obtained is unsatisfactory.

Fractures of the medial malleolus are often associated with type I or II fractures separations of the distal fibula or avulsion fractures of the tip of the

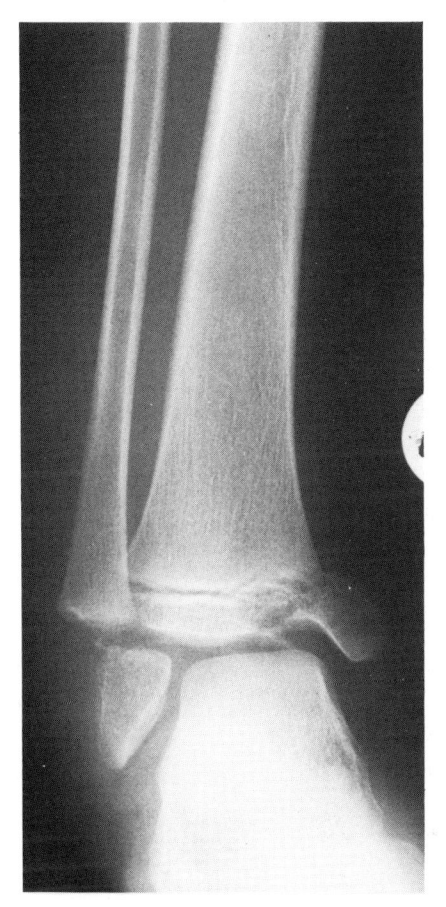

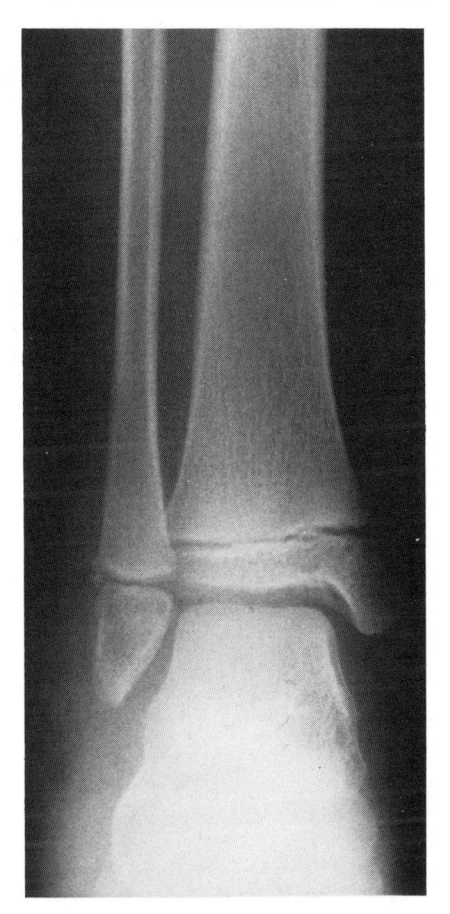

Figs 6.90 & 6.91 Displaced type II fracture of the distal fibular epiphysis and type III fracture of the medial malleolus. A small metaphyseal fragment is attached to the displaced fibula. (*Right*) An accurate closed reduction has been achieved.

lateral malleolus (Figs. 6.90–6.93). Fractures of the medial malleolus are usually either type III or IV injuries but severe compression injuries may also produce a type V lesion with permanent impairment of growth. The type III and IV fractures of the medial malleolus require accurate reduction which may be achieved by closed manipulation or by open reduction and Kirschner wire fixation if this is not achieved (Fig. 6.94). A below-knee plaster cast is applied for six weeks.

FOOT

Fractures of the talus and calcaneum—which are uncommon injuries in childhood—are treated by plaster cast immobilisation for 3–4 weeks. Avulsion

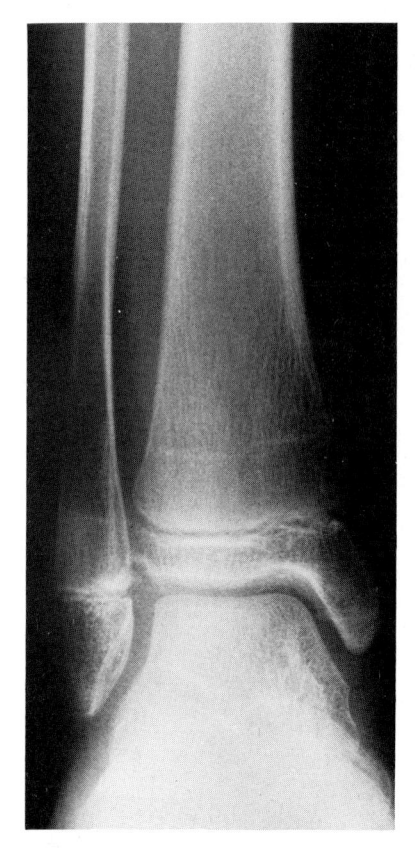

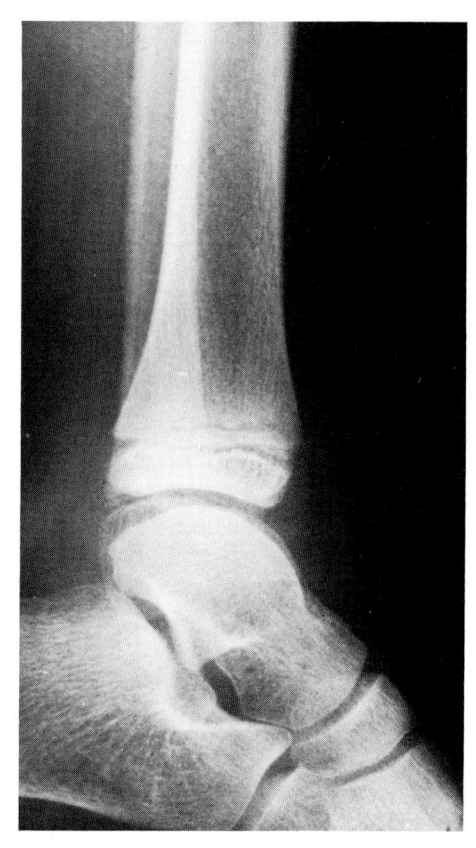

Figs. 6.92 & 6.93 Same case as Fig. 6.90. X-ray taken two years later. The anatomy and growth of the ankle are normal.

fractures of the styloid process of the fifth metatarsal are relatively common and often require a below-knee walking cast for three weeks.

Children may complain of pain over the tubercle of the navicular following a foot injury and difficulty is often encountered in distinguishing between the accessory navicular bone and an avulsion fracture of the tubercle of the navicular. However, persistent pain is treated with a below-knee plaster cast for three weeks and, after this, a Thomas heel will tip the foot over during walking and relieve pressure on this area.

SPINE

Cervical spine

Injuries of the cervical spine are uncommon in children. Although most involve the upper cervical vertebrae, the normal appearance of pseudosubluxation between the second and third cervical vertebrae in young children is a frequent source of diagnostic error (Figs. 6.95 & 6.96). This appearance is due to the large

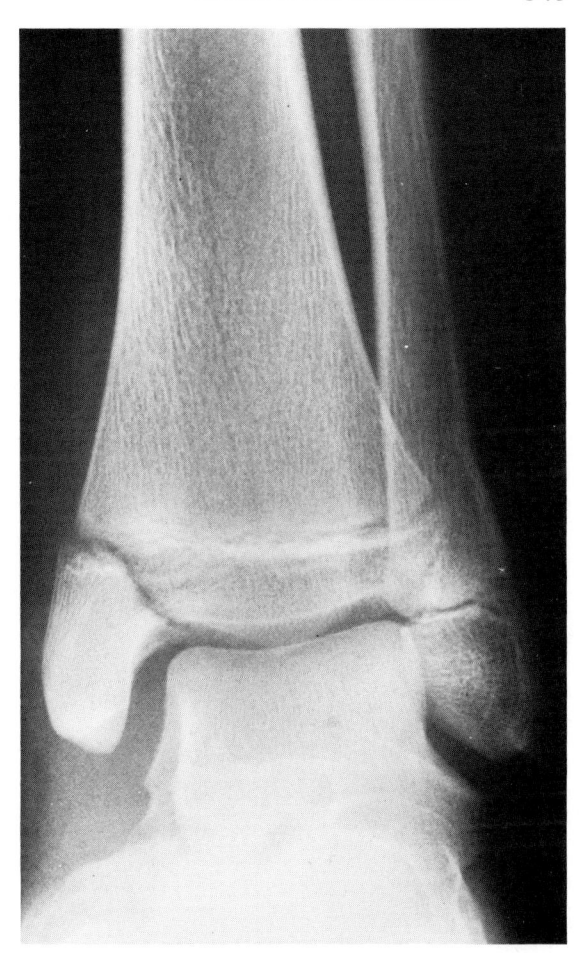

Fig. 6.94 Type III fracture of the medial malleolus. Solid union with normal growth was achieved using a plaster cast.

amount of flexion that is possible between these vertebrae in young children. A true subluxation is indicated by a greater degree of motion and is usually associated with fractures of the body of C2 or of its posterior elements. In addition a retropharangeal soft tissue mass will be present. Furthermore, dislocations without fracture do not occur at any level of the normal spine in childhood as the ligaments are stronger than the bone. However, atlanto-axial instability and dislocations due to ligament laxity are seen in Down's syndrome, and occasionally in cases of ligament softening associated with pharyngitis (Fig. 6.97).

Fractures of the odontoid frequently occur as a result of diving and trampoline accidents. The fracture usually passes through the growth plate between the dens and the body of the second cervical vertebra. The child usually has a painful neck or torticollis with normal spinal cord function. The neck is initially supported by halo or skull tong traction and later by a halo cast or Minerva jacket. Union of the fracture is assessed by x-rays taken six weeks later. Excessive movement between the first and second cervical vertebrae is an indication for a posterior fusion between these vertebrae.

346   Chapter 6

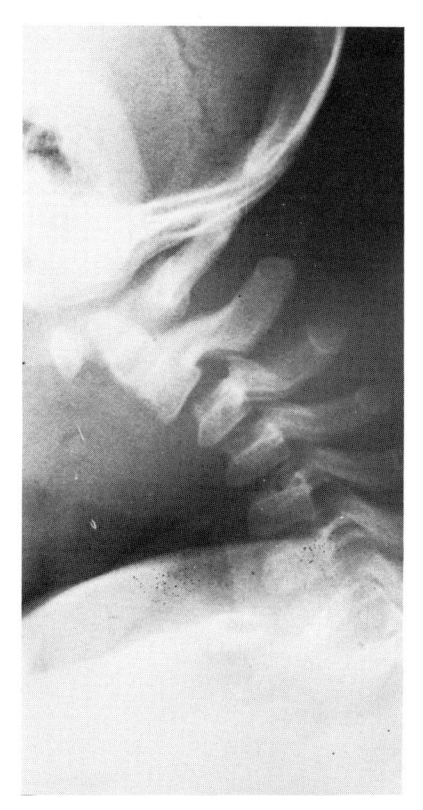

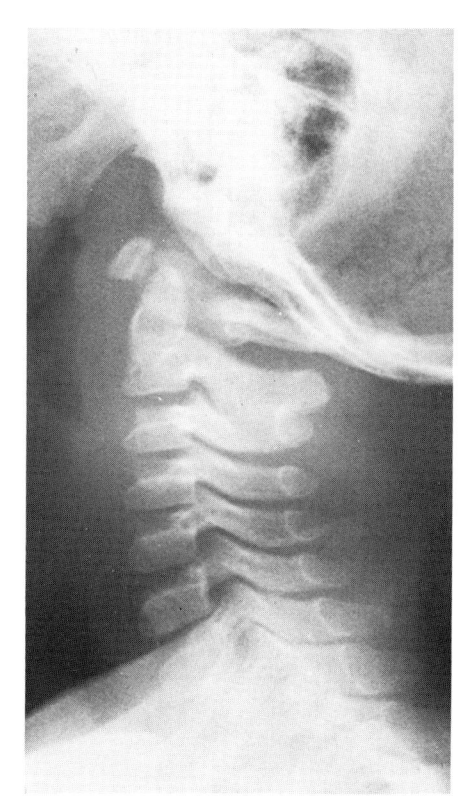

Figs. 6.95 & 6.96   Pseudosubluxation of C2 and C3. Lateral x-ray of the flexed cervical spine of a 4-year-old child. The appearance of subluxation of C2 on C3 is normal at this age. (*Right*) There is no pre-vertebral swelling and the shape of the body of C3 is normal. The reduced amount of lordosis is also common at this age.

Fig. 6.97   Atlanto-axial dislocation and tetraplegia in a 2-year-old child with ligament laxity. There is marked anterior displacement of C1 on C2. The spinal canal is grossly narrowed with the posterior arch of C1 jamming the spinal cord against the back of the dens. The anterior arch of C1 is displacing the pharyngeal air shadow forwards. The dislocation was reduced by halter traction and reduction was maintained by a posterior C1/C2 fusion supported by a Minerva jacket.

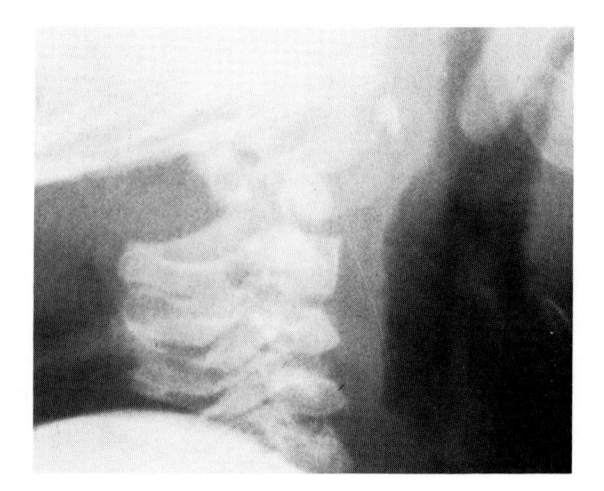

Relatively minor injuries may produce gross instability of the atlas on the axis with compression on the spinal cord when there are developmental anomalies of the odontoid process. These anomalies are seen frequently in children with skeletal dysplasias involving the spine such as spondyloepiphyseal dysplasia and pseudoachondroplastic dwarfism. Posterior fusion is required to stabilise these segments of the cervical spine.

Thoracic and lumbar spine

Wedge compression fractures of the thoracic and lumbar vertebrae are seen in children who fall from a height. Bed rest is used until the pain is improved and then ambulation is commenced with a spinal support; future growth of the spine is usually normal.

Fracture dislocations at the thoraco-lumbar junction with transection of the spinal cord may follow motor vehicle accidents. As with adults, children with spinal cord injuries are best managed in spinal injury units. In addition to the problems seen in adults with spinal cord injuries, the growing child rapidly develops progressive scoliosis and kyphosis requiring early fusion (Fig. 6.98). Anterior fusion with Dwyer instrumentation and posterior fusion with Harrington rod support is usually required to prevent progression of these spinal deformities. Deformities of the lower limbs resulting from spasticity are also common and often require surgical correction.

FRACTURES IN SPECIAL CIRCUMSTANCES

Compound fractures

These fractures are uncommon in childhood and usually consist of a small puncture wound produced by a spike of the underlying bone. Careful debridement of the soft tissues and skin is required. For low velocity injuries it is appropriate, following debridement, to primarily close the wound and treat the fracture as a closed injury. In children with severely compound injuries, the wound is excised and closed by delayed primary suture or skin graft. There is rarely any need for internal fixation as stability can usually be achieved with an external fixateur.

Fractures associated with arterial injuries

The treatment of ischaemia associated with supracondylar fractures of the humerus has already been described (p. 297). Injuries to the major arteries in the lower limb are rare but are seen with high velocity accidents. The circulation must be restored as early as possible by vascular reconstruction in order to reduce the likelihood of permanent neuromuscular damage to the limb. The adjoining fracture may be stabilised by an external fixateur or internal fixation, although some fractures of the shaft of the femur can be satisfactorily immobilised by skeletal traction.

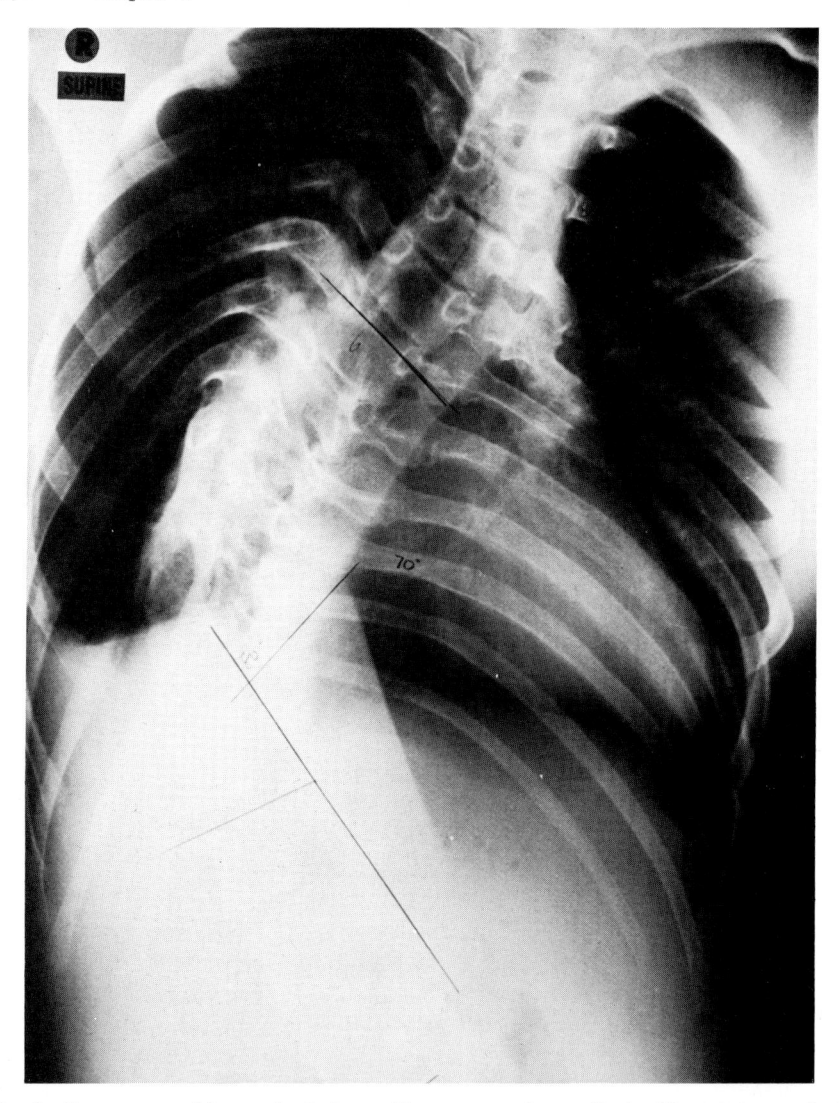

Fig. 6.98 12-year-old paraplegic boy with a progressive scoliosis. The total paraplegia occurred at the age of 2 years as a result of vascular damage to the spinal cord following a rupture of the thoracic aorta.

Child abuse

Child abuse is an important cause of orthopaedic injuries. The children are frequently less than 3 years of age and have previously attended their doctor with bruises, fractures, or head injuries. Multiple fractures at different stages of healing and metaphyseal fractures with extensive bone formation are common (Fig. 6.99). Whenever child abuse is suspected, the child is admitted to hospital for further investigation. Care is always required in order to distinguish this disorder from fragile bone conditions such as osteogenesis imperfecta.

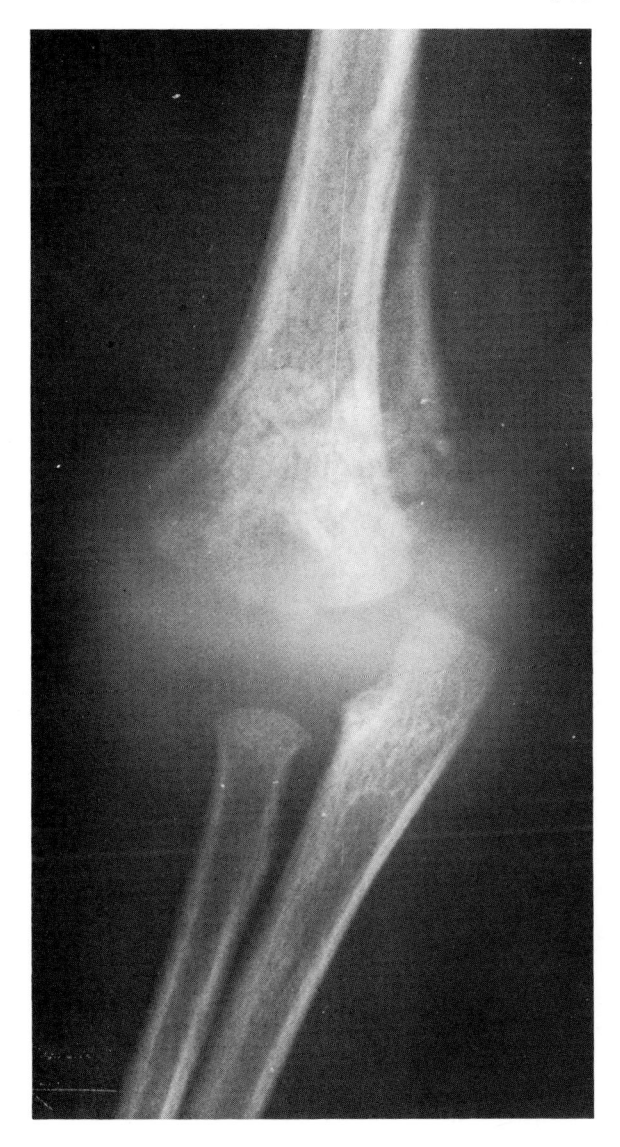

Fig. 6.99 Infant with multiple fractures at varying stages of healing and a subdural haematoma. This displaced type I injury of the condyle of the humerus is common in child abuse.

Pathological fractures

Lytic lesions, in particular simple bone cysts, may first become evident as a result of a fracture. The treatment is determined by the nature of the lesion. Fractures are also common in children with generalised osteoporosis either from osteogenesis imperfecta or various paralytic disorders. These fractures heal rapidly with simple forms of external immobilisation, but occasionally hyperplastic callus results which may be confused with an osteosarcoma.

Stress fractures

These fractures occur particularly in the upper-third of the tibia, the lower-half of the fibula, and occasionally in the necks of the metatarsals. They may resemble an osteosarcoma or osteomyelitis. Typical stress fractures are treated by decreased activity and, occasionally, a plaster cast. Serial x-rays are required to show that the lesion is healing. A biopsy is indicated whenever the appearance or the behaviour of the lesion is not typical of a stress fracture.

Appendix

ROYAL CHILDREN'S HOSPITAL
Melbourne, 3052

_____ 19__

Instructions to Out-patients with Fractures (broken bones), Injuries or Diseases, treated in a Plaster of Paris Cast

Name of Patient:

1 For the next . . . . hours you must lie down.

2 During the time in the case of a fracture of any bone in the upper limbs, have the hand raised so that it is the most elevated part of the body. In the case of the lower limbs (for example, a broken ankle), raise the foot off the bed and place the plaster cast on a pillow.

You should report to the Casualty Department or Fracture Clinic next day to see the Orthopaedic Surgeon, and at once if you notice any tightness of the plaster cast, indications of which you will find in the fingers and toes as follows:

- (a) Marked swelling.
- (b) Marked blueness.
- (c) A tight severe pain that is not eased by elevating the limbs.
- (d) Inability to move the fingers or toes.
  (You should continually move them even while resting.)
- (e) Numbness or loss of sensation.

Surgeon-in-Charge

CHAPTER 7

Bone Tumours

Classification, 353

Diagnosis, 354
Clinical; Radiology; Radio-isotope bone scanning; Haematology; Biochemistry; Biopsy

Treatment, 383
Benign tumours; Primary malignant bone tumours; Treatment of osteosarcoma; Treatment of Ewing's sarcoma

A multidisciplinary approach is required in order to provide optimal management of bone tumours. The orthopaedic surgeon, radiologist, and pathologist work together to establish the correct diagnosis as early as possible. The plan of treatment can then be formulated but it is preferable with malignant tumours to seek the advice of other medical and paramedical staff in a combined therapy clinic. In this way a co-ordinated programme of care can be discussed with the patient and family.

CLASSIFICATION

Most classifications of bone tumours, including that of the World Health Organisation, are based upon histological patterns. However, a classification based upon the radiological appearance of bone tumours is of more practical value to the clinician. This type of classification is given in Table 7.1. A further advantage of this classification is that lesions with similar appearances to primary bony tumours can be included. For example, simple cysts, non-ossifying fibromas, and fibrous dysplasia are not true tumours but they are the most common disorders to produce a cystic appearance. Osteomyelitis and other non-neoplastic lesions such as stress fractures, exuberant callus, and heterotopic calcification are also important as they may resemble primary malignant bone tumours. The possibility that osteomyelitis might be confused with a primary bone tumour is the major reason for always establishing the diagnosis of the lesion before commencing treatment.

Table 7.1 Radiological classification of bone tumours and related lesions.

Lesions protruding from the bone	Striated lesions
Osteochondroma	Haemangioma
Osteoma	
	Aggressive lesions
Cystic lesions	Primary tumours
Simple bone cyst	Osteosarcoma
Aneurysmal bone cyst	Ewing's sarcoma
Osteoblastoma	Histiocytosis X
Non-ossifying fibroma	Fibrosarcoma
Fibrous dysplasia	Chondrosarcoma
Enchondroma	Chordoma
Chondroblastoma	Malignant lymphoma
Chondromyxoid fibroma	Secondary tumours
Eosinophilic granuloma	Neuroblastoma
Congenital fibromatosis	Leukaemia
Neurofibroma	Non-neoplastic lesions
	Osteomyelitis
Sclerotic lesions	Stress fractures
Osteoid osteoma	Exuberant callus
	Heterotopic calcification

DIAGNOSIS

Biopsy of the lesion is required to establish the histological diagnosis but this procedure can best be planned and carried out if a list of the most likely diagnoses is made beforehand. The diagnosis is therefore established by considering the clinical and radiological features, the results of other investigations, and finally the macroscopic and histological appearances of the lesion.

CLINICAL

The clinical suspicion of a bone tumour is the first step towards making a diagnosis. It is usually suspected immediately whenever there is a mass or a fracture resulting from a trivial fall. A mass may be produced by an osteochondroma, osteoid osteoma, expansile cyst or malignant bone tumour while pathological fractures frequently occur through benign cysts and, less commonly, through malignant tumours. However, in most instances, the nature of the tumour cannot be determined from the clinical features but they do localise the region to be x-rayed.

A tumour may not be suspected when the child only complains of a mild, deep, aching pain which may initially be relieved by salicylates but later becomes persistent and is often worse at night. An x-ray of the painful area is always required even when there are no abnormal physical signs. Failure to carry out an x-ray under these circumstances is the usual reason for the delayed diagnosis of osteoid osteomas and Ewing's sarcomas.

RADIOLOGY

Radiological studies are carried out in order to study the local lesion and to determine whether lesions exist in other parts of the body. The radiological techniques, the terminology used to describe bone tumours, and the radiological features of specific tumours will be considered.

Radiological techniques

The *initial assessment* of the local lesion is made using plain x-rays. These should always include a standard antero-posterior and lateral view of the whole of the involved bone. Should the x-rays be normal, the possibility of referred pain should be considered and more proximal regions examined. If, despite these measures, nothing unusual is found but the pain persists, then the x-rays should be repeated.

Tomograms are useful to define the intra-osseus and soft tissue extent of tumours, particularly when they are located within the spine or pelvis. Computerised tomography provides more detail about the tumour than can be obtained using standard tomograms. Angiography does not provide sufficient additional information to warrant its use.

Assessment of lesions at other sites. Bone sarcomas characteristically metastatise to the lungs and to other parts of the skeleton. A search for metastases within the lungs is made using plain x-rays and tomograms. Computerised tomography is a valuable technique as it provides more detailed information about the size, location and number of metastases in the lungs.

A skeletal survey, in which plain x-rays are taken of each bone, can also be used to detect metastases but this has largely been replaced by radio-isotope bone scans which are a more sensitive method of detecting metastases. However, skeletal surveys are useful in polyostotic benign disorders such as fibrous dysplasia.

Terminology used in describing bone tumours

Many of the terms that are used to describe the gross pathological features of a bone tumour can also be used to describe the radiological features. In both instances particular note is taken of the site, size, shape, margin, contents, and soft tissue extension of the tumour. As when examining the gross pathology, these features are used to determine whether the lesion is benign or malignant and a short list of most likely diagnoses is produced.

Benign tumours usually have the radiological features of a slowly growing lesion. Benign lesions protruding from the bone, such as osteochondromas, have well defined margins and contain a well organised trabecular bone pattern (Fig. 7.1). It is common for benign lesions within the bone to have a cystic appearance which is produced by the slow replacement of normal bone with the contents of the tumour (Fig. 7.2). The fluid in a simple bone cyst produces a structureless appearance; a 'ground glass' appearance is common in fibrous dysplasia, whilst spotty calcification is characteristic of tumours containing cartilage.

The margin of the lesion also needs to be carefully examined: in benign lesions the margin (which is also referred to as the transition zone) is well defined with

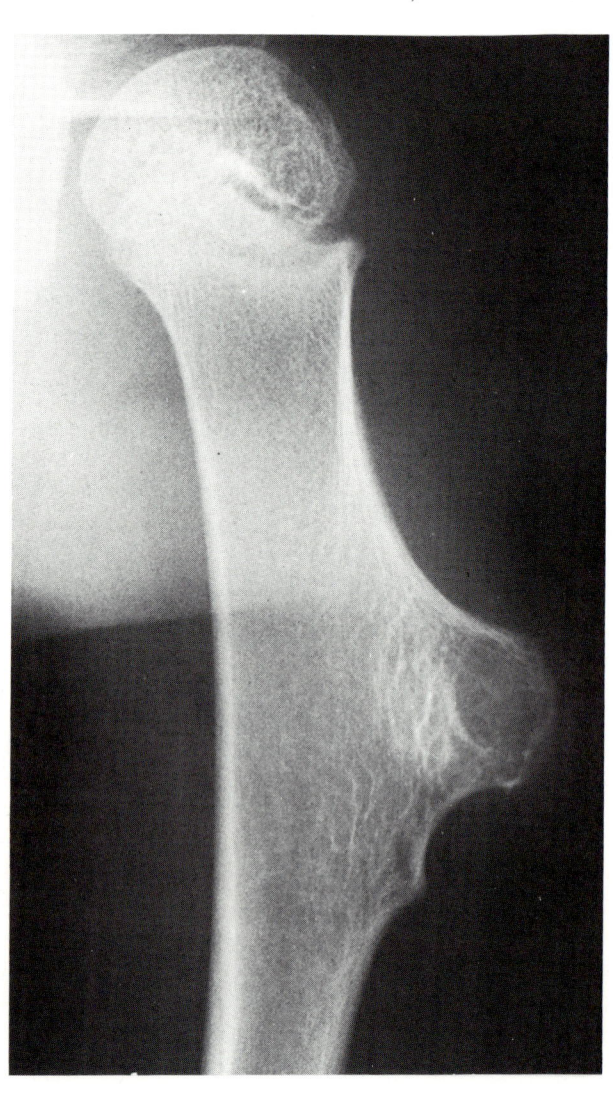

Fig. 7.1 A typical pedunculated osteochondroma protruding from the upper humerus.

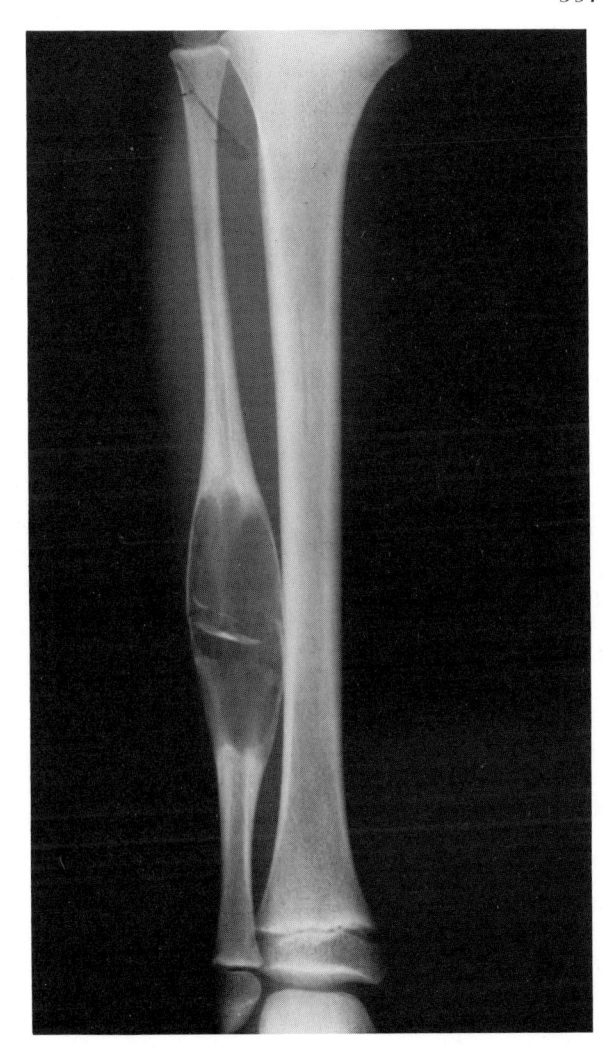

Fig. 7.2 Simple cyst of the fibula. Note the typical features of a benign lesion: the cyst has a well defined margin and a thin layer of subperiosteal new bone. This cyst contains greenish water fluid but the lower half is more opaque as a result of bleeding from a fracture. The fracture fragments within the cyst produce the 'fallen fragment sign' which is typical of this cyst.

clear demarcation between the lesion and the normal bone. The margin may also be scalloped or undulating—as in chondromyxoid fibromas and fibrous cortical defects. The overlying subperiosteal bone also requires careful examination: with benign lesions there is a well defined layer of subperiosteal bone which is laid down as the lesion gradually enlarges. However, the subperiosteal bone may be thick and sclerotic, as in osteoid osteomas, but its uniform nature distinguishes it from the patchy sclerosis seen with osteosarcomas. Some benign lesions also show hypertrophy of remaining trabeculae which produces the thickened septa in the chondromyxoid fibromas and the vertical striations which are commonly seen in haemangiomas of the vertebral bodies.

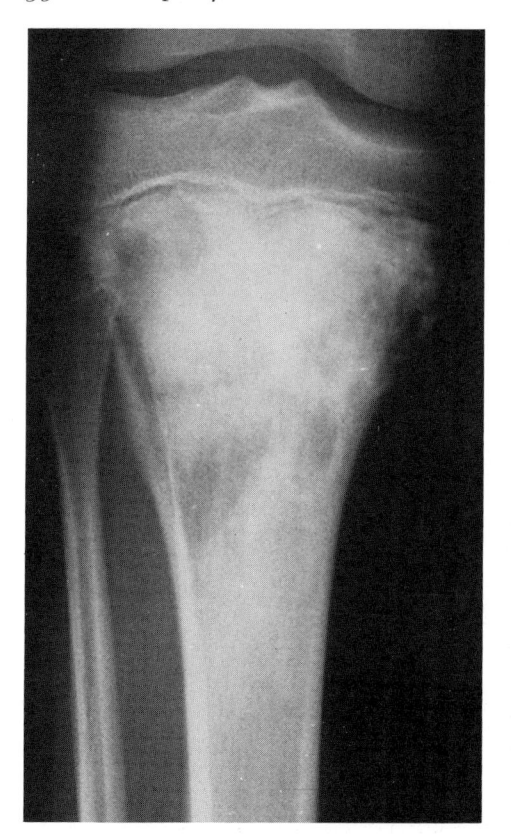

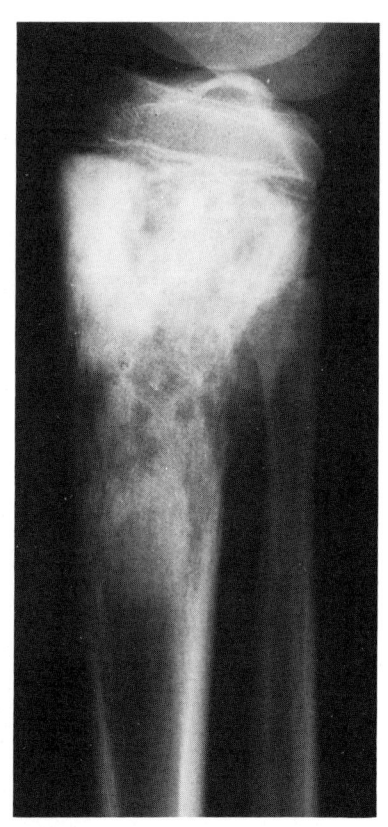

Figs. 7.3 & 7.4 Osteosarcoma of the proximal tibia in a 10-year-old boy. Note the typical features of an aggressive lesion. The tumour has poorly defined margins and there is loss of the normal trabecular bone pattern in the metaphysis and destruction of the overlying cortex with extension of the tumour into the soft tissue. There is patchy sclerosis due to tumour bone and there is a pathological fracture extending obliquely across the middle of the tumour. There is also subperiosteal new bone on the lateral side. The lateral view shows extensive destruction of the normal bone with a soft tissue mass posteriorly.

Aggressive lesions show a poorly defined margin often with evidence of infiltration of the tumour into the normal bone and into the soft tissue (Figs. 7.3 & 7.4). The aggressive nature of the tumour also produces a different pattern of periosteal reaction to that seen with benign lesions (Fig. 7.5). Repeated elevations of the periosteum by the rapidly growing tumour produces the characteristic 'onion skin' laminations of subperiosteal bone as seen in Ewing's sarcoma. More rapidly growing tumours, such as osteosarcomas, frequently produce radially directed bone spicules aligned along Sharpey's fibres and radially directed blood vessels producing the characteristic 'sunburst' pattern. The Codman's triangle is also another feature of rapidly growing lesions and is produced by subperiosteal new bone at the site where the periosteum becomes detached from the bone at the margins of the tumour

Bone Tumours 359

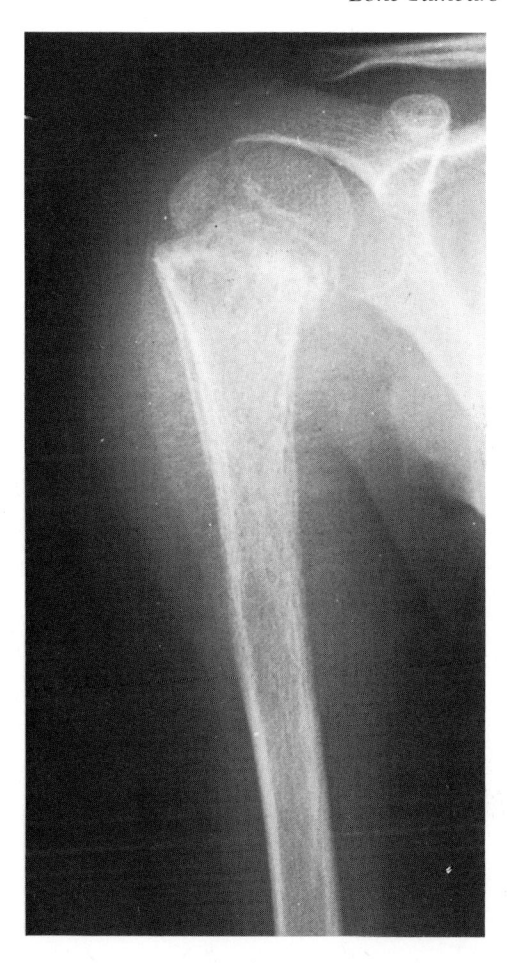

Fig. 7.5 Ewing's sarcoma of the proximal humerus. This lesion has the typical features of a primary malignant bone tumour. There is destruction of the metaphyseal and diaphyseal bone with a fracture through the proximal metaphysis. There is a 'sunburst' pattern of new bone formation on the medial and lateral sides of the humerus as well as laminated new bone formation on the lateral side. There is also a large soft tissue swelling.

The contents of an aggressive lesion frequently show evidence of rapid bone destruction with loss of the overlying cortex and extension of the tumour into the soft tissues. Areas of patchy sclerosis due to the formation of tumour bone are a common feature of osteosarcomas.

Radiological features of specific bone tumours

The radiological features of some of the more common bone tumours and related lesions will be considered.

LESIONS PROTRUDING FROM THE BONE

Osteochondromas. These lesions have a characteristic appearance: they protrude from the metaphysis adjacent to the growth plate; they are either pedunculated or

360 Chapter 7

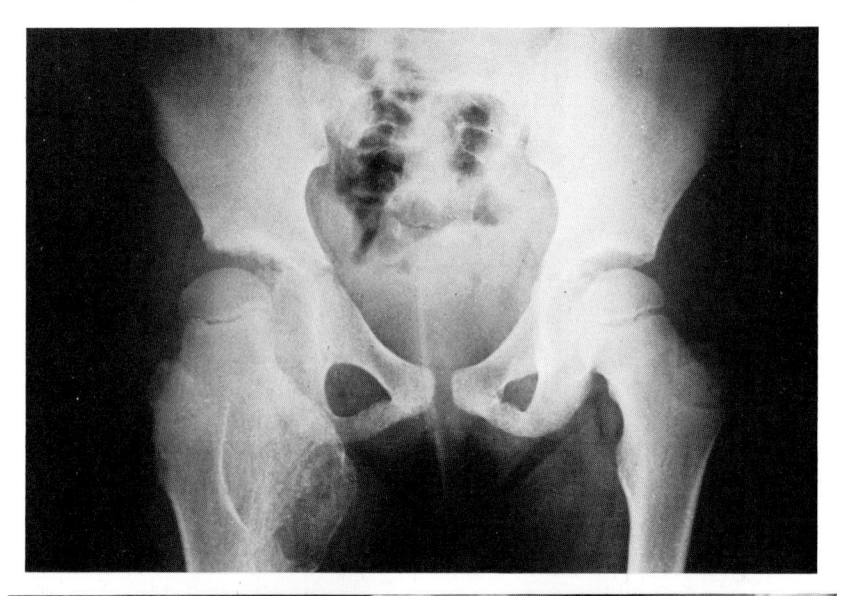

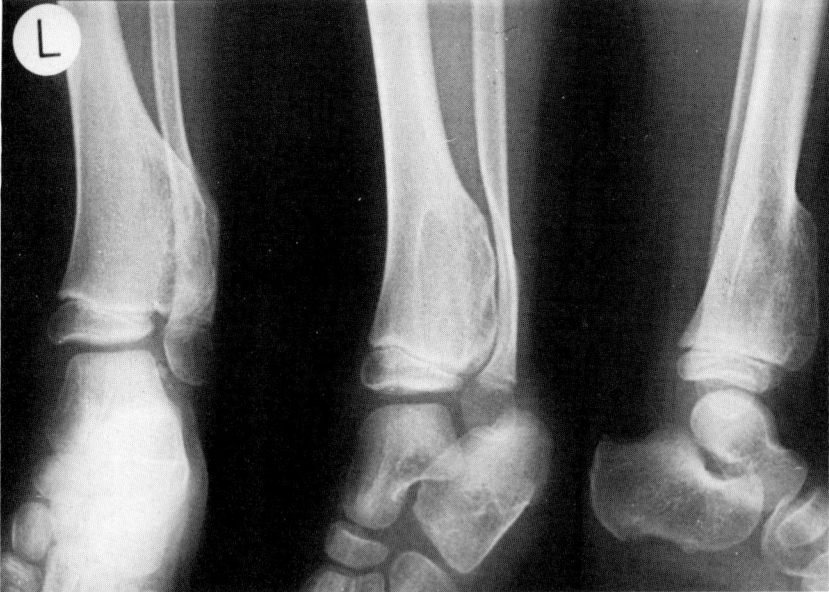

Figs. 7.6 & 7.7 Multiple osteochondromas in a child with diaphyseal aclasis. (*Top*) A large sessile osteochondroma on the medial side of the neck and upper femur. There is a coxa valga and the head of the femur is displaced laterally because of impingement of the osteochondroma against the pelvis. Progressive subluxation was prevented by excision of the lesion. (*Bottom*) A typical sessile osteochondroma of the distal tibia with characteristic deformation of the fibula. The tibial lesion frequently requires excision because of deformity, pain and ankle dysfunction but it is preferable to wait for the lesion to grow away from the growth plate.

sessile but the overlying cartilage cap is not visible on the x-ray; they grow away from the growth plate and cease growing at skeletal maturity; and they are often solitary, although children with the autosomal dominant disorder diaphyseal aclasis have osteochondromas on almost every bone (Figs. 7.6 & 7.7).

Osteomas. This bony lesion produces a hemispherical protrusion from the calvarium.

CYSTIC LESIONS

Simple bone cyst. This cyst contains greenish watery fluid. It is usually found as a concentric lesion in the metaphysis of the proximal humerus or the neck of the femur (Figs. 7.8–7.10). It often occupies the entire metaphysis and may produce

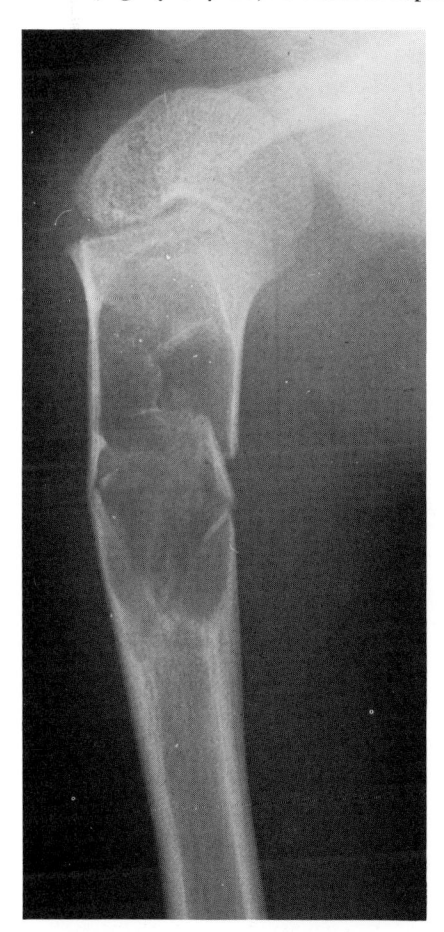

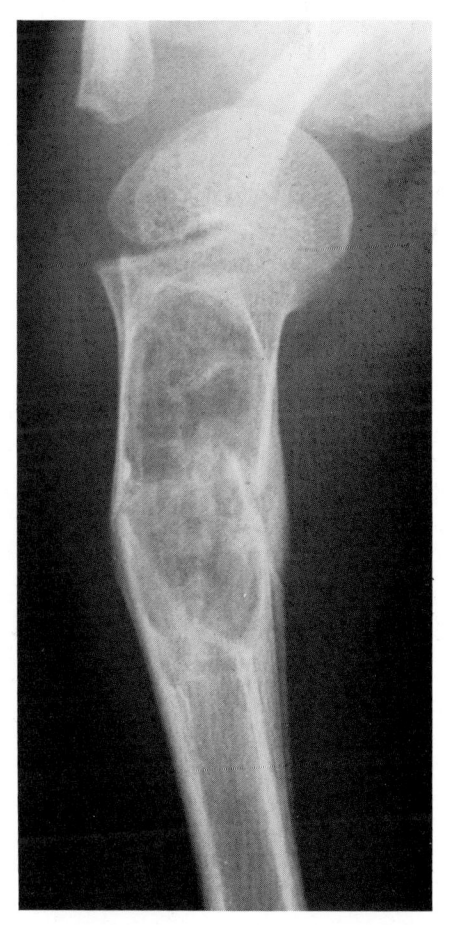

Figs. 7.8 & 7.9 A typical simple bone cyst of the proximal humerus with a fracture. (*Right*) Appearance of the cyst following healing of the fracture six weeks later. The lesion was not biopsied or surgically treated.

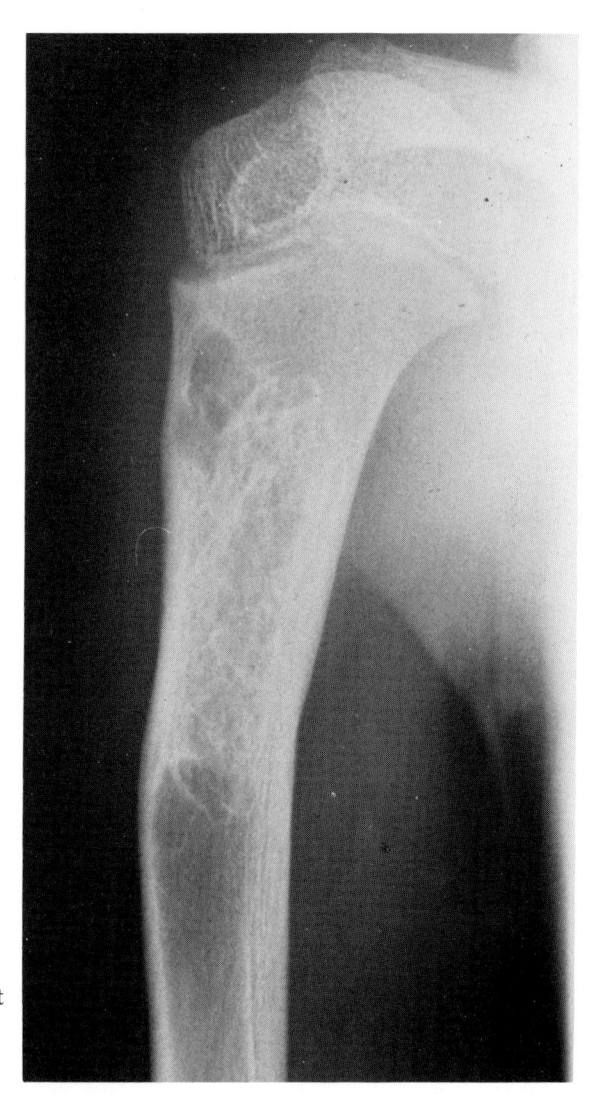

Fig. 7.10 Same patient as Fig. 7.8. Healing continues six months later.

some expansion of the bone. The fluid contents account for the structureless appearance of the cyst and the wall consists of a fine sclerotic line with rapid transition to bone of normal density. Fractures of the wall of the cyst are common and fragments of bone often fall to the bottom of the cyst.

Aneurysmal bone cyst. This cyst has a number of important distinguishing features from the simple bone cyst. It is more common in the proximal tibia and the pelvis, it is often eccentrically placed in the metaphysis, and it may become

Bone Tumours 363

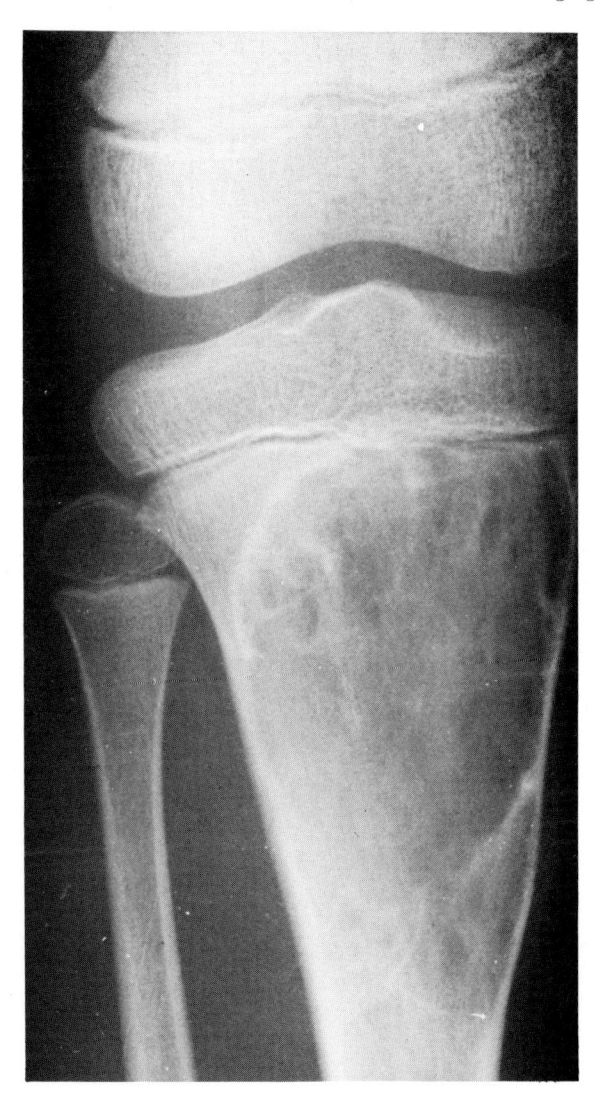

Fig. 7.11 Aneurysmal bone cyst of the proximal tibia. The cyst expanded rapidly.

large with marked expansion of the bone (Fig. 7.11). It usually has a multilocular appearance and the overlying subperiosteal bone may be deficient where the contents have extended into the adjoining soft tissue. Rapidly expanding cysts and cysts where the contents have spread into the soft tissues are features indicating that the cyst is behaving in an aggressive manner (Fig. 7.12).

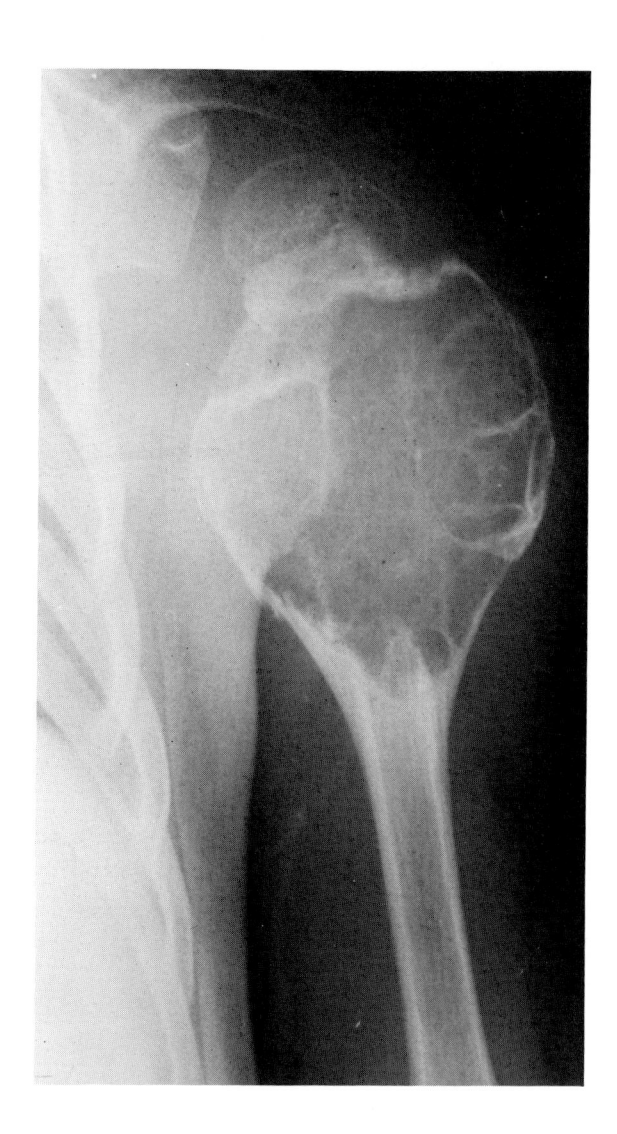

Fig. 7.12 Rapidly growing aneurysmal bone cyst of the proximal humerus.

Osteoblastoma. This tumour resembles the aneurysmal bone cyst. It occurs most commonly in the posterior elements of the spine.

Non-ossifying fibroma. This cystic lesion is located in the cortex of the metaphysis of the long bones, in particular the femur and the tibia. The internal margin of the lesion is sclerotic and the overlying cortical bone is thin and bulging. Small lesions are often referred to as fibrous cortical defects or metaphyseal fibrous defects and larger lesions as non-ossifying fibromas (Figs. 7.13 & 7.14).

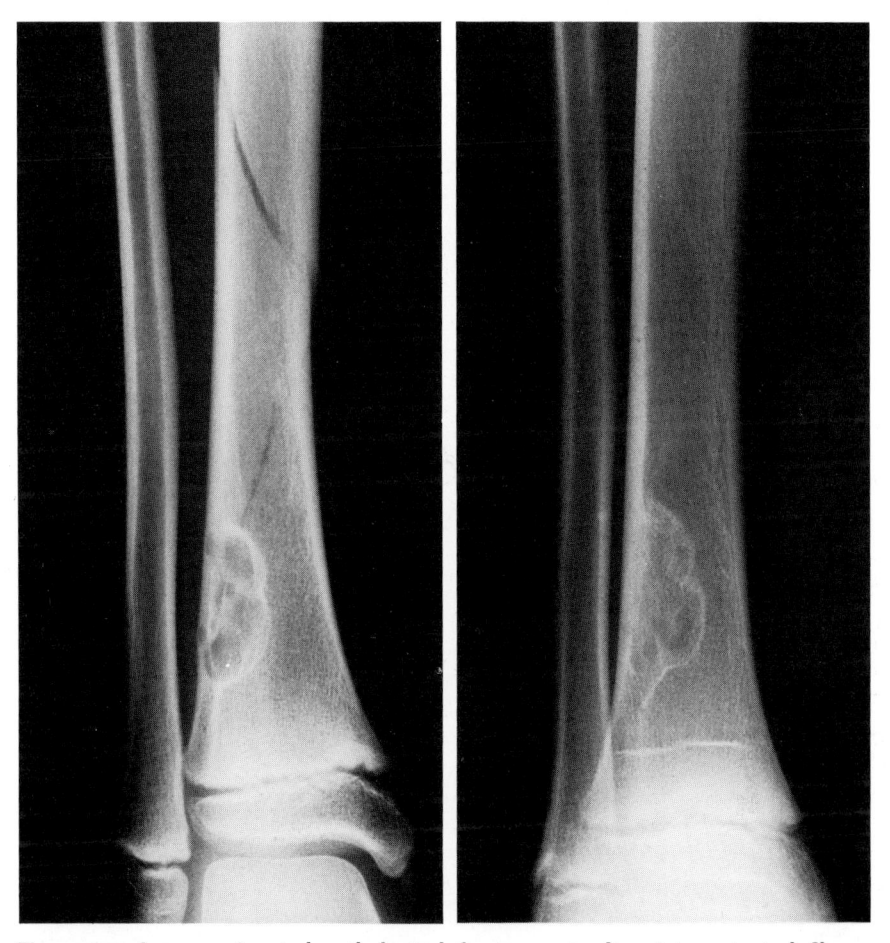

Figs. 7.13 & 7.14 A spiral pathological fracture extending into a typical fibrous cortical defect of the lower tibia. It is eccentrically placed in the cortex and has a scalloped, well defined, inner margin. (*Right*) Two years later the overlying cortex is returning to normal and the contents of the cyst are undergoing ossification indicating that the lesion is healing.

Fibrous dysplasia. This lesion in bone produces a 'ground glass' appearance due to the mixture of fibrous tissue and small pieces of trabecular bone. The margins of the lesion are frequently undulating and there may be mild expansion of the bone. Fibrous dysplasia may occupy the full length of a bone such as the femur and produce progressive bowing with a 'shepherd's crook' deformity and repeated fractures. It may also be localised to the metaphysis or to the diaphysis.

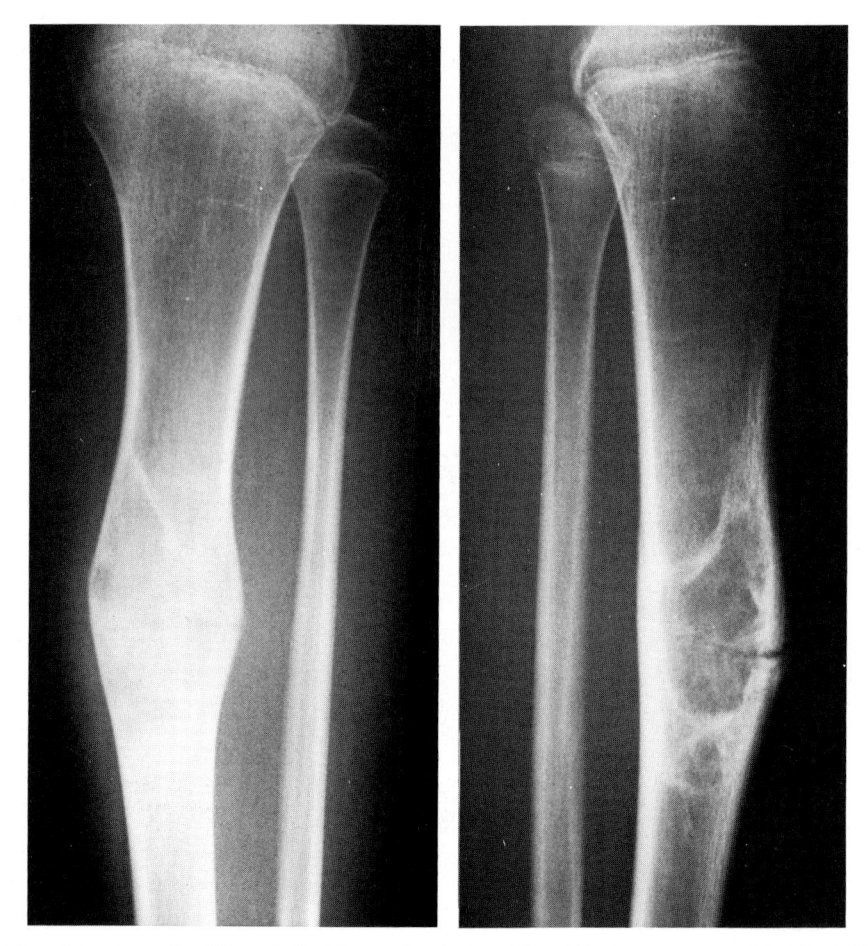

Figs. 7.15 & 7.16 Monostotic fibrous dysplasia of the tibia in a 12-year-old girl. A–P x-ray of the lesion in the tibia. The central part of the diaphysis is expanded and contains lucent and sclerotic areas. The inner border of the cortex has an undulating appearance. The lateral view shows the stress fracture and the typical ground glass appearance of fibrous dysplasia. This lesion was first noted at the age of 4 years and the diagnosis confirmed by biopsy, but curettage and bone grafting at the age of 5 years was unsuccessful.

Lesions in the diaphysis of the tibia frequently produce a marked forward bow of the tibia (Figs. 7.15 & 7.16). Fibrous dysplasia may also be polyostotic in which case it is often associated with skin pigmentation and endocrine abnormalities such as precocious puberty and is then designated as the Albright's syndrome (Figs. 7.17 & 7.18).

Enchondroma. These lesions are commonly seen in the phalanges, metacarpals and metatarsals. They usually have an oval appearance and are located in the

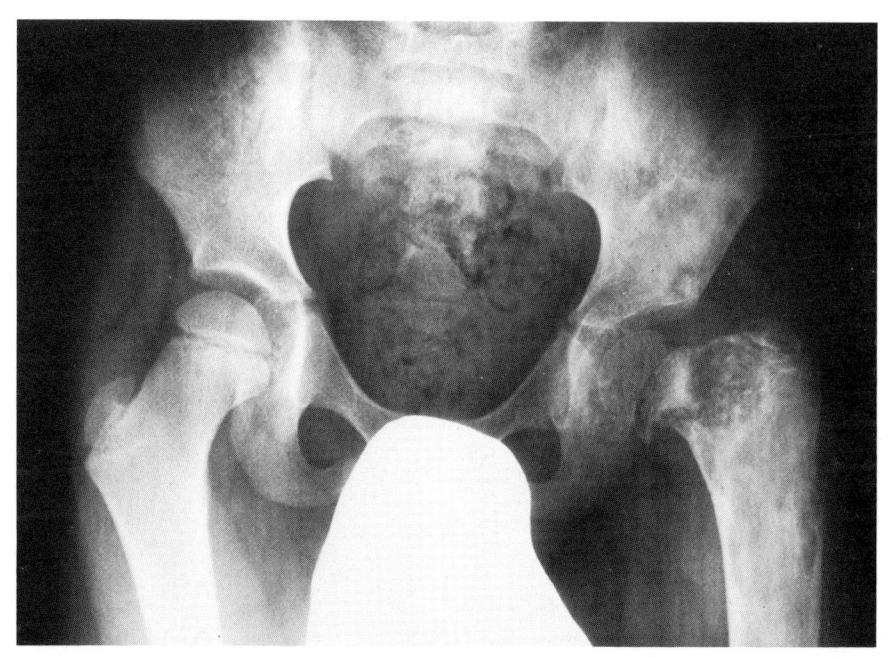

Fig. 7.17 Polyostotic fibrous dysplasia in an 8-year-old boy. Note the unilateral involvement of the pelvis and femur. There is a marked coxa vara with a pathological fracture through the lucent lesion in the neck of the femur.

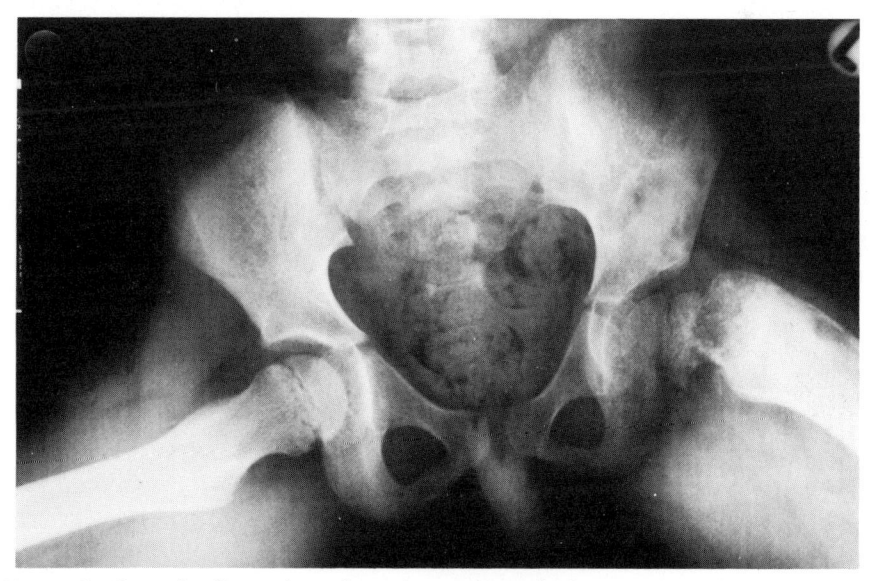

Fig. 7.18 Lateral radiograph confirms the presence of a fracture through this area. The fracture united following restoration of the normal neck shaft angle using a Pauwel's osteotomy of the proximal femur.

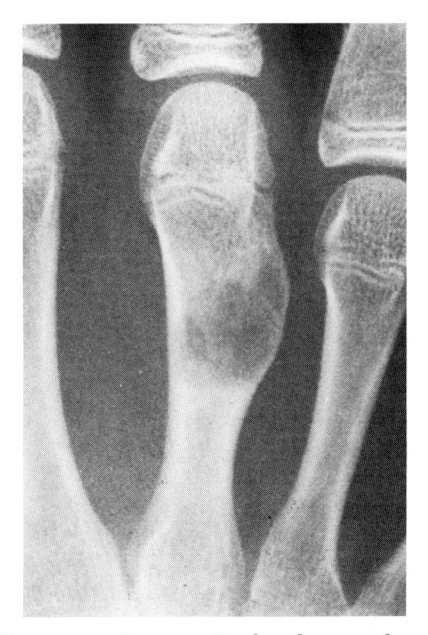

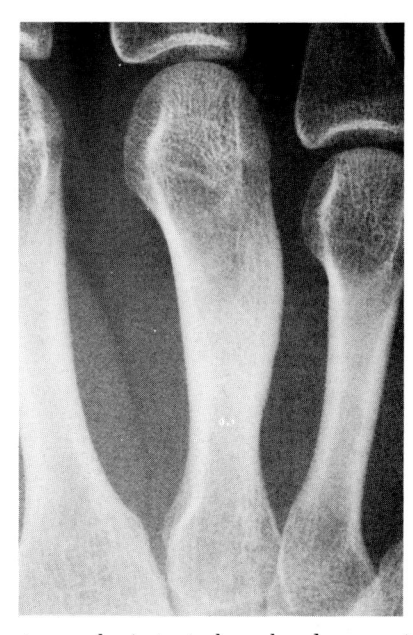

Figs. 7.19 & 7.20 Enchondroma of a metacarpal. A typical enchondroma with expansion and thinning of the cortex and stippled calcification of the matrix. (*Right*) Film taken two years later. The lesion healed following curettage.

Fig. 7.21
Chondroblastoma of the proximal humerus. A cystic lesion is present in the greater tuberosity and extends across the growth plate into the epiphysis; there is also loss of the overlying bone. The matrix shows a small amount of spotty calcification. A cure can usually be achieved by curettage and bone grafting. However this lesion recurred on two occasions and, because of its locally aggressive nature, the proximal end of the humerus was excised.

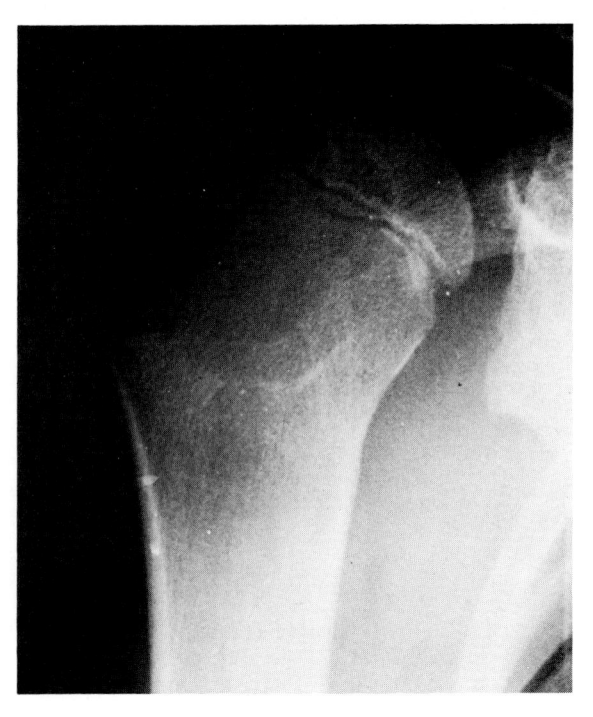

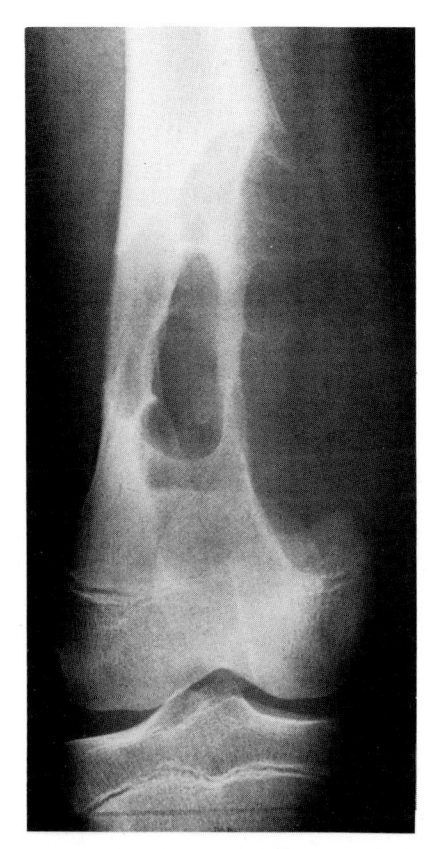

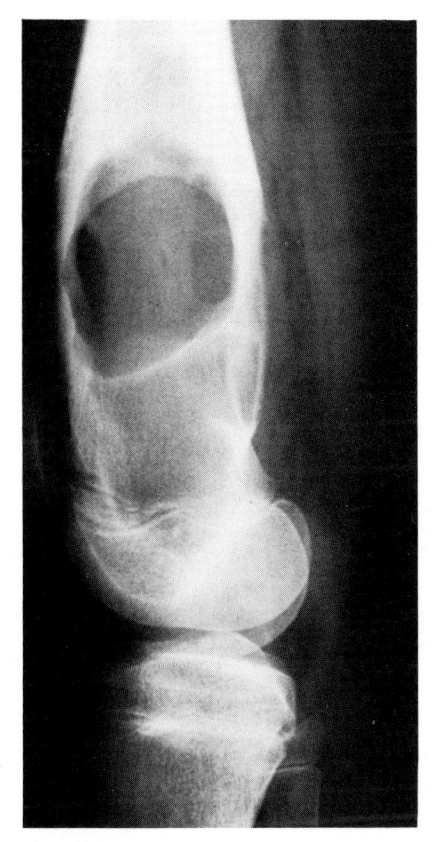

Figs. 7.22 & 7.23 Chondromyxoid fibroma of the lower femur. Antero-posterior appearance of a multiloculated cyst with complete absence of the medial cortex and displacement of the soft tissues by the tumour. The lateral view shows expansion of the distal femur. At operation the periosteum was intact but the medial cortex was absent and there were several other holes in the cortex. The intervening cortical bone was hypertrophied. A cure was achieved by curettage and packing with homograft bone.

metaphysis and diaphysis of these bones (Figs. 7.19 & 7.20). The contents have a characteristic speckled appearance due to spotty calcification within the cartilage. The overlying cortex is often thin and bulging and pathological fractures are common.

Chondroblastoma. This tumour occupies the epiphysis of long bones and may extend to the subchondral bone plate and can also extend across the epiphyseal plate into the adjacent metaphysis. It is common in the greater tuberosity of the upper humerus where the lesion is found to be round or ovoid and is usually eccentrically placed (Fig. 7.21). The contents of the lesion have a fuzzy, mottled appearance due to spotty calcification of the cartilage within the lesion. The

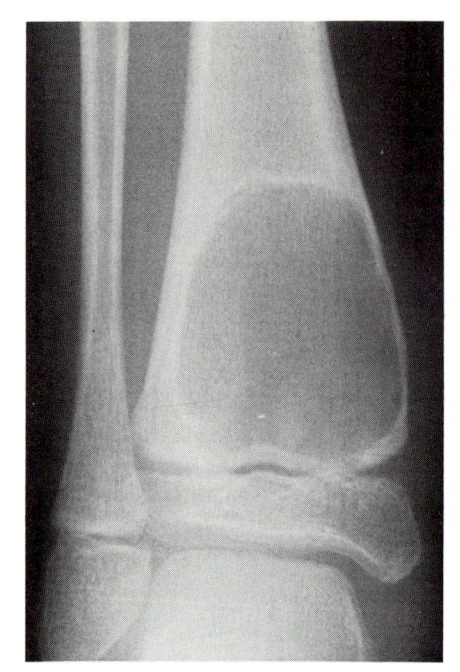

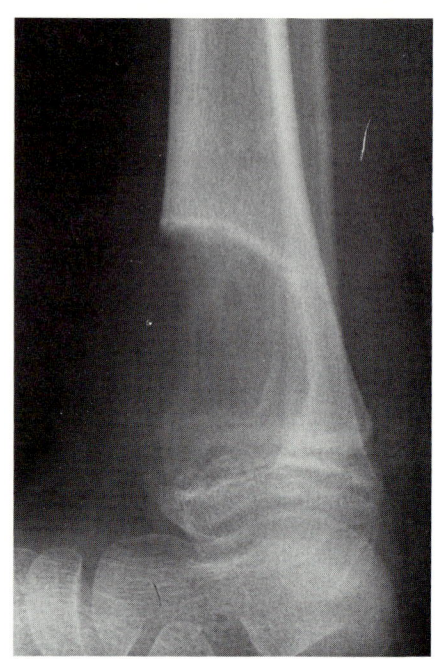

Figs. 7.24 & 7.25 Chondromyxoid fibroma of the distal tibia. A unilocular cystic lesion with a well defined margin and slight expansion of the medial cortex. The lateral view shows that the anterior cortex is absent. At operation the anterior periosteum was intact. A cure was achieved by curettage and bone grafting and the lower tibial growth plate continued to grow normally.

margin is often sclerotic and, where the cortex has been expanded, a thin layer of subperiosteal bone usually remains.

Chondromyxoid fibroma. This is an eccentrically placed cystic lesion in the metaphysis of the long bones, in particular the lower femur and upper tibia (Figs. 7.22 & 7.23). The cyst is often large and expands the bone; it has a trabeculated appearance due to the corrugations on the inner surface of the wall of the lesion. The margin is well defined and may be sclerotic and scalloped though defects in the cortex are common (Figs. 7.24 & 7.25).

Eosinophilic granuloma. This localised form of histiocytosis X is particularly common in the flat bones and ribs where it produces a punched-out appearance without marginal sclerosis (Fig. 7.26). Eosinophilic granulomas also occur in the long bones but they frequently have a more aggressive appearance and may resemble a Ewing's sarcoma. In the vertebral column they characteristically produce a vertebra plana (Figs. 7.27 & 7.28).

Bone Tumours 371

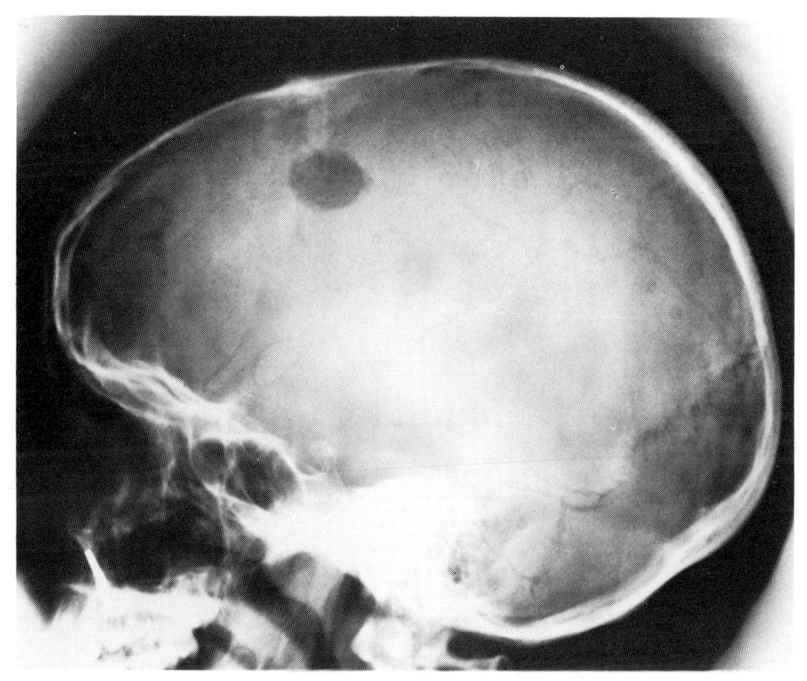

Fig. 7.26 Typical eosinophilic granuloma of the skull with a punched-out appearance.

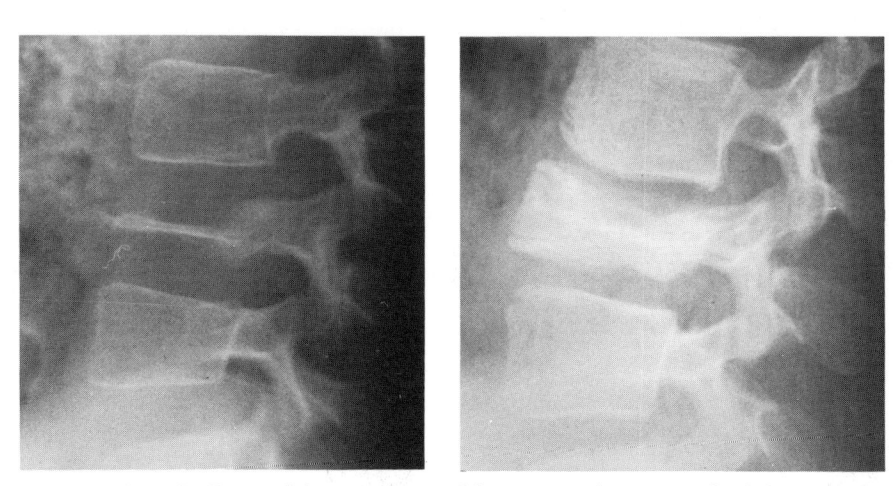

Figs. 7.27 & 7.28 Eosinophilic granuloma of the spine producing vertebral plana. (*Right*) Three years later there has been partial re-growth of the vertebra involved. No specific treatment was given.

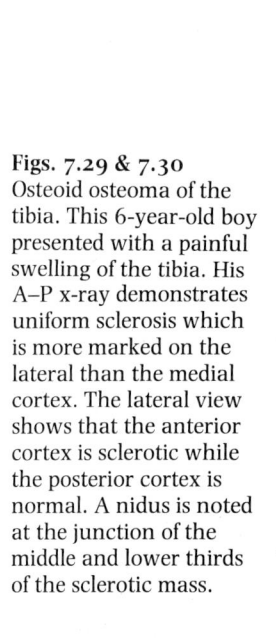

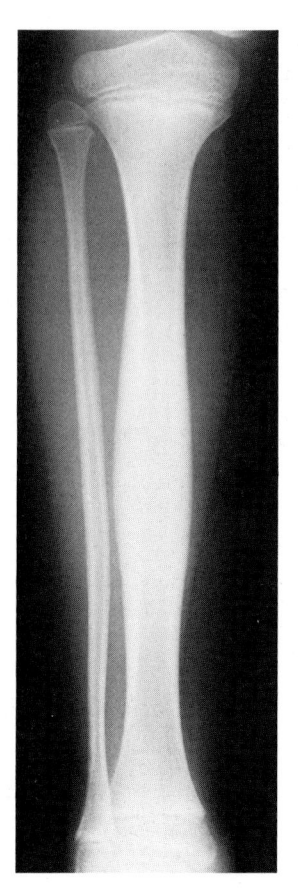

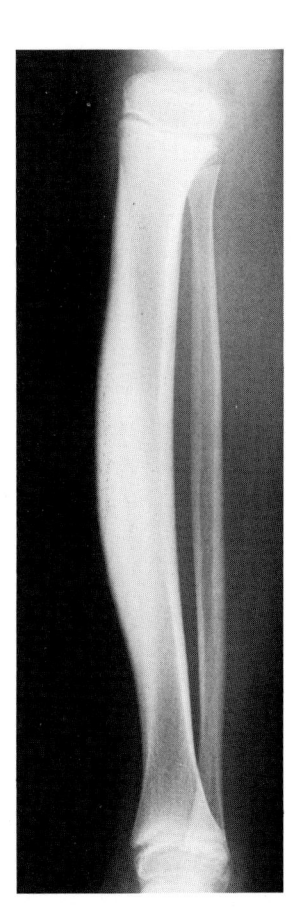

Figs. 7.29 & 7.30
Osteoid osteoma of the tibia. This 6-year-old boy presented with a painful swelling of the tibia. His A–P x-ray demonstrates uniform sclerosis which is more marked on the lateral than the medial cortex. The lateral view shows that the anterior cortex is sclerotic while the posterior cortex is normal. A nidus is noted at the junction of the middle and lower thirds of the sclerotic mass.

SCLEROTIC LESIONS

Osteoid osteoma. This lesion frequently gives rise to an eccentrically placed area of dense sclerosis in the cortex of the long bones (Figs. 7.29 & 7.30). The sclerotic bone has a uniform appearance and is a reaction to the osteoid osteoma which is best seen on tomograms as a small lucent nidus (Fig. 7.31). Sclerosis and enlargement of the pedicle of a vertebra is also suggestive of an osteoid osteoma and is best defined using computerised tomography. In addition, these lesions produce an intensely hot spot on radio-isotope bone scans.

STRIATED LESIONS

Haemangioma. This hamartomatous lesion is most commonly found in the vertebral bodies and in the calvarium. The striated appearance of the vertebral haemangiomas is due to hypertrophy of the vertical trabeculae. In the skull, the haemangiomas may have a honeycombed appearance or may show striations of bone radiating out from the centre of the lesion.

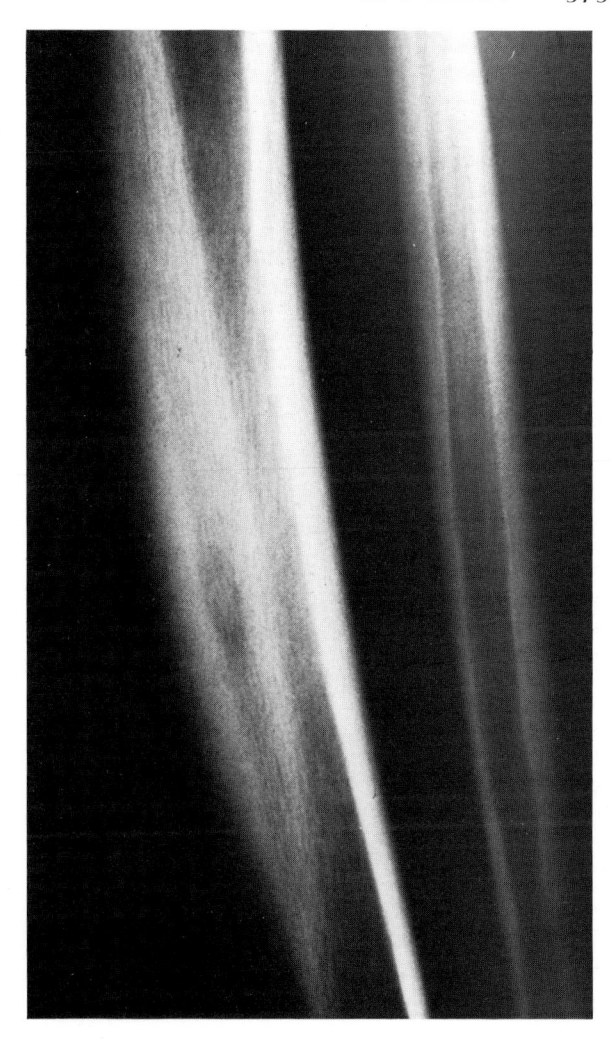

Fig. 7.31 Same case as Fig. 7.29. The nidus is well demarcated in this lateral tomogram. The boy's pain was immediately relieved by excision of the nidus.

AGGRESSIVE PRIMARY BONE TUMOURS

Osteosarcoma. This malignant bone tumour is commonly found in the metaphysis of the lower femur or upper tibia. It shows all the radiological features of a rapidly growing aggressive tumour (see p. 357). There is destruction of bone with invasion of normal bone extending into the subperiosteal layer and into the soft tissues. There are often patchy areas of tumour bone within the mass and there may be a 'sunburst' or 'onion skin' periosteal reaction and a Codman's triangle

374 Chapter 7

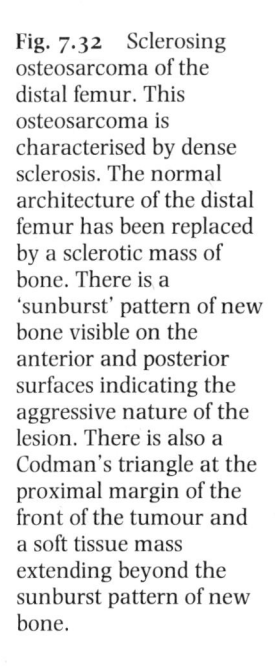

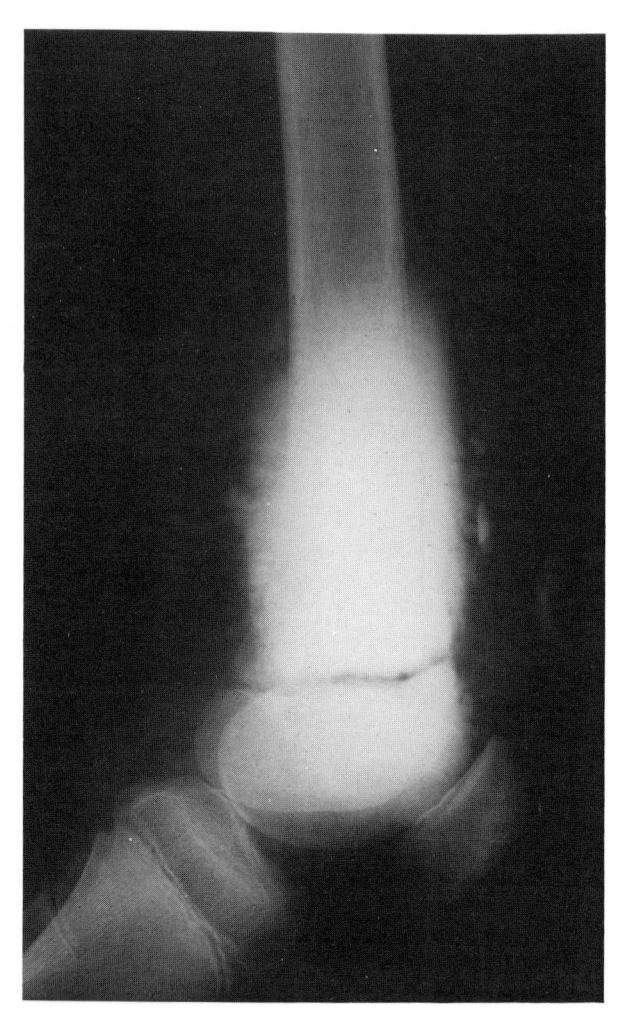

Fig. 7.32 Sclerosing osteosarcoma of the distal femur. This osteosarcoma is characterised by dense sclerosis. The normal architecture of the distal femur has been replaced by a sclerotic mass of bone. There is a 'sunburst' pattern of new bone visible on the anterior and posterior surfaces indicating the aggressive nature of the lesion. There is also a Codman's triangle at the proximal margin of the front of the tumour and a soft tissue mass extending beyond the sunburst pattern of new bone.

(Fig. 7.32). However, there is considerable variation in the appearance of osteosarcomas depending on the composition of the matrix (Figs. 7.33 & 7.34). Periosteal and parosteal osteosarcomas are located on the outer surface of the bone but, with time, they invade the underlying cortex. They are frequently sclerotic but there are usually features which indicate its aggressive nature.

Ewing's sarcoma. Ewing's sarcoma may also occur in the metaphysis but is more common in the diaphysis. It also has the characteristic features of an aggressive lesion with destruction of bone and infiltration of the tumour into normal bone (see p. 357). In addition there is frequently an 'onion skin' type of periosteal reaction and extension of the tumour into the soft tissue (Figs. 7.35 & 7.36).

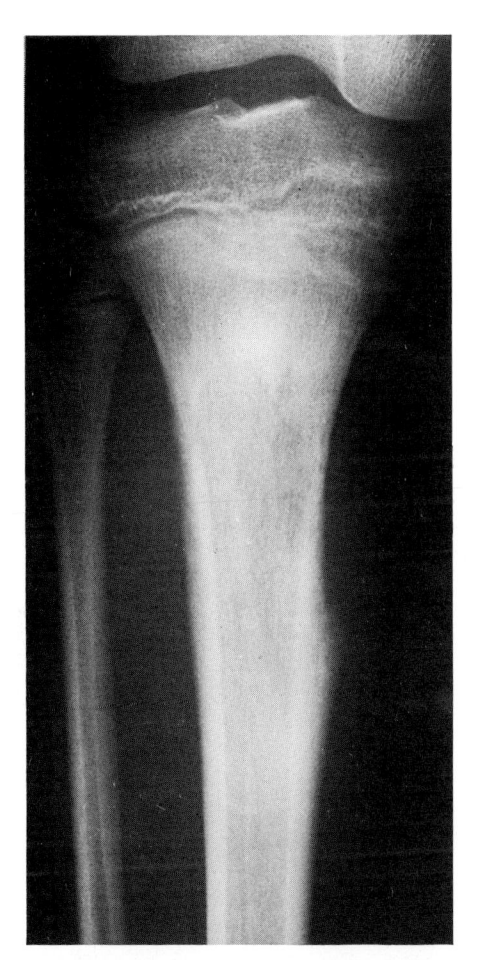

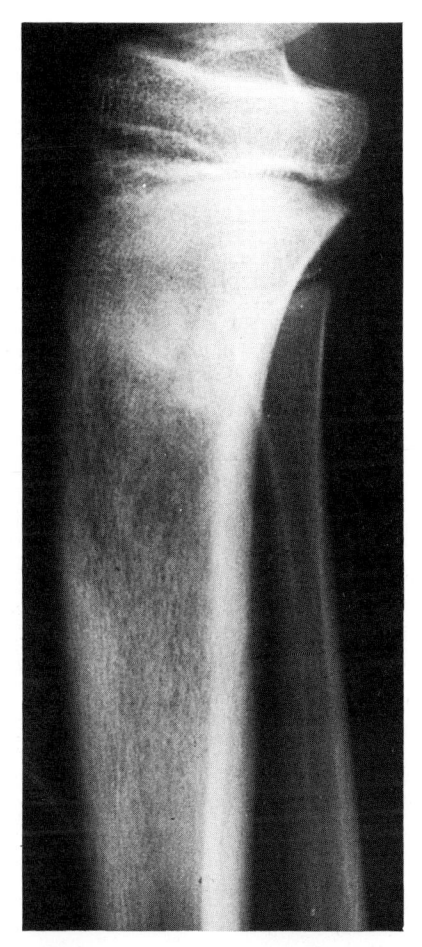

Figs. 7.33 & 7.34 Osteosarcoma of the proximal tibia in a 9-year-old boy. The poorly defined A–P view shows that the cortices are partially destroyed and there are areas of patchy sclerosis within the lesion. The medial cortex of the tibia is thickened at the distal end of the lesion due to subperiosteal new bone formation. On the lateral view, note the cortical erosions and patchy sclerosis. This lesion did not show the degree of destruction, sclerosis or subperiosteal new bone formation often seen with osteosarcomas.

Histiocytosis X. As this lesion may produce destruction of bone with an 'onion skin' type of periosteal reaction, it always needs to be considered as an alternative diagnosis to Ewing's sarcoma (Figs. 7.37 & 7.38).

Fibrosarcoma. This primary malignant bone tumour produces extensive destruction with invasion of the adjoining bone but there is frequently little reactive bone formed.

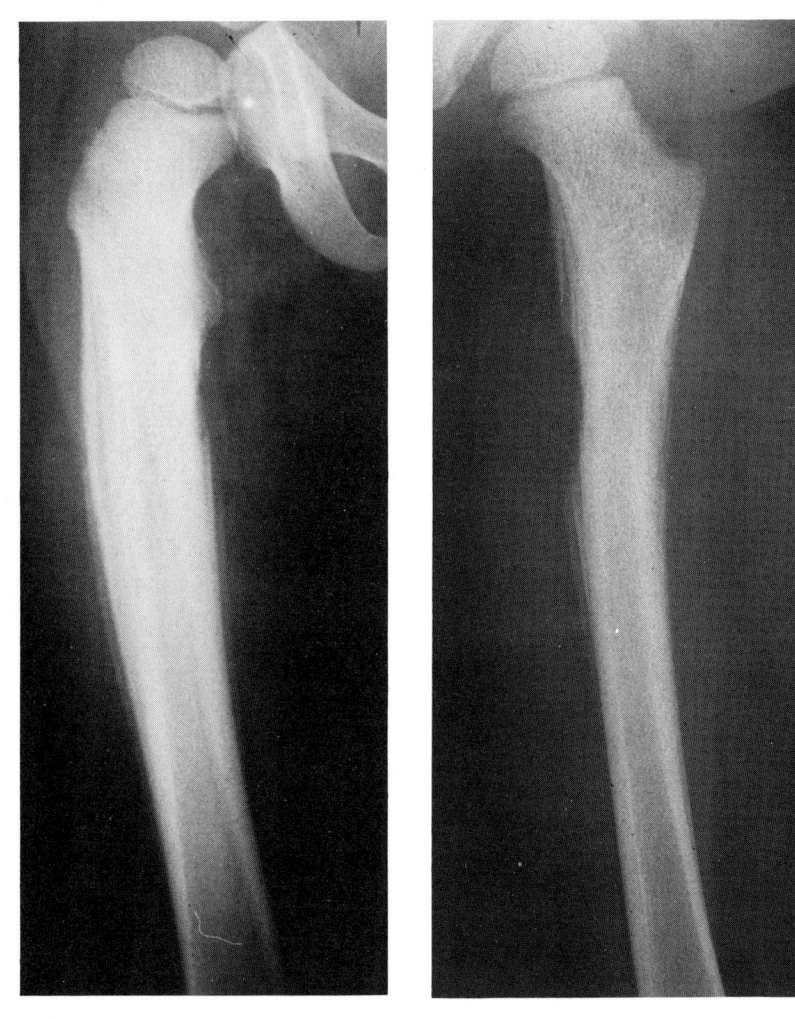

Figs. 7.35 & 7.36 Typical Ewing's sarcoma of the shaft of the femur. There is destruction of cortical bone and typical 'onion skin' new bone formation. In the lateral view the onion skin laminations of new bone are interrupted by an area of 'sunburst' reaction.

AGGRESSIVE SECONDARY BONE TUMOURS (FIG. 7.39, see p. 378)

Neuroblastoma. Neuroblastoma commonly produces multiple punched-out lesions in the skull and may produce destructive lesions in the peripheral skeleton (Fig. 7.40, see p. 379).

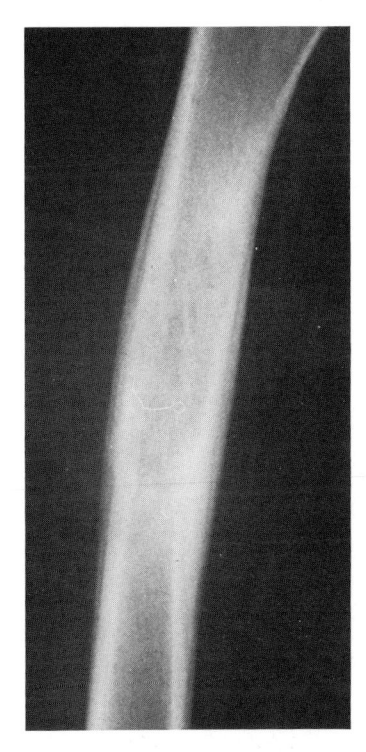

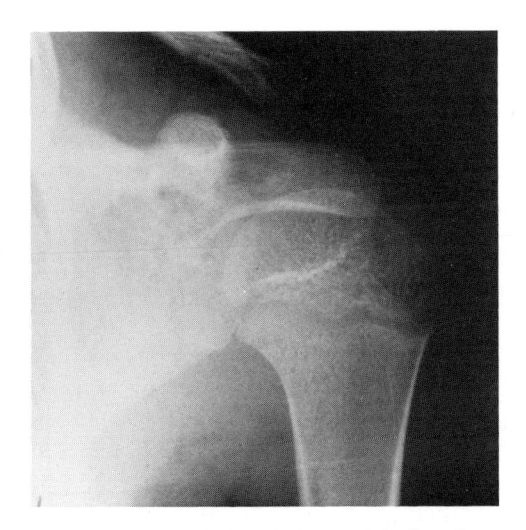

Figs. 7.37 & 7.38 Typical appearance of histiocytosis X in the diaphysis of the long bones in a 9-year-old girl. It is an aggressive poorly defined lesion with destruction of the cortex and shows laminated subperiosteal new bone. (*Right*) Same patient as Fig. 7.37. A destructive lesion in the neck of the scapula extending into the coracoid process and the acromion. Laminated subperiosteal new bone was also present on the acromion. Cure can usually be achieved by curettage or with curettage and bone grafting. However the scapular lesion recurred and, because of its rapid growth, the child was treated with chlorambucil which led to complete healing of the lesion.

Leukaemia. A line of metaphyseal rarefaction adjoining the growth plate is a characteristic feature of acute leukaemia but extensive areas of bone destruction with periosteal new bone formation may also occur (Fig. 7.41, see p. 379).

NON-NEOPLASTIC LESIONS

Osteomyelitis, stress fractures, exuberant callus and heterotopic ossification may give rise to aggressive features suggesting an oesteosarcoma (Figs. 7.42–7.46, see pp. 380–3).

378   *Chapter 7*

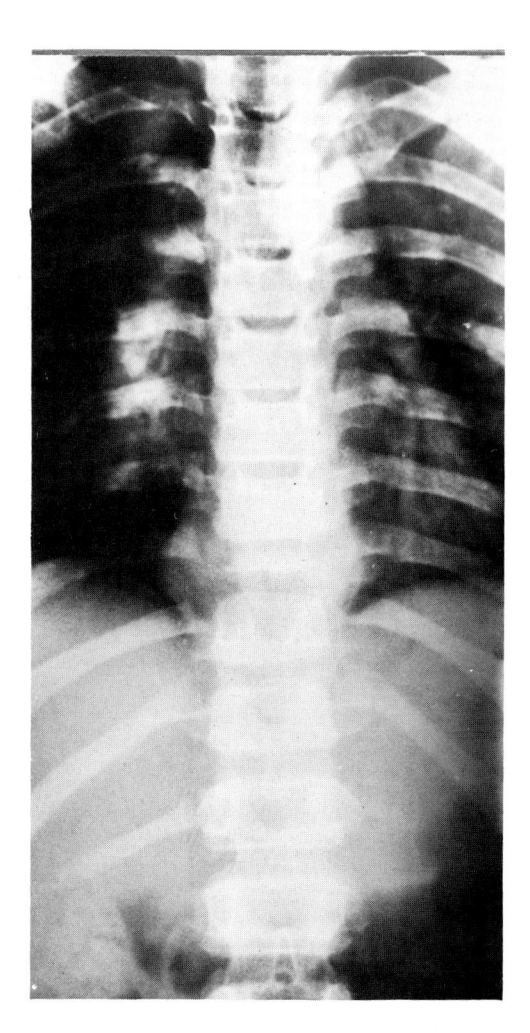

Fig. 7.39 Complete collapse of the 9th thoracic vertebra due to metastatic synovial sarcoma. The malignant nature of the lesion producing the collapse is indicated by the extensive soft tissue swelling. Eosinophilic granulomas also produce vertebra plana but rarely soft tissue swelling.

RADIO-ISOTOPE BONE SCANNING

The skeleton may be scanned following the injection of radio-isotopes such as ^{99m}technetium polyphosphate. The exact mechanism of uptake of these complexes by the bone has not yet been determined. The agent may interchange with the surface of the hydroxy apatite crystal or bind to newly formed collagen. Increased uptake of the radio-isotope is observed wherever there is increased bone formation.

Most primary malignant bone tumours have a markedly increased uptake of the isotope but there is also frequently an increased uptake beyond the radiological confines of the tumour. Patchy areas of increased activity may

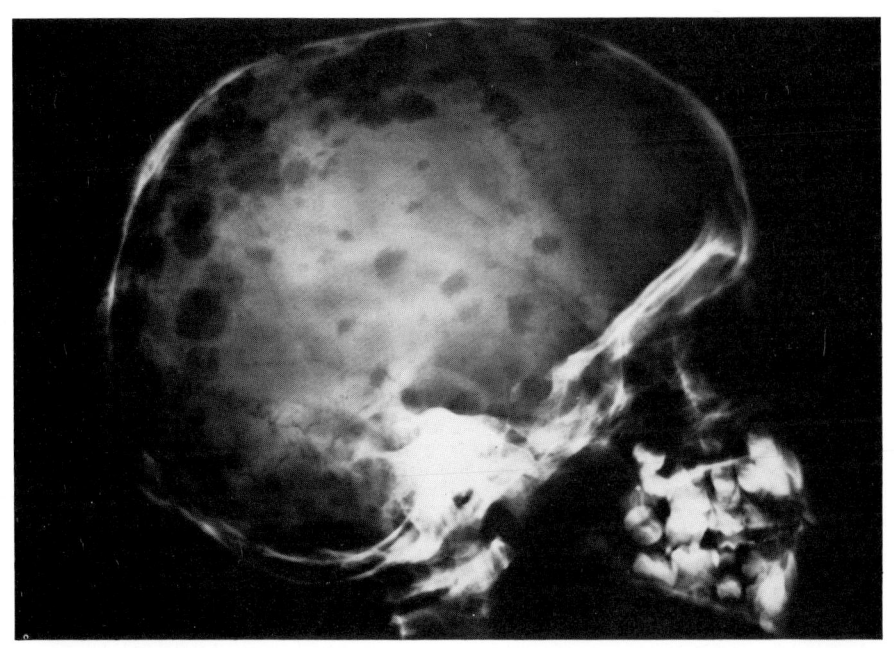

Bone Tumours 379

Fig. 7.40 Secondary neuroblastoma producing typical punched-out lesions within the skull.

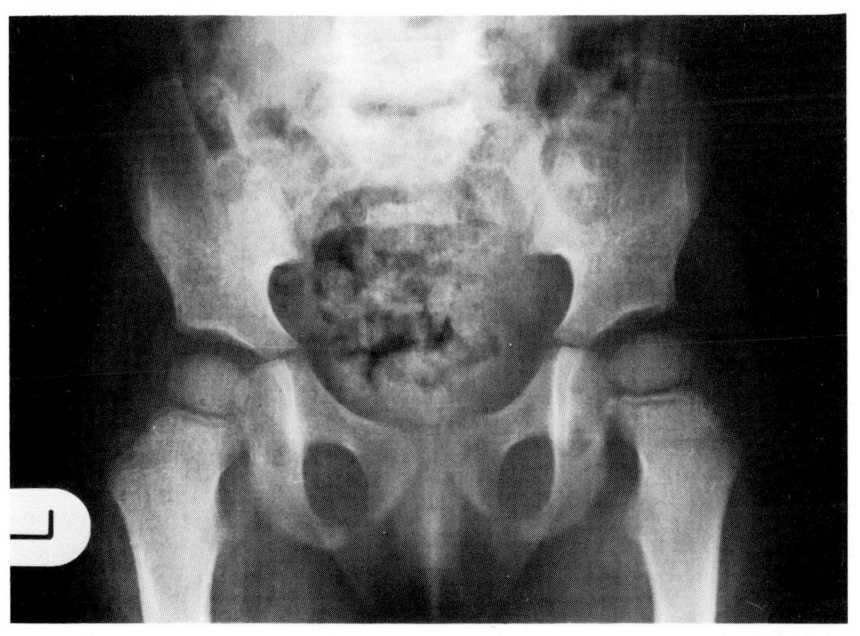

Fig. 7.41 Acute leukaemia. There is generalised osteoporosis. Lucent lines in the metaphysis noted here in the upper femora and iliac crest are typical of acute leukaemia.

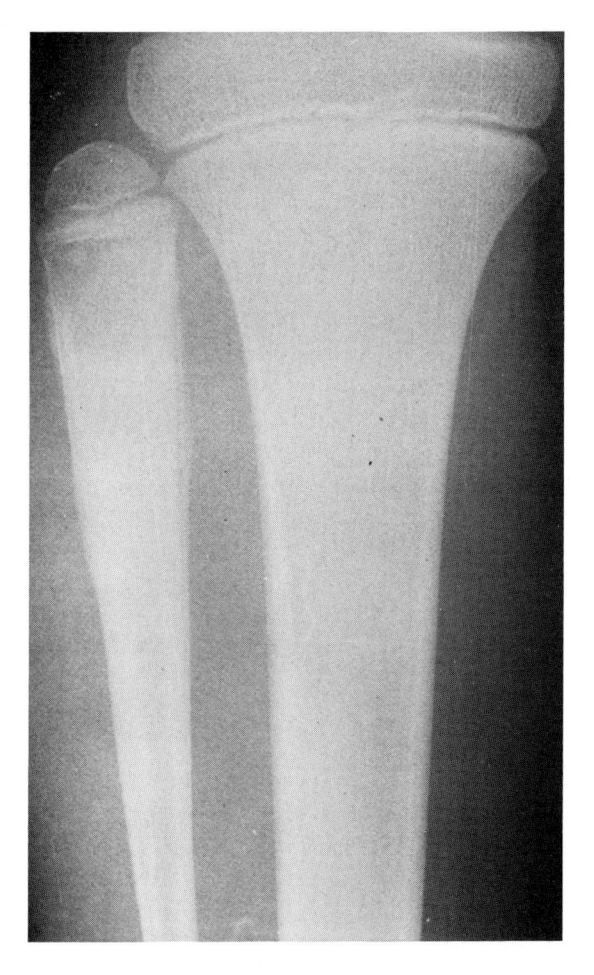

Fig. 7.42 Osteomyelitis of the proximal fibula. This child was thought to have Ewing's sarcoma because of a large swelling and the aggressive radiological features. At operation the upper fibula was expanded with subperiosteal new bone and the lucent area in the metaphysis contained granulation tissue and trabecular bone. Histology showed chronic osteomyelitis but the cultures were negative. The lesion has completely healed with antibiotic therapy.

indicate metastases while more uniform uptake reflects osteoporosis and increased bone turnover. This procedure has been shown to be a more sensitive method of detecting skeletal metastases than the standard skeletal radiological survey.

HAEMATOLOGY

A full blood examination and erythrocyte sedimentation rate are performed in all patients suspected of having a primary malignant bone tumour or histiocytosis X. The prognosis is usually worse in patients with primary malignant bone tumours who have an elevated erythrocyte sedimentation rate, anaemia, or a high white cell count. However, in many instances, the haematology investigations are normal but serve as a baseline for future reference.

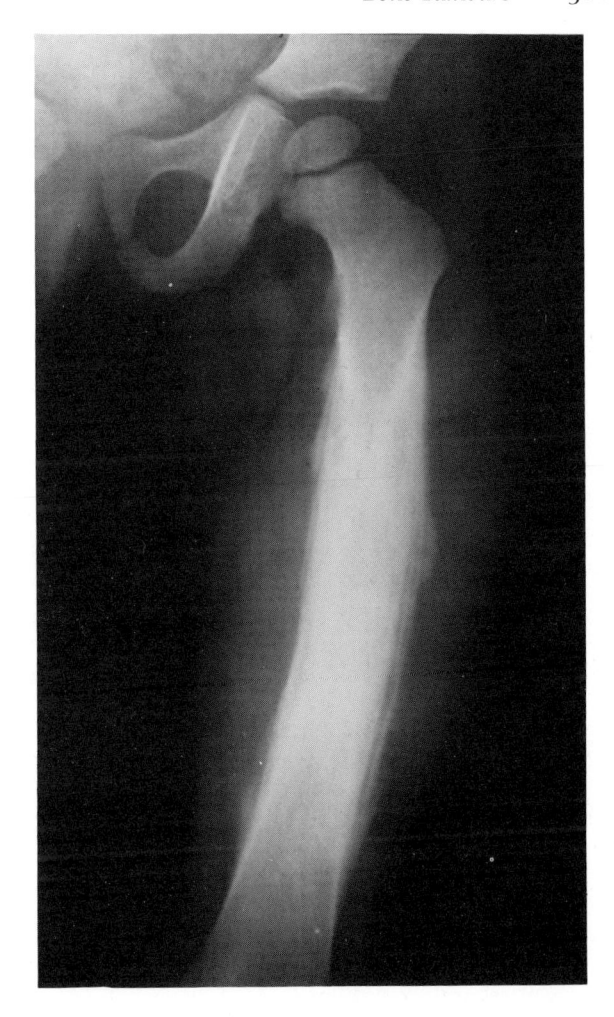

Fig. 7.43 Chronic osteomyelitis of the femur. This lesion of the diaphysis has aggressive features with a large soft tissue mass, patchy, laminated subperiosteal new bone with some areas of bone destruction but extensive sclerosis. These features are similar to those produced by Ewing's sarcoma but the extensive sclerosis of the shaft is unusual with that tumour.

BIOCHEMISTRY

Biochemical tests of liver function are always performed as a screening test for metastases within the liver. Urinary 3-methoxy, 4-hydroxy, mandelic acid levels are measured in children suspected of having neuroblastoma. In these children the bone marrow is also examined in order to stage the disease.

BIOPSY

While bone biopsy may seem to be a trivial procedure it needs to be carefully planned as all subsequent treatment will depend on a correct histological diagnosis. Pre-operative discussion with the pathologist and radiologist will enable the surgeon to plan his biopsy. This also ensures that the incision is placed

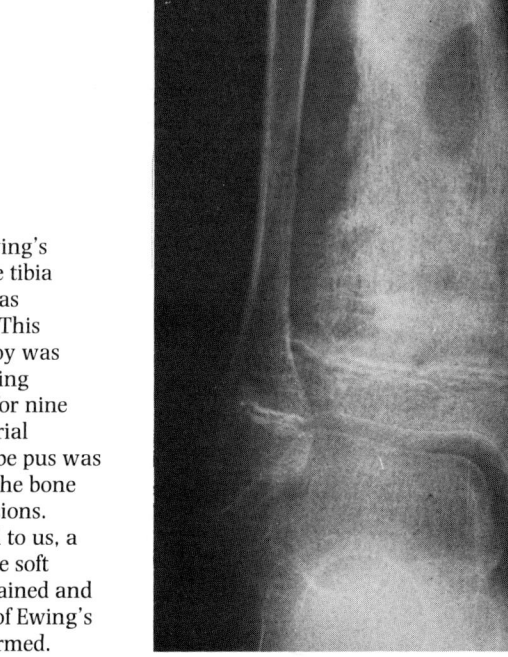

Fig. 7.44 Ewing's sarcoma of the tibia misdiagnosed as osteomyelitis. This 13-year-old boy was treated as having osteomyelitis for nine months. Material considered to be pus was drained from the bone on three occasions. When referred to us, a biopsy of viable soft tissue was obtained and the diagnosis of Ewing's sarcoma confirmed.

in a site which is appropriate for any further treatment that may be required. Whenever possible the biopsy is carried out in the hospital where further care can be given regardless of the nature of the lesion.

Open biopsy under general anaesthesia is the preferred method. It ensures that adequate material is collected for the pathologist as the macroscopic appearance of the tumour can be assessed and different regions of the tumour can be biopsied. In most instances an incisional biopsy will be carried out but, on occasions, such as with lesions in the rib or in the fibula, an excisional biopsy is carried out.

It is preferable for the pathologist to be present in the operating theatre during the biopsy. The aim of the procedure is to provide him with viable soft tissue which can be used for standard frozen and paraffin section histology, imprint cytology, and electron microscopy. The frozen sections are useful as they ensure the adequacy of the specimen although the pathologist may not wish to give a final diagnosis until he has examined the paraffin sections. Imprint cytology is an important procedure in the diagnosis of Ewing's sarcoma as glycogen can be

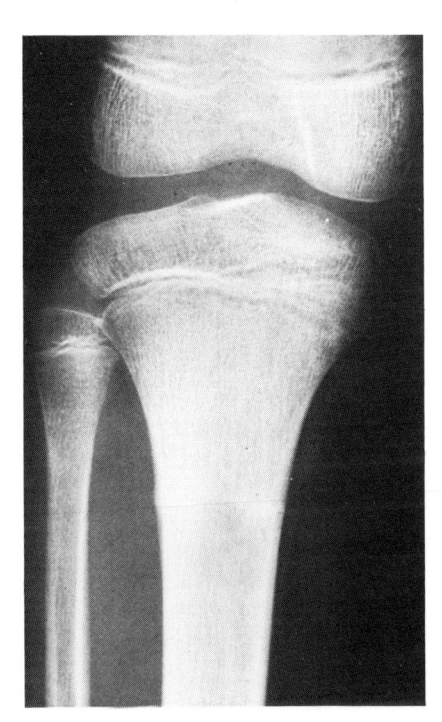

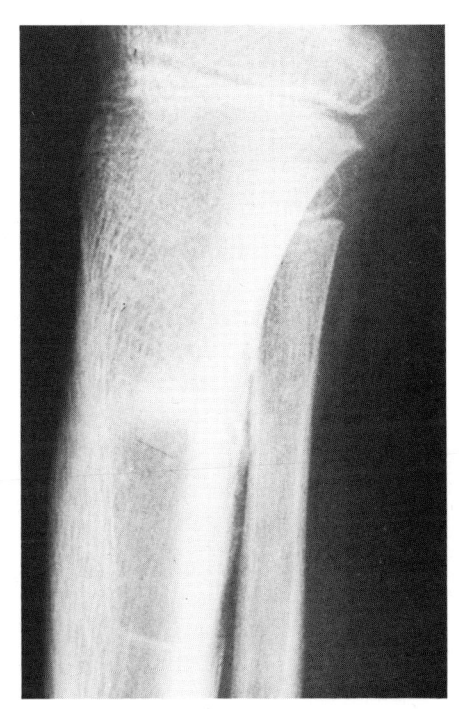

Figs. 7.45 & 7.46 Stress fracture of proximal tibia. Transverse sclerosis with a small amount of subperiosteal new bone on the lateral side. The lateral view shows an area of irregular subperiosteal new bone formation on the posterior surface of the tibia. These aggressive features often lead to confusion with malignant bone tumours such as osteosarcomas. If there is doubt about the nature of the lesion a biopsy is required.

readily demonstrated in the tumour cells with this technique. Ultrastructural examination of the tumours may also be helpful in arriving at a final diagnosis. However, for many tumours, the histological diagnosis will be made using the paraffin sections and the pathologist's opinion is usually available within a day following the biopsy—as long as he has been provided with an adequate soft tissue specimen. If the tumour contains a lot of bone, it will be necessary to decalcify the specimen which will often take four or five days. The pathologist should not be given reactive new bone, necrotic tissue, or tissue that has been diathermied or roughly handled.

Some lesions are obviously benign such as simple bone cysts, aneurysmal bone cysts and non-ossifying fibromas. It is reasonable, after scraping out the contents of the cyst and giving it to the pathologist, to proceed with packing the cavity with autogenous bone chips. It is also appropriate to excise the nidus of an osteoid osteoma completely. However, for lesions of uncertain nature and for lesions with malignant features, further treatment should await the histological diagnosis. Necrotic material resembling pus as well as material resembling granulation tissue is also collected for bacteriological examination.

TREATMENT

The principles of treatment of benign and malignant bone tumours and the protocols of treatment used for osteosarcoma and Ewing's sarcoma will be considered separately.

BENIGN TUMOURS

Several benign lesions that resemble bone tumours can be observed but the majority of bone tumours require surgical treatment. In the past, radiotherapy was frequently used to treat benign lesions as they usually regressed rapidly with relatively low dosages. However surgery should now be used instead of radiotherapy because of the risk of malignant transformation of benign tumours which is almost exclusively confined to children who have received radiotherapy.

Observation

Typical osteochondromas need not be excised unless they enlarge and produce discomfort or dysfunction. This also applies to children with diaphyseal aclasis as it is impractical to remove all the osteochondromas. Small typical fibrous cortical defects which are frequently a coincidental finding on an x-ray can also be observed and will usually heal spontaneously (see Figs. 7.13 & 7.14).

Surgery

CURETTAGE AND BONE GRAFT

As many benign tumours have a characteristic macroscopic appearance it is reasonable to carry out the definitive treatment at the time of biopsy. Simple bone cysts usually contain greenish fluid; aneurysmal bone cysts bleed excessively since they contain material like a blood-filled sponge; enchondromas contain bluish hyaline cartilage; and non-ossifying fibromas often contain a yellow mass of fibrous tissue. The contents of these cysts are removed by curettage and the cavity is packed with bone chips. It is unnecessary to graft small cysts and large cysts present many problems because of the amount of bone required to fill them. In very young children it is more convenient to use bank bone. Other materials—such as plaster balls—have been used to overcome the difficulty of obtaining sufficient bone graft.

Benign bone tumours may recur despite careful curettage and bone grafting. A second curettage is usually successful but difficulties are often encountered with simple bone cysts and aneurysmal bone cysts. Simple bone cysts will frequently persist despite repeated curettages and bone grafts. The reason for the persistence of the cyst and the resorption of the bone graft is unclear. Because of these difficulties it is often better to observe typical simple bone cysts in non-weight-bearing bones such as the proximal humerus. It is known that the cyst may heal following a fracture and it is also known that the cyst grows progressively towards the diaphysis and becomes surrounded by a thicker wall which decreases the susceptibility to fracture (see p. 361). It has been suggested that the injection of corticosteroids into this cyst may hasten its repair but this method requires further evaluation. If this cyst gives rise to repeated fractures or is located in important weight-bearing areas, such as the neck of the femur, then curettage and bone grafting is required as the first procedure and, if the cyst recurs, total excision of the cyst is carried out followed by the insertion of corticocancellous bone struts beneath the periosteum (Fig. 7.47).

Recurrence of aneurysmal bone cysts may present additional problems because of rapid growth and locally aggressive features. Total excision of rapidly growing aneurysmal bone cysts is often the only practical way of achieving a cure (Figs. 7.48–7.51). Longer lengths of corticocancellous bone are required than with simple bone cysts, but the rapid re-modelling of children's bones will lead to the rapid incorporation of the graft. Radiotherapy is contraindicated (Figs. 7.52–7.54).

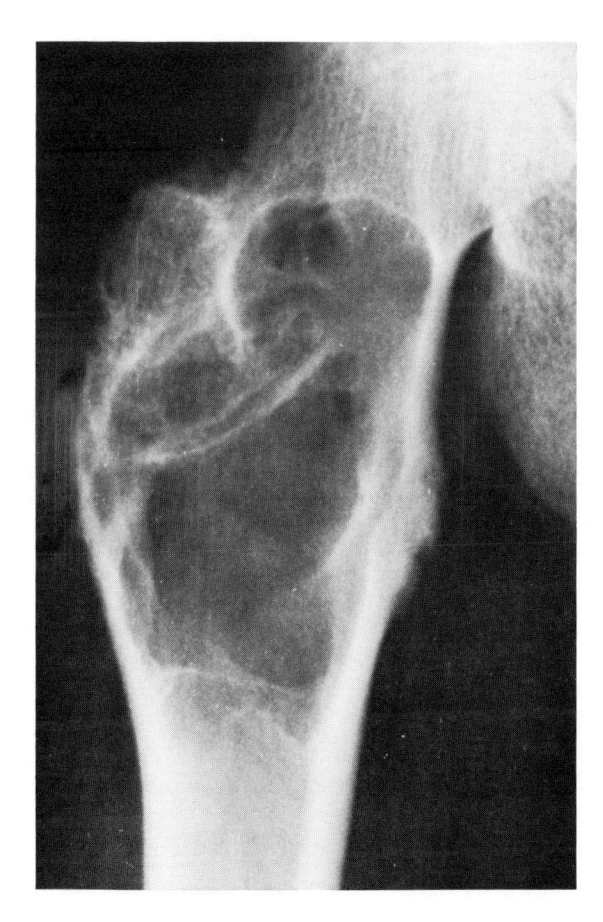

Fig. 7.47 Simple bone cyst of the neck of the femur in a 7-year-old boy. Because of the risk of repeated fractures, the cyst was curetted and bone grafted and corticocancellous grafts were laid beneath the periosteum on the medial side of the neck. The cyst recurred but the thickened medial cortex prevented further fracture.

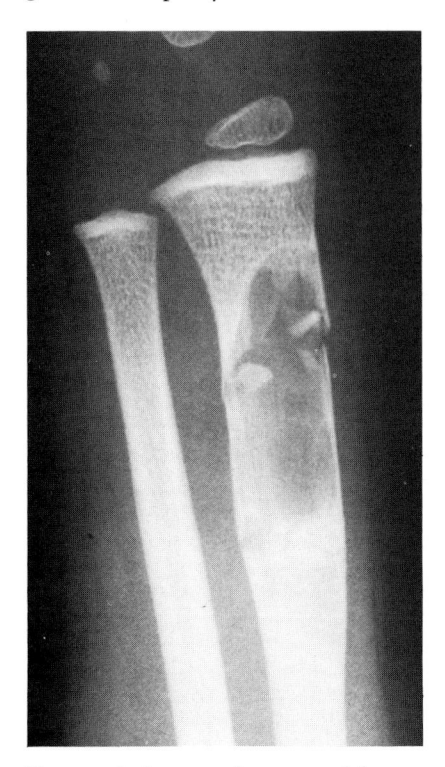

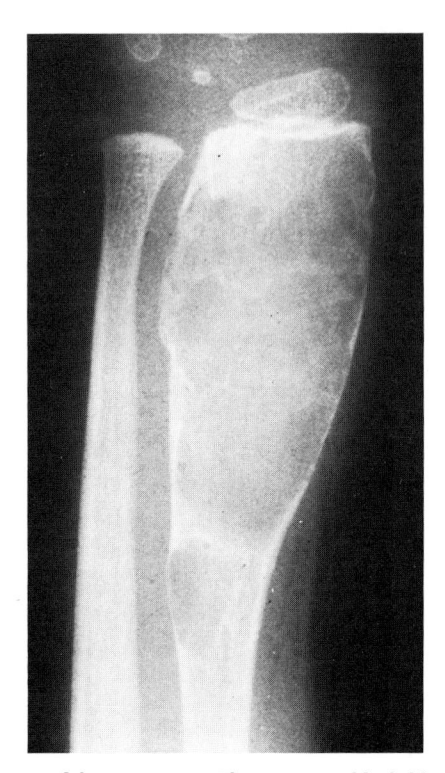

Figs. 7.48 & 7.49 Aneurysmal bone cyst treated by resection. This 2-year-old child presented with a fracture through an eccentrically placed cyst of the distal radius. It was not treated surgically. (*Right*) At the age of $3\frac{1}{2}$ years the forearm rapidly expanded. The lesion now has the typical features of an expansile aneurysmal bone cyst. The cyst was resected subperiosteally. The radius was divided transversely proximal to the cyst but distally the cyst was transected through the metaphysis; the remainder of the cyst was curetted from the growth plate. A corticocancellous graft from the tibia was inserted into the defect.

EXCISION

Osteochondromas are treated surgically by total excision. Care must be taken to remove the cartilage growth cap completely in order to prevent recurrence. Extra bone is removed from the base so that the normal shape of the bone is restored. The nidus of osteoid osteomas are also treated by excision (Figs. 7.55 & 7.56). To ensure that the lesion has been excised, the specimen is x-rayed and split for macroscopic examination (Fig. 7.57).

Benign lesions located in bones that can be resected without functional loss (such as the ribs, fibula, or posterior elements of the spine) are normally best treated by excision. Bone grafting of the defect is usually unnecessary. Benign lesions in other bones are often easier to treat initially by curettage, reserving

Bone Tumours 387

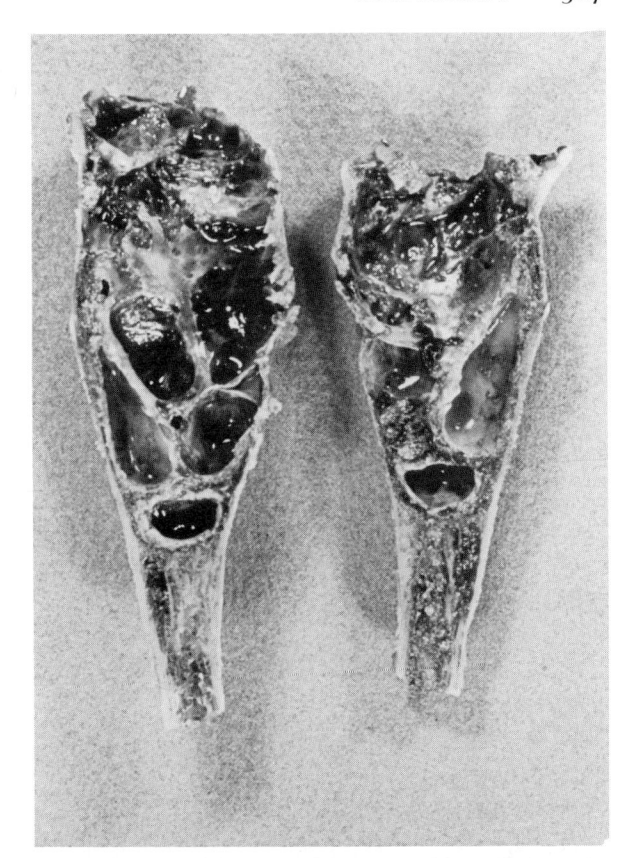

Figs. 7.50 & 7.51
Same patient as Fig. 7.48. The typical multilocular appearance with areas of haemorrhage are seen on the cut surface of the resected specimen. (*Bottom*) Ten months later the radius has undergone considerable re-modelling and continues to grow normally.

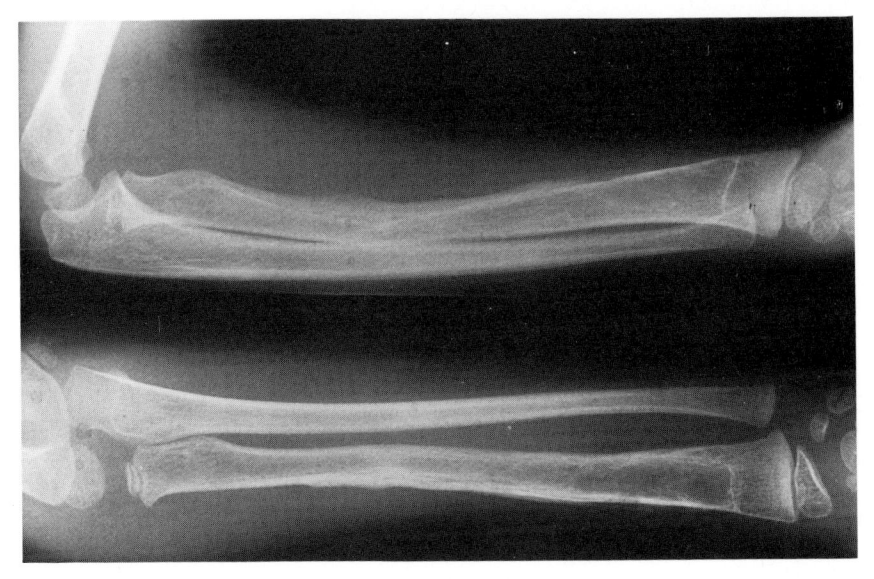

388   Chapter 7

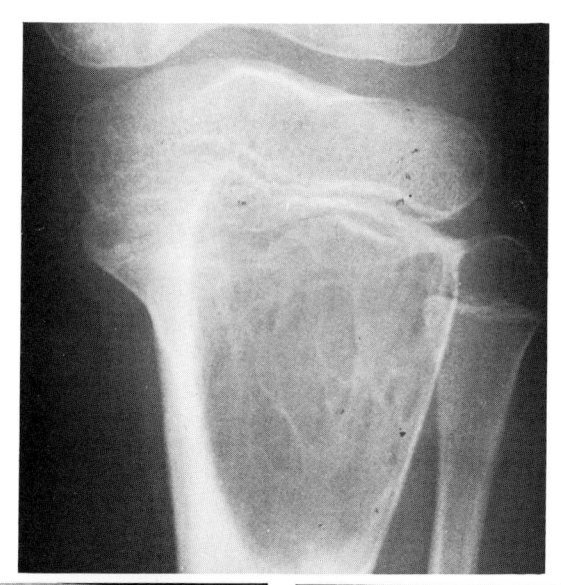

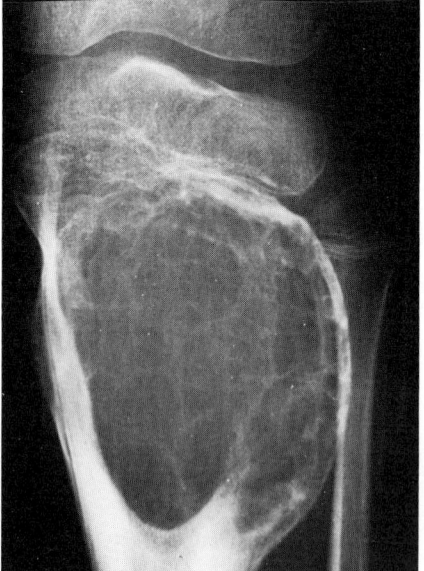

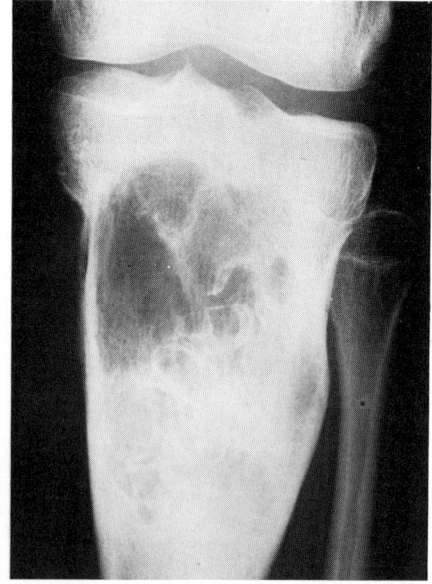

Figs. 7.52–7.54 Aneurysmal bone cyst with radiation-induced fibrosarcoma of the proximal tibia. The cystic lesion is eccentric with expansion and thinning of the overlying cortex. The remainder of the margin is sclerotic but not as clearly defined as with a simple bone cyst. The lesion was treated by curettage and bone grafting but the cyst rapidly recurred and showed more aggressive features. (*Bottom left*) X-ray of the recurrent cyst. The cyst has undergone further expansion and shows fine septa throughout, indicating its multilocular nature. There is also laminated subperiosteal new bone both medially and laterally. A further curettage and bone graft procedure was carried out but, two months later, it was obvious that the cyst had recurred and radiotherapy was given to the area. (*Bottom right*) Four years later there was a recurrence of pain due to a radiation-induced fibrosarcoma producing a lytic area in the tibial metaphysis.

Bone Tumours 389

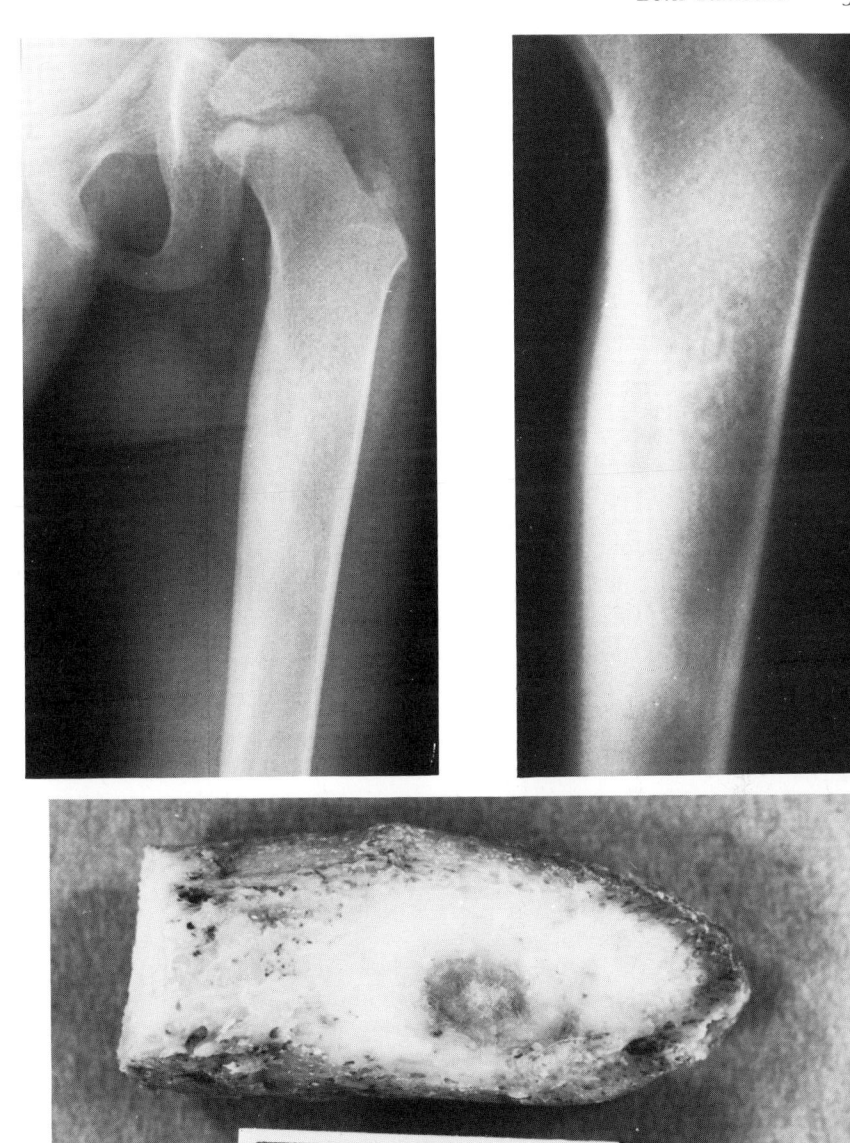

Figs. 7.55–7.57   Osteoid osteoma of the femur in a 6-year-old boy. This boy had chronic pain with quadriceps wasting and loss of knee jerk thought to be due to a neurological disorder. (*Top left*) Eccentric sclerosis of the shaft of the femur. This sclerosis is uniform with a benign appearance and a nidus is noted near the region of the lesser trochanter. (*Top right*) A tomogram of the nidus consisting of a lucent area with central calcification. The pain was immediately relieved following excision of the lesion. (*Bottom*) The nidus is surrounded by dense sclerotic bone.

bone grafting and excision for recurrences. Excision is also indicated whenever the lesion is rapidly growing with aggressive features (see above).

PRIMARY MALIGNANT BONE TUMOURS

The treatment of primary malignant bone tumours is complex and requires careful planning and co-ordination. This section will describe the role of the multidisciplinary combined therapy clinic in planning and co-ordinating the treatment and give details concerning the methods of treatment.

Combined therapy clinic

To provide optimal care for a child with a primary malignant bone tumour, it is necessary for the family to have access to a wide variety of medical, paramedical, and nursing personnel with expertise in this field. The combined therapy clinic provides a forum for all parties who are likely to take part in the treatment to express their opinion and to help formulate the plan of treatment.

The doctor who is primarily in charge of the care will co-ordinate the activities of different groups and will be directly responsible to the child and his family. It is the role of this doctor to discuss the plan of treatment with the parents and to introduce them to the different people who will be involved in the treatment. The medical social workers and nursing staff play an important role in assisting the families throughout this difficult period.

Methods of treatment

There are two main types of treatment available for malignant bone tumours: the first type includes surgery and radiotherapy and is directed towards the primary tumour; the second type includes chemotherapy and immunotherapy and is directed towards the metastases. Surgery, radiotherapy and chemotherapy will be considered in detail.

SURGERY

Surgery is the principal method of treating the primary tumour. In most instances this will consist of amputation. Radical local resection of malignant tumours is being evaluated as an alternative procedure in several centres. It has the advantage that it avoids amputation but is only feasible when total resection of the tumour can be guaranteed and where reconstruction is feasible. It may also be a reasonable alternative in low grade tumours located in bones that can be resected without significant functional loss.

The disadvantages of amputation are obvious. The loss of function and the alteration of body image are of particular concern to the adolescent. In general, good function can be expected with amputations in the lower limb which preserve the knee joint. While many above-knee amputees can walk well, the loss of the knee joint is a considerable disability. Hip disarticulations and hind quarter amputations produce a very severe functional disability. It is always preferable to carry out a trans-femoral amputation above the tumour as the patient will function better than with a hip disarticulation. An added difficulty with hip disarticulations and hind quarter amputations is that the more proximally located tumours generally have a poor prognosis. Other cosmetic and functional problems are encountered with amputations in the upper limb. Unfortunately the available prostheses are unable to restore normal hand and arm function. The elbow joint is also of critical importance as children with below-elbow amputations can frequently learn to use a prosthesis without difficulty, but an above-elbow amputee has more difficulty, and a child with a shoulder disarticulation will rarely make use of a prosthesis.

Careful preparation of the family is required before the amputation. After the diagnosis has been established and the plan of treatment has been formulated, discussions are held with the parents. It is of considerable benefit to the family if the medical social worker and head nurse are included in these discussions as they can provide important continuing support for the family. It is also important that these discussions are carried out in a private setting and with both parents present. Once the plan of treatment has been finalised with the parents it is necessary to discuss the need for amputation with the child or adolescent. These discussions should be carried out 1–2 days before the amputation in order to give the child sufficient time to adapt to the proposed treatment, and also sufficient time to ask questions.

Is is essential to have a rehabilitation programme for these children which includes the early provision of a prosthesis. This will enable the prosthetic programme to be detailed to the parents and the child before the amputation. It is extremely helpful if the family can meet another child who has had an amputation at the same level and wears the type of prosthesis which the child will use later. This enables the family to obtain realistic information and usually helps them to feel more optimistic about the future.

The amputations can usually be carried out using standard procedures. It is probably better to do the amputation without a tourniquet as experimental evidence indicates that pulmonary metastases may be more readily established in the presence of fibrin and platelet aggregates released following removal of the tourniquet. The amputation needs to be carried out in a meticulous manner in order to ensure primary wound healing as wound complications are a particular problem if the child is to receive chemotherapy. It also interferes with their prosthetic programme.

Although immediate prostheses can be used following amputations in the lower limb, it is difficult to align the prosthesis with the patient supine on the operating table. However a prosthesis can be fitted and aligned correctly on the tenth day when the wound is healed and the child is comfortable. For below-knee amputations, an interim prosthesis can be readily made using a plaster socket assembled onto the shank and SACH foot units normally used in the manufacture of a permanent prosthesis. An adjustable polypropylene quadrilateral socket assembled onto a reclaimed wooden knee shank and SACH foot unit can be provided in one hour to the above-knee amputee (Figs. 7.58 & 7.59). The adjustable sockets are commercially available; they therefore avoid the need to cast the painful stump and can be adjusted to accommodate the fluctuations in stump volume. Gait training is begun on the tenth day and most children and adolescents rapidly regain their confidence and learn to walk well. Definitive prostheses are provided when the stump has reached a constant size. Most adolescent girls prefer to have an endoskeletal prosthesis with a cosmetic cover.

Upper limb amputations are required less often. The overall management is

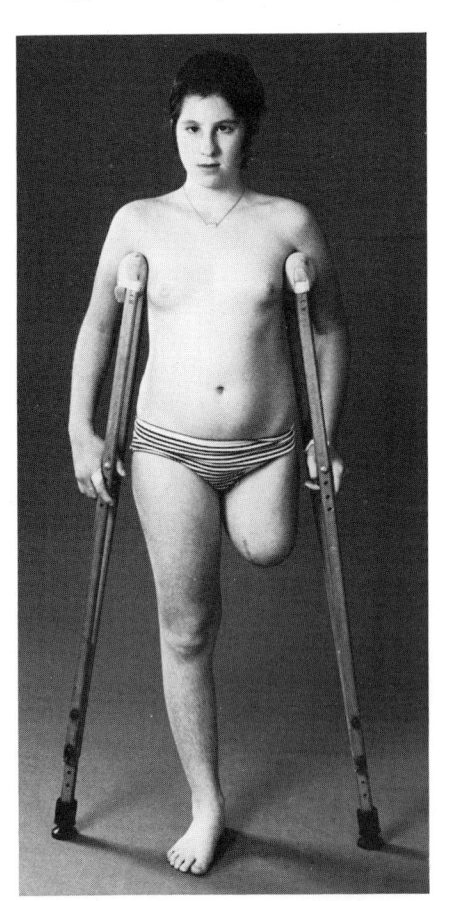

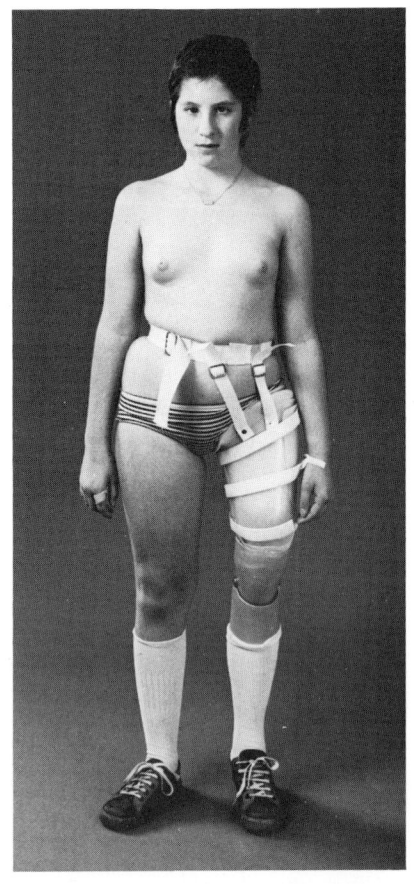

Figs. 7.58 & 7.59 Trans-femoral amputation for osteosarcoma of the distal femur. (*Right*) Interim prosthesis provided ten days following the amputation. It consists of an adjustable polypropylene quadrilateral socket suspended from a waist band and assembled onto reclaimed prosthetic components.

carried out along the same lines as for amputations in the lower limb. Immediate or interim prostheses can also be provided using reclaimed prostheses. A reclaimed prosthesis with a slightly larger socket can be fitted to the child's stump using an elastamer lining.

The surgical treatment discussed so far has been directed towards achieving a cure. However, palliative surgery needs to be considered when metastases are already present. It may be necessary to carry out palliative amputations because of chronic pain or pathological fractures. Resection of solitary or small numbers of lung metastases from osteosarcoma may prolong the patient's survival but is obviously impractical where there are large numbers of metastases.

RADIOTHERAPY

Primary malignant bone tumours frequently recur locally when radiotherapy is used as the sole method of controlling them. The inability of radiotherapy to cure the local tumour is readily apparent with the relatively resistant tumours such as osteosarcoma, chondrosarcoma, and fibrosarcoma. Ewing's sarcoma is sensitive to radiotherapy but there is a high recurrence rate particularly in the pelvis. This indicates that the degree of sensitivity of the tumour to radiotherapy does not correlate directly with the ability of the radiotherapy to cure the sarcoma.

A further problem with radiotherapy is that the dosages used to treat the primary tumour produce severe trophic changes in the surrounding tissues. The susceptibility of the cornea, gonads, bone marrow, intestine and thyroid are well known and efforts are always made to shield these areas. Serious lung and kidney damage results when dosages in excess of 2000 rads are given to these areas. However, in the limbs, doses as low as 1000 rads will usually damage the epiphyseal growth plate leading to a leg length discrepancy. Joint stiffness and soft tissue fibrosis also lead to dysfunction and the accompanying osteoporosis may result in fracture. The severity of these changes is greater when high doses of radiotherapy are used and this may produce such functional impairment that amputation will be required. A further concern is the production of radiation-induced malignant tumours in the irradiated connective tissues.

It is clear that radiotherapy cannot be considered to be a curative method of treatment when dosages are used that are compatible with good function and growth. Although high doses of radiotherapy may control the primary tumour more frequently there are so many added problems that it is preferable to use alternative methods, i.e. surgery or a lower dosage of irradiation that enables the tumour to be surgically resected.

Radiotherapy has an important role in the palliative treatment of symptomatic metastases.

CHEMOTHERAPY

The late appearance of metastases after the complete removal of the primary tumour has led to the concept that micrometastases are present at the time of presentation. To achieve a cure, systemic chemotherapy is included in the protocols of treatment of primary malignant bone tumours. It should be noted however that the chemotherapeutic agents are unable to control large primary tumours.

There are different classes of cytotoxic agents. There are the alkylating agents such as cyclophosphamide, anti-metabolites such as methotrexate, plant derivatives such as vincristine, and antibiotic derivatives such as adriamycin.

The selection of the cytotoxic agent to treat any particular malignant tumour is largely empirical. As many malignant bone tumours have only a small fraction of their cells undergoing mitosis, the alkylating agents which act on resting as well as dividing cells are frequently used. Vincristine (which leads to an arrest in the metaphase) is frequently used in the treatment of Ewing's sarcoma; adriamycin (which interferes with the transcription of DNA and protein synthesis) is frequently used in the treatment of Ewing's sarcoma and osteosarcoma.

There are several important principles in the use of cytotoxic agents. Combination chemotherapy is usually recommended. Several agents are selected which act at different sites in the cell cycle. This provides a broader action and prevents the cumulative side effects which arise when several drugs acting on the same phase of the cell cycle are used. Intermittent therapy is used as it has been shown to be less toxic than continuous therapy because it allows the normal tissues time to recover. There are no clear guidelines as to how long it takes the chemotherapy to eradicate the micrometastases but periods from 18 months to two years are commonly used.

A two year course of chemotherapy has a profound effect on the child and the family. Home activities and schooling are interrupted by attendances at hospital and by periods in which the child feels extremely ill. It is important to reduce the number of attendances as far as is possible and to arrange for others involved in the treatment to review the child during their attendances for chemotherapy. Although there are many complications that can occur, most are predictable and can be prevented by careful clinical and haematological monitoring. This applies particularly to patients who also receive radiotherapy as they are more sensitive to the side effects of the chemotherapy. Alopecia, which frequently occurs with the use of vincristine and cyclophosphamide, is of particular concern to the adolescent and, although it can be reduced by using a scalp tourniquet, most of the children will wear a wig.

Chemotherapy directed against micrometastases is being used to achieve a cure. The use of chemotherapy in this adjuvant manner appears to have produced a dramatic improvement in the survival of patients with primary malignant bone tumours but there is now some uncertainty as to whether it increases the survival of patients with osteosarcoma.

Chemotherapy can also be used in a palliative role when the patient has widespread metastases. Chemotherapy may reduce both the tumour bulk and the pain, particularly in patients with Ewing's sarcoma. However, if the widespread metastases are giving few symptoms, chemotherapy is unlikely to be of benefit as the possibility of a cure is remote.

TREATMENT OF OSTEOSARCOMA

There has been a recent upsurge of interest in the treatment of osteosarcoma because of dramatically improved results. Many centres now report survival rates of up to 60% two years after presentation. This is in marked contrast to the expected survival rates of less than 20%.

There is little controversy about the need for surgery to treat the primary tumour. Amputation is the standard procedure while radical local resection is undergoing evaluation in many centres. An above-knee amputation is the commonest procedure as over 50% of the osteosarcomas occur in the lower end of the femur and upper tibia. Trans-femoral amputation at the junction of the middle- and lower-thirds of the femur is carried out for osteosarcomas of the proximal tibia. The bone marrow is curetted from the proximal fragment and frozen sections are examined by the pathologist. We have not observed any skip lesions in this material. Controversy surrounds the most appropriate level of amputation for osteosarcomas situated in the distal femur. Studies of amputated specimens show that the primary tumour does not extend above the radiological upper limit of the lesion and, for this reason, we recommend amputation through the femur at least 5 cm above the radiological limit. The bone marrow is also curetted from the proximal shaft and examined by the pathologist; however, we have not observed skip lesions nor have we observed local stump recurrences except in patients with advanced metastatic disease. For these reasons hip disarticulation is not warranted.

Meticulous surgical technique is important. The amputation is preferably carried out without a tourniquet because of the experimental evidence indicating that metastases are more likely to develop in the lungs if a tourniquet has been used. Careful closure of the muscles and fascia over the end of the bone is required to prevent adhesion of the bone to the skin scar. Careful wound closure is also required to ensure primary healing. On the tenth day the dressings are removed, an interim prosthesis is fitted, and training in the use of the prosthesis is begun.

One of the most controversial aspects of the treatment of osteosarcoma is the role of adjuvant chemotherapy. Following the introduction of adjuvant chemotherapy there have been numerous reports of dramatically improved results with at least 60% of the patients surviving without apparent disease for at least two years. The commonly used agents include methotrexate with citrovorum rescue, vincristine, and adriamycin. Interest has been mainly centered on the relative effectiveness of the different drug protocols and, in particular, on whether the very high doses of methotrexate were more effective than the lower doses. Against this, similar results have been achieved at the Mayo Clinic using amputation alone. These discrepancies indicate that further evaluation of the role of the chemotherapy agents using concurrent controls is required. This also applies to other systemic forms of therapy such as immunotherapy and interferon.

Some patients at presentation or later develop a small number of lung metastases which can be resected surgically. Improvement in the period of survival has been reported following such procedures. However, the presence of multiple lung metastases or metastases elsewhere in the body usually indicates that the disease is incurable. Under these circumstances, palliative treatment such as radiotherapy may be used to alleviate pain.

TREATMENT OF EWING'S SARCOMA

As with osteosarcoma there has been a recent upsurge of interest in Ewing's sarcoma because of dramatically improved survival rates. These were attributed to the combination of radiotherapy to the whole of the involved bone and the use of adjuvant chemotherapy. However greater experience with this therapy has shown that although Ewing's sarcoma is sensitive to radiotherapy, approximately 30% of the tumours, particularly those involving the pelvis, recur at the primary site. It has also become clear that surgical treatment at that stage is not able to prevent the appearance of widespread metastases that follow soon afterwards. A further 30% of patients have significant functional disabilities associated with the use of radiotherapy such as growth plate arrest, soft tissue fibrosis, and decreased joint motion.

The role of surgery in the treatment of the primary lesion is being re-evaluated because of the problems of local recurrence and functional disability following the use of radiotherapy. Surgery may take the form of an *en bloc* resection of a small tumour localised to a bone which can be resected without functional loss, such as the fibula. If the tumour is large, such a resection would be technically difficult or impossible, unless the size of the mass was reduced beforehand by radiotherapy. The resection is then carried out 4–6 weeks after the completion of the radiotherapy. This has proven to be a worthwhile approach for Ewing's sarcoma of the pelvis in which there is a high local recurrence rate when radiotherapy is used alone (Figs. 7.60 & 7.61). Resections of large parts of the pelvis are compatible with good function. Amputation is the preferred method of treating primary tumours in the limbs. This particularly applies to lesions below the knee where fibrosis, joint stiffness, and deformity are common.

Ewing's sarcoma is more sensitive to chemotherapy than osteosarcoma and this treatment has played a major role in the dramatic improvement in results. The actuarial disease-free five year survival rate is between 60 and 70%. A variety of chemotherapy protocols are used including vincristine, actinomycin D, and cyclophosphamide. Other protocols use VM-26, imidazole carboxamide, and adriamycin. These agents are given in cycles over a two year period.

Bone Tumours 397

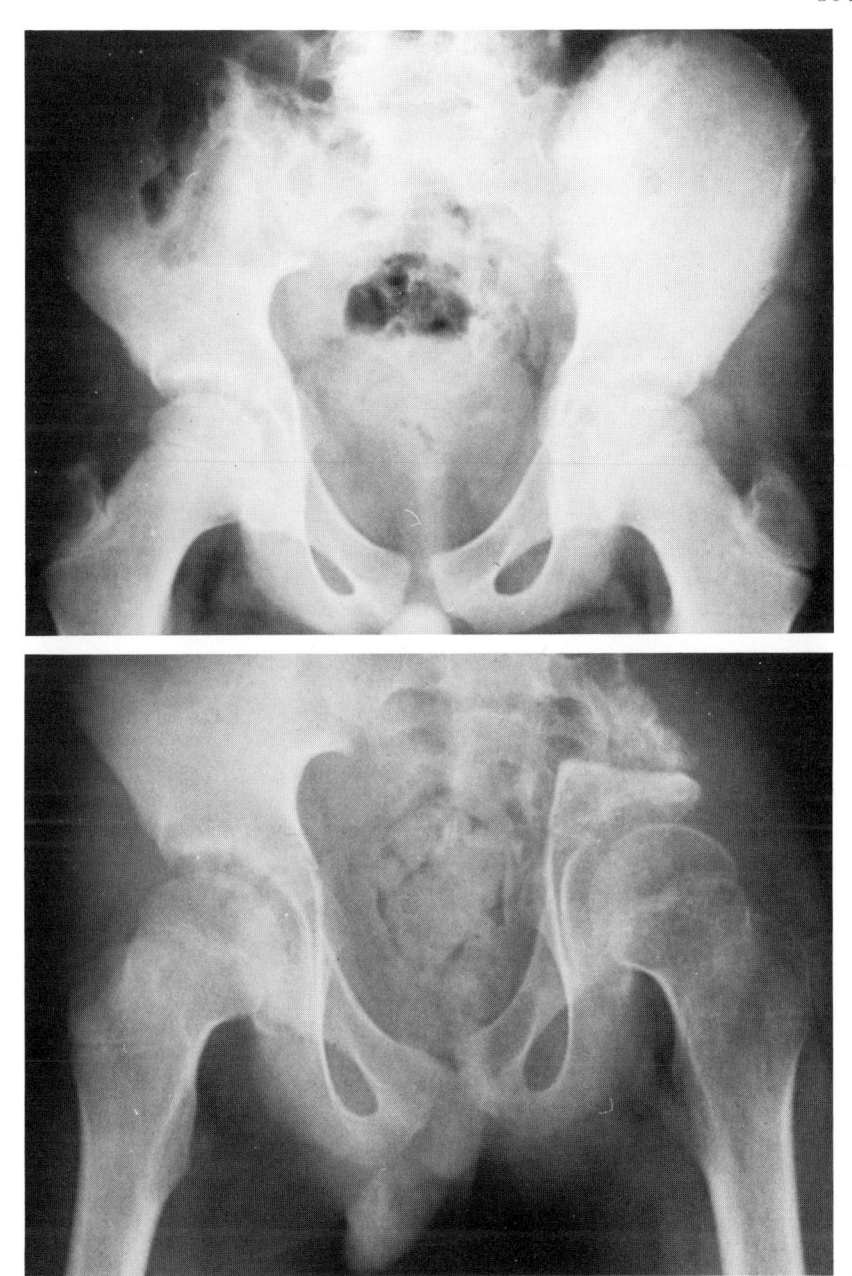

Figs. 7.60 & 7.61 There are areas of bone destruction and sclerosis due to a Ewing's sarcoma in the left ilium. (*Bottom*) Six weeks following the completion of a course of 5000 rads to the left ilium and chemotherapy, the left ilium was resected from the sacro-iliac joint to the acetabulum. Bone graft was placed between the sacrum and the remaining pelvis. The patient continues to be free of disease two years following the resection.

Palliative radiotherapy or chemotherapy are required when children have metastatic Ewing's sarcoma producing pain or neurological abnormalities. The metastases frequently respond rapidly to small doses of radiation and to cytotoxic agents, with relieve of pain.

CHAPTER 8

Some Generalised Disorders with Orthopaedic Implications

Arthrogryposis, 400
Principles of treatment; General management; The foot in arthrogryposis; The knee in arthrogryposis; The hip in arthrogryposis; The spine; Management of the upper limb

Osteogenesis imperfecta, 410
Classification; Management

Neurofibromatosis, 418
Diagnosis; Clinical features; Management

Muscular dystrophy, 426
Classification; Clinical features; Diagnosis; Management

Marfan's syndrome (arachnodactyly), 431
Clinical features; Management

Down's syndrome (mongolism), 432

Thalassaemia, 434

Hereditary neuropathies, 434
Peroneal muscular atrophy (Charcot-Marie-Tooth disease); Friedreich's ataxia; Congenital indifference to pain

Haemophilia, 438
Classification; Orthopaedic implications of haemophilia; Management

Chronic arthritis in childhood, 445
Juvenile chronic arthritis (JCA); Arthritis related to infectious disease; Arthritis related to malignancies; Arthritis of non-inflammatory cause; Ankylosing spondylitis; Rheumatic fever; SLE; dermatomyositis; scleroderma and polyarteritis nodosa; Henoch-Schönlein purpura; The arthritis of inflammatory bowel disease; Reiter's syndrome; Management of the child with JCA; Treatment

Poliomyelitis, 454
Clinical features; Management

ARTHROGRYPOSIS

Arthrogryposis means literally a curved joint; it is a congenital disorder characterised by multiple rigid joint deformities (Fig. 8.1).

Aetiology

There is no evidence that the condition is genetic in origin. That arthrogrypotic deformities are sometimes seen in association with meningomyelocele and that, in other cases, sections of the cord have shown a paucity of anterior horn cells have influenced some authorities to believe that the condition is neurogenic in origin. Certainly the muscle lesions are those characteristic of neurogenic muscular atrophy. It is of considerable interest that an identical condition occurs in sheep, cattle, and horses and there is very good circumstantial evidence that it

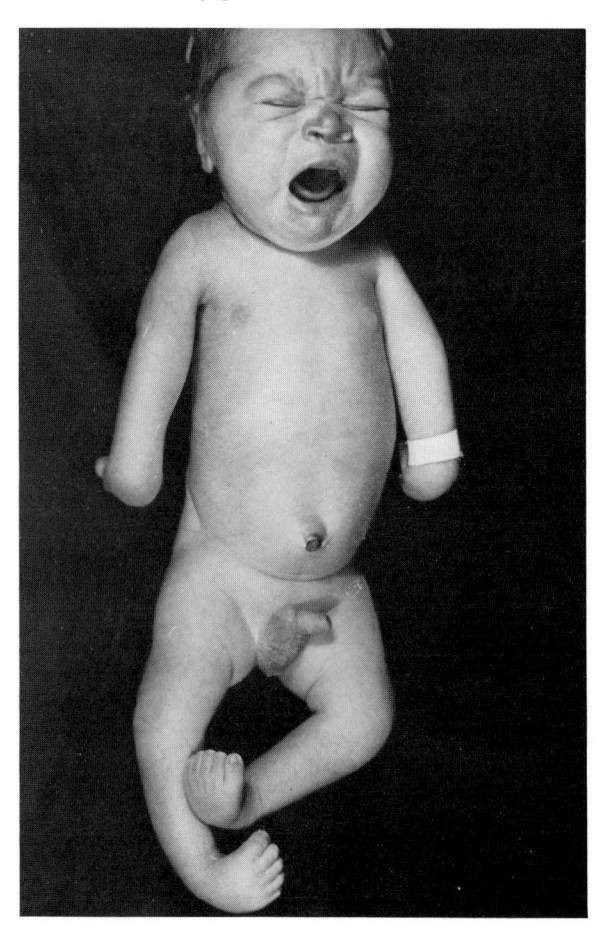

Fig. 8.1 A typical case of arthrogryposis multiplex with involvement of all four limbs.

is caused by infection of the mother by the Akabane virus during early pregnancy. This virus has not yet been isolated in man. The aetiologic hypothesis is well described by Whittem on the basis of his study of the condition occurring in animals. He suggests that the primary condition is a degeneration of the anterior horn cells occurring in the early months of gestation. As a result of the early destruction of muscle fibres in utero, certain muscles are affected earlier or more severely than others: they lose their tone and fail to counterbalance the normal tone of their antagonists. This tends to restrict the normal movement of muscles and joints during the period of their rapid growth and leads to partial fixation of joints, producing the clinical changes of arthrogryposis.

Clinical features

The clinical features vary widely in extent, but most cases have several features in common: 1 Featureless extremities—the normal skin creases are absent and deep skin dimples are often present in the vicinity of joints. 2 Rigidity of several joints. 3 Dislocation of joints, most commonly the hip. 4 Absence or fibrosis of muscles or muscle groups. 5 Normal intellectual development. Quite commonly all four extremities are affected; less often the changes may be confined to one limb or even to part of one limb.

Pathology

In the affected joints, the actual articulation is normal or nearly normal at birth and remains so for a number of years. The obstruction to motion is almost wholly extra-articular and, when this is freed, the joint moves through a range close to that of normal. The muscles vary greatly. One muscle may be of normal size and colour while an adjacent one may be small, pale, contracted or completely absent. Ligaments and capsules are always found to be contracted in affected joints and the strength and density of these contractures are such that forceful methods of correction are not only ineffective but are likely to be harmful in causing pressure necrosis of articular cartilage.

PRINCIPLES OF TREATMENT

Early surgical release

Experience has shown that forcible stretching or manipulation under anaesthesia is either ineffective or produces fracture—especially in the foot where correction is obtained at the expense of crushing the fragile tarsal bones. Similarly, osteotomy is unsatisfactory as a means of obtaining correction as subsequent growth cancels out any gain obtained.

Prolonged plaster fixation

Prolonged plaster fixation followed by physiotherapy and splinting is necessary to obtain correction made possible by surgical release.

Tendon transfer

Tendon transfer should be carried out whenever possible to replace absent or ineffective muscles, and there is special scope for this at the elbow.

GENERAL MANAGEMENT

At a very early stage the parents should be brought into contact with an orthopaedist experienced in the management of these infants. Only he can give an accurate prognosis and adequately reassure them that all is not as bad as it may appear. The surgical treatment is outlined and it is almost always possible to say that the child will be of above-average intelligence and will be able to walk and be independent. Treatment presents tremendous difficulties in these children but most can be brought to adulthood as happy and resourceful individuals.

THE FOOT IN ARTHROGRYPOSIS

The foot presents as a rigid deformity in equinovarus and should have first priority in treatment which should be commenced immediately after birth (Figs. 8.2 & 8.3). Serial casting is used to correct the adductus and varus without any attempt being made to overcome the equinus deformity. At about 4–6 weeks a radical posterior release is carried out in which a segment of the tendo-Achilles is removed and the posterior capsule of the ankle and subtalar joints is divided. Radical medial release may also be indicated if complete correction of the inversion has not been obtained by closed means. Carefully applied plasters are used for many months to maintain the correction. After this, retentive splinting is indicated for a number of years.

Talectomy should only be used as a last resort because of the high relapse rate.

THE KNEE IN ARTHROGRYPOSIS

The knee is seen in two main varieties, stiff in full extension and stiff in various degrees of flexion.

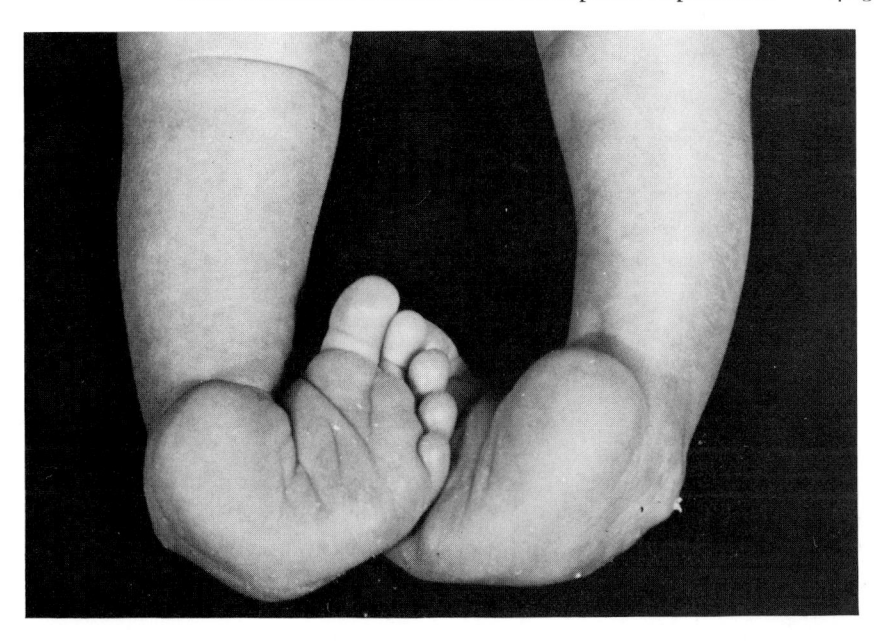

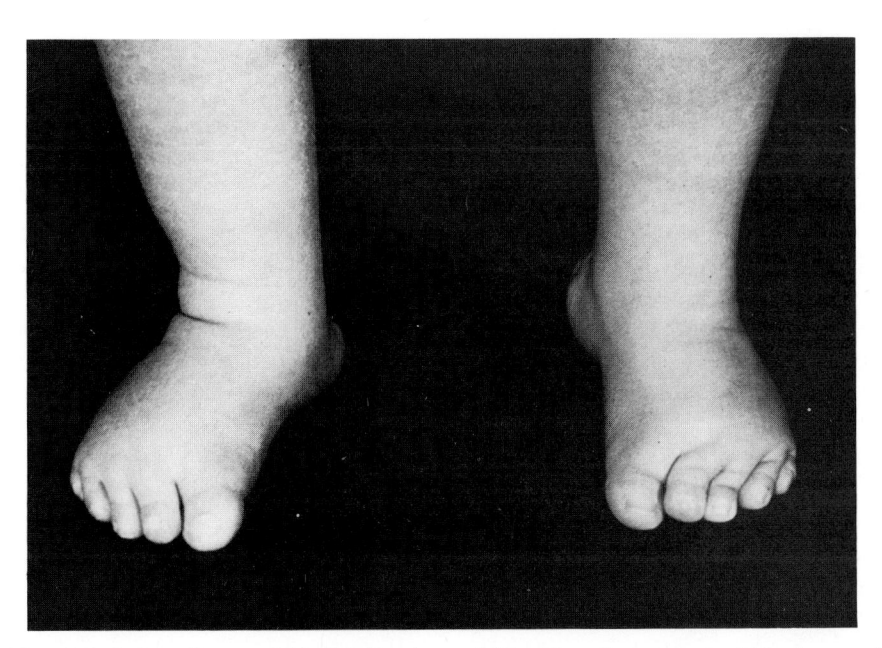

Figs. 8.2 & 8.3 Severe rigid club feet in a child with arthrogryposis. This degree of deformity is rarely seen in 'ordinary' club feet. (*Below*) The same feet after treatment—an initial period in serial plaster casts followed by radical posterior release.

Extended or hyperextended knee

Here there is usually a severe contracture of the quadriceps, often associated with fixation of the patella to the femur (Fig. 8.4). Serial splinting can be tried in the first few months and, in a few cases, will succeed. However, most of these will require surgical release of the quadriceps contracture after the age of 4 months (Fig. 8.5). Although the stiff knees are best treated at a very early age, mobilisation is still possible after some years although the range of motion obtained is considerably less.

Flexed knee

The flexed knee is more common and here the hamstrings and posterior capsule are contracted. Serial splinting in the early months rarely succeeds and open release of the hamstrings and posterior capsule should be employed at an early age. Sometimes it is necessary to explore the front of the joint at the same time in order to remove a fibro-fatty plug which blocks movement. If early treatment is

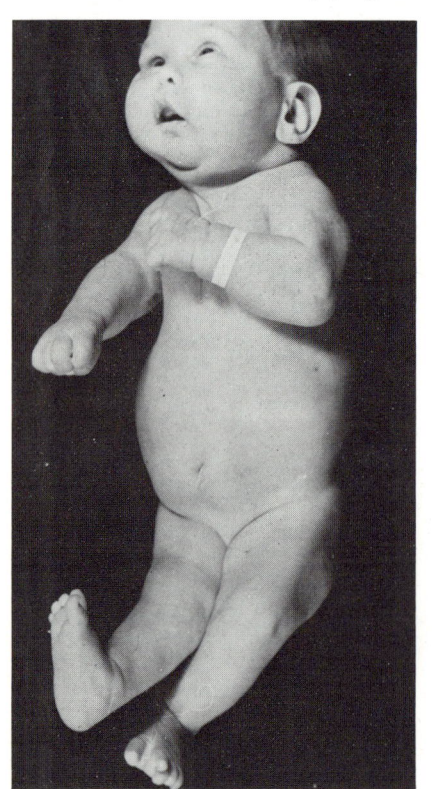

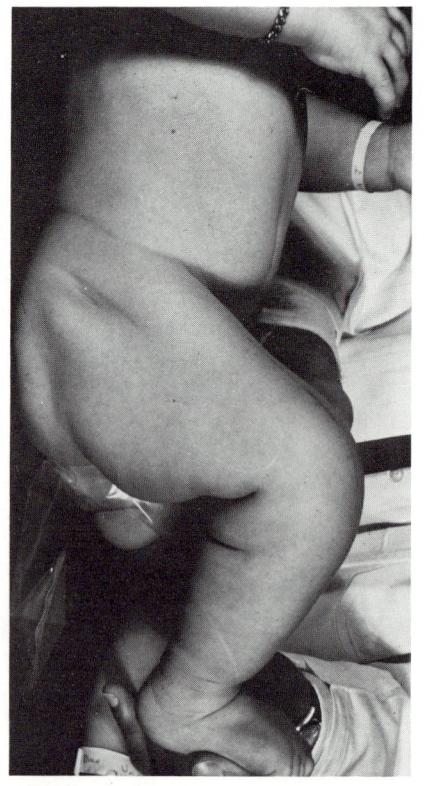

Figs. 8.4 & 8.5 Hyperextended right knee in arthrogryposis. (*Right*) Quadricepsplasty carried out at the age of 6 months produces a range of movement from 0 to 90°.

deferred until the child is at least 2 or 3 years old, correction can only be obtained by supracondylar osteotomy of the femur and this may have to be repeated during the growth period.

THE HIP IN ARTHROGRYPOSIS

Involvement of the hip can also be classified into two varieties: deformity without dislocation, and dislocation without deformity. In the first group, the problem is usually one of flexion deformity; this is rarely severe and will often respond to simple splinting in infancy. When dislocation of one or both hips is present, deformity is usually absent although associated stiffness may be a feature. For all practical purposes closed methods of reduction never succeed and should not be attempted. Open reduction should be deferred until the child is about 6 months old and should not be attempted until the knee—if previously stiff in extension—has already been treated. If the hips are stiff and dislocated, open reduction should not be attempted for, although this can be achieved, the hips remain stiff in their new position and no advantage is gained (Figs. 8.6 & 8.7).

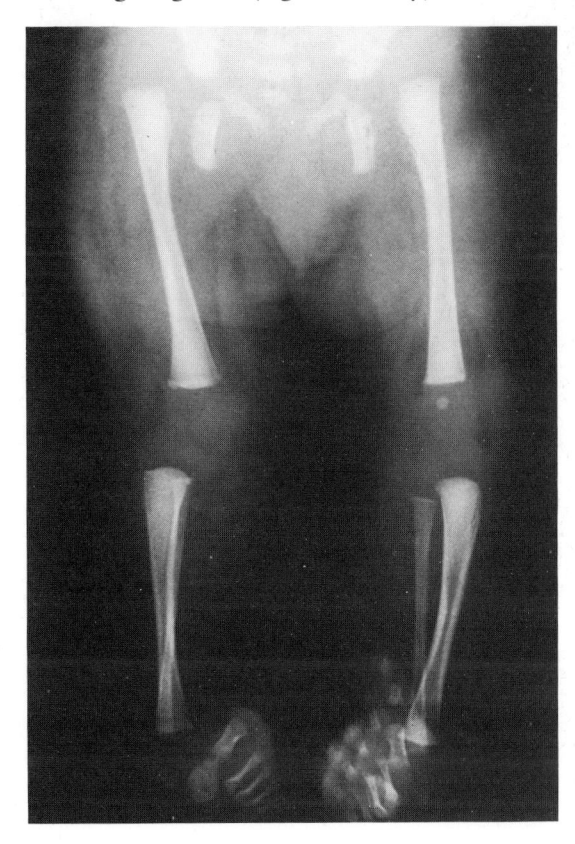

Fig. 8.6 Bilateral teratological dislocations of the hip in a babe with generalised arthrogryposis. These hips were very stiff clinically and were mistakenly submitted to open reductions.

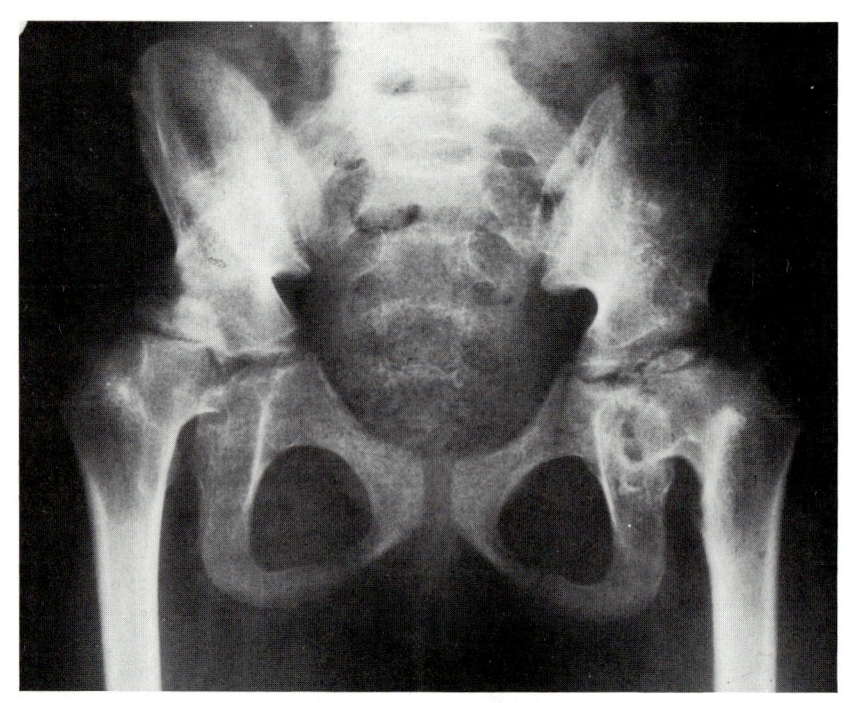

Fig. 8.7 The same patient as Fig. 8.6. After open reductions the hips are enlocated and remain stiff so that no advantage has been gained. Eventually some form of arthroplasty will be required to facilitate sitting.

THE SPINE

Spinal deformity is uncommon in arthrogryposis and is only seen in severely affected children with involvement of all four limbs.

Lordosis

Lordosis may be secondary to hip flexion deformity but usually occurs in its own right. Although the deformity is rigid, treatment is not required.

Scoliosis

Long paralytic-like C-shaped curves are seen which rapidly become rigid and tend to progress during the growth period. Bracing is not usually possible but if, at maturity, the degree of the curve is unacceptable, correction can be obtained by instrumentation. The Dwyer procedure is particularly useful in this regard.

MANAGEMENT OF THE UPPER LIMB

In the upper limb the classic deformity consists of limitation of abduction of the shoulder together with a medial rotation deformity (Fig. 8.8). The elbow is fixed either in flexion or full extension. The wrist, when affected, is invariably flexed and there is a wide variation in involvement of the fingers and thumb. Stiffness of the interphalangeal joints is almost invariably present, and the total hand function is often poor.

Shoulder

If medial rotation at the shoulder is present bilaterally, the hands oppose each other back to back. Although surprisingly good function can be obtained by a crossover grasp (Fig. 8.9), there are difficulties in using crutches and holding onto devices. In the circumstances, rotation osteotomy of each humerus will occasionally be indicated.

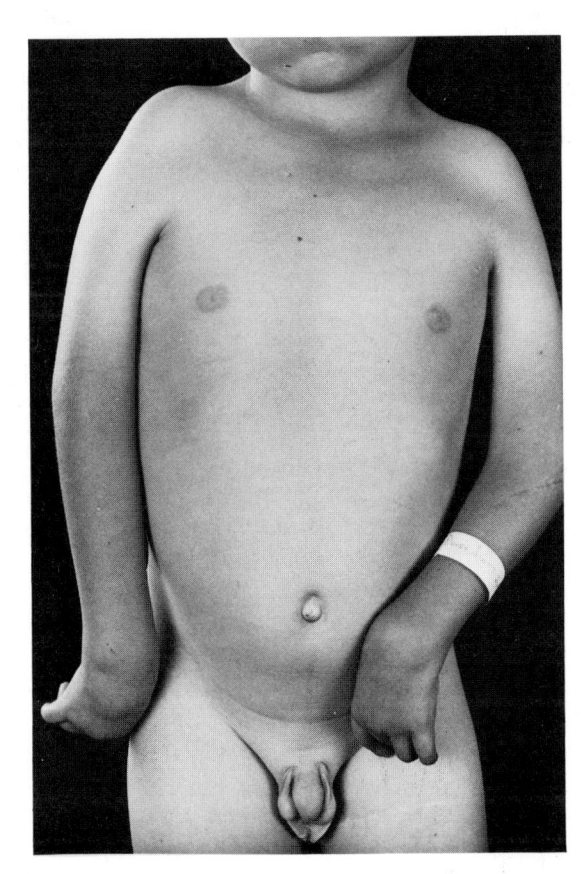

Fig. 8.8 Upper limb involvement in arthrogryposis. The arm is internally rotated at the shoulder, extended at the elbow, and the wrist is flexed. On the left side a triceps transfer has been carried out.

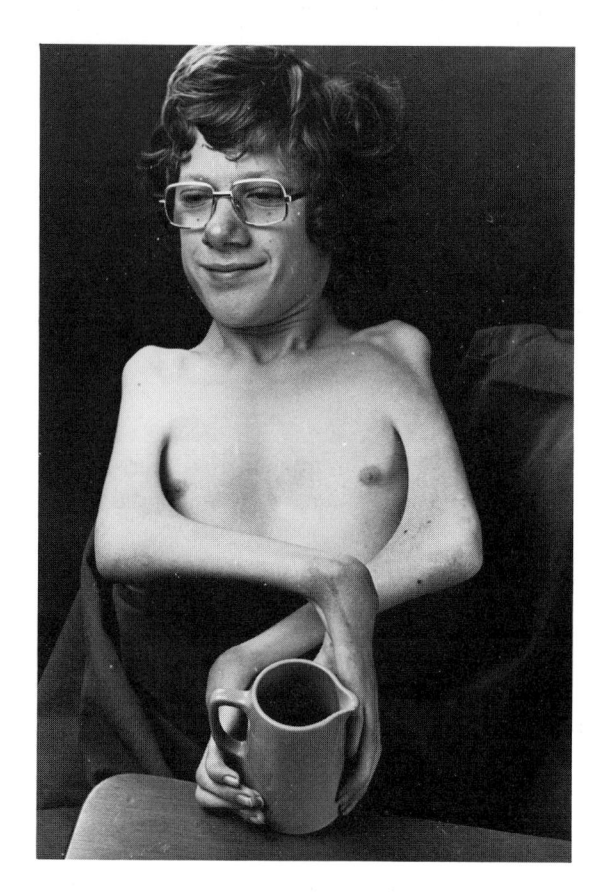

Fig. 8.9 A 12-year-old boy severely affected with arthrogryposis. Despite very poor musculature he has achieved remarkable function. The crossover grip is demonstrated.

The elbow joint

The elbow joint is a rather neglected field but great improvement can be gained here. Like so many other joints the elbow presents two distinct types of deformity. The first type is the elbow that is stiff in flexion: here the elbow usually has a useful range around the right-angle position and treatment is not necessary. The second and most important type is the elbow that is stiff in extension: only a few degrees of movement occur as a rule; the triceps is always strong and the biceps and brachialis usually completely absent. These rigid elbows can be considerably helped by a posterior release operation on the elbow and, at the same time, the triceps is transferred forward to act as a flexor motor. It is best to select one arm to be used for feeding and for this a triceps transfer is very satisfactory. Transfer however always produces a flexion deformity so that this arm cannot be used for toilet purposes. The other elbow is therefore mobilised by tricepsplasty only and this hand is then used for toileting. The elbow may be passively bent so that the two hands oppose each other. If the lower limbs are not involved, this type of surgery can be carried out at an early age but, if the lower limbs are involved, treatment of the arm should be deferred at least until the child is agile on crutches.

The hand

The hand in arthrogryposis is often severely affected by a combination of stiff joints and the absence of motor muscles. Despite this, most of these children learn ways of managing their feeding, toileting, dressing and other essential activities. The surgeon will be severely taxed in deciding not only what can be done to help but whether it should be done; the balance is often so critical that altering one feature may upset the whole system.

The wrist

The wrist presents a fairly standard deformity of fixed flexion and ulnar deviation. This deformity should not always be corrected because, if there is severe finger involvement, these children rely on the hooking effect of bent fingers and a flexed wrist. If there is any doubt the wrist can be corrected by serial casting and the new position tried out. If it is unacceptable, it can be allowed to relapse to the original deformity. If it is agreed that the corrected position of the wrist improves function, arthrodesis should be considered. If done before maturity, some permanent intramedullary fixation is essential. The position most favoured for arthrodesis is in 10–15° of palmar flexion.

The thumb

The thumb is often hypoplastic and clasped into the palm so that it cannot contribute much to function. Correction of this deformity requires release of the web, a skin supplement, and a tendon transfer to the dorsum to replace the absent extensors and abductors. A sublimis tendon usually provides the best transfer. Results on the whole are somewhat disappointing because of the small size of the digit and the relative weakness of the available motors.

The fingers

The fingers are affected more often than not with a combination of stiff metacarpophalangeal and interphalangeal joints and absent or weak long flexors and extensors. If the hand has some pinch and some grasp, no matter how distorted, it is often best left alone. Occasionally some of the stiff finger joints can be released. Perhaps the most rewarding is the finger flexed at the interphalangeal joint where sublimis release is indicated. Some badly affected hands have long spindly fingers stiff in extension and the function of these can be improved by releasing the interphalangeal joints and allowing them to become stiff again in the flexed position.

Summary

Arthrogryposis has an evil reputation amongst orthopaedic surgeons, for the deformities are known to be resistant to correction and relapse during growth is common. On the basis of our experience it is suggested that many of these difficulties have been due to a delay in initiating treatment, to the use of unsuitable methods such as manipulation, and to a lack of appreciation of the pathological changes. Aggressive surgical treatment in infancy and early childhood is more successful than previously accepted methods of care.

OSTEOGENESIS IMPERFECTA

Osteogenesis imperfecta (OI) is a congenital disorder causing generalised bone fragility. It was first described about 250 years ago in Germany and 120 years later the histology was studied in von Recklinghausen's laboratory. One of the earliest sufferers was the Scandinavian King, Ivar the Boneless. Despite his disability, Ivar went on to conquer England and became King of Northumberland until he died in about 800 AD.

The disease is seen in all races and at all levels of society. Although the skeletal manifestations are the most striking and the most important, it is well to remember that changes also occur in the skin, ligaments, tendons, sclera, and the inner ear. The latter commonly leads to deafness in early adult life. Numerous other congenital malformations, particularly cardiac and hip anomalies, have been described in association with osteogenesis imperfecta and the presence of these should not be overlooked.

The basic pathological change is the failure of collagen to maturate. This produces a typical thin skin and lax ligaments. Osteoblasts produce defective osteoid so that both spongiosa and cortical bone is poorly developed.

CLASSIFICATION

Various attempts have been made to classify this disease into types, but the two most useful classifications are those based on radiology and genetics.

Radiological classification

From the viewpoint of surgical treatment a radiological classification is preferable and that suggested by Fairbanks is commonly used. Three types are distinguished.

Thick bone type. Those affected are usually dwarfed and have other severe manifestations. At birth the bones are short and wide, the cortex being thin and the spongiosa expanded (Fig. 8.10). Fractures are common but deformity is less severe than in the slender bones. The majority in this category have the potential for learning to walk.

Slender bone type. This is the most common and is characterised by diffuse osteoporosis and slender shafts, often with no apparent medullary cavity in the middle (Fig. 8.11). Bending occurs without fractures and gross deformity is often seen. The ends of the long bones are sometimes expanded to an extraordinary degree and have a honeycombed and whirled appearance, the so-called 'pop corn' epiphysis. This is a poor prognostic sign and few, if any, of these children will walk.

Cystic type. This type is extremely rare. The whole of the shafts of the long bones are honeycombed. The natural history is similar to the thick boned type.

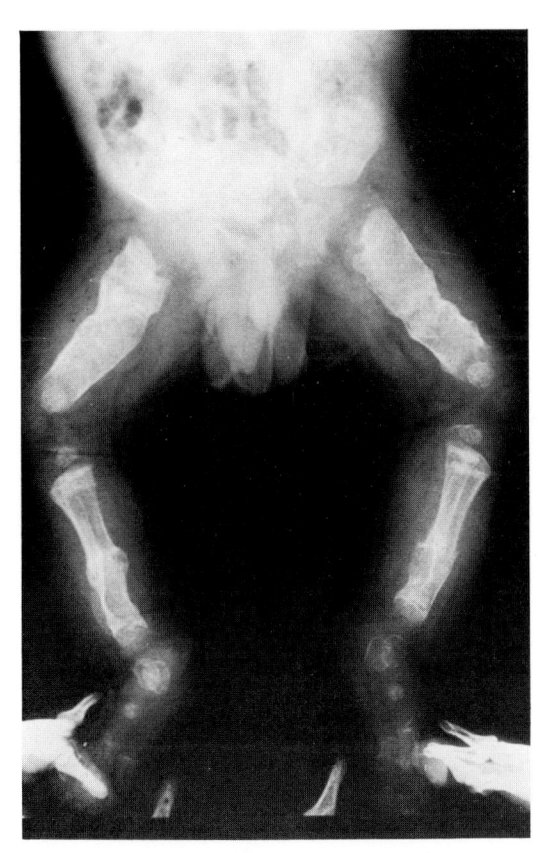

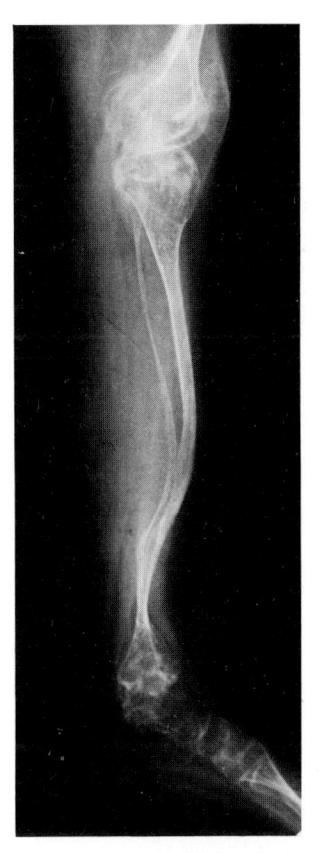

Figs. 8.10 & 8.11 Osteogenesis imperfecta. (*Left*) Thick bone type. (*Right*) Thin bone type.

Genetic and clinical classification

Dominantly inherited OI with blue sclera. These are usually mild cases and, although they may have many fractures in childhood, resolve at maturity. The prognosis is good for ambulation and achieving independence.

Lethal perinatal OI. Multiple fractures and gross deformity present at birth. Usually stillborn.

Progressive deforming OI with normal sclera. Severely affected cases who rarely achieve walking.

Dominantly inherited OI with normal sclera. Similar to those with progressive deforming OI but mostly familial.

Clinical features at birth

All types may be born with multiple intra-uterine fractures and this is usually an indication that the disease is present in a severe form; the prognosis is then usually poor. However, it is not always so; cases have been observed where all birth fractures have healed and very few, if any, have occurred subsequently. If the babe is born alive and survives the neonatal period, long term survival is the rule. Multiple fractures will be apparent from the deformity and the crepitus noted when handling. The fontanelles are widely open and the skull has a characteristic appearance with bitemporal bossing.

Childhood

The child soon develops a large flat head (Fig. 8.12), rather like a sunflower and, when teeth appear, they are transparent and discoloured. Excessive sweating is common. Progressive deformity of the long bones occurs with or without fractures (Fig. 8.13). The affected children are usually bright, intelligent and outgoing, although a few remain fearful and withdrawn.

Adulthood

During early adult life most of the blue eyed variety become deaf due to otosclerosis but this can be relieved by appropriate surgery. Progressive kyphosis with or without scoliosis usually develops and may become very disabling (Fig. 8.14).

MANAGEMENT

When an affected baby is born to parents one or both of whom have the condition

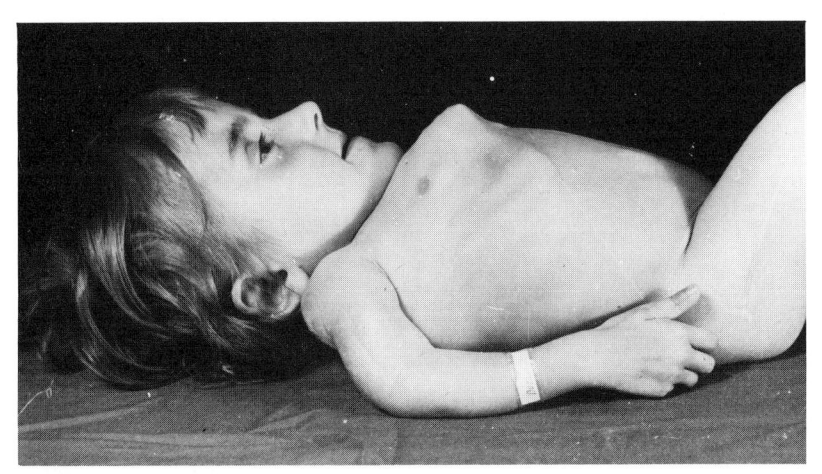

Some Generalised Disorders with Orthopaedic Implications 413

Fig. 8.12 Chest deformity in osteogenesis imperfecta. This degree of deformity is only seen in those children who are very dwarfed, have white sclerae, and nearly all of whom are non-walkers.

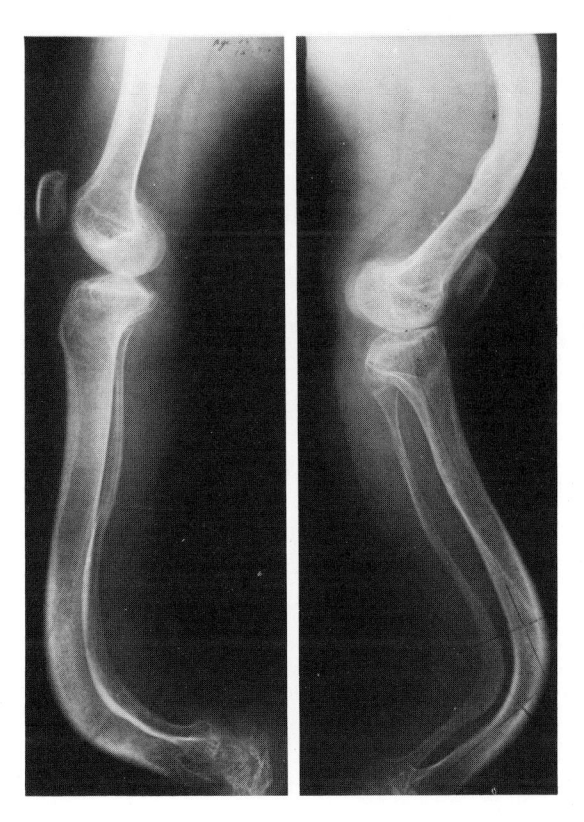

Fig. 8.13 Radiographs of a previously untreated 16-year-old girl. The deformities are nearly all due to gradual bending rather than to malunion following fracture.

414   Chapter 8

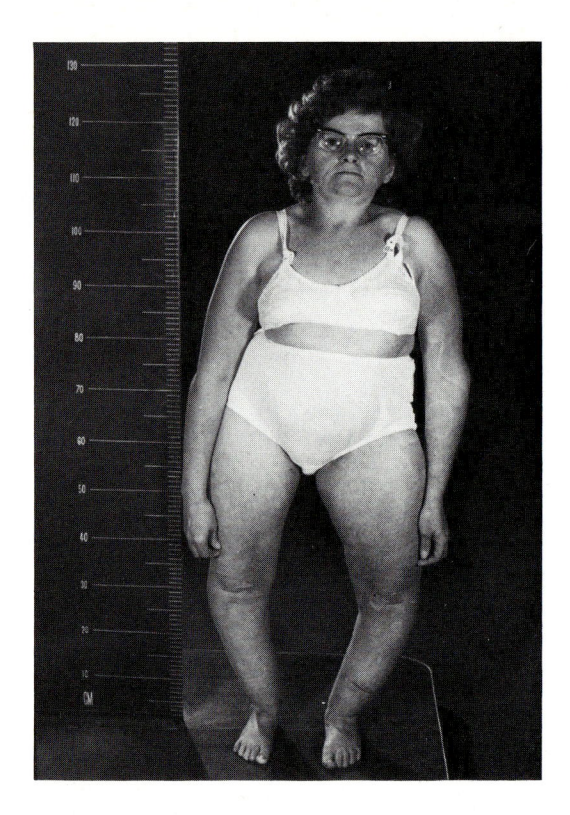

Fig. 8.14 A 30-year-old woman with osteogenesis imperfecta. She had a previous history of more than 100 fractures—all treated conservatively. Tibial osteotomies were required to relieve knee pain.

they know only too well all the implications. The surgeon can help by classifying the disease into a particular type and should be able to give a fairly accurate prognosis. However, over half of those born with OI are due to mutations and the parents are normal. In these circumstances, it is necessary to explain the condition in some detail, to relate in simple terms how it happened, and what is the likely outcome. The details of treatment are not sought at this stage, and it is usually desirable for the surgeon to be rather more optimistic than he might feel.

The infant with multiple fractures presents a problem in nursing which may be eased by constructing a wooden tray with sides. This is filled with soft foam rubber covered with ultra thin plastic (e.g. 'Gladwrap'). The baby is nursed in this and can be easily transported around the nursery and the home. Actual splinting of the fractures is usually not indicated.

Medical treatment

Drugs do not greatly influence this condition. However, two drugs can be used to effect.   1   Sodium fluoride, given in massive doses (10–15 mg daily), undoubtedly improves the dental condition. It may also diminish sweating and there is some evidence that the incidence of fractures is reduced.   2   Magnesium oxide

(10 mg per kilogram per day) is mainly of value in controlling excessive sweating. The mode of action of magnesium is probably a direct one on the sweat glands (the magnesium ion is a common ingredient of anti-perspirants).

Conservative treatment

The prevention of fracture and deformity by the use of braces is extremely difficult and, in severe cases, is probably impossible. Considerable advances have been made in recent years using the technology of plastics. This has revolutionised the construction of devices that accurately fit the limb or trunk, while at the same time allowing mobility. When fractures do occur they can be treated as any other fracture in childhood—by reduction and plaster cast immobilisation. This works reasonably well for the isolated fracture, but immobilisation causes increased porosis so that a vicious circle may be initiated. It is for this reason that surgical methods of care have been developed.

Surgical treatment (Figs. 8.15 & 8.16)

The modern era of operative treatment was ushered in by Sofield when he described his method of fragmentation and rodding in 1952. This basic method has stood the test of time, although various minor improvements and modifica-

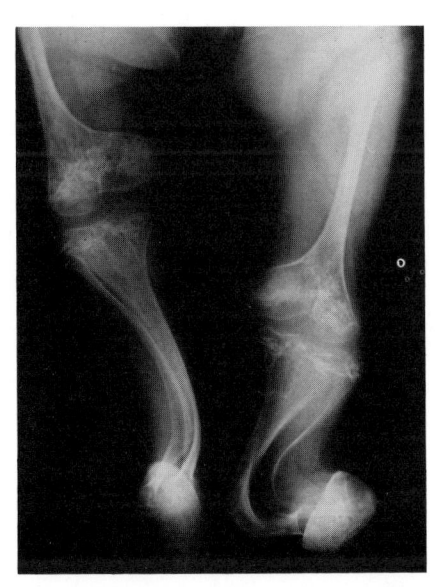

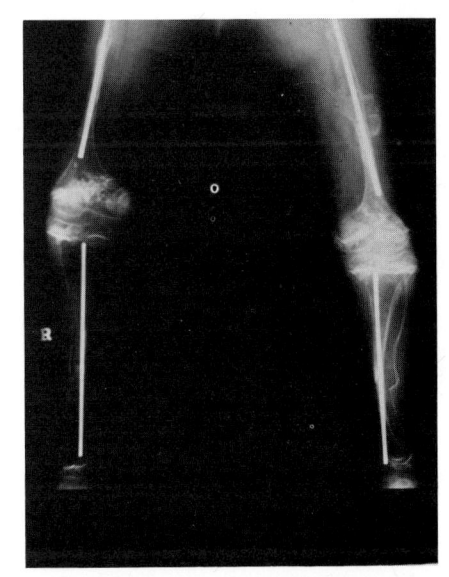

Figs. 8.15 & 8.16 X-rays of the lower limbs of a 14-year-old boy with osteogenesis imperfecta. Most of the deformity occurred by gradual bending rather than from malunion following fractures. The 'popcorn' epiphyses are well shown. (*Right*) After fragmentation and rodding, walking was achieved but, because of muscular weakness, this was abandoned two years later in favour of a motorised wheelchair.

tions have been made since. It consists essentially of removing the whole of the diaphysis of the long bone and dividing it up into a number of segments each of which is reasonably straight. After restoring the medullary cavity by drilling, all the segments and the two ends are immobilised with an intramedullary steel rod. The placement of this rod is facilitated by the method of threading them together.

INDICATIONS FOR OPERATIVE TREATMENT

No hard and fast rules can be laid down as to when or if rodding should be carried out. In any given child the decision will be influenced by the following general considerations.

Age. Although rodding can be carried out in infancy, the effect is quickly dissipated by growth (Figs. 8.17 & 8.18) so that, unless repeated fractures are occurring, operation is best postponed until after the third or fourth year when most of those severely affected will be making some effort to crawl and stand.

Type of bone. Both thick bone and thin bone types can be rodded, and each presents its own peculiar difficulty. In general, the thin bones will require earlier rodding while the thick bones can often be left for a fairly long time as their tendency to produce deformity and to fracture is less.

Prognosis for walking. Most children affected with OI will either walk or can be aided to do so. There are two variants with a poor prognosis: those with thin bones having expanded honeycombed ends and all cases with extreme dwarfism, especially if accompanied by severe chest deformity. Those with white sclera rarely become walkers.

Development of deformity. There is a wide variation in the rapidity with which deformity develops but, if it does occur early, then rodding should be done earlier and repeated as necessary to allow walking braces to be fitted and to minimise shortening. Even neglected cases which have developed severe deformity can be salvaged at the expense of significant loss in length.

Incidence of fracture. If fractures are occurring repeatedly in the one bone, rodding is indicated and in many instances children themselves will ask that it be done.

THE ROLE OF RODDING IN THE UPPER LIMB

For a variety of reasons the upper limb presents a much less attractive field for operative treatment. Fractures occur less frequently and deformity, even of fairly

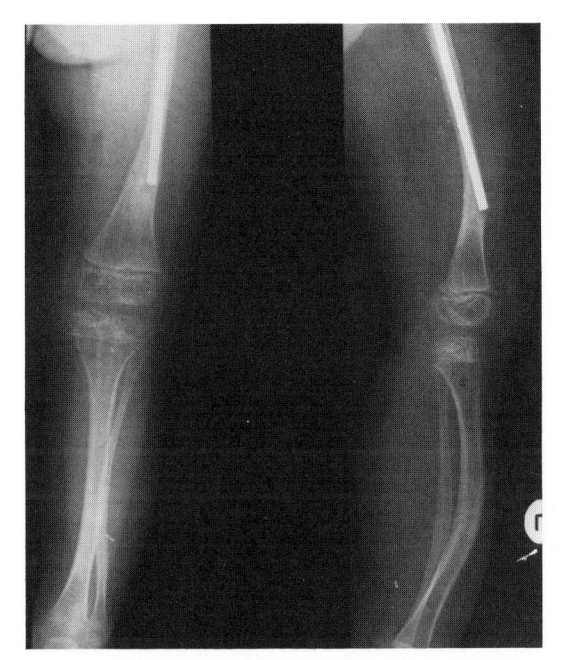

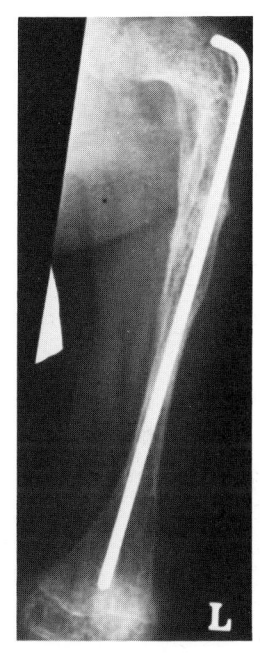

Figs. 8.17 & 8.18 The effect of growth: the femur is gradually binding around the end of the rod and eventually re-fracture will occur at this site. (*Right*) Migration of rods: with growth the rod has migrated sideways and the femur is becoming bowed again.

gross degree, can often be accepted. The humerus is difficult to approach safely and the bone is either devoid of a medullary cavity throughout most of its length or the cavity is so wide that a rod offers little rigidity (Fig. 8.19). Similarly, the forearm bones are difficult to rod and these tend to migrate quickly. In any case, most severe deformities in the young are best treated by manual osteoclasis and plaster immobilisation.

Summary

In clinical practice osteogenesis imperfecta is seen in a wide range of severity and many children are so minimally affected that special treatment is unnecessary. However, at the other end of the scale, the disease is extremely crippling and conventional methods of treatment do little to alleviate the problem. There can be no doubt that those who do require intramedullary rodding have less fractures and less hospitalisation, are happier, less apprehensive, and arrive at maturity with limbs that are reasonably straight. It must be said, however, that the operation of rodding these fragile bones requires a great deal of experience and technical skill if good results are to be achieved.

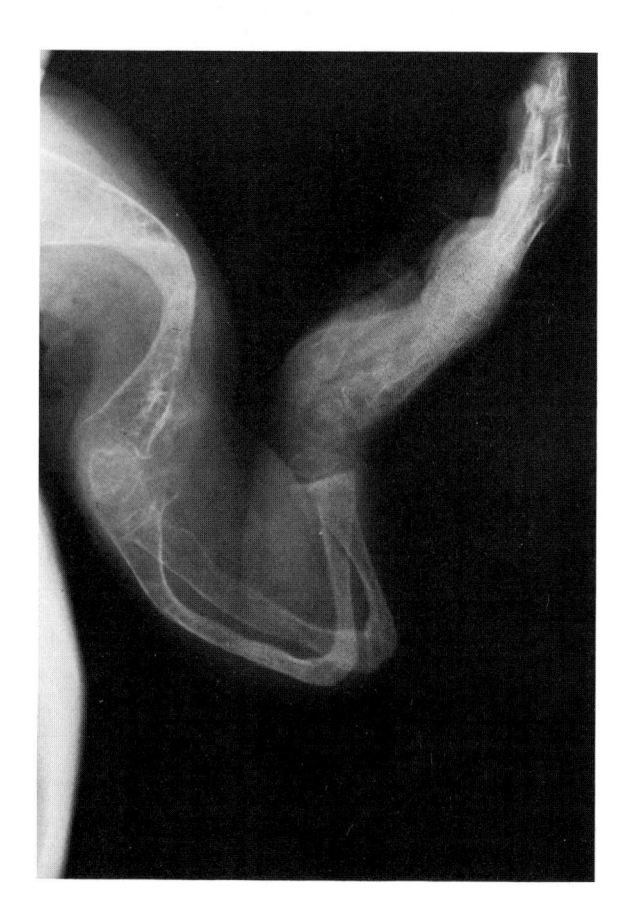

Fig. 8.19 Gross upper limb deformity in osteogenesis imperfecta.

NEUROFIBROMATOSIS

In 1882, von Recklinghausen described a genetically based disease in which an autosomal dominant inheritance pattern was evident in half the patients while the other half resulted from spontaneous mutations. It is still not known how the genetic abnormality leads to the wide variety of manifestations observed in this disease.

DIAGNOSIS

The diagnostic hallmark of neurofibromatosis is the 'café-au-lait' skin spot (Fig. 8.20). As these spots are also seen in otherwise normal individuals, Crowe and his colleagues concluded that more than six café-au-lait spots, each measuring more than 1.5 cm in diameter, were required to make the diagnosis of neurofibroma-

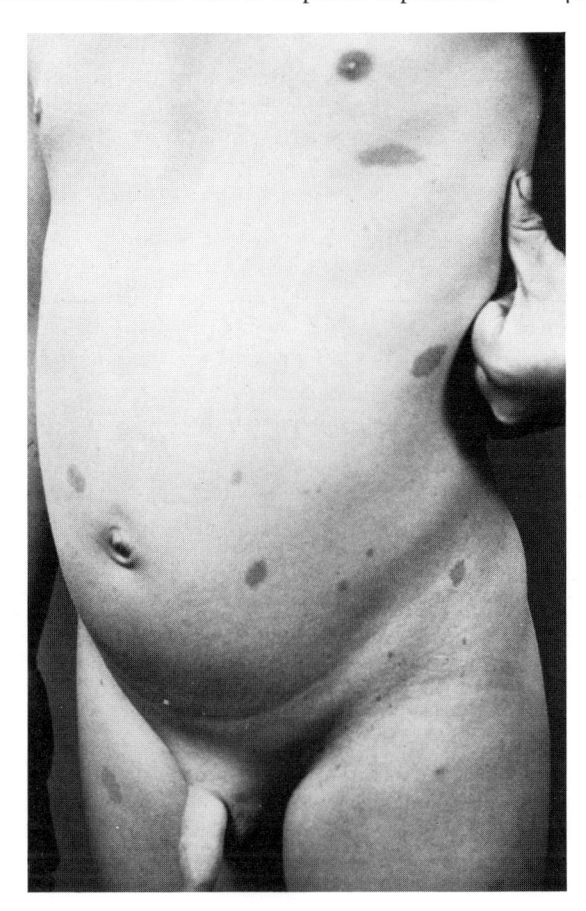

Fig. 8.20 Typical café-au-lait pigmentation in neurofibromatosis.

tosis. However, fewer spots can be accepted when there is a family history of this disease. The diagnosis can also be made by histological examination of neurofibromas.

CLINICAL FEATURES

There is a wide range of manifestations which do not appear at the same time or in any predictable manner.

Skin lesions

Café-au-lait spots are the most frequent skin lesions. They vary considerably in number and in their degree of pigmentation. They are occasionally present at birth but become more numerous as the child grows older. The distribution of the spots is unrelated to the site of any internal manifestation of this disease. Other skin lesions are also observed including intradermal neurofibromas, large hairy pigmented patches, bathing trunk naevi, and occasionally vitiligo. The large hairy patches and bathing trunk naevi are very disfiguring.

Neurofibromas

They are also characteristic of this disorder and are either clinically discrete or plexiform. The discrete lesions are frequently seen in subcutaneous nerves as ovoid tumours with the nerve fibrils distributed throughout the mass. The capsule frequently consists of compressed tumour tissue and, although the lesion is clinically discrete, it frequently has plexiform histological features.

The plexiform neurofibromas are also characteristic and consist of a worm-like mass of tissue. They are frequently seen in the cervical and cervicothoracic regions and tend to spread from one anatomical area to another, such as from the thoracic cavity into the neck (Fig. 8.21) or the intervertebral

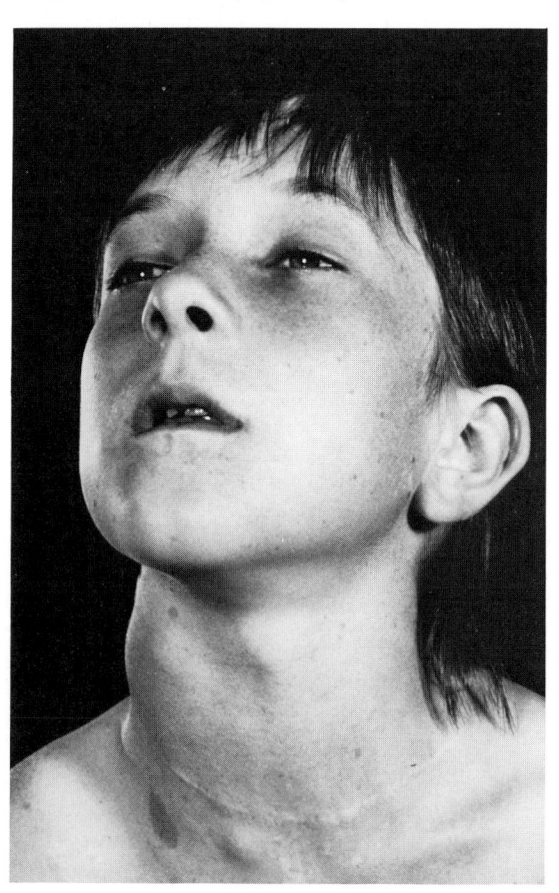

Fig. 8.21 Extensive tumour formation in the neck and mediastinum in a case of neurofibromatosis. Subtotal removal had been carried out previously. The infiltrating nature of the tumour is similar to a malignancy and a fatal outcome from involvement of the spinal canal is usual.

Some Generalised Disorders with Orthopaedic Implications 421

foramina and spinal canal. They are frequently large and invade neighbouring tissues (Fig. 8.22). In the limbs, they are commonly associated with gigantism (Fig. 8.23). The limb is enlarged in all directions with hypertrophy and

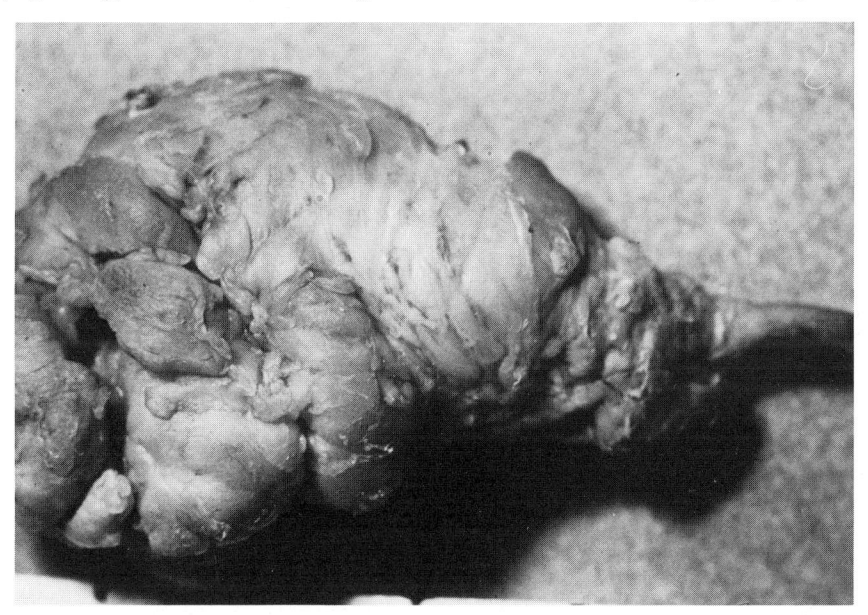

Fig. 8.22 This tumour, the size of a coconut, was removed from the loin of a child with neurofibromatosis. The spinal nerve from which the tumour arose is seen on the right of the photograph.

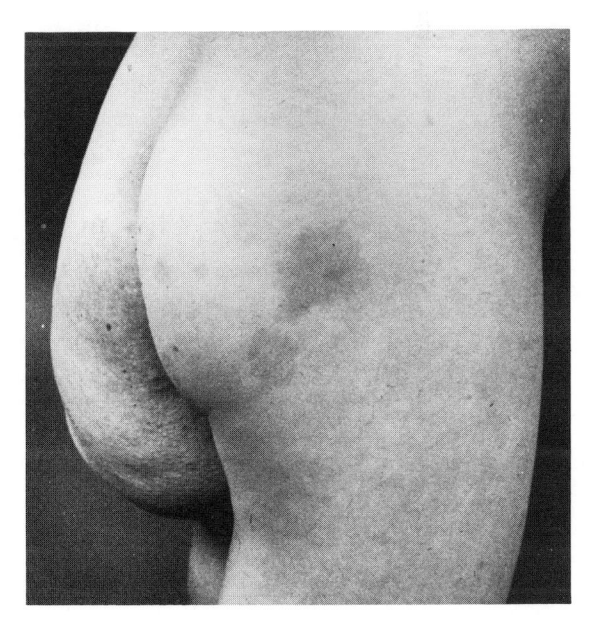

Fig. 8.23 Café-au-lait pigmentation and plexiform neurofibromatosis of the left buttock.

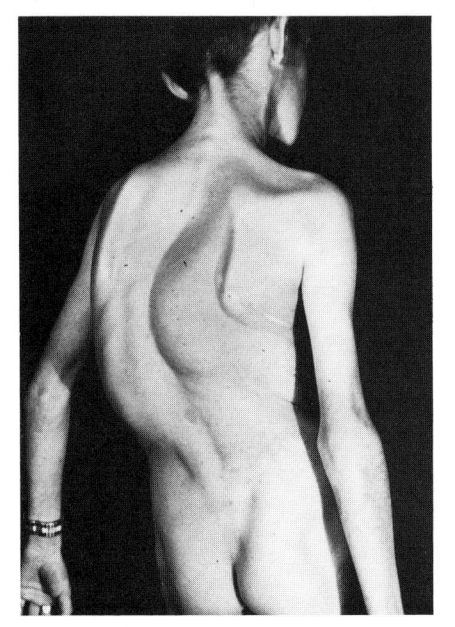

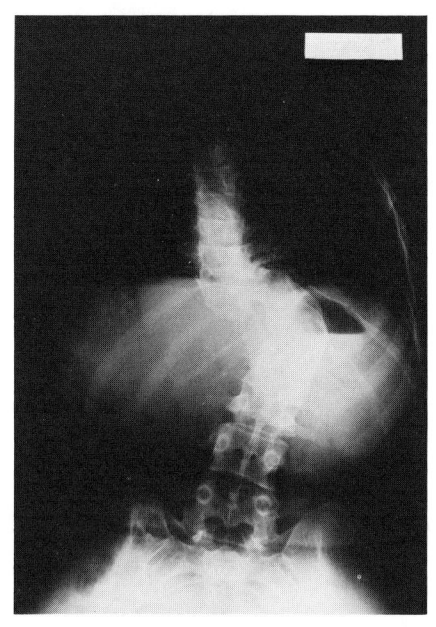

Figs. 8.24 & 8.25 (*Left*) Severe rigid scoliosis typical of neurofibromatosis. (*Right*) Radiograph of a 10-year-old boy with a severe thoracolumbar scoliosis associated with neurofibromatosis.

hyperplasia of all the tissues including the bone and the skin. The skin is frequently redundant, hangs in folds, is often heavily pigmented, and may give rise to pain. Sarcomatous transformation of neurofibromas is uncommon in childhood but occurs increasingly with age.

Skeletal—spine

Spinal deformities are important because they frequently progress to severe deformity and paraplegia (Fig. 8.24). The deformity consists of a rigid kyphoscoliosis with gross vertebral abnormalities of apical vertebra deformation, scalloping of the vertebral bodies, and a 'twisted ribbon' deformity of the ribs (Fig. 8.25). Neurofibromas are occasionally found in association with the vertebral abnormalities but, in many cases, there is no evidence of neurofibromatous tissue. It has been claimed that many of the vertebral abnormalities are the result of vertebral dysplasia.

Vertebral anomalies are also seen in children who do not have spinal deformities. These abnormalities include scalloping of the vertebral bodies which may be associated with meningoceles, erosions of hypertrophy adjacent to plexiform neurofibromas, and congenital anomalies to the spine.

Peripheral

The peripheral skeletal changes are common in children who have hypertrophy of a limb. In most instances a plexiform neurofibroma will be evident in some part of the limb but most of the enlargement is due to hypertrophy and hyperplasia of other tissues. The long bones are frequently elongated and spindly but may show areas of sclerosis. Subperiosteal bone cysts are relatively common and give rise to cortical defects; occasionally large subperiosteal cysts will result from a haemorrhage beneath the periosteum with secondary calcification in the wall of the cyst.

Pseudarthrosis of the long bones, in particular the tibia and the radius, is a very important manifestation of neurofibromatosis (Figs. 8.26 & 8.27). It is not usually present at birth but the bone will be bowed and x-rays will show that the medullary cavity in the bowed area is absent and the cortex is sclerotic. In some instances a cyst is present at the apex of the bow. With time, the bowing and sclerosis will increase and a fracture will result which is very difficult to treat and frequently results in pseudarthrosis. Even if the pseudarthrosis does heal, there is often severe shortening of the affected bone.

CNS manifestations

These manifestations can be broadly divided into progressive lesions (i.e. tumours) and non-progressive lesions (i.e. dysplasias). Optic neuromas are the commonest type of tumour in the central nervous system: children frequently present with decreased vision, strabismus, oscillatory eye movements, or occasionally with ptosis, proptosis or hydrocephalus. At the time of presentation there is usually severe deterioration of the visual acuity.

Brain tumours such as astrocytomas and gliomas frequently present with headaches, vomiting, ataxia, and cranial nerve palsies. Acoustic neuromas are rare in children although frequently seen in the adult.

Spinal cord tumours such as astrocytomas and ganglioneuromas frequently present with spastic paraparesis, spinal scoliosis, and back pains. These abnormalities are also seen in children with plexiform neurofibromas which have invaded the spinal canal.

The non-progressive dysplastic conditions of the brain present with mental retardation, behavioural disturbances, epilepsy, and cerebral palsy.

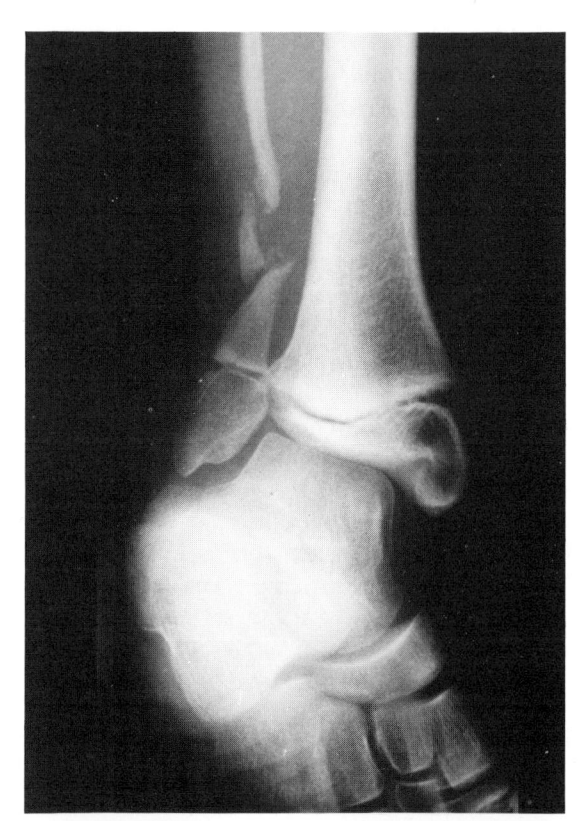

Figs. 8.26 & 8.27
Pseudarthrosis of the fibula in a boy with neurofibromatosis. Progressive valgus deformity of the ankle resulted.

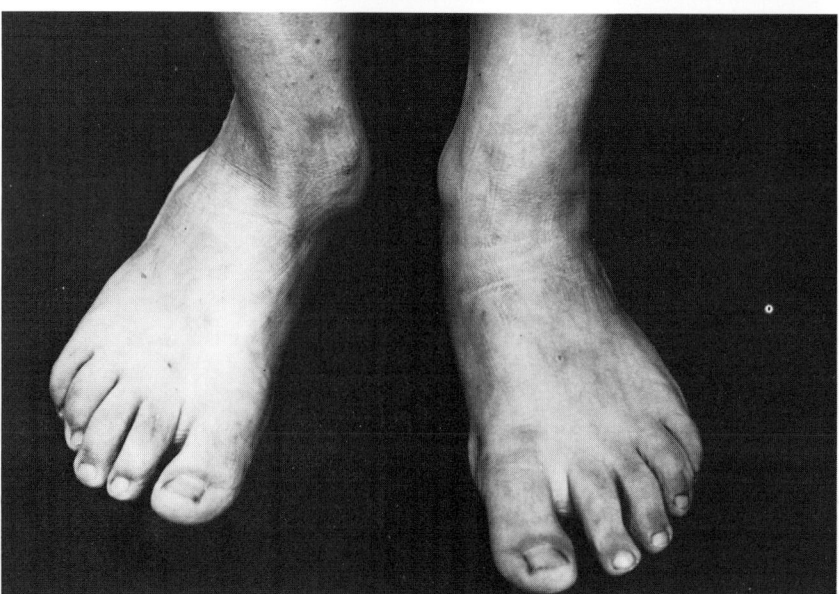

MANAGEMENT

Because of the wide variety of manifestations of this disease it is important to consider it as a diagnosis in many clinical situations. Once a diagnosis has been made, a careful search should be made for the manifestations which frequently present at an advanced stage, i.e. optic neuromas, intrathoracic neurofibromas, and spinal deformities. It should also be remembered that spinal cord tumours frequently present in the early stages with scoliosis, back pain, and abnormalities of gait and posture.

Many of the manifestations of neurofibromatosis such as café-au-lait spots do not require treatment. However, specific attention needs to be given to progressive disorders, e.g. optic neuromas, spinal cord and brain tumours, spinal deformities, and pseudarthrosis. Progressive spinal deformities require early arthrodesis of the spine. Progressive bowing of the tibia requires bone grafting in order to prevent progression and careful treatment will be required for an established pseudarthrosis. Leg length discrepancies are another problem which often progresses and requires a combination of epiphyseal arrest and bone shortening for its correction. The feet are frequently different in size which gives rise to problems of buying footwear. On occasions it may be feasible to make the feet more equal in size by exercising the outer ray of the enlarged foot. In many instances this is not sufficient and either shoes of dissimilar size will need to be worn or a slipper can be made for the normal foot to make it the same size as the enlarged foot.

Careful judgement is required in making a decision regarding the treatment of neurofibromas. Discrete neurofibromas situated on subcutaneous nerves can be excised if they are giving trouble; however, neurofibromas of major nerves usually cannot be excised without producing significant neurological dysfunction. Plexiform neurofibromas are even more difficult to treat because of their extent and infiltrating nature. As a result it is usually impossible to excise these tumours completely so that subtotal resection is reserved for children who are having chronic pain.

Genetic counselling is important as there is no specific treatment available for neurofibromatosis. In families with an autosomal dominant inheritance pattern, the risk of further affected children is 50%, while in families with normal parents it is likely that the affected child has a new mutation and further pregnancies are unlikely to produce another child with neurofibromatosis. However, future children of the affected child would have a one in two chance of inheriting this trait. Although predictions can be given for the likelihood of other children being affected by neurofibromatosis, it is difficult to predict the type of manifestations that other children will develop as it is the trait that is inherited rather than the tendency to a particular manifestation.

MUSCULAR DYSTROPHY

The term muscular dystrophy is reserved for those cases of progressive weakness of skeletal muscle which are genetically determined and in which the primary pathological change is in the muscle itself and is not secondary to disease of the central or peripheral nervous system.

CLASSIFICATION

Many attempts at classification have been made based on genetics or on clinical characteristics but, since there is a wide variation in types, an accurate classification is difficult to devise. The histological changes in the muscle are similar in all types although varying in severity.

The following clinical classification is usually accepted: 1   Duchenne type (pelvic girdle, severe form, sex linked, autosomal recessive variety);   2   limb girdle—either pelvic girdle (mild form, sex linked recessive) or scapulo-humeral (autosomal recessive);   3   facio-scapulo-humeral (autosomal dominant).

CLINICAL FEATURES

The various types differ with respect to age onset, the actual muscle groups involved, and the rate of progression. However, in most types, the course is progressive with periods of remission until the patient becomes bed-ridden.

Duchenne type

This is the commonest type and occurs in boys in early childhood. Symmetrical weakness of the pelvic girdle is followed by shoulder girdle involvement. Pseudohypertrophy—especially of the calf musculature—is a feature (Fig. 8.28). The condition usually presents before the age of 5 years, walking commonly ceases at about 10 years, and death is common before 20 years from respiratory infection. The child presents because of frequent falls, inability to keep up with his peers, and inability to climb stairs or rise from the floor.

The appearance of the child is very characteristic. He stands with a lumbar lordosis with extended knees, enlarged calves and may have difficulty in standing plantigrade due to the development of equinus. When rising from the floor he 'climbs up his legs' (Gowers' sign—Fig. 8.29). Later, wasting of the shoulder muscles occurs and, with further progression, deformities appear—especially equinus at the ankle (triceps surae) and flexion at the hip and knee (iliotibial band). Scoliosis and kyphoscoliosis may become severe and present great difficulties in sitting.

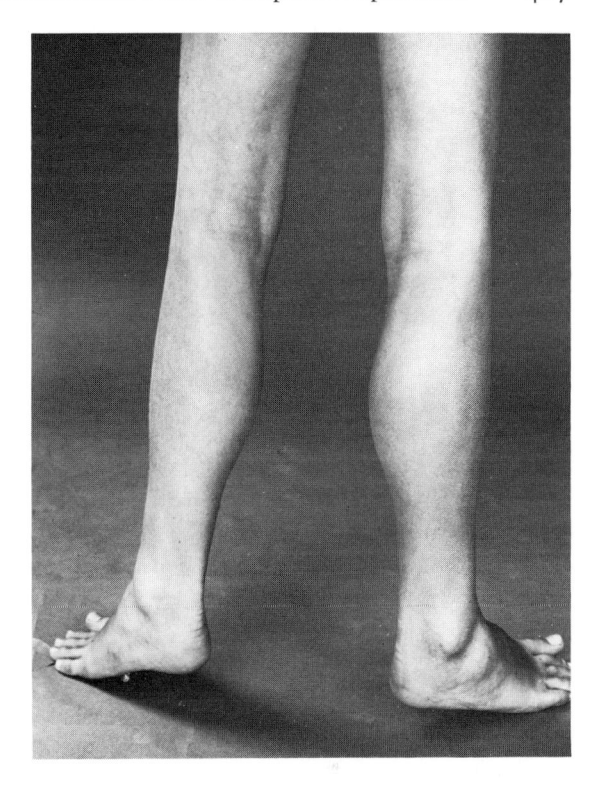

Fig. 8.28
Erb–Duchenne or pseudohypertrophic dystrophy. Note the bulky calves and equinus deformity.

Limb girdle muscular dystrophy

Less common than Duchenne type, the onset in this variety is also delayed and may present between the ages of 10 and 50 years. Weakness of muscles in either the shoulder, the pelvic girdle, or both develops slowly. Pseudohypertrophy of the calf is present in less than one-third of cases. Contractures develop late. Severe disability has usually developed within 20 years of the onset and most die of the disease.

Facio-scapulo-humeral muscular dystrophy

Males and females are affected with equal frequency in this variety, the usual onset being in the second decade. There is a wide variation in the degree of severity but, in most cases, the facial muscles are affected first which gives the characteristic deadpan expression and later may interfere with speech. The muscles of the shoulder girdle are next involved. Pseudohypertrophy is rare and contractures are mild. Most patients remain ambulant and live a normal life span.

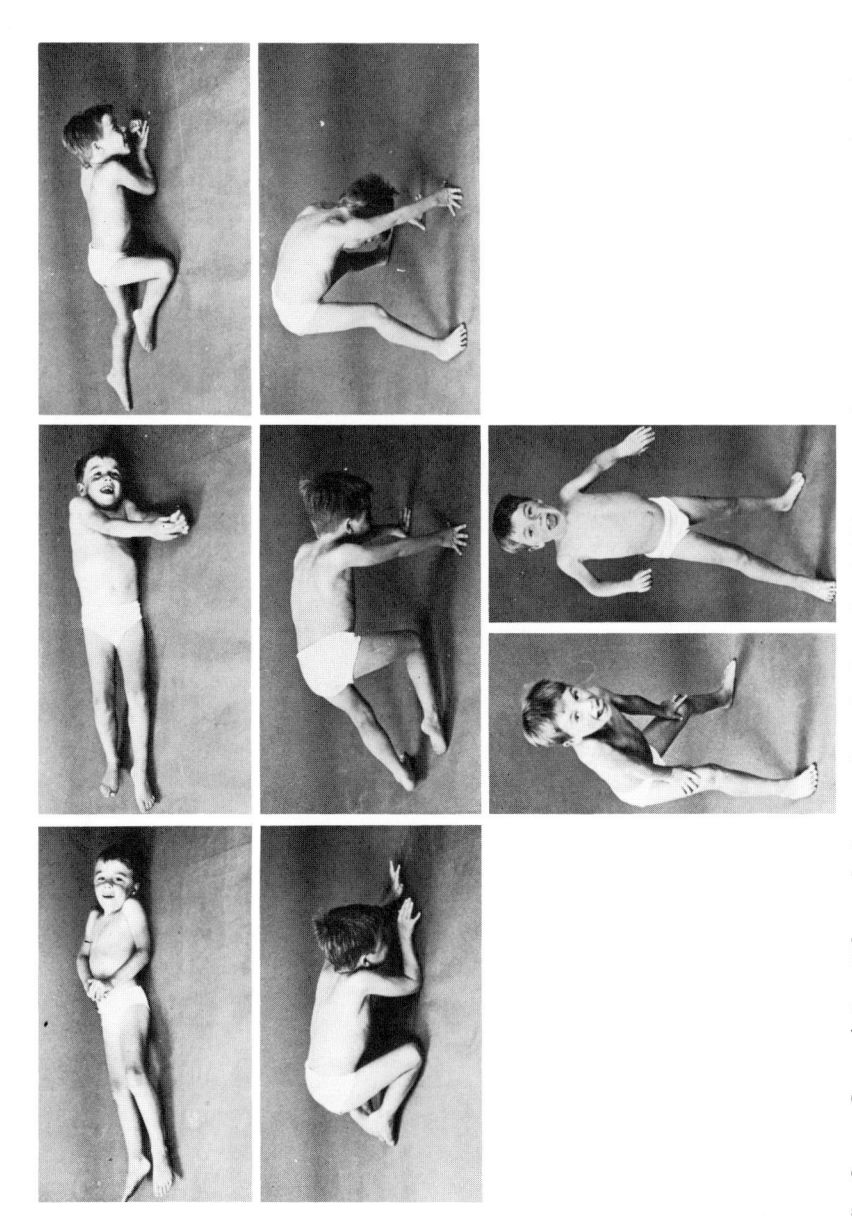

Fig. 8.29 Gowers' sign. When asked to rise from the floor the child has to use his arms to overcome trunk weakness.

DIAGNOSIS

Diagnosis is based on:

Recognition of the clinical signs. This is easy in the established case but may present difficulties in the early stages.

The genetic history.

Neurological examination. When a child presents with muscle weakness it should first be determined whether the primary cause is myopathic or neuropathic. In neuropathic disorders, distal weakness is the first indication, whereas proximal involvement is the rule in early muscular dystrophy. Deep tendon reflexes are preserved for a long time in dystrophies but are affected early in neuropathic disorders.

Serum enzymes. Creatinine kinase—the level of this enzyme is always increased in the serum of patients with muscular dystrophy. Aldolase—high levels occur especially in the Duchenne type of muscular dystrophy and in the early stages of all types. In adult types the level may be much less and may even be normal.

Muscle biopsy. Histological examination of specimens removed at operation will show characteristic degenerative changes but will not distinguish between the various types.

MANAGEMENT

Once the diagnosis is established, the parents should be given an account of the condition with a somewhat more optimistic bias than the subsequent course might justify. They should also be acquainted with any genetic considerations which may apply and arrangements made for them to consult a clinical geneticist. It is usual to explain the immediate situation to the child without discussing any future implications. Most of these affected children are soon frustrated at their inability to play with their friends, become withdrawn and passive. As they slowly but remorselessly deteriorate, their morale is affected and it becomes increasingly difficult for parents, teachers, and therapists to kindle a spark of happiness. Nevertheless, every effort should be made to maintain optimism and to provide a range of interests and activities which is as wide as possible.

Specific treatment

There is no specific treatment available for muscular dystrophy.

Physical treatment

ACTIVITY

Since inactivity aggravates the muscle atrophy, activity to the point of fatigue is encouraged. However it is important to be realistic and to recognise when an activity has become too difficult to be enjoyable. When ill from any cause, bed rest is restricted to a minimum and, should fractures occur, early weight-bearing in the cast is carried out wherever possible.

PASSIVE MOTION

Since walking will finally be abandoned due to the combination of muscle weakness and contractures, the latter are minimised by regular passive motions particularly at the knee and ankle and this may be carried out at home by the parents. Night splintage may be used but is not well tolerated.

NUTRITION

Because of decreased activity, overeating, and pampering, obesity is common and further increases the difficulties of ambulation in the early stages and later of nursing. Every effort should therefore be made to prevent obesity.

BRACING

Since contractures occur very quickly once walking is abandoned, every effort within reason should be made to prolong the walking period. Lightweight braces may be indicated to control quadriceps weakness.

SURGERY

Soft tissue surgery has a dual small role to play: firstly, to relieve contractures—subcutaneous section of the heel cord and tensor fasciae latae are useful in this regard and should be followed by as early ambulation as possible. Secondly, to achieve muscle balance. In some children confined to chairs, the feet become fixed in equinovarus so that weight is born on the dorsum of the foot. The tibialis posterior muscle remains active for a number of years and it has been found useful both to correct the deformity by elongation of the heel cord and manipulation under anaesthesia and to prevent recurrence by transfer of the tibialis posterior forwards. The foot will usually remain corrected until the child is bed-ridden.

WHEELCHAIR

Once ambulation is impractical, an electric wheelchair will provide these unfortunate children with a much appreciated degree of independence.

HOME CARE

Muscular dystrophy is a particularly distressing condition for the parents and they will require continual advice and support, particularly from the physiotherapist and occupational therapist. A programme of home physiotherapy should be organised and the mother instructed how to carry out the various passive movements and stretching exercises. Once the wheelchair phase has started there is an increasing risk of contractures and more effort will be required to prevent them. Not all contractures are preventable but at least they can be minimised. The importance of good seating, both in the wheelchair and at other times, is to be stressed as spinal curvatures tend to develop quite rapidly. Swimming should be encouraged but at all times should be supervised. Parents are instructed that, as long as possible, the boy should retain independence in daily living skills, and particularly in such things as dressing, feeding and bathing himself. School work can be carried out by correspondence and hobbies and crafts are encouraged to alleviate the boredom which is inevitable in a wheelchair existence. Regular home visits by the occupational therapist will help in this regard and also determine whether any alterations are required to the home such as special rails and ramps to facilitate home care.

MARFAN'S SYNDROME (ARACHNODACTYLY)

This is an inborn error of development in which there is excessive cartilage growth at all epiphyseal plates. It is inherited as a simple Mendelian or autosomal dominant trait.

CLINICAL FEATURES

The affected child is tall and thin with remarkable elongation of the fingers and toes. Ligamentous laxity and muscular underdevelopment are the rule and the posture is poor—often with a funnel chest and dorsal round back. Other changes occur frequently such as aortic dilatation, dissecting aneurysm of the aorta, and dislocation of the lens in the eye.

MANAGEMENT

From an orthopaedic point of view the two most common areas of concern are the feet and the spine. The feet, which are very long and thin, develop gross plano-valgus deformity which later becomes rigid and painful. A fearsome footwear problem is presented by these feet on account of their size, shape, and posture. Conservative treatment with boots and arch supports is usually ineffective and eventually triple arthrodesis is demanded; this is best done by inlay rather than joint excision.

The spinal surgery is usually a kyphosis and may be progressive and severe. A Milwaukee brace is indicated in these severe cases and is most effective. In tall girls approaching maturity, premature growth arrest by oestrogen therapy is a useful adjunct to treatment and allows the brace to be discontinued at an earlier stage.

DOWN'S SYNDROME (MONGOLISM)

One of the most widely known forms of mental retardation, Down's syndrome has been identified as trisomy 21, a condition in which the child has an extra G chromosome. The risk is particularly high in older mothers. Children with Down's syndrome may present to the orthopaedic surgeon with a wide variety of conditions most of which are secondary to ligamentous laxity. These conditions are set out below roughly in the sequence in which they might occur.

POLYDACTYLY

Polydactyly of the hand is common and should be corrected because it is unsightly and also because the child should be able to wear gloves in the winter since peripheral circulation is poor and chilblains are a common complaint.

GENU VALGUM

The mongoloid toddler rapidly develops quite severe knock knee but this will usually resolve if obesity is kept under control. Most adults, and especially the females, have rather more knock knee than normal.

SUBLUXATION OF THE CERVICAL SPINE

Spontaneous subluxation of the atlas on the axis is common in Down's syndrome. Symptoms may be absent or be insidious and overlooked, and some will present with progressive quadriplegia. The incidence of spine involvement may be as high as 25% and some of these will have an associated hypoplasia of the odontoid.

Some Generalised Disorders with Orthopaedic Implications 433

Early detection is important and stabilisation by spinal fusion should always be carried out.

DISLOCATION OF THE HIP AND ACETABULAR DYSPLASIA (FIG. 8.30)

Hip dislocations are easily reduced but are very unstable due to the extreme ligamentous laxity; for this reason they do not respond well to conservative treatment. Surgery is not often required as a second class result can be accepted in view of the limited use expected. Occasionally capsule reefing and correction of the femoral anteversion will be required so as to gain stability. The various forms of pelvic osteotomy are hardly ever indicated. All forms of surgery on the hip should be avoided wherever possible as the complication rate is staggeringly high.

DISLOCATION AND SUBLUXATION OF THE PATELLA

Recurrent dislocation and subluxation of the patella is common, especially in girls, and may become very disabling. Treatment is similar to that carried out in the normal child although the medial capsule must also be reefed and the vastus medialis advanced forward across the front of the patella. This is, of course,

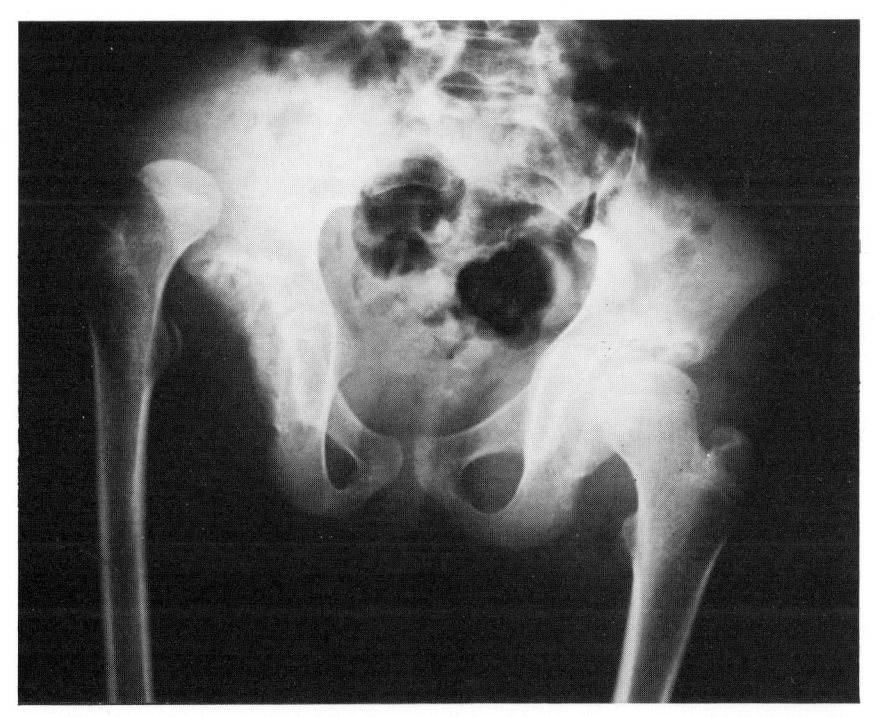

Fig. 8.30 Radiograph of a child with Down's syndrome. She presented at the age of 12 years with a recent dislocation of the right hip which occurred spontaneously.

additional to transfer of the patella tendon medially and distally. Even so the results are not always satisfactory. If surgery fails or if pain from chondromalacia patellae becomes a problem in older children, patellectomy is advisable.

FLAT FEET

Severe flat foot is the rule but most can be managed with adequate boots and long arch supports.

HALLUX VARUS AND VALGUS

In Down's syndrome the real abnormality is usually in the metatarsal and the hallux may be varus or valgus in association with this deformity. Surgical correction is effective and consists of a proximal metatarsal osteotomy with either reefing or releasing of the medial capsule of the metatarsophalangeal joint.

SCOLIOSIS

This is rarely a problem and, when it is, can be treated by standard methods.

THALASSAEMIA

Thalassaemia is a genetically determined disease transmitted by adult carriers whose ancestry can be traced to the Mediterranean area. It is inherited as a single autosomal incompletely dominant gene. An abnormal haemoglobin is formed leading to a severe haemolytic anaemia which demands frequent transfusion of whole blood. Skeletal changes, commonly seen in x-ray examination, are caused by a combination of hypertrophy of the bone marrow and faulty protein metabolism (Figs. 8.31 & 8.32). These changes include osteoporosis, widening of the medulla, and thin cortices with coarse reticulations. Clinically, many affected children show premature fusion of epiphyses of the long bones and increased tendency to fracture (Fig. 8.33), synovitis due to haemosiderosis, and the development of deformities in the lower limbs. Fractures heal slowly and need prolonged periods of protection. Early ambulation—using walking casts, cast braces, and braces—should be employed wherever possible. Open surgery for fractures or their complications should be avoided.

HEREDITARY NEUROPATHIES

Although there are a number of familial neuropathies with overlapping pathology, only two varieties are seen with any frequency in orthopaedic practice. These are peroneal muscular atrophy and Friedrich's ataxia and both

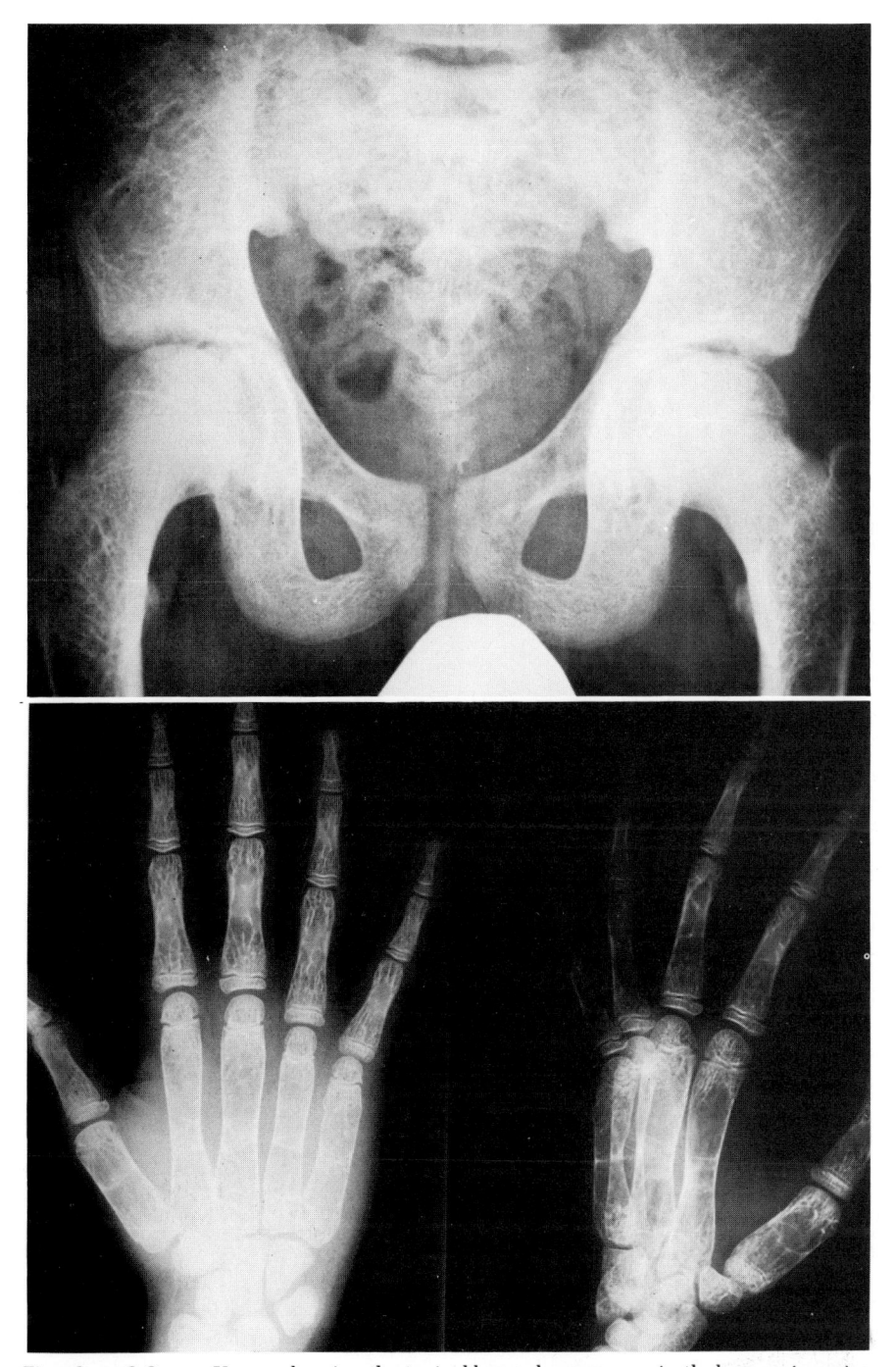

Some Generalised Disorders with Orthopaedic Implications 435

Figs. 8.31 & 8.32 X-rays showing the typical bone changes seen in thalassaemia major.

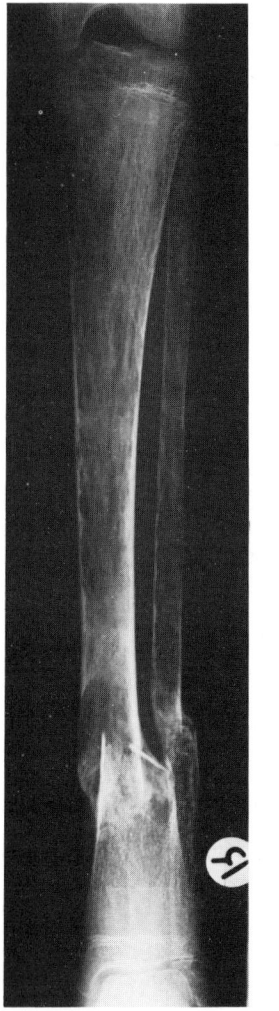

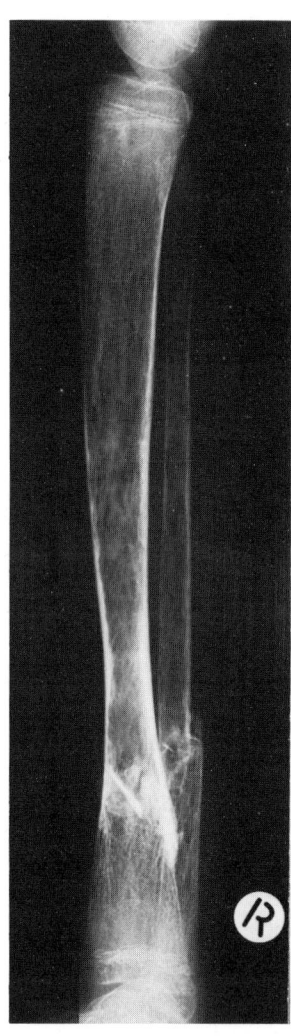

Fig. 8.33 Thalassaemia major. A pathological fracture has occurred in the tibia.

commonly present to the orthopaedic surgeon with pes cavus in childhood. In most cases the diagnosis has not been known or suspected at presentation

PERONEAL MUSCULAR ATROPHY (CHARCOT–MARIE–TOOTH DISEASE)

This condition is probably the commonest neurological disorder encountered in childhood and is characterised by a progressive symmetrical weakness of the lower limb muscles. The disease is inherited in either dominant or recessive form.

Clinical features

Pes cavus develops early and usually presents in the age group 5–10 years. Because the weakness starts in the intrinsic muscles and soon involves the peroneals, the foot becomes cavo-varus and recurrent instability of the ankle is common. There are nearly always complaints about footwear. Muscle atrophy gradually extends proximally but does not involve the proximal thigh so that the so-called 'stork leg' appearance is developed. Much later, muscles of the hand and forearms are involved but progress is very slow so that the final disability is never severe and longevity is not affected.

Management

The first step in management is to confirm the diagnosis with a neurologist and to arrange genetic counselling for the parents.

From an orthopaedic point of view a number of measures will prove helpful. In the early stages of peroneal weakness the shoes can be fitted with heels slightly raised on the outer side and floated out. Later, when this becomes ineffective, a below-knee brace (outside iron, inside T strap or ankle–foot orthosis) will be indicated. The tibialis posterior is usually found to be strong even when the peroneal and anterior tibial muscles have lost all strength. It is tempting to advise transfer of this muscle forwards but our experience is that, while this is most effective initially, the effect rarely lasts more than two years after which time the disease process begins to involve the transferred muscle.

After maturity, correction by triple arthrodesis is usually indicated. In severe cases it may be wise to correct some of the deformity first by plantar release as this will minimise the amount of bone to be removed. If the tibialis posterior is still active at the time it should be divided to restore muscle balance and so prevent recurrence of deformity.

FRIEDREICH'S ATAXIA

This condition has similar genetic implications to peroneal muscular atrophy and, although the most important effect is cerebellar ataxia, pes cavus and scoliosis are also features. Survival over the age of 30 years is unusual.

Clinical features

Ataxia may commence in early childhood and pes cavus is also an early manifestation. Scoliosis occurs in a few cases somewhat later. Neurological examination will show loss of deep reflexes, nystagmus, inco-ordination, and extensor plantar responses.

Management

Although the result is less satisfactory, the management of this condition is along similar lines to that in peroneal muscular atrophy.

Scoliosis is treated using conventional methods according to the degree and rapidity of change.

CONGENITAL INDIFFERENCE TO PAIN

A rare anomaly of unknown cause in which there is a complete sensory loss to pain. This leads to important changes due to injury affecting mainly the skin and joints.

Clinical features

These patients present in early childhood with multiple sores due to minor injuries or burns, mutilated fingertips from chewing and deformity of the limbs due to malunion from unrecognised fractures. Later, swollen joints are the rule as Charcot-like changes become established.

Management

The main aim of treatment is the prevention of injuries and this is extremely difficult in young children who feel no pain and are often very difficult to control. The reason for the latter feature is not clear but may be related to the fact that the parents are unable to punish the child physically. When repeated injuries to the skin result in chronic ulceration, plaster immobilisation and protection may be the only way of securing healing. When a joint is injured it may suggest the presence of pus as it is swollen, hot, and red; if any doubt exists a diagnostic aspiration is advisable. When such joints are opened, the excess joint fluid will contain thousands of snowflakes which are fragments of articular cartilage. At this stage it may be necessary to provide a permanent ankle–foot orthosis in an attempt to limit further destruction. However such a joint will eventually succumb and the classical Charcot changes ensue (Fig. 8.34). By the time these children have grown to adulthood they are usually crippled by multiple Charcot joints in the lower limbs and are eventually reduced to a wheelchair existence.

HAEMOPHILIA

Haemophilia is a sex-linked inherited disorder of blood clotting which affects males and is due to a deficiency of coagulation factors. The condition is usually not manifest until the first year of life when multiple bruising appears and is

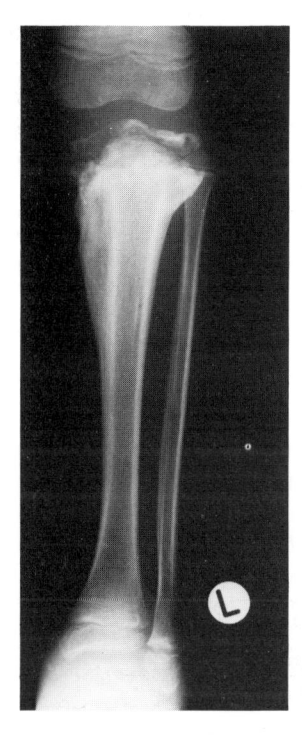

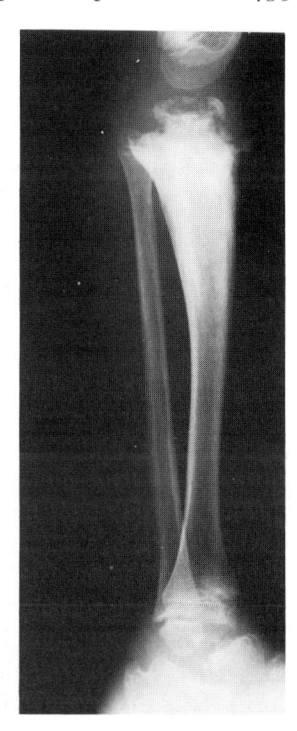

Fig. 8.34 An x-ray of the tibia of a 10-year-old boy with congenital indifference to pain. Note the excess bone production proximally following a fracture and the disappearance of the body of the talus.

followed by bleeding into body cavities, especially joints. Bleeding can be prevented and the effused blood rapidly resorbed by the administration of Factor VIII.

CLASSIFICATION

There are three types of haemophilia: *haemophilia A*—the commonest type, due to Factor VIII deficiency; *haemophilia B* (Christmas disease)—due to Factor IX deficiency; and *haemophilia C*—an uncommon form due to Factor XI deficiency which is inherited as an autosomal dominant trait and is seen in both sexes.

ORTHOPAEDIC IMPLICATIONS OF HAEMOPHILIA

Haemarthrosis

Haemophiliacs are particularly susceptible to joint bleeding which originates from the synovial membrane and produces considerable pain and muscle spasm. Once this membrane has been exposed to blood for a prolonged period there is uptake of iron, leucocyte, and platelet enzymes and this results in synovial damage and hypertrophy. The hypertrophied synovium will bleed readily so that a vicious cycle is established which eventually leads to loss of articular cartilage, adhesion formation, and chronic irreversible joint damage. Haemorrhages also occur into the subchondral bone causing necrosis of cartilage and exposure of the underlying bone. The knee is the most frequent site of haemarthroses and commonly develops disabling arthritis later in life (Figs. 8.35–8.37). Haemarthrosis of the ankle may also result in symptomatic degenerative arthritis (Fig. 8.38). The third most common joint to be involved is the elbow but this does not usually lead to late disability.

RADIOGRAPHIC CHANGES

Initially radiographs are normal. As the number of haemarthroses increases, narrowing of the joint space occurs with subchondral rarefaction. In the knee joint there is characteristically a squared off appearance to the femoral condyle. Erosions similar to those seen in rheumatoid arthritis may occur.

Haemorrhage into muscle

Minor bleeding into muscle is common but serious bleeding occasionally occurs especially in the iliopsoas, calf, and forearm. Bleeding may produce secondary pressure on nerves, vessels or skin and, after resorption, fibrosis may produce serious contracture. Even relatively minor trauma to the forearm should be

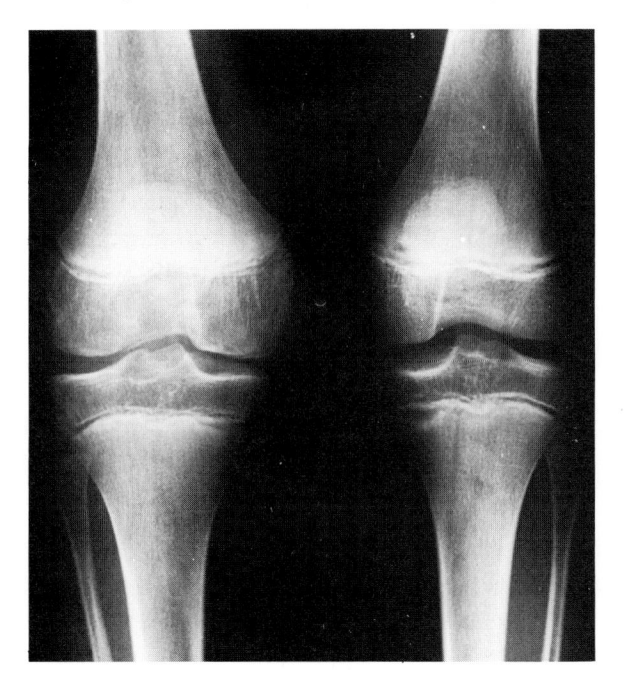

Fig. 8.35 Early arthropathy. A–P radiograph of both knees of a boy who has had frequent haemarthroses in the right knee. Note the increased size of femur, patella and tibia, the coarser trabeculation, the squaring of the shape of the femoral condyles, and the irregular loss of joint space.

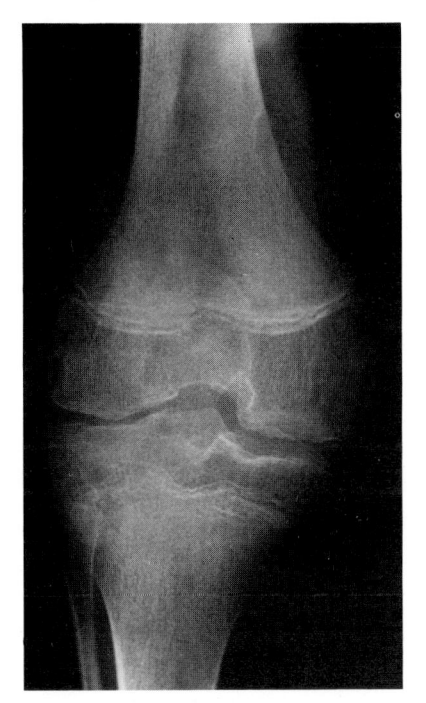

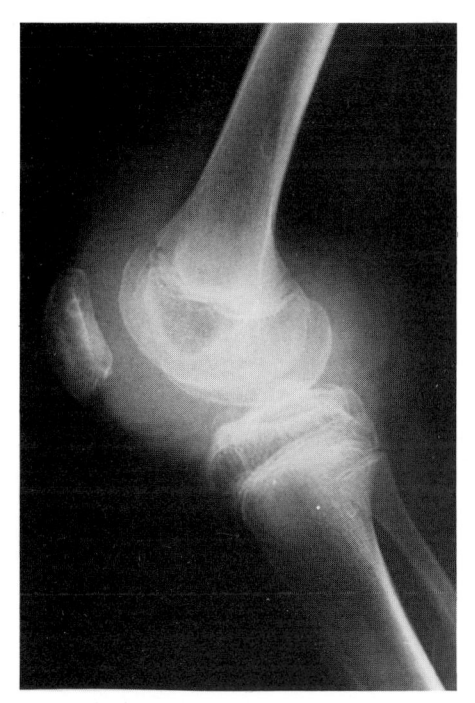

Figs. 8.36 & 8.37 Late arthropathy. A–P and lateral radiographs of the knee of a boy who had suffered frequent haemarthroses and who had developed antibodies to Factor VIII thus precluding adequate therapy. Note the fixed flexion deformity, posterior subluxation of the tibia, increased bulk of the condyles, and irregular articular surfaces.

regarded as potentially serious in the haemophilic patient. If any features of ischaemia occur, then extensive decompression should be performed immediately. The most frequent nerve lesion seen affects the femoral nerve when bleeding has occurred into the iliacus muscle sheath.

Fractures

Complications from fracture are surprisingly uncommon but should be forestalled by the use of padded plasters which are split longitudinally, hospital observation, and anti-haemophilic treatment.

Pseudotumours or haemophilic cysts

The term pseudotumour is to describe a progressive cystic swelling due to recurrent haemorrhage into muscle. An adjacent bone may be involved. They occur very rarely but should not be mistaken for a tumour.

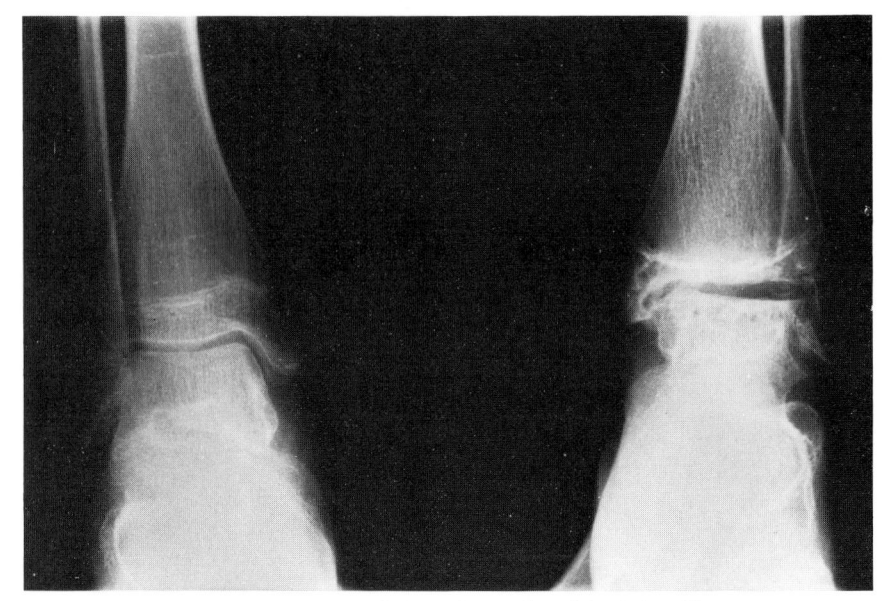

Fig. 8.38   Haemophilic arthropathy of the left ankle.

Soft tissue haematoma

Even minor direct injury may cause massive collections of blood which can ulcerate overlying skin.

MANAGEMENT

Children suffering from haemophilia should be managed at a haemophilic clinic within a children's hospital. A suitably staffed clinic is attended by a haematologist, orthopaedic surgeon, dentist, physiotherapist and social worker.

Prophylaxis

The parents of children who have had more than one haemarthrosis are given an advice sheet. This contains lists of appropriate toys and games. The child is later advised to avoid contact sports and is encouraged to take part in swimming and other activities less likely to cause injury.

Home treatment of haemophilia

The availability of freeze-dried Factor VIII concentrates has made home treatment of haemophilia feasible. Such programmes have been established throughout all major haemophilia centres and are functioning successfully.

Home treatment consists of training the family or patient to infuse Factor VIII intravenously at home. This is suitable for all severe haemophiliacs (Factor VIII level less than 1%) who are having bleeds at least twice per month. The basic prerequisites are co-operation of the child and the family, and veins which can be readily venepunctured. Children as young as 4 years may be more co-operative to treatment administered by the parents than to that given in hospital. There is a thorough training programme for the parent or child who is to administer the Factor VIII at home.

The indications for home infusion are early treatment of joint and soft tissue bleeding. It is hoped that early treatment will prevent sizeable haemorrhages into the joint cavity and the secondary changes to synovial membrane that follow its exposure to blood for long periods. Parents are instructed to treat the bleed as soon as pain has become apparent and not to wait for the appearance of swelling.

In order to administer a home treatment programme efficiently it is necessary to ask the parents or the patient to complete a questionnaire which describes each bleed, the dose of Factor VIII given, and the ease with which the procedure was accomplished.

Management of acute haemarthrosis

The management is aimed at rapid pain relief, early mobilisation of the affected joint, restoration of normal joint function, and the prevention of late arthritis.

There are three phases in the management of a haemarthrosis. 1 Factor VIII replacement and analgesia. 2 The local management of a haemarthrosis. 3 Physiotherapy.

FACTOR VIII REPLACEMENT

This should be given as soon as possible after the haemarthrosis has been diagnosed. If the patient is on the home care programme then the child knows that he is developing a harmarthrosis because of the pain; he has immediate Factor VIII replacement and generally no further treatment is necessary.

If a decision to aspirate the joint has been made (for reasons that will be considered below), Factor VIII replacement should be given immediately before aspiration and repeated 12 hours later. Subsequent doses depend on the patient's response. Factor VIII concentrates are the most preferred form of replacement therapy but, if the patient has antibodies to Factor VIII, then Factor IX is infused.

Analgesics. Paracetamol is the analgesic of choice. Aspirin is always contraindicated because of its effect on blood coagulation. Potent analgesics are avoided as being likely to lead to drug addiction in adult life.

Chapter 8

THE LOCAL MANAGEMENT OF A HAEMARTHROSIS

Indications for aspiration. The principal reason for aspirating a haemarthrosis is to reduce pain so that early use and early exercise are possible. Whether or not to aspirate a haemarthrosis will depend on a number of other factors: the degree of pain; the duration of the haemarthrosis; the joint involved—the knee is more likely to require aspiration than other joints; previous history of haemarthroses in the affected joint; previous experience with the management of haemarthroses at other joints and of other bleeding episodes in that particular child; and the presence of antibodies to Factor VIII.

Technique of aspiration. The aspiration is usually performed under general anaesthesia, although local anaesthesia may be used in co-operative children over the age of 14 years. The procedure should be performed gently by inserting the needle in one place and passing its point to the back of the patella. The needle should not be moved about more than is absolutely necessary. The suprapatellar pouch should not be pumped and vigorous flexion of the knee is to be avoided.

Post-operative management. Usually a plaster back slab is preferable to a cylinder as it enables the patient to view their quadriceps muscle (which in turn facilitates early static quadriceps exercises) and it allows ready removal for exercises. In general, the physiotherapist should begin static quadriceps exercises and gentle knee flexion exercises 1–2 days after aspiration. If there have been frequent recent haemarthroses of the joint or if the last haemarthroses required prolonged immobilisation, then a plaster cylinder is applied and retained for up to two weeks.

PHYSIOTHERAPY

24–48 hours after the joint has been immobilised (whether or not it has been aspirated), the physiotherapist gently removes the back slab and the pressure dressing about the knee. Static quadriceps exercises commence and gentle mobilisation follows at a rate depending upon the degree of discomfort. Pain is avoided at all costs as these children become very apprehensive and will not co-operate if the treatment is painful.

Generally, mobilisation will continue over the next 1–4 days with a number of treatment sessions each day until the patient is at least partially weight-bearing on crutches. He must have gained enough strength and range of movement to provide support and be safe when weight-bearing. Physiotherapy is then continued on an out-patient basis. Occasionally Factor VIII infusions may be necessary to facilitate physiotherapy and the physiotherapist should be informed of the time and frequency of these injections.

As soon as possible the back slab is removed and the child returned to gentle swimming as this is the most enjoyable and most effective form of physiotherapy.

Management of the child who has frequent haemarthroses

Children who have frequent knee haemarthroses should see the physiotherapist monthly so that they can be encouraged in their quadriceps exercises and swimming activities. Such visits also enable the range of motion of the knee and the circumference of the thigh to be recorded.

Some have such frequent haemarthroses that a removable polypropylene knee support with velcro fasteners is employed. It supports the knee in full extension and is worn to school and at other times when trauma to the knee is likely to occur. At other times, active exercises are encouraged to prevent quadriceps wasting. If there is established quadriceps wasting with knee instability and frequent haemarthroses, then a knee–ankle–foot orthosis is worn for the greater part of each day. Children who have frequent ankle haemarthroses should wear boots and if these are ineffective then an ankle–foot orthosis is worn as well.

Fixed flexion deformity at the knee, if progressive, should be treated by a period of reverse dynamic traction. The limb is supported in a Thomas' splint with Pearson attachment; in addition a padded canvas sling is applied to the anterior aspect of the suprapatellar pouch and is threaded underneath the metal bars on either side of the splint. A cord is attached to the ends of this sling and a weight of 3 kg is applied; this is increased over a period of two days. The patient is encouraged to flex and extend the knee frequently. The knee is gradually extended and when it is straight the Pearson attachment is removed.

Rarely is synovectomy of the knee justified. It should be considered for those children who have several bleeds into the knee each month for a period of at least a year, those who have a chronically swollen knee between bleeding episodes, and those who have no degenerative changes in their x-rays. Naturally the presence of antibodies to Factor VIII contraindicates surgery.

CHRONIC ARTHRITIS IN CHILDHOOD

With the marked decline in rheumatic fever in recent years, the most common type of subacute arthritis seen in paediatric practice is that due to viral infection, but joint sepsis, malignancy, and juvenile chronic arthritis are frequently seen in orthopaedic practice. In this section some of the common causes of chronic arthritis listed in Table 8.1 are discussed briefly. For each of these conditions the main clinical features and special investigations which are helpful in diagnosis will be emphasised and the principles of management of a child with juvenile chronic arthritis (JCA)—formerly known as Still's disease or juvenile rheumatoid arthritis—will be discussed. Although many of these conditions are primarily managed in the medical sphere, they may present to the orthopaedic surgeon as a problem of subacute or chronic synovitis in one or more joints.

Table 8.1 Conditions causing or simulating chronic arthritis in childhood.

Infectious diseases
septic arthritis
viral related arthritis
reactive arthritis
sympathetic effusions of osteomyelitis

Childhood malignancies
leukaemia
neuroblastoma

Non-inflammatory conditions of bones and joints
limb pains (growing pains)
psychogenic musculoskeletal dysfunction

Rheumatic diseases
juvenile chronic arthritis
rheumatic fever
ankylosing spondylitis
Henoch-Schönlein purpura
polyarteritis nodosa
systemic lupus erythematosus
dermatomyositis
scleroderma
inflammatory bowel disease
Reiter's syndrome
psoriatic arthritis

Miscellaneous
foreign body synovitis
villo nodular synovitis
disorders of coagulation

JUVENILE CHRONIC ARTHRITIS (JCA)

The term JCA is used to describe that form of arthritis in children under the age of 16 which persists for more than three months and where other causes of chronic arthritis have been excluded. In JCA, affected joints are swollen, stiff, and warm; movement is usually limited, particularly after periods of immobility. Different degrees of joint disturbance are seen; some children have a marked effusion with a rich proliferative synovium, but with surprisingly little functional impairment; others may show a minimal effusion with quite severe limitation in movement. This latter group have a dry restrictive arthritis which is particularly prone to cause longstanding functional impairment.

In the past children with JCA have been classified on the basis of their clinical presentation into three groups: those with a primary systemic disorder characterised by fever, hepatosplenomegaly and relatively mild arthritis initially; those with polyarthritis involving multiple joints; and those with pauci-articular arthritis where less than five joints are affected. Long term follow up of these three groups of children have demonstrated the limitations of this approach. The current classification recognises the role of probable immune response genes which are linked to the major histocompatibility antigens, and the significance of different antibodies in the serum of affected children.

The major histocompatibility antigen in man is the human leucocyte antigen or HLA, which is located on the short arm of the sixth chromosome. There is some evidence that this is important in controlling immune response to various antigens and in particular that it may account for the strong association between HLA B27 tissue type and ankylosing spondylitis. Just as in adult rheumatoid arthritis where the disease is diagnosed on the presence or absence of the rheumatoid factor—an anti-IgG antibody of the IgM class—this factor is sought in childhood although it is infrequently seen. More often, an antibody against nuclear antigens, the anti-nuclear factor (ANF), can be detected. At present these three factors (the presence of HLA B27, rheumatoid factor, and ANF) form three of the sub-groups of JCA which are increasingly being recognised. Other sub-groups of children with JCA are discussed below.

Systemic onset JCA

This pattern of onset of disease is common in young children although it may occur at any age. Characteristically the child looks sick and has a high fever which is irregularly intermittent. In addition rashes, hepatosplenomegaly, lymphadenopathy, polyserositis with leucocytosis, and ultimately growth retardation are common. Most patients develop chronic polyarthritis within the first months of the illness and up to a quarter of them go on to have a severe deforming arthritis. When first seen in an orthopaedic department there may be difficulty in differentiating the condition from septic arthritis with septicaemia.

Rheumatoid factor positive JCA

This is characterised by severe destructive arthritis in many joints and a poor prognosis. It is really an adult type rheumatoid arthritis developing in childhood and usually occurs in girls, particularly in late childhood. Less than 10% of children with JCA fall into this group.

Polyarticular JCA (rheumatoid factor negative)

Overall about a quarter of children with JCA have this pattern of disease and about 10% of them will develop significant destructive arthritis in the long term. Many of these children run a rather protracted course with low grade fever, mild anaemia, malaise and hepatosplenomegaly with lymphadenopathy being prominent before ultimate remission of their disease. Although it is unlikely that children with polyarthritis will present to an orthopaedic department, a significant number with only a few joints affected in the early stages may present as an orthopaedic diagnostic problem.

Where the arthritis is largely confined to a single joint, three further groups of JCA are recognised.

Pauci-articular arthritis (ANF positive)

This is particularly common in young girls with JCA. Invariably a major joint is affected with one or two smaller joints being involved also. Severe joint disease is rare and the prognosis for joint recovery is excellent. The major problem arises because of chronic iridocyclitis which affects half the patients in this group in the first ten years of their disease. Iridocyclitis is potentially serious and may cause blindness; in its early stages it may be quite asymptomatic and only formal ophthalmological assessment by slit lamp examination will enable its detection. Early therapy is crucial if vision is to be preserved.

Pauci-articular arthritis (ANF negative)

This is the group of children which will often be seen by orthopaedic surgeons. The prognosis of their disease is excellent although initial concern may be aroused because of the possibility of joint sepsis or even tuberculosis.

Pauci-articular arthritis associated with HLA B27

Nearly 90% of adults with ankylosing spondylitis have tissue type HLA B27. A significant number of these patients when seen in adulthood have a prior history of pauci-articular arthritis, particularly affecting the knees, ankles, and hips. Commonly symptoms of sacro-iliitis, with or without radiological demonstration of this, may be seen. Although these children may have remission of their peripheral arthritis, long term follow up is essential to allow the early detection of ankylosing spondylitis, adequate treatment, and prevention of deformity. Between 5 and 10% of these patients may show acute iritis during childhood which is readily diagnosed because of its acute pain and clinical appearance. It requires urgent ophthalmological treatment. This type of eye disease is to be contrasted with insidious chronic iritis which is seen commonly in young girls with pauci-articular joint disease and positive ANF.

ARTHRITIS RELATED TO INFECTIOUS DISEASES

These include septic arthritis, osteomyelitis with sympathetic effusion in adjacent joints, viral related and reactive arthritis. The diagnostic problems of septic arthritis and osteomyelitis are considered elsewhere (p. 138). Many viral infections including rubella, mumps, chicken pox, arbor virus, infectious mononucleosis, and hepatitis B have all been associated with arthritis. Generally joint symptoms follow some days or up to four weeks following the infection, although they may precede the onset in hepatitis B infection. In these arthritides joint swelling usually resolves in a few weeks with salicylate treatment. In the acute phase, the diagnosis may be confused with acute sepsis, most commonly seen after chicken pox, and later with JCA. It is important that children with viral related arthritis should not be mistaken for JCA patients because the prognosis in the former is excellent; only when joint swelling persists for more than three months can the diagnosis of JCA be seriously entertained in the absence of other diagnostic criteria. Symptoms are usually well controlled with salicylates.

One reactive arthritis is a sterile synovitis which is associated with bacterial infection, often in the gastrointestinal tract; Shigella, Salmonella and Yersinia have all been implicated. These diseases may affect one or several joints and are usually self-limiting; the diagnosis is suspected by preceding gastroenteric illness. Symptomatic treatment with salicylates will usually control symptoms.

ARTHRITIS RELATED TO MALIGNANCIES

Although it is uncommon for malignancies to present as a primary arthritis, this can occur. Leukaemia, neuroblastoma, lymphoma, Hodgkin's disease, histiocytosis and sarcomas can all cause musculoskeletal complaints which mimic arthritis; however, frank arthritis—the result of infiltration of malignant cells into structures around the joint—is most frequently seen in leukaemia and neuroblastoma. The patient is usually extremely ill and the affected joints are painful, swollen, and red. The diagnosis is usually suggested both by the severe bone and joint pain, and by the demonstration of hepatosplenomegaly, lymphadenopathy or other abnormal masses. A diagnosis of malignancy should be considered if a child with suspected rheumatic disease does not respond to salicylate therapy.

ARTHRITIS OF NON-INFLAMMATORY CAUSE

Although many orthopaedic conditions discussed elsewhere in this book give joint pain, they do not cause joint swelling and will not be considered in this section. Limb pains, or growing pains of childhood, are a common complaint. Although most pains are localised to the calf region, occasionally symptoms are localised to the joints; joint swelling and morning stiffness are not seen. Therapy relies entirely on parental reassurance. Persistent nocturnal limb pain always arouses concern of local malignancies and osteoid osteoma.

Psychogenic musculoskeletal dysfunction is occasionally seen in children with primary psychiatric disorders where repeated trauma can cause joint swelling. Diagnosis, however, usually rests on there being a significant degree of disability inappropriate to the clinical findings and laboratory investigations. There are some children with recurrent or persistent joint pain who have normal clinical, laboratory and radiological investigations and who appear emotionally adequate; their symptoms, which have been termed arthromyalgia, appear to resolve with reassurance.

ANKYLOSING SPONDYLITIS

Whilst the presentation of ankylosing spondylitis in childhood may be identical to that seen in adults with back ache and sciatic-like pain, the first symptoms of this disease in childhood are usually the result of peripheral arthritis. 95% of these patients are HLA B27 positive and the importance of this tissue type, particularly in males with peripheral arthritis, has been indicated. Some children are troubled with attacks of acute iridocyclitis which is clinically apparent and readily controlled with topical treatment. Medical management of the disease is similar to that in adults.

RHEUMATIC FEVER

Rheumatic fever is a disease occurring after a group A beta-haemolytic streptococcal infection and is associated with arthritis, although carditis is the most concerning complication. The rash of erythema marginatum is the characteristic skin lesion but subcutaneous nodules and chorea may also be seen. Although this arthritis can be confused with JCA, it is usually migratory and acutely painful but rarely persists for more than a few days in any one joint. Several joints may be affected, predominantly knees, ankles and wrists in that order. The diagnosis rests on the demonstration of appropriate criteria and a history of a preceding streptococcal infection. Unlike the arthritis of JCA, salicylates in adequate dose rapidly control joint symptoms. The most important aspect of rheumatic fever is its recognition and the prevention of recurrent infection by appropriate antibiotic prophylaxis. The significance of a preceding beta-haemolytic streptococcal infection has been indicated and a rising anti-streptococcal (AST) titre is a marker of this; however it should be appreciated that nearly a third of children with JCA show high levels of this antibody. The significance of this is not clear.

SLE, DERMATOMYOSITIS, SCLERODERMA AND POLYARTERITIS NODOSA

Detailed discussion of these conditions is beyond the scope of this book. The arthritis of SLE can be confused with JCA and a positive ANF titre is often seen;

today, demonstration of antibodies to double stranded DNA is diagnostic of SLE. Characteristically, the arthritis of SLE is not destructive and is usually transient although avascular necrosis of bone is seen and can cause joint pain. In the early stages of both scleroderma and that form of dermatomyositis where the muscular or cutaneous manifestations are poorly developed, the joint stiffness may be mistaken for the dry restrictive arthritis of JCA.

HENOCH-SCHÖNLEIN PURPURA

This is the most common type of vasculitis in childhood and may be difficult to recognise when the arthritis symptoms precede the onset of the characteristic rash. Suspicion of this disease may be aroused if there is retention of joint mobility despite the discomfort. Furthermore, a skin rash (which may be maculopapular, purpuric, or urticarial) over the ankles and buttocks may suggest this diagnosis. A fully developed clinical picture associated with abdominal pain, patchy angioneurotic oedema of the hands, feet and genital area as well as nephritis, will not usually present to the orthopaedic surgeon.

ARTHRITIS OF INFLAMMATORY BOWEL DISEASE

Both ulcerative colitis and regional enteritis may be associated with arthritis which may affect either peripheral joints or resemble ankylosing spondylitis. In the peripheral arthritis only a few large joints are involved and the arthritis is often transient and settles once the underlying bowel disease is controlled. Joint destruction is uncommon and the prognosis is good.

Inflammatory bowel disease should be considered in all children presenting with arthritis where weight loss, poor growth, recurrent fevers, anaemia, erythema nodosum and bowel symptoms occur. Sometimes, however, the arthritis precedes recognisable bowel symptoms by several years.

REITER'S SYNDROME

The triad of urethritis, conjunctivitis, and arthritis is occasionally seen in childhood although sometimes the syndrome is incomplete. It is seen most commonly after Shigella infections but, in adolescence, may follow sexual exposure with gonococcal infections and other sexually transmitted diseases. The arthritis may be transient or chronic and usually affects only a few joints. The response to salicylates is usually satisfactory but other non-steroid and anti-inflammatory drugs may be required.

MANAGEMENT OF THE CHILD WITH JCA

History

The history of onset of joint disease is of major importance. It is important to ascertain the extent of joint involvement and whether a significant past history of joint disease has occurred. Recent illnesses, particularly those associated with exanthems, might suggest a viral basis to the arthritis, as recent contact with boils or other staphylococcal infection might suggest a septic arthritis. When there is a preceding history of gastroenteritis-like illnesses, the possibility of a reactive arthritis, Reiter's syndrome, or the arthritis of inflammatory bowel disease may all warrant consideration.

Examination

The child should be thoroughly examined to ascertain the extent of joint involvement. The routine physical examination should specifically exclude cardiac murmurs which might suggest rheumatic fever, the buttock or foot rash indicative of Henoch-Schönlein disease, or other rashes to suggest viral arthritis. While hepatosplenomegaly and lymphadenopathy may be seen in the systemic form of JCA, the question of malignancy arises in this situation. Where the blood pressure is elevated, the possibility of a collagen disorder with vasculitis warrants consideration. Although the chronic iritis seen in young girls with JCA cannot be detected in its early stages by routine ophthalmological examination, the acute iritis associated with HLA B27 is usually painful and clinically obvious.

Investigations

A routine *analysis of urine* is essential to exclude the proteinuria and haematuria suggestive of a vasculitis. The extent of laboratory investigation will be determined by the clinical picture. Where there is real concern about the possibility of septic arthritis, a *full blood examination* may indicate leucocytosis with mild anaemia but this is often seen in systemic rheumatoid disease; a normal haemoglobin and white cell count will usually preclude the possibility of childhood leukaemia. *Radiological investigation* is usually necessary to exclude pathology. Where there is concern about joint sepsis, many patients will require joint *aspiration* after these preliminary tests and in some circumstances a *synovial biopsy* may be warranted. Although the joint fluids from septic joints may be clearly purulent, have low viscosity, and form a fibrin clot, similar features can be seen in children with JCA. Bacteriological identification of micro-organisms may establish the diagnosis of septic arthritis.

Where the need for joint aspiration and synovial biopsy is not indicated, further laboratory and ophthalmological data may be sought; less than 10% of children with JCA have a positive *rheumatoid factor*, but it should be sought in view of its prognostic value. The importance of detecting *anti-nuclear factor* and *tissue typing* has been discussed. All children who have JCA in any form should have a *slit lamp examination* for identification of clinically inapparent chronic iridocyclitis; this should be continued for at least two years at 3–6 month intervals.

TREATMENT

General

All children with arthritis should be placed on a normal diet. During the acute phase of their arthritis they will limit their activities of their own accord. Where hospitalisation has been required, joint pain may warrant immobilisation. Once acute symptoms have resolved, joint movement should be encouraged and mobilisation effected at the earliest opportunity. In lower limb arthritis, this may be with the assistance of crutches but, with the help of the physiotherapist and adequate medical treatment, prolonged use of crutches should not be required. No child with chronic arthritis should be rested in bed for a prolonged period because of the risk of joint contractures developing. It is important that schooling should be maintained at all costs and, in the rare instances where hospitalisation or prolonged absence from school is required, appropriate educational facilities should be arranged. Occasionally where JCA is not adequately explained to parents or where family resources are inadequate, the impact of this illness on a family can be catastrophic. In these cases psychiatric counselling from the outset may be indicated if an effective regime of treatment is to be instituted.

Local

The main aim of local treatment is to restore joint function as soon as possible. Adequate joint function may well be achieved soon after control of the disease but a full range of movement may not be restored for months or even years. During the early phases of the illness, night splints are useful for the prevention of joint deformity or for joint comfort. Many children will reject the use of splints but where the disease is progressive, difficult to control medically, or particularly where it is of the dry restrictive type, splinting is essential to prevent joint deformity. Where joint deformity has developed, serial plaster casting, prolonged periods of prone lying to treat hip joint contractures, and even traction may be necessary. Rarely intra-articular steroids and manipulation under a general anaesthetic are necessary, if one or two joints are involved and do not respond to simple treatment. Manipulation carries a significant risk of fracture.

Drugs

Drug treatment for JCA is based on the use of salicylates in effective doses. The usual starting dose for salicylates is 60–80 mg per kg per day, but these doses should be subsequently developed until an effective therapeutic serum level is achieved and joint disease controlled. Most children tolerate salicylates well, although occasionally they may need to be discontinued or reduced in dosage because they cause gastrointestinal discomfort, irritability, hepato-toxicity or bleeding disorders due to interference with platelet function or hypoprothrombinaemia. Indocid is a useful alternative drug. Where these measures fail, penicillamine or parenteral gold may be warranted, and in rare cases low dose oral prednisolone may be necessary to control severe systemic disease, severe iritis or the pericarditis of JCA. Where iridocyclitis is detected (and evidence of it should be sought every 2–3 months) local installation of atropine drops and steroids may be warranted to prevent the onset of glaucoma and cataracts with permanent visual impairment.

Surgery

The role of surgery in JCA is mainly to perform a diagnostic *synovial biopsy*. Not all children with JCA require this but it is indicated with single joint involvement when other disorders cannot reasonably be excluded. Although *synovectomy* has enjoyed some popularity in the past, it is rarely indicated today unless there is extensive synovial proliferation which is mechanically interfering with joint function. The place of reconstructive joint surgery in JCA is under investigation.

In some cases of arthritis no diagnosis can be made on the basis of the investigations above, and joint biopsy findings are usually inconclusive; serial clinical evaluation and assessment of response to medical treatment will usually define the specific type of JCA a child is suffering from, and the long term prognosis.

POLIOMYELITIS

Poliomyelitis is an infectious disease caused by one of a group of neurotrophic viruses. These viruses have a special affinity for the anterior horn cells in the cord and motor nuclei in the brain stem. The nerve cells undergo acute inflammatory changes which may lead to necrosis. Those cells suffering only minor damage may recover and this recovery will be complete within weeks. An accurate prognosis for the future can be made within three months of the onset—when it can be taken that muscles which have not recovered to 30% of their normal strength will never be useful.

CLINICAL FEATURES

A child or adult will complain of malaise and headache on the first day and then will develop a fever and a sore throat. Pain in the neck and low back follows and, after a day or two, paralysis is noted. Neck and spine stiffness and muscle tenderness are characteristic features. Atypically, the onset may occur with respiratory and swallowing difficulties if the bulbar region only is affected. Lumbar puncture usually reveals an increase in protein and cells, initially polymorphs but later almost exclusively lymphocytes.

MANAGEMENT

It is convenient to consider the course of the disease in three phases: *acute phase*—lasting 5–10 days and culminating in paralysis; *convalescent phase*—lasting about twelve months this is the period in which a variable degree of recovery of muscle power occurs; *aftermath*—following the period of recovery, this final stage encompasses the residual disability which the patient must bear for the rest of his life.

Acute phase

The management in the acute phase is influenced by the important observations that both muscle fatigue and certain injections increase the severity of paralysis. It is therefore necessary for the patient to take complete physical rest once symptoms have developed. A firm bed is used and suitable sedatives and analgesics prescribed. Once paralysis appears, sandbags, slings, pillows and removeable splints are used to relieve pain in affected muscles and to prevent deformity. As the pain and spasm diminish passive movements can be instituted and soon a Hubbard bath will be found useful. A watch is kept for the development of bulbar paralysis as this may necessitate ventilation or tracheostomy or both. After about three weeks some recovery will be evident and at this stage a complete muscle chart should be recorded using the MRC (1942) grading:

0 no contraction
1 flicker
2 active movement with gravity eliminated
3 active movement against gravity
4 active movement against gravity and resistance
5 normal power

This muscle charting will be repeated at intervals and will provide a valuable record of recovery.

Convalescent phase

This phase is characterised by progressive but patchy recovery of muscle power. The aims of treatment are to restore muscle power and to prevent deformity.

RESTORATION OF MUSCLE POWER

Recovering muscles require a combination of rest and activity. Rest is required because fatigue inhibits recovery and exercise is needed to overcome weakness from disuse. Once neurological recovery is complete, hypertrophy of surviving muscle cells is encouraged by resistance exercises. Thus, there will be a progressive programme of physical activity monitored at intervals by muscle charting. Walking may be commenced once this can be performed either with or without support.

PREVENTION OF DEFORMITY

Deformity may occur due to: muscle spasm in the acute phase, muscle imbalance, unprotected weight-bearing, improper splinting, or abnormal growth. It may therefore be prevented by: adequate physiotherapy, correct splinting, or resumption of normal activity.

This phase can be considered to occupy about one year when any disability still present must be considered to be permanent. Further benefit will not accrue from continued physiotherapy and a decision may be required as to whether surgery is now indicated.

Aftermath phase

The final disability may be considered under four main headings.

INSTABILITY

A joint is said to be unstable if it collapses under weight-bearing and, in the context of poliomyelitis, this is due to muscle paralysis. it may be overcome by: 1   *Progressive resistance exercises* which may convert a weak muscle to one sufficiently strong to produce stability.   2   *Trick movements*, e.g. the gluteus maximus acting as an extensor of the hip may stabilise a weak knee.   3   *Bracing* will be required in most cases of instability affecting the lower limb. A long leg caliper controls knee, ankle and subtalar joint. An unstable hip may require the use of a stick or crutch.   4   A wide range of *surgical procedures* has been devised and, although many of these have been discarded, a solid core remains and these can be most helpful. Surgical procedures to overcome instability fall into three groups.

Tendon transfer. Any tendon whose rating is greater than 4 on the MRC scale can be transferred but the muscle must be strong enough to carry out the task in the new situation and it must be possible to spare it from its original location. Tendon transfers are very useful to improve function in the hand and the foot, but have much less value in more proximal joints.

Tenodesis. Tenodesis of paralysed tendons has very little, if any, use as the anchored tendons soon stretch and become ineffective.

Arthrodesis. Arthrodesis is rarely indicated at the hip or knee but is often used both to correct deformity and overcome instability in the foot. Triple arthrodesis as described by Dunn is the technique most commonly used but the modification of Lambrinudi is useful for drop foot. If no deformity is present, stability may be achieved by the inlay technique (see p. 125).

DEFORMITY

Fixed deformity may be seen early following muscle spasm but mostly occurs slowly and insidiously as a result of muscle imbalance. At first the deformity is produced by contracture of soft tissues but later bone growth and joint alignment are affected and this will continue until growth ceases. Passive stretching and splintage may slow down the rate of development of deformity but will rarely prevent it. Often the deformity can be predicted by the pattern of muscle imbalance present and prevented by an appropriate tendon transfer or tenotomy. Occasionally some deformity is beneficial and should be preserved, e.g. a little equinus will help stabilise a weak quadriceps. Once developed, fixed deformity may be corrected by the following methods:
   continuous traction, e.g. in the knee
   serial or wedged plaster casts
   tenotomy—if the tendon is dispensable
   tendon lengthening if the tendon is not dispensable
   osteotomy or arthrodesis.

SHORTENING

Shortening in the lower limb is not necessarily proportional to the degree of paralysis. Minor degrees of shortening, say up to one inch, are often beneficial in a weakened limb as less effort is required in the swing phase of gait. However, when shortening is or is expected to be in excess of one inch, every effort should be made to produce equality. The need to wear a heavy raised boot is an added strain for a badly weakened limb.
   The management of leg length discrepancy is considered on p. 153.

CIRCULATORY DEFICIENCY

Paralysed limbs feel uncomfortably cold especially in winter and are liable to develop dependent oedema and chilblains. The lower leg should be protected with woollen stockings and fur lined boots and a peripheral dilator prescribed by the winter months. Lumbar ganglionectomy is indicated in severe cases and is very effective in relieving symptoms.

CHAPTER 9

Reflections on the Practice of Surgery

Defining objectives; Conservative versus operative treatment; Planning the operation—type, timing, sequence; The operation; Physiotherapy

Anaesthesia in paediatric orthopaedic practice, 465
Pre-operative assessment; Pre-operative medication; The anaesthetic administration; The recovery period; Intravenous therapy and blood transfusion; Consideration of special procedures

The details of surgical practice are usually learnt by our system of apprenticeship but some teachers are better than others, and some do not teach at all. In the event a trainee may not be exposed to some important details. This chapter is an attempt to define some of the many principles which govern successful and harmonious surgical practice.

DEFINING OBJECTIVES

Before any treatment is proposed it is necessary to define its objective. Are we expecting to improve function or appearance or both? If function is to be improved, are we aiming to have the child walk further or faster? Do we expect to convert a non-walker into a walker or into one who can be walked a few steps for transfer? Once decided, this objective should not only be discussed with the patient or his parents but recorded in the clinical history. Most medico-legal actions have as their basis a failure on the part of the surgeon to inform his patient what he is proposing to do and what can reasonably be expected from this treatment.

CONSERVATIVE VERSUS OPERATIVE TREATMENT

It has been traditional to use simple and conservative methods of treatment in the first instance and, should they be found wanting, then surgery would be advised. This sequence was based on a philosophy that first we must do no harm and also, originally, on the various dangers attached to open surgery. Although these dangers have largely been eliminated, the philosophy persists in many quarters.

Conservatism is still regarded as something sacred so that surgery is still preceded by long periods in casts and braces, and by physical therapy. It should be recognised that this sequence is time consuming, uneconomical and unsound if there happens to be—as there now usually is—a surgical solution which is safe, quick, and effective. An excellent example is seen in the relapsed or resistant club foot where surgery in skilled hands can produce full correction in one operation in contrast to many months of wedged or serial casts.

PLANNING THE OPERATION—TYPE, TIMING, SEQUENCE

It is not sufficient simply to recommend an operation without any qualification. It may be necessary, especially in more complex problems, to introduce some important modification to the standard technique. If the condition is bilateral it must be decided whether both sides should be corrected at the one operation or whether they should be staggered and, if so, at what interval. An operative programme may involve three or more separate procedures and the timing and sequence of these will need much thought. Finally, when all the decisions have been made and discussed they should be recorded. If any departures have been made from the usual routine, the reason for this should be stated. (Many orthopaedic procedures are planned months ahead of their execution; when the patient arrives in hospital the reasons for previous decisions may be difficult to remember.)

On arrival of the patient in hospital, a cross check of all previous decisions is made and the limb destined for surgery marked in some indelible way.

The operating room

Having checked the side and site of operation, the surgeon's next responsibility is to supervise the posturing of the patient on the operating table. This must be done personally—verbal instruction to a theatre attendant after scrubbing up is a very poor substitute. The chosen posture is maintained by sandbags and adhesive strapping and must receive the approval of the anaesthetist before the operation commences. It is always wise to discuss each proposed operation with the theatre sister well in advance of the starting time so that any special instruments can be procured and sterilised. This saves both time and embarrassment if the deficiency is discovered during the operation.

The incision

While it remains true that decisions are more important than incisions, most surgeons can afford to spend more time planning the latter. The patient expects improvements in function—not an ugly scar. Most of the practical surgical approaches were designed to give a surgeon adequate exposure but cosmesis was rarely considered. With present day knowledge of skin healing, it is always possible to design a skin incision which will give an acceptable scar. All proposed incisions should be drawn on the skin first. An ideal pen is a sharpened wooden swab stick and best ink is gentian violet. In general, incisions should be straight rather than curved or S shaped, not only because they look better but also because they heal better. In the upper limb, incisions can often be placed on the inner side, e.g. the axillary approach to the shoulder and the medial approach to the humerus. Around the hip, the Smith-Petersen approach should be modified as described by Salter, that is the vertical component is deleted as it is this part which makes such a bad scar and one which is impossible to hide in any conventional type of swimming costume. All wounds are best closed with a subcuticular suture which does not need to be removed: children fear removal of sutures far more than their insertion.

THE OPERATION

It is outside the scope of this volume to cover all the details of operative technique. Instead, several important points will be discussed.

Atraumatic surgery

Gentle handling of tissues is the hallmark of good surgery. The skin edges require particular care and should not be undermined superficial to the deep fascia or grasped with tissue forceps. The exposure should be wide enough so that muscles do not need to be retracted with great force and at all times articular cartilage must be regarded as sacred. At the conclusion of any operation, debridement of the wound is carried out and all tags of tissue and damaged muscle excised. If dead tissue is included in the wound closure, the chances of sepsis are greatly increased.

Haemostasis

It is important to control bleeding during the operation not only to conserve blood but also to make it possible for the surgeon to see what he is doing. Even if the wound is dry before closure suction drainage should be instituted if it is considered that further oozing is likely, e.g. from the cut surface of cancellous bone after innominate osteotomy. In the limbs, if a tournique has been used it should not be necessary to remove this prior to closure provided the wound is sutured in such a way that blood may escape into the dressings.

Internal fixation or not

The modern trend to fasten everything together with metal should be strongly resisted in the case of children. Although the use of metal in certain circumstances is almost mandatory (for example in the fixation of slipped upper femoral epiphysis), metallic implants are rarely required in fracture treatment and are usually unnecessary in routine orthopaedic operations. The insertion of plates and screws usually demands a bigger exposure, a longer operation, and a second operation later to remove the implants. It is often desirable to slightly modify the position following operation so as to obtain the best result and, if internal fixation has been used, this is usually not possible. Triple arthrodesis is a good example and the use of staples in lieu of good carpentry is to be condemned.

Surgical speed

Whilst surgery performed in haste is obviously wrong, some account should be taken of the advantages of speedy surgery. The surgeon who is able to complete an operation quickly usually knows what he is doing and how to do it, the post-operative course is normally more comfortable, there is less swelling, and less likelihood of sepsis. Speed in surgery is not only due to manual dexterity: it starts with good planning and is helped by an efficient anaesthetic service. More importantly, it is largely due to forward thinking on the part of the surgeon and his assistant. The surgeon should ask for the next instrument before he actually needs it and should forewarn the theatre staff of any special instruments or equipment likely to be needed during the operation.

Bandage or plaster

In general, soft tissue wounds can be dressed with a crepe bandage while operations on bones and joints demand plaster cast fixation. Children, however, do not respect bandages and the surgeon should use a plaster cast as a post-operative dressing in most cases. Even with such minor procedures as the release of a trigger thumb, healing will be better and there will be less drama if the hand is immobilised in plaster. The plaster applied in the operating room should be as thin as possible so that if it requires splitting or removal in the immediate post-operative period, this will be relatively easy. Before the child goes home, the plaster can be repaired or made stronger as the case may be. Crepe bandages applied at operation must be used very carefully, as each layer increases the pressure in geometrical progression. When swelling occurs the bandage may become dangerously tight.

The operation record

Having completed the operation, the surgeon should now dictate the operation record in some detail, even though he may consider the procedure to have been routine. The record should consist of four parts: exposure, the findings, the procedure, and the closure.

Finally, the after-care is laid down: how long in bed, whether to get up on crutches, any special precautions, how long in plaster, and how long before he will be seen again or re-admitted and so on. The importance of the after-care instructions is that all concerned with the care of this child—whether nurses, residents, or social workers—will be able to give the same version to the parents. It is obvious that the operation note must be typed into the clinical record as a matter of urgency.

Post-operative pain

In orthopaedic surgery, post-operative pain is due to one or more of the following causes: 1 Tightly tied skin sutures: it is only necessary to appose the skin edges not to strangle them. 2 Lack of immobilisation by cast, traction or frame. 3 Swelling inside a rigid dressing or cast. If swelling is anticipated, such as after foot stabilisation or arthrodesis of the wrist, the cast should be split longitudinally with a knife before the child leaves the operating room. Elevation of the limb in the ward is essential after any surgery. 4 Inadequate analgesia: analgesics are always required in the first 24 hours regardless of other factors. 5 Ischaemia: continuous, severe, generalised pain especially in the upper limb is likely to be caused by ischaemia and, if there is any suspicion of this, the plaster cast should be removed completely as the first step.

PHYSIOTHERAPY

The physiotherapist has long been recognised as an essential member of the orthopaedic team yet most residents and many surgeons have only a rudimentary knowledge of the details of this form of treatment or of its scope and limitations. Physiotherapy in childhood bears little resemblance to its adult counterpart and the therapists working in this field require special qualities of patience, understanding, and sensitivity. They also must understand the nature, growth and development of the child and be able to communicate not only with children but also with their parents so that a high level of trust is established.

Physical treatment

This represents only a small proportion of physiotherapy and can be broken down into a number of parts.

Exercise is the backbone of physical treatment in childhood. A distinction must at once be drawn between exercises and exercise. Exercises are virtually useless in childhood: the child cannot see the point and, after an initial effort, they are simply not done. Much greater effort can be obtained by exercise which will often be disguised as play or as some form of sport which the child enjoys. It is really a matter of tricking the child into doing something she can enjoy and which happens to have a therapeutic value. Following trauma and operation, the therapist will be called up to get the child ambulant often on crutches. This will be more a matter of allaying the child's fears of hurting himself and gaining his trust than of actually teaching him how to walk. In cerebral palsy, a wide range of differing techniques is used to teach affected children skills such as head control, sitting, crawling, walking—skills which develop naturally in the normal child. Following severe head injuries with brain damage, similar techniques are of inestimable value in controlling spasticity and in eventual rehabilitation.

Hydrotherapy has been used extensively in the past but has tended to go out of fashion with the changing pattern of disease. However hydrotherapy is still very useful for improving circulation, re-educating muscle, and mobilising stiff joints. It is also used for general exercise and enjoyment, particularly following severe injury and burns. The Hubbard type of above-ground pool is preferable to the more conventional swimming pool as it enables treatment to be supervised by the therapist from outside the pool.

Electrotherapy is hardly ever used in childhood and in fact most departments do not even possess the equipment.

Parent–therapist relationship

A large part of physiotherapy in children is aimed at the parents and involves training them in a home therapy programme for their child. Periodic visits to the department will be needed for supervision and changes in the routine, but the majority of the treatment will be carried out at home by the mother. As the child becomes older the need for physiotherapy will diminish as greater emphasis is placed on education and daily living activities. At all times the therapist will have an invaluable role in parental advice, support, and reassurance. The physiotherapy session will often provide a better climate than the clinic for the parents to voice their concerns, fears, and doubts and to receive adequate answers. If the therapist is unable to answer any important queries, appropriate referral can be arranged.

The doctor–therapist relationship

It is important that the surgeon appreciates the possible contribution of the therapist and selects appropriate cases for referral. Children with flat feet and poor posture may need help, but the physiotherapist cannot be expected to provide it. Likewise, children with undiagnosed aches and pains need a diagnosis, not a physiotherapist.

The referral letter must contain all relevant information so that the therapist can approach the problem intelligently. This information will include the diagnosis, the specific problem requiring treatment, and the aim of treatment. Previous treatment, especially surgery, needs to be outlined, as does whether the child is having any drugs and whether any special precautions are required in treatment.

During the course of treatment it may become apparent to the therapist that there are other problems, e.g. visual or auditory defects which need attention and this information can be given to the surgeon so that appropriate referrals can be arranged. As soon as possible after any surgery—particularly in cerebral palsy—the child needs to be re-united with the therapist, for the recovery from surgery is likely to be more protracted without this support.

It will be seen from what has been described that a basic knowledge of the role of the physiotherapist is required of those who may wish to prescribe this form of treatment. Any orthopaedic resident should regard it as part of his training to spend some time in a department to see at first hand the techniques used.

ANAESTHESIA IN PAEDIATRIC ORTHOPAEDIC PRACTICE

Although the success of paediatric orthopaedic operations is mainly related to the surgical procedures performed, the memory and acceptance of the treatment is to a large extent concerned with the anaesthetic, particularly the induction and recovery periods. This is especially so in the common situation in which orthopaedic management requires many anaesthetics. If successive procedures are not to become increasingly difficult, each anaesthetic must be handled in the most pleasant manner possible.

The following description of anaesthetic methods represents, in the main, the current practice at the Royal Children's Hospital, Melbourne.

PRE-OPERATIVE ASSESSMENT

The aim of the pre-operative visit and examination is to enable the anaesthetist to decide if there are any factors present likely to influence the choice of the anaesthetic agent or the method of administration. It also gives the anaesthetist an opportunity to gain the friendship and trust of the patient and, if possible, of the parents as well.

One is particularly concerned with any present illness or any relevant past illnesses. Adverse reactions to previous anaesthetics are important and a predisposition to haemorrhage is noteworthy. It is also important to know of current drug therapy and any abnormal reactions to drugs which are likely to be used.

The psychological state of the patient is important but is not always easy to assess. Most children behave in a predictable and satisfactory manner at the time of induction of anaesthesia. Children under 3 years of age often cry at the needle puncture but, above this age, crying or struggling is unusual. Certain types of children who are likely to present difficulties are recognisable. Some children struggle, cry or scream when anyone approaches to carry out even the simplest detail of medical or nursing care and these react in the same way to the induction of anaesthesia. The child who is abnormally bright is frequently unstable and has a reversal of behaviour shortly before anaesthesia is commenced. In cases where the mother refuses to be separated from the child one can usually anticipate trouble. These children with behaviour problems form an important group because pre-operative medication with a variety of drugs is often disappointing and makes little or no improvement in the situation. An attempt to gain rapport with the child is the only measure likely to be successful.

It is assumed, and seems reasonable, that the administration of an anaesthetic to a sick child will have an adverse effect on the illness. However statistics indicating the degree of risk are not available. The problem centres largely around acute respiratory tract infections and acute gastro-enteritis. The magnitude of the operation is also relevant for one is more likely to defer a major procedure (such as an arthrodesis of the hip or a spine fusion) than a minor procedure. It is usual to postpone an operation if the patient shows objective signs of illness such as fever, purulent nasal discharge, otitis media, husky voice, severe cough, physical signs of lung disorder, diarrhoea, or vomiting.

A different problem is presented by the child with multiple congenital abnormalities. Here, in addition to orthopaedic problems, there may be congenital anomalies of heart, lungs, or central nervous system. Experience suggests that children with multiple severe anomalies present a greatly increased degree of anaesthetic risk. This factor must be taken into consideration when decisions regarding anaesthesia and surgery are made.

PRE-OPERATIVE MEDICATION

It is customary to administer a premedication consisting of atropine or hyoscine together with a sedative or a narcotic drug. The intention is both to make the child pleasantly sleepy and to gain a depression of the central nervous system which will add to the effects of a general anaesthetic. Experience has shown that it is important for the staff to establish good relations with the patient. It must also be noted that premedication can have adverse effects such as giddiness, vomiting, fall in blood pressure, sweating, and a prolonged period of post-operative unconsciousness. Caution is therefore necessary and, in the case of out-patients in whom a quick recovery is desirable, the amount of sedative or narcotic drug must be reduced or omitted.

The calculation of premedication dosages in terms of micrograms or milligrams per kilogram of body weight has resulted in fewer adverse results, and the use of the tuberculin syringe for measuring small volumes has increased the accuracy of administration.

The value of pre-operative preparation and medication can be nullified if well intentioned but misguided people excite children by playing with them in the pre-anaesthetic period.

THE ANAESTHETIC ADMINISTRATION

General anaesthesia is the method of choice for most surgical procedures in children. Currently anaesthesia is most frequently induced with the intravenous injection of an anaesthetic agent. This method has achieved almost universal acceptance in adults because it is much more pleasant than an inhalational induction. The same applies in children where two additional factors have influenced the increasing use of intravenous anaesthesia: the availability of sharp disposable needles, and the recognition that intravenous agents may be given to patients of all sizes provided the dose is suitably adjusted. When veins are small or absent, resort may be had to intramuscular injection. Ketamine is a suitable drug for use in this way in that it does not sting at the time of administration or cause pain later; if mixed with hyaluronidase, ketamine will frequently cause unconsciousness in less than one minute.

In children under 3 years of age, the administration of certain drugs per rectum will produce deep sleep. Thiopentone sodium is one of these and, if given rectally in a dosage of 40 mg/kg body weight, will cause deep sleep to supervene in about six minutes. The method is an excellent one but it has fallen into disuse mainly because of the time involved in instilling the thiopentone and in waiting for it to act. Children in this age group are accustomed to having their temperatures taken per rectum and therefore do not find this procedure unusual.

Induction of anaesthesia by inhalational methods is commonly used in babies and children under one year of age. Older children consider the method as unpleasant although some dislike injections so intensely that they are prepared to breathe the anaesthetic instead.

Once unconsciousness has supervened, anaesthesia may be continued either with a face mask or with an endotracheal tube. It is customary to use an endotracheal tube when the operation is on the head or neck or the patient is to be placed in an unusual position, prone, or on the orthopaedic frame. Endotracheal intubation is easy in normal children, difficult in Pierre Robin's syndrome, arthrogryposis, cleft lip and cleft palate, and virtually impossible in the rare Gargoyle deformity.

Ketamine administered either intravenously or intramuscularly has now lost some of the favour it enjoyed when first introduced, but it still has a use for manipulation of fractures and the application of plasters.

Local and regional analgesic techniques may be employed in paediatric orthopaedic practice, particularly with older children. The techniques employed include local infiltration of the operation site, nerve blocks (e.g. the brachial plexus block), and the intravenous injection of local analgesic agents into an exsanguinated limb. The latter method is valuable for children with forearm fractures. If the local analgesic technique is accompanied by overall sedation with ketamine or a benzodiazepene drug (e.g. diazepam (Valium)) the whole procedure is usually satisfactory to all concerned. Such methods have a considerable potential application but are particularly indicated where difficulty is anticipated in regard to an inhalation anaesthetic.

Although the matter of internal body temperature is not strictly a part of the anaesthetic technique it must be considered every time an anaesthetic is administered to a child. Because children present a larger surface area in proportion to their size than adults, the internal body temperature is more prone to variation. General anaesthesia largely abolishes temperature regulation so that the patient becomes poikilothermic. If the operating room temperature is 25°C internal body temperature tends to remain at the pre-operative level. If the room temperature exceeds 25°C the internal body temperature tends to rise. Prior to the installation of air conditioning equipment in operating theatres this was a common problem during summer time. At a normal theatre ambient temperature of 20–21°C there is a tendency to progressive heat loss during an operation. This is most marked in children under 2 years of age for whom the use of a warming blanket is beneficial. Older children do not need a warming blanket but should be adequately covered. An interesting cause of body temperature variation relates to the use of the tourniquet. If a mid-thigh tourniquet is in place for one hour, the exposed limb below the tourniquet becomes cool from contact with the air. When the tourniquet is released, blood circulates through the cold limb resulting in a fall of internal body temperature of 0.5–0.75°C over the next five minutes. If two mid-thigh tourniquets are employed simultaneously the total fall in body temperature is 1–1.5°C.

If a patient has a low internal body temperature at the end of an operation he tends to have cold, blue extremities and shiver on awakening. The application of plaster casts has not been found to have a measurable effect on internal body temperature.

THE RECOVERY PERIOD

One of the most significant developments in recent years has been the establishment of recovery rooms in hospitals with consequent improvement of care in the important early post-anaesthetic period.

It is a fundamental observation that general anaesthesia abolishes many of the protective reflexes of the body especially those relating to respiration so that the airway may be partly or completely obstructed. Moreover if foreign material, such as vomitus or blood, is present in the mouth it may be aspirated into the lungs with harmful effects. At a certain point in the recovery period the protective reflexes return and from then on the patient is considered to be in a safe state. Before then the patient must be placed in the lateral position if possible and should be carefully and constantly attended. Depending on the duration of anaesthesia and the drugs used, consciousness returns after different lengths of time. Although a quick return results in a more rapid attainment of a safe state, a slower recovery is often preferable as it gives more time for haemorrhage to cease before the child starts moving again and is often associated with a persisting analgesia.

Since respiratory safety is largely related to oxygenation, it is desirable to administer some added oxygen in the post-operative period.

In most substantial operations pain appears during the recovery period. Unnecessary moving of patients should be avoided and they should be nursed in the most comfortable position. If this does not relieve pain, an intramuscular injection of an analgesic drug should be given. Maximum doses of the commonly used analgesics are: morphine 0.2 mg/kg of body weight, omnopon 0.3 mg/kg, and pethidine 1 mg/kg. It is customary to give only three-quarters of the full dose as the first post-operative injection. Vomiting is a frequent complication of surgery and anaesthesia during the first two post-operative days. There are now a number of potent anti-emetic drugs available: prochlorperazine maleate (Stemetil) is usually effective. If vomiting persists despite the administration of an anti-emetic drug, the case should be reviewed as the vomiting may be due to a drug idiosyncrasy or to a surgical complication.

One should be especially cautious of post-operative pain that is not readily relieved by an adequate dose of analgesic drug. The cause may be a surgical complication such as haemorrhage, ischaemia, a tight plaster, or an unreduced dislocation.

INTRAVENOUS THERAPY AND BLOOD TRANSFUSION

Most major orthopaedic operations result in either a significant blood loss or a delay in the resumption of the oral intake of fluid. For these reasons intravenous therapy and blood transfusion form an important part of the overall management. It is desirable that one should estimate the probable blood loss and fluid requirements in advance so that a suitable intravenous line can be established either before or early in the operation. As blood may take some time to obtain and cross-match, arrangements should be made sufficiently early to avoid haste.

Intravenous equipment has been greatly improved in recent years so that the placement of the line is easier and its life expectancy is increased. As many patients will have numerous operations and infusions it is desirable to conserve veins. Cut down procedures should be avoided and the size of the cannulae used should be as small as possible for the expected blood loss. The forearm is the best site for an intravenous infusion but the back of the hand is frequently the most practical one. At times the cubital fossa and the foot may be used. Usually the limb should be splinted. If this is difficult with ready made splints, a well fitting splint can be made with a plaster bandage.

Blood loss during operation may be measured by inspection of the suction bottle and by weighing the blood-stained swabs and packs. These are now available in standard weights so that any increase in weight represents blood. As some blood cannot be measured because it is on the drapes, the measured loss will

470   Chapter 9

always be less than the actual loss and allowance must be made for this. It should also be remembered that the blood provided by a blood bank is diluted by anti-coagulant. Thus a unit of whole blood contains 400 ml of blood and 100 ml of anti-coagulant solution.

An approximate estimation of the blood volume of the patient can be made by calculating that there are 80 ml of blood per kilogram of body weight. Assuming that the patient is not dehydrated or anaemic pre-operatively, the indication for blood transfusion is the loss of 10% of the calculated blood volume or the appearance of circulatory signs of blood loss such as falling blood pressure or rising pulse rate.

An important factor in managing blood replacement is a knowledge of the variation in haemoglobin levels which occurs in normal healthy children. A newly born baby has a haemoglobin level of 22 g/100 ml of blood. At the end of two weeks this has fallen to 16 g/100 ml. Thereafter a slower fall occurs till the age of 2 years when the haemoglobin level is 11 g/100 ml. From that age the level rises and, in adolescence, reaches the adult levels of 14 g/100 ml for females and 16 g/100 ml for males. These figures are noteworthy as a great deal of surgery is performed on children approximately 2 years of age and it is important to recognise that a 2-year-old child with a haemoglobin level of 11 g/100 ml of blood is not anaemic and that nothing is to be gained by transfusing beyond this point. Overinfusion and overtransfusion should be avoided and, if the patient is small, a burette should be interposed between the large container of blood or fluid and the patient.

In operations where much blood loss is anticipated, it is good practice to commence with 6% Macrodex or Haemaccel. In this way one can maintain the blood volume during the operation and give the precious supply of blood after haemostasis has been secured.

In operations involving bone, post-operative bleeding may constitute a substantial problem. If a suction bottle or similar device is used, this must be exposed for all to see and watched closely. It may happen that so much blood flows into the suction bottle that circulatory failure follows due to loss of blood volume. This is a desperate situation which should be dealt with by turning off the suction bottle, applying pressure over the operation site, and giving appropriate fluids intravenously.

As a point of policy, every effort is made to minimise blood loss by meticulous surgery and by the injection of vasoconstrictors at the operating site. Transfusions are avoided if possible, particularly in girls in whom the development of antibodies could adversely affect a subsequent pregnancy.

CONSIDERATION OF SPECIAL PROCEDURES

Manipulation and plaster: changes of plaster

Procedures for orthopaedic manipulations and plaster applications form part of most paediatric orthopaedic operating lists. While plaster removals are usually done without anaesthesia, manipulation and plaster application commonly require a general anaesthetic and light surgical general anaesthesia is usually employed. At one time it was thought unwise to use repeated thiopentone, halothane, nitrous oxide anaesthesia for this because of the possibility of precipitating hepatitis. This fear appears to be unfounded and this form of anaesthesia continues to be commonly used. Ketamine has frequently been given since it was first introduced, but its use both for this and other procedures has diminished, mainly because of the possibility of causing hallucinations. Ketamine, however, does have one outstanding advantage: the ability to be injected intramuscularly.

Reduction of fractures

The problem associated with the treatment of recent fractures or dislocations relates mainly to the undigested food in the stomach at the time of accident. It is feared that the food will be vomited or regurgitated at some time during or after the anaesthetic administration with the possibility of aspiration into the respiratory tract. Digestion usually ceases when an accident has occurred so that waiting does not ensure an empty stomach. In addition it is generally desirable to reduce a fracture or dislocation without too much delay. The alternatives include a carefully given general anaesthetic, either with a face mask or an endotracheal tube, or a local analgesic technique. Local analgesic techniques are especially applicable to fractures of the forearm or hand. A brachial plexus block may be used or the intravenous injection of 0.5% lignocaine given into an exsanguinated limb.

Spine surgery

Extensive surgery on the spinal column to straighten abnormal curvatures or to stabilise the spine below the affected area in some cases of spina bifida has become an established part of orthopaedic practice. For the anaesthetist, blood loss is the greatest problem in the anaesthetic management of these cases. It is possible to measure blood loss progressively during the operation and replace it at the same rate: this was the method initially used when such operations were first performed. More recently the artificial induction of hypotension by the intravenous infusion of sodium nitroprusside has been used with great success to reduce haemorrhage. However meticulous care of the hypotensive patient is essential if complications are to be avoided.

Osteogenesis imperfecta

Despite their small size and many deformities, children afflicted with osteogenesis imperfecta are good subjects for general anaesthesia. However specific difficulties do exist. Because of the shape of the jaws and tongue, respiratory obstruction above the level of the larnyx is apt to occur more often than in normal children and calls for extra care. When endotracheal intubation is necessary, it is desirable to have a selection of tubes available as the size of the larynx is not predictable either from the age or weight of the patient. Increased metabolic rate and heat production necessitate the pre-operative measurement of body temperature and the intra-operative monitoring of internal body temperature with an oesophageal thermometer. Any tendency for internal body temperature to rise above pre-operative levels during the operation is countered by exposing more of the patient to the air, thereby increasing heat loss. The excessive sweating which many of these patients show is responsible for a greater tendency to develop dehydration, especially if the child vomits post-operatively or is slow in resuming oral intake of fluids. It is therefore necessary to administer intravenous fluids to most patients suffering from osteogenesis imperfecta who come to operation.

From the time when intramedullary rodding of the long bones was first commenced at the Royal Children's Hospital 20 years ago, it has been recognised by all concerned that, if consistently good results are to be obtained, blood loss should be minimised and the total operating time should be as short as possible. The application of these principles has resulted in few complications.

Spina bifida

Orthopaedic operations on patients suffering from spina bifida present certain difficulties for the anaesthetist. Because of numerous previous intravenous injections and cannulations, these patients frequently have few accessible veins. Even the external jugular veins are frequently not available because they have been employed for shunt procedures. Apart from previous intravenous therapy many of these patients would have inaccessible veins in any case because of obesity. On the psychological side, most have had so much surgery and other treatment that they are unusually apprehensive of any future operations. The older children, particularly those with normal intelligence, often have an insight into their own insoluble problems which increases the difficulty. While the actual mechanism of administering an anaesthetic does not usually present any great difficulties, the patients frequently require smaller doses of drugs than normal for their weights. Blood loss tends to be less well tolerated, so that blood and fluid replacement must be carefully handled.

Arthrography with contrast media

This procedure consists of the injection during general anaesthesia of a radio-opaque iodine-containing medium into a joint, usually the hip. Rapid absorption of the compound occurs so that further x-rays taken some time later show radio-opaque urine in the bladder. As with the intravenous injection of such compounds those who are sensitive to the compound are apt to develop circulatory failure or cardiac arrest.

In order to minimise the danger, about 25 years ago the practice was adopted of diluting the radio-opaque compound before injecting it and of leaving the needle in the joint so that, after the x-rays had been taken and developed, the compound could be removed by aspiration. Since these precautions have been taken, complications of arthrography have vanished.

Blood disorders

From time to time anaesthetists are required to administer anaesthetics to patients suffering from blood disorders including haemophilia, Christmas Disease, von Willebrand's disease, thalassaemia, and sickle cell anaemia. It is essential to obtain the advice and co-operation of the haematology department concerning the use of blood and blood products. Such patients do not usually present any specific anaesthetic problems, and are well served with a conventional anaesthetic administered with a higher concentration of oxygen than usual.

It has been our experience that complications are rare if procedures on these patients are carefully planned.

Anaesthetic management of out-patients

Because of the high cost of in-patient care and the fact that out-patient treatment minimises the disturbance of life for the patient and family, there is now a tendency for an increasing amount of surgical work to be conducted in this manner.

The prerequisites for out-patient care of surgical conditions include the following: the patient should be in good health; the procedure should not be of a type likely to be associated with surgical or anaesthetic complications; post-operative pain which will not be relieved by aspirin or a similar drug should be unlikely; and the patient should be given clear instructions, preferably in a printed form, with emphasis on the necessity of reporting any serious complication. As a general rule, long periods of travel should be avoided and the rest of the day should be spent in bed.

Index

Abscess
  Brodie's, 145–6
  in osteomyelitis, 14, 142, 143, 145–6
Accident to child, effect on parent and child, 3
Acetabulum
  dysplasia
    in cerebral palsy, 112
    congenital, 33–40, 179, 180, 181–3
    in Down's syndrome, 433
  fractures, 317
Aclasis, diaphyseal, 359, 384
Acquired conditions in neonate, 11–15
Adolescence, characteristics of, 248–9
Albright's syndrome, 364
Amputation
  in congenital absence of fibula, 75–6
  in gigantism, 86
  in leg length inequality, 71 (Fig. 2.51), 72, 75–6
  in primary malignant bone tumour, 390–3, 395, 396
  in supernumerary toes, 85
  Syme's, 71 (Fig. 2.51), 72, 75–6
Anaesthesia in surgery, *see under* Surgical practice, principles of
Anderson technique in tibia lengthening, 162
Ankle
  fractures, 336
    fibula, distal growth plate, 337
    tibia, distal growth plate, 338–40
    tibia, metaphyseal, distal, 337
  Gruca reconstruction, 73–5
  instability, recurrent, 278–9
  movements and deformities, terminology, 10–11
Ankylosing spondylitis, 446 (Table 8.1), 447, 448, 450
Anti-nuclear factor (ANF), 447
Arachnodactyly, 431–2, *see also* Marfan's syndrome
Arthritis, chronic
  and ankylosing spondylitis, 446 (Table 8.1), 447, 448, 450
  conditions causing or simulating, 445–6
  and dermatomyositis, 446 (Table 8.1), 450–1

Arthritis, chronic (*cont.*)
  and Henoch-Schönlein purpura, 446 (Table 8.1), 451
  and infectious diseases associated with, 448–9, *see also* Arthritis, septic; Osteomyelitis
  of inflammatory bowel disease, 446 (Table 8.1), 451
  and malignancies associated with, 449
  of non-inflammatory cause, 449–50
  and polyarteritis nodosa, 446 (Table 8.1), 450–1
  and Reiter's syndrome, 446 (Table 8.1), 451
  and rheumatic fever, 446 (Table 8.1), 450
  and scleroderma, 446 (Table 8.1), 450–1
  and systemic lupus erythematosus, 446 (Table 8.1), 450–1
  treatment, 453–4
  see also Juvenile chronic arthritis (JCA)
Arthritis, septic, 138, 141, 149–53, 196, 448
  in infancy, 14–15, 141, 149, 154
Arthrodesis
  of hip, 70, 183
  of knee, 71 (Fig. 2.51), 72
  of wrist, 83, 114–15
  see also Triple arthrodesis
Arthrogryposis, 400–1, 410
  foot, 402
  hip, 405
  knee, 174, 402–5
  management, general, 402
  and quadriceps contracture, 174, 404
  and spina bifida, 46–7, 400
  spine, 406
  treatment, principles of, 401–2
  upper limb, management, 407–10
Ataxia, 99, 122
  Friedreich's, 122, 163, 434–6, 437–8
Athetosis, 98–9, 100, 101, 102
  surgery in, 103, 115

Back knee, 11, 18, 56
Backache in adolescence, 249–50
  hysterical, 255
  lumbago, 255–6

474

Index 475

Backache in adolescence (*cont.*)
  lumbar disc syndrome, 254–5
  osteoblastoma, 256
  osteochondritis, 250
    dorsal, 250–1
    lumbar, 252
  postural, 250
  spinal metastasis, 256
  spondylolisthesis, 253–4
  spondylolysis, 253
Baker release of calf aponeurosis, 105
Baker's cyst, 176
Biopsy of bone, 354, 380–3
Birth defects
  classification, 15–16
  see also specified defects
Birth fractures, 12
Blount's disease, 77
Bone cysts, *see under* Cysts
Bone graft, 384, 385, 386, 390
Bone scan, 209, 375–6
Bone shortening in leg length inequality, 159–61
Bone tumours, 353
  classification, 353–4
  diagnosis, 354
    biochemistry, 377
    biopsy, 354, 380–3
    clinical, 354–5
    haematology, 376–7
    radio-isotope bone scanning, 375–6
    radiology, *see* Radiology of bone tumours and related lesions, in diagnosis
  terminology, 355–8
  treatment, 383
    benign tumours, 384–90
    Ewing's sarcoma, 396–8
    osteosarcoma, 395–6
    primary malignant tumours, 390–5
Boston brace, 209, 211–12
Bowlegs, 11, 118, 128, 131
  and prone sleeping, 89
  tibial, 77, 89, 90 (Fig. 3.1), 91
Brodie's abscess, 145–6
Broomstick cast
  and hip, adduction, spastic, 109–11
  and hip, dislocation, congenital, 95
  and Perthes' disease, 192
Butler procedure in fifth toe deformities, 171

Café-au-lait pigmentation, 204, 269 (Figs. 5.12–13), 418–20, 422 (Fig. 8.23), 425
Calvé's disease, 148
Cast brace, femoral, 327–8
CAT scan in scoliosis, 207, 209
Catterall's classification in Perthes' disease, 190–1

Cerebral palsy, 96, 154
  assessment of child, 101
  ataxic, 99
  athetoid, 98–9, 100, 101, 102, 103, 114–5
  causes, 96–8
  classification, 98–9
  diagnosis, 99–101
  floppy infant, 99
  gait in, 100, 109, 112–13, Fig. 3.17, 122
  gluteal weakness, 113
  hospitalisation, 116
  leg length inequality, 115–16
  rigid, 99
  spastic, 98
    diplegia, 100
    hemiplegia, 100
    quadriplegia, 100–1
  spinal deformity, 116
  surgery, 102, 103
    in athetosis, 103, 115
    for hands, 113–15
    in hip adduction, spastic, 109–11
    in hip dislocation and subluxation, 111–12
    in hip internal rotation, 112–13
    in knee flexion, 109
    in spastic equinovalgus, 105–6
    in spastic equinovarus, 106–9
    in spastic equinus, 104–5
  treatment, 102
    bracing, 102, 104
    drugs, 103
    physiotherapy, 102
    surgery, *see* Cerebral palsy, surgery
  upper limb in, 113–15
Charcot-Marie-Tooth disease (peroneal muscular atrophy), 163, 434–7
Chemotherapy in bone tumours, 390, 393–6, 398
Chiari osteotomy, 45 (Fig. 2.31), 53 (Table 2.4), 112, 176–8, Fig. 4. 36–7, 182–3
Child abuse, and orthopaedic injuries, 349–50
Child development, 88–9
Child psychology, 2
Chondroblastoma, 365–6
Chondrolysis, in slipped upper femoral epiphysis, 259
Chondromalacia patellae, 261–3, 264, 265, 273, 434
Clavicle
  fractures, 294–5
  pseudarthrosis, congenital, 83–4
Claw toes, 163, 164, 165, 169
Club foot, congenital, *see* Talipes equinovarus, congenital
Club hand, radial, 80–3

Cobb technique of spinal curvature
        measurement, 207–8, 235
Cocked up fifth toe, 171–2
Codman's triangle, 358, 372
Collar and cuff sling, 13, 246, 290–1
    and fractured humerus, 12, 295, 296, 297, 300
Communication with parents, 6–7, 69, 249
Congenital dislocation of hip, see Hip, dislocation, congenital
Congenital indifference to pain, 438
Congenital malformation, 10–11, 15–16
    definition, 8
    see also specified malformations
Consultation, aims and method, 2, 4–7
Coronal traction, 39, 95, 178
Cottrell traction, 217
Coxa magna, 11
Coxa valga, 11
Coxa vara, 11, 37, 69, 153, 196, 256
    causes, 196
    in fractures of femur, 322, 325
    infantile, 196–200
Cubitus varus deformity, 301–2
Curly toe, 169–71
Cysts
    Baker, 176
    of bone
        aneurysmal, 362, 384–5
        in neurofibromatosis, 422–3
        simple, 351, 361, 384–5
    haemophilic, 441
    popliteal, 176

Defect, definition of, 8
Deformity, definition of, 8
Denis Browne splint, 24–8, 40, 91
Deprived child, definition, 8
Dermatomyositis, 446 (Table 8.1), 450–1
Diagnosis and examination, 5
    in neonatal period, 11–12
Diastematomyelia, 42, 163, 164, 231, 237, 239
Disability, definition of, 8
Disadvantaged child, definition, 8
Discitis, 146–9
Discoid meniscus, 174–5
Dislocations, 280, 293, 344
    see also under Elbow; Hip; Patella; Radius; Shoulder; Thumb; Ulna
Down's syndrome (mongolism), 344, 432–4
Dunlop traction, 299–300
Dwyer's osteotomy of os calcis, 32, 165–6, 279
Dwyer's procedure in scoliosis, 58, 217, 225–30, 346, 406

Dysplasia
    acetabular, 33–40, 112, 179, 180, 181–3, 433
    fibrous, 154, 268, 364
Dysraphism, spinal, 163, 164, 236–40

Elbow
    in arthrogryposis, 408–9
    dislocation, 303–4, 308
        of radial head, 13, 309
    fractures of humerus
        lateral condyle, 302–3
        lateral epicondyle, 305
        medial epicondyle, 304–5
        supracondylar, 297–302
    fractures of olecranon, 308
    fractures of radius, proximal, 305–8
    pulled, 94–5
    release in cerebral palsy, 115
    in valgus and in varus, 11
Enchondroma, 364–5, 384
Epilepsy in cerebral palsy, 103
Epiphyseal arrest, see Epiphysiodesis in leg length inequality
Epiphysiodesis in leg length inequality, 71, 85, 86, 87, 159
Epiphysiolysis, femoral, upper, 256–9
Equinovalgus, spastic, in cerebral palsy, 105–6
Equinovarus
    spastic, in cerebral palsy, 106–9
    and spina bifida, 54
Equinus deformity, 10, 54
    spastic, in cerebral palsy, 104–5
Erb-Duchenne paralysis, 12–13
Ewing's sarcoma, 141, 355, 381–2, 393
    radiology in diagnosis, 358, 359 (Fig. 7.5), 372–3, Fig. 7.44
    treatment, 396–8
Examination of patients, 5
    neonates, 11–12
Extension prostheses in proximal femoral focal deficiency, 71–2

Factor VIII, 439, 442–3, 444, 445
Factor IX, 439, 443
Femur
    derotation osteotomy, 179–80
    epiphysis, lower, ossification abnormalities, 172
    epiphysis, upper, slipped, 256–9
    fractures
        distal growth plate injuries, 330–2
        intra-articular, distal, 332–3
        midshaft, 325–9
        of neck, 319–25
        subtrochanteric, 325
        supracondylar, 329–30
        upper-third, 325

Index   477

Femur (*cont.*)
  proximal focal deficiency, 65–6
    classification, 66–9
    management, 69–72
  surgical shortening of, 160, 176–8, 179
Fibroma
  chondromyxoid, 366–9
  non-ossifying, 363, 384
Fibrosarcoma, 373–4
Fibula
  absence, congenital, 72
    classification, 72–3
    management, 73–6
  fractures, 335, 337
  pseudarthrosis, 79
  surgical shortening of, 161, Fig. 4.25
Fingers
  in arthrogryposis, 409
  fractures, 315
  mallet, 315
Flat foot, 10–11
  in children, 118, 123–6, 131
  congenital, 59–64
  in Down's syndrome, 434
  peroneal spasmodic, 274–6
  in toddlers, 93
Floppy infant, 99
Foot
  fractures, 341
  movements and deformities, terminology, 10–11
  muscle hypertrophy, 86
  normal, 134–5
  see also specified deformities and malformations affecting foot and Footwear
Footwear, 134–8
  in flat feet, 125
  in leg length inequality, 158–9
  in pes cavus, 164–5
Forearm, fractures and dislocations, *see under* Radius *and* Ulna
Fractures, 280–1
  and arterial injuries, 293–4, 347–9
  birth, 12
  buckle, 281, 288, 293, 310, 329
  characteristic features, 281–5
  in child abuse, 349–50
  complications
    arterial injury, 293–4, 347–9
    in haemophilia, 441
    nerve injury, 293
  compound, 346–7
  diagnosis, principles of, 286–8
  diaphyseal, 281
  follow up, in treatment, 291–3
  greenstick, 281, 289
  growth plate injuries, 281–5, 288

Fractures (*cont.*)
  healing of, 285–6
  immobilisation of, 289–91
  metaphyseal, 281
  pathological, 351
  reduction of, 289
  stress, 351, 374, 383 (Figs. 7.45–6)
  treatment, principles of, 289–93
  see also under specified bones, joints, regions
Friedreich's ataxia, 122, 163, 434–6, 437–8

Gait
  in childhood
    antalgic limp, 120
    ataxic, 122
    calcaneus, 121
    in cerebral palsy, 122
    drop foot, 121–2
    flat feet, 123–6, 131
    footwear, 125, 134–8
    gluteus maximus weakness, 121
    hysterical, 123
    inset hips, 128–32
    in-toeing, 128–33
    knock knees, 127–8, 131
    limp, 120–3
    metatarsus adductus, 128, 132–3
    normal, 118–20
    obesity, 128, 133–4
    in quadriceps weakness, 121
    'scissors', 122
    short leg limp, 120
    stiff hip, 122
    stiff knee, 122
    unstable hip limp, 120
  in toddlers, 89
    ataxic, 99
    in cerebral palsy, 100, 109, 112–13, Fig. 3.17
    in congenital dislocation of hip, 95
    in-toeing, 89–92
    out-toeing, 92–3
    Trendelenburg, 95, 120
Galeazzi fracture dislocation, 310
Gallows traction, 39, 291, 325
Genetic counselling, 7
  in cerebral palsy, 96
  in congenital dislocation and dysplasia of hip, 34
  in neurofibromatosis, 425–6
  in peroneal muscular atrophy, 437
  in spina bifida, 48
Genu recurvatum (back knee), 11, 18, 56
Genu valgum, *see* Knock knee
Genu varum, *see* Bowlegs
Gigantism, 85–6, 421
Gower's sign, 427
Granuloma, eosinophilic, 148, 369

Grice's operation, 53 (Table 2.4), 55, 64
Growth plate
 excision of bone bridge at, 161
 injuries, 281–5, 288
Gruca ankle reconstruction, 73–5
Gunstock deformity, 301–2

Haemangioma, 370
Haemarthrosis, 288, 333
 in haemophilia, 439–40, 442, 443–5
Haemophilia, 438–9
 classification, 439
 management, 442–5
 orthopaedic implications, 439–42
Hallux, supernumerary, 84–5
Hallux rigidus, 277–8
Hallux valgus, 11, 105, 434
 in adolescence, 276–7
Hallux varus, 11, 16, 434
Halo traction, 217, 344
Hamilton Russell traction, 291, 317, 325–7
Hammer toes, 169, 171
Hand
 in arthrogryposis, 409
 and cerebral palsy, treatment, 113–15
 dislocation, metacarpophalangeal joint of thumb, 314–15
 fractures
  metacarpal, 312–14
  phalangeal, 315
Handicaps of children
 definition, 8
 effect on child, 3–4
 effect on parents, 2–3, 69
Harrington techniques on spine, 58, 214, 217–24, 226–30, 236, 346
Head injuries in childhood, 246–7
Heels, sore, 168
Hemiatrophy, congenital, 85
Hemihypertrophy, 85–7
Hemivertebra, 201, 231
Henoch-Schönlein purpura, 446 (Table 8.1), 451
Hip
 adduction, spastic, in cerebral palsy, 109–11
 arthritis, septic, 149, 151, 154
 arthrodesis, 70, 183
 in arthrogryposis, 405
 dislocation, 317–19
  in arthrogryposis, 405
  in cerebral palsy, 111–12
  in Down's syndrome, 433
 dislocation, congenital, 33–4
  as cause of leg length inequality, 153
  in first year of life, 34–40
  presenting at ages one and two, 95–6
  presenting after age two, 176–8

Hip
 dislocation, congenital (cont.)
  surgical management, 178–84
  teratological, 36
 dysplasia, congenital, 33–40
  see also Acetabulum, dysplasia; Hip, dislocation, congenital
 external rotation, 18–19
 inset, 91–2, 112–13, Fig. 3.17, 128–32
 internal rotation, 92, 112–13, 128–32
 and in-toeing, 91–2, 112–13, 128–33
 irritable, 189, 194–6, 259
 joint re-surfacing of, 184
 limp, in instability of, 120
 observation, 189, 194–6, 259
 replacement, 183–4
 in spina bifida, 56–7
 subluxation
  in cerebral palsy, 111–12
  congenital, 33, 38, 95, 179–81
 tuberculosis, 189–90
Histiocytosis X, 369, 373, 377
Holdsworth procedure in fifth toe deformities, 171, 172
Homocystinuria, 231
Horner's syndrome, 13
Hospitalisation
 adolescent patient, 249
 effect on child, 4, 116
Human leucocyte antigen (HLA), 447
Humerus, fractures of
 of lateral condyle, 302–3
 of lateral epicondyle, 305
 of medial epicondyle, 304–5
 proximal, 295–6
 shaft, 296
 supracondylar, 297–302
 upper metaphysis, 296
Hydrocephalus, 42, 43, 49
Hydrotherapy, 464
Hypertrophy of limbs, 85–7
Hysterical back pain in adolescence, 255
Hysterical gait, 123

In-toeing
 in childhood, 128–33
 in toddlers, 89–92, 93, 112–13
Irritable hip, 189, 194–6, 259

Juvenile chronic arthritis (JCA), 152, 268, 445, 446–7, 449
 management, 452–3
 pauci-articular
  ANF negative, 448
  ANF positive, 448
  associated with HLA B27, 448
 polyarticular (rheumatoid factor negative), 447–8

Juvenile chronic arthritis (*cont.*)
　rheumatoid factor positive, 447
　systemic onset, 447
　treatment, 453–4
Juvenile rheumatoid arthritis, *see* Juvenile chronic arthritis

Kernicterus, 96, 97
Klisic procedure in congenitally dislocated hip, 176–8
Knee
　arthrodesis, 71 (Fig. 2.51), 72
　in arthrogryposis, 174, 402–5
　discoid meniscus, 174–5
　flexion in cerebral palsy, 109
　haemarthroses, 445
　meniscus
　　discoid, 174–5
　　injuries to, 272–4
　Osgood–Schlatter disease, 259–61
　ossification abnormalities, lower femoral epiphysis, 172
　osteochondritis dissecans, 172, 262, 269–72, 274
　osteochondritis of tibial tubercle, 259–61
　penetrating wounds, 274
　popliteal cyst, 176
　quadriceps contracture, 172–4, 265, 404
　in spina bifida, 55–6
　see also Knock knee; Patella
Knock knee, 11, 118, 127–8, 131, 268, 432
Knowles' pins
　in fractures of femur, 321, 322, 323 (Figs. 6.54–5), 324 (Fig. 6.59)
　in fractures of tibia, 336
　in upper femoral epiphysiolysis, 258
Kyphoscoliosis
　in cerebral palsy, 116
　of neurofibromatosis, 232, 421
Kyphosis
　spinal, 57, 201 (Table 4.2), 205, 207, 208, 345–6
　　adolescent, 250–1
　　in cerebral palsy, 116
　　juvenile, 233–6
　　in Marfan's syndrome, 432
　　tibial, 76–8, 79, 153

Landau reaction, 100
Langenskiöld's excision of bone bridge at growth plate of bones, 161
Larsen's syndrome, 245
Leg length inequality
　calculation of matured discrepancy, 157–8
　causes, 153–4
　in cerebral palsy, 115–16
　in congenital hemiatrophy and hemihypertrophy, 85

Leg length inequality (*cont.*)
　examination, 154–7
　limp, 120
　management, 71–2, 85, 87, 157–62
　measurement, 155–7
　in osteomyelitis, 140
　in poliomyelitis, 457
　in proximal femoral focal deficiency, 71–2
　timing of arrest, 157–8
Leg lengthening, 71, 162
Leukaemia, 256, 374, 446 (Table 8.1)
Limp in childhood, 120–3
Locomotion, development of, 88–9
Lordosis, 51 (Fig. 2.34), 201 (Table 4.2), 205, 207, 208
　in arthrogryposis, 406
　in Scheuermann's disease, 233, 234
Lumbago, 255–6
Lumbar disc syndrome in adolescence, 254–5
Lymphatic anomalies causing hypertrophy, 87

McMurray's sign, 273
Malalignment syndrome of knee, 261
Malformation, congenital, 10–11, 15–16
　definition, 8
　see also specified malformations
Mallet finger, 315
Mallet toe, 169
Marfan's syndrome, 231, 431–2
Meniscus
　discoid, 174–5
　injuries to, 272–4
Metatarsus adductus
　in childhood, 128, 132–3
　in infancy, 16–17, 128
　and prone sleeping, 16, 89, 90
　in toddler, 89, 90
Metatarsus primus elevatus, 277
Metatarsus primus varus, 276, 277
Metatarsus varus, 17, 90–1, 133, 167
Milestones in child development, 88–9
Milroy's disease, 87
Milwaukee brace
　in Marfan's syndrome, 432
　in Scheuermann's disease, 235–6, 251
　in scoliosis, 209–12, 213, 214, 226, 231
Minerva jacket, 344, 348
Moe sacral hook, 230 (Figs. 4.103–4)
Mongolism (Down's syndrome), 344, 432–4
Monteggia fracture dislocations, 309–10
Moro reflex, 100
Muscular dystrophy, 163, 426
　classification, 426
　clinical features, 426–9
　　Duchenne, 426–7
　　facio-scapulo-humeral, 427–9
　　limb girdle, 427

480 Index

Muscular dystrophy (cont.)
    diagnosis, 429
    management, 429–31

Necrosis, avascular
    femoral, 189, 319, 321, 322, 323 (Figs. 6.56–7), 325
        in Perthes' disease, 184, 185
        in slipped upper epiphysis, 256, 257, 258
    vertebral, 250–2
Neuroblastoma, 256, 374, 446 (Table 8.1)
Neurofibromatosis, 85, 154, 268, 418
    clinical features, 419
        CNS manifestations, 423–5
        neurofibromas, 420–1
        skeletal, 232, 268, 269 (Figs. 5.12–13), 421–3
        skin lesions, 419–20
    diagnosis, 418–19
    management, 425–6

Obesity, 128, 133–4
Observation hip, 189, 194–6, 259
O'Connor boot, 71, Fig. 2.51, 159
Olecranon, fractures of, 308
Ortolani's sign, 36, 198
Osgood–Schlatter disease, 259–61
Osteoblastoma, 256, 363
Osteochondritis
    in adolescence, 250
        dorsal spine, 250–1
        lumbar spine, 252
    dissecans, 172, 262, 269–72, 274
    juvenilis, 184
    of tibial tubercle, 259–61
Osteochondromas, 356, 359, 384, 386
Osteochondrosis in adolescence, 250–2
Osteogenesis imperfecta, 12, 350, 351, 410, 417
    classification, 410–12
    clinical features, 412
    management, 412–17, 471–2
Osteoma, 361
    osteoid, 355, 370, 386
Osteomyelitis, 14, 138, 351, 374, 448
    acute, 138
        bacteriology, 140
        chronicity of infection, 139–40
        clinical features, 140
        complications, 142
        differential diagnosis, 141
        investigations, 140–1
        management, 141–2
        spread of infection, methods, 138–9
    chronic, 142, 380 (Fig. 7.42), 381 (Fig. 7.43)
        of insidious onset, 145–6

Osteomyelitis
    chronic (cont.)
        as sequel to acute infection, 143–5
        discitis, 146–9
        tuberculous, 146
Osteosarcoma, 351, 372, 374
    treatment, 395–6
Out-toeing, 92–3
Overlapping fifth toe, 171–2

Pain, congenital indifference to, 438
Paralysis
    Erb-Duchenne, 12–13
    obstetrical, 12–14
    sciatic, neonatal, 13–14
Parents
    anxieties of, 2–3, 6–7, 464
    communication with, 6–7, 69, 249
    of handicapped children, 2–3, 69
    treatment of child by mother, 7, 464
Patella
    adherence to femur, 174, 404
    chondromalacia, 261–3, 264, 265, 273, 434
    dislocation
        congenital, 265, 268
        habitual, 174, 265
        recurrent, 263–5, 433
        traumatic, 263
    in Down's syndrome, 433–4
Patient
    in adolescence, 248–9
    attitude to, 1–2, 3, 249
    examination of, 5
    neonates, 11–12
    psychology of, 2, 249
Pattens, 71, 159
Pauwels' osteotomy in infantile coxa vara, 200
Pavlik harness, 36, 38–9
Pelvis, fractures, 315
    of acetabulum, 317
    outside of ring, 317
    of ring, double, 316
    of ring, single, 315–16
Peroneal muscular atrophy (Charcot-Marie-Tooth disease), 163, 434–7
Peroneal spasmodic flat foot, 274–6
Perthes' disease, 154, 184, 196
    aetiology, 184
    bone scan, 189
    Catteralls' classification, 190–1
    clinical features, 186
    differential diagnosis, 189–90
    incidence, 184
    management, 191–3
    natural course of, 190
    pathology, 185–6
    prognosis, factors indicating, 190–1

Index 481

Perthes' disease (cont.)
  radiological features, 187-9, 190
  types, 186, 190-1
Pes cavus, 11, 162-3
  aetiology, 163
  clinical features, 164-5
  congenital convex, 59-64
  in Friedreich's ataxia, 436, 437
  investigation, 163-4
  management, 164-5
  pathogenesis, 163
  in peroneal muscular atrophy, 436, 437
  surgery, 165-7
Pes planus, see Flat foot
Phemister's technique in epiphyseal arrest, 159
Physiotherapy, 463-5
  in cerebral palsy, 102, 114
  and fractures, 293
  in haemophilia, 444-5
  in muscular dystrophy, 431
Plagiocephaly, 19, 212, 244
Poliomyelitis, 154, 163, 454
  clinical features, 455
  management, 455-8
Polyarteritis nodosa, 446 (Table 8.1), 450-1
Polydactyly
  fingers, in Down's syndrome, 432
  toes, 84-5
Popliteal cyst, 176
Posture, normal, at birth, 16
  variations of, 16-19
Posture and gait, 123
  cerebral palsy, 122
  flat feet, 118, 123-6, 131
  footwear, 125, 134-8
  inset hips, 91-2, 112-13, Fig. 3.17, 128-32
  in-toed gait, 128-33
  knock knees, 118, 127-8, 131
  metatarsus adductus, 128, 132-3
  obesity, 128, 133-4
Proximal femoral focal deficiency, see under Femur
Pseudarthrosis
  of clavicle, (congenital), 83-4
  femoral, 69-70
  fibular, 79
  in neurofibromatosis, 422-3
  post-operative, in scoliosis, 229
  of tibia, 79-80
Pseudohypertrophy in muscular dystrophy, 426, 427, 429
Pseudotumours in haemophilia, 441
Pugh's traction, 196
Putti-Platt operation, 246

Quadriceps contracture, 172-4, 265, 404

Radiology of bone tumours and related lesions, in diagnosis, 355
  aggressive lesions, 357-8
  benign tumours, 356-7
  chondroblastoma, 365-6
  cysts of bone
    aneurysmal, 362
    simple, 361
  dysplasia, fibrous, 364
  enchondroma, 364-5
  Ewing's sarcoma, 141, 358, 359 (Fig. 7.5), 372-3, 382 (Fig. 7.44)
  fibroma
    chondromyxoid, 366-9
    non-ossifying, 363
  fibrosarcoma, 373-4
  granuloma, eosinophilia, 369
  haemangioma, 370
  histiocytosis X, 369, 373
  leukaemia, 374
  neuroblastoma, 374
  osteoblastoma, 363
  osteochondromas, 356, 359
  osteoma, 361
    osteoid, 370
  osteosarcoma, 372, 374
  techniques, 355
Radiotherapy in bone tumours, 384, 390, 393, 396, 398
Radius
  absence, congenital, 80-3
  dislocation of head, 13, 309
  fractures
    metaphyseal, distal, 310-12
    proximal, 305-8
    of shaft, 309, 310
  Galeazzi fracture dislocation, 310
  growth plate injuries, distal, 312
  Monteggia fracture dislocation, 309-10
Reiter's syndrome, 446 (Table 8.1), 451
Reverse club foot, 60
Rheumatic fever, 141, 151, 446 (Table 8.1), 450
Rheumatoid factor, 447
Rickets, 77, 268, 283
Risser cast, 226
Risser's sign, 208
Robert Jones procedure, 167
Rotation-plasty in proximal femoral focal deficiency, 71 (Fig. 2.51), 72

Salter innominate osteotomy, 178, 179, 195 (Figs. 4.51-3), 461
Scheuermann's disease, 233-6, 250-1
Schmorl's nodes, 235
'Scissors gait', 122
Scleroderma, 446 (Table 8.1), 450-1
Scoliosis, 202

Scoliosis (*cont.*)
  adult, natural history of, 203
  in arthrogryposis, 406
  of childhood, natural history, 202
  clinical assessment, 203-9
  congenital, 216, 217, 230-1
  and Down's syndrome, 434
  in Friedreich's ataxia, 437, 438
  idiopathic
    adolescent, 214, 215-16
    infantile, 212-13, 217
    juvenile, 214
  and Marfan's syndrome, 231
  and neurofibromatosis, 232, 421, 423
    (Figs. 8.24-5)
  neuromuscular, 227-30
  non-structural, 201 (Table 4.2)
  postural, infantile, 19
  in Scheuermann's disease, 233
  in spina bifida, 58-9
  structural, 201 (Table 4.2)
  surgery in, 216-17, 226-7
    Dwyer's procedure, 58, 217, 225-30, 346, 406
    Harrington's techniques, 58, 214, 217-24, 226-30, 346
  terminology, 202
  treatment, conservative, 209-12, 213, 214, 216
Shelf arthroplasty for acetabular dysplasia, 181-2, 182-3
Shoulder
  in arthrogryposis, 407
  dislocation, 245-6
Sinus formation
  in osteomyelitis, 143, 145
  in spinal dysraphism, 237, 238, 240
Skeletal injuries in childhood, characteristic features, 280-1
Sleeping posture, 16, 89, 90
Smith-Petersen approach in hip operations, 178, 181, 461
Spasticity in cerebral palsy, 98, 100-1, 103, 114
Spica cast
  in arthritis, septic, of hip, 15, 153
  in congenital dislocation of hip, 40, 95, 179
  in discitis, 149
  in fractures of femur, 320, 321, 322, 325-6, 327
  in Pauwels' osteotomy, 200
Spina bifida, 40, 239
  anaesthesia in operations for, 471, 472
  bone fragility, 48
  causes of deformity, 43-7
  chilblains, 48
  definitions of forms of, 40-2

Spina bifida (*cont.*)
  management, 48-52
    antenatal diagnosis, 48-9
    foot deformity, 52-5
    genetic counselling, 48
    hip deformity, 56-7
    knee deformity, 55-6
    scoliosis, 58-9, Figs. 4.101-4, 227-30
    spinal surgery in, 57-9, Figs. 4.101-4, 227-30, 471, 472
  meningocele, 40, 41 (Fig. 2.26(2)), 47
  multiple system involvement, 42-3
  myelocele, 40, 42 (Fig. 2.26(4))
  myelomeningocele, 42 (Fig. 2.26(3)), 43-4, 48-9, 52 (Fig. 2.35), 55, 62-3 (Figs. 2.42-4)
  definition, 40
  occulta, 41, Fig. 2.26(1)
  pressure sores, 48
Spine
  in arthrogryposis, 406
  deformities, classification of, 200-1
  in Down's syndrome, 432-3
  dysraphism, 163, 164, 236-40
  embryology and early development, 201-2
  injuries
    cervical, 342-4
    thoracic and lumbar, 345-6
  in neurofibromatosis, 421-2
  see also Spina bifida
Spondylolisthesis in adolescence, 253-4
Spondylolysis in adolescence, 253
Sprains, 280
'Statue of Liberty' position, 13, 245
Steinmann pins, 325, 329
Still's disease, *see* Juvenile chronic arthritis
Stryker frame, 226
Surgical practice, principles of, 459
  anaesthesia
    administration, 467-8
    in blood disorders, 473
    in fractures and dislocations, 471
    in orthopaedic manipulation and plaster application, 470-1
    in osteogenesis imperfecta, 471-2
    outpatients, 473
    pre-operative assessment and medication, 465-6
    recovery period, 468-9
    in spina bifida, 471, 472
    in spine surgery, 471
  arthrography, 472-3
  blood loss and transfusion, 469-70, 471-2
  conservative versus operative treatment, 459-60
  defining objectives, 459
  intravenous therapy, 469-70
  operation, 461-3

Surgical practice, principles of (*cont.*)
    planning of, 460–1
    outpatients, 473
    physiotherapy, 463–5
Syme's amputation, 71 (Fig. 2.51), 72, 75–6
Syndactyly, toes, 85
Synovitis, 274, 445, 446 (Table 8.1), 449
    transient (hip), 194–6
Systemic lupus erythematosus (SLE), 446 (Table 8.1), 450–1

Talipes calcaneovalgus, 60
    postural, 17
Talipes equinovarus, congenital
    anatomical features, 19–20
    bone and joint changes, 20–1
    clinical features, 21
    differentiation from metatarsus varus, 133
    incidence, 19
    and leg length inequality, 153
    radiological features, 21–3
    soft tissue changes, 21
    treatment, 23–4
        Denis Browne splintage, 24–8
        serial casting, 28
        surgical, 28–33
Talipes equinovarus, postural, 17
Talocalcaneal angle, 22–3
Talus, congenital vertical, 55, 59–64
Tarsal coalition, congenital, 274–6
Taylor brace, 226
Tendo-Achilles, lengthening of, 31, 64, 105, 106, 125
Thalassaemia, 434
Thalidomide, 80
Thomas heel, 137, 341
Thomas splint, 330, 445
Thumb
    in arthrogryposis, 409
    dislocation of metacarpophalangeal joint, 314–15
    trigger, 94
Tibia
    bowing of, 76–8, 79, 89, 90 (Fig. 3.1), 91
    derotation osteotomy, 33
    fractures
        diaphyseal, 335–6
        growth plate, distal, 338–40
        growth plate, proximal, injuries, 334
        metaphyseal, distal, 337
        metaphyseal, proximal, 334
        of spine of, 333–4
        Tillaux, 338–9, 343
    internal torsion, 89, 90 (Fig. 3.1), 91, 118, 128
    kyphosis, 76–8, 79, 153
    lengthening, 162
    osteochondritis of tubercle, 259–61

Tibia (*cont.*)
    pseudarthrosis, 79–80
    surgical shortening, 160–1
Toe(s)
    claw, 163, 164, 165, 169
    curly, 169–71
    fifth, cocked up or overlapping, 171–2
    hammer, 169, 171
    mallet, 169
    in pes cavus, surgery, 167
    supernumerary, 84–5
    syndactyly, 85
Toe nails, ingrowing, 278
Torticollis, 240
    neonatal, 240
    secondary, 241–2
    sternomastoid (or infantile), 19, 240, 243–5
Traction, 289, 291, 325
    coronal, 39, 95, 178
    Cottrell, 217
    Dunlop, 299–300
    gallows, 39, 291, 325
    halo, 217, 344
    Hamilton Russell, 291, 317, 325, 327
    Pugh's, 196
Trendelenburg gait, 95, 120
Trendelenburg sign, 95, 120, 121 (Fig. 4.2), 257
Trethowan's sign, 257, 258 (Fig. 5.4)
Trigger thumb, 94
Triple arthrodesis, 462
    in cavo-varus, 167
    in cerebral palsy, 106, 109
    in club foot, 32–3
    in flat foot, 125, 276
    in Marfan's syndrome, 432
    in metatarsus varus, 91, 167
    in peroneal muscular atrophy, 437
    in poliomyelitis, 457
    in spina bifida, 54
Tschirkin's sign, 254 (Fig. 5.3)
Tuberculosis
    of hips, 189–90
    osteomyelitis, 146

Ulna
    fractures
        growth plate, distal, injuries, 312
        metaphyseal, distal, 310–12
        olecranon, 308
        of shaft, 309–10
    Galeazzi fracture dislocation, 310
    Monteggia fracture dislocation, 309–10

Van Nes' rotation-plasty, 71 (Fig. 2.51), 72
Vascular anomalies, causing hypertrophy, 86–7

Vertebra(e)
  and discitis, 146–9
  embryology and early development, 201–2
  in neurofibromatosis, 421–2
  plana, 369
  in spinal injuries, 342–6
  wedge, 201, 231, 235, 250, 345
Volkmann's ischaemic contracture, 291, 293

Von Recklinghausen's disease, *see* Neurofibromatosis

Warts, plantar, 278
Wrist
  arthrodesis, 83, 114–15
  in arthrogryposis, 409
  fractures, 312